# Lymphatic Imaging

## Lymphography, Computed Tomography and Scintigraphy

**Second Edition**

# Volumes of
# Golden's Diagnostic Radiology Series
# published or in preparation

| | |
|---|---|
| **Taveras & Wood:** | Diagnostic Neuroradiology |
| **Dodd & Jing:** | Radiology of the Nose, Paranasal Sinuses and Nasopharynx, *Second Edition in Preparation* |
| **Rabin & Baron:** | Radiology of the Chest |
| **Cooley & Schreiber:** | Radiology of the Heart and Great Vessels |
| **Edeiken:** | Roentgen Diagnosis of Diseases of Bone |
| **Sussman & Newman:** | Urologic Radiology |
| **Campbell et al:** | Radiologic, Ultrasonic, and Nuclear Diagnostic Methods in Obstetrics |
| **Littleton:** | Tomography—Physical Principles and Clinical Applications |
| **Martin:** | Atlas of Mammography: Histologic & Mammographic Correlations |
| **Gottschalk, Hoffer, Berger, & Potchen** | Diagnostic Nuclear Medicine, *Second Edition in preparation* |
| **Dreyfuss & Janower:** | Radiology of the Colon |
| **Hatfield & Wise:** | Radiology of the Gallbladder and Bile Ducts |
| **Friedman:** | Radiology of the Liver, Biliary Tract, Pancreas and Spleen |
| **Jing & Dodd:** | Radiology of the Oropharynx, Hypopharynx and Larynx |
| **Castaneda:** | Interventional Radiology |
| **Bryan et al:** | Diagnostic Neuroradiology |

# Lymphatic Imaging

## Lymphography, Computed Tomography and Scintigraphy

**Second Edition**

**Edited by**

## Melvin E. Clouse, M.D.

Associate Professor of Radiology, Harvard Medical School;
Chairman, Department of Radiology,
New England Deaconess Hospital,
Boston, Massachusetts

## Sidney Wallace, M.D.

Professor of Radiology, M.D. Anderson Hospital and Tumor Institute
University of Texas Medical Center
Houston, Texas

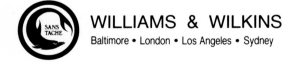

**WILLIAMS & WILKINS**
Baltimore • London • Los Angeles • Sydney

# GOLDEN'S DIAGNOSTIC RADIOLOGY

JOHN H. HARRIS, JR., M.D., SERIES EDITOR

*Editor:* George Stamathis
*Associate Editor:* Victoria M. Vaughn
*Copy Editor:* Deborah K. Tourtlotte
*Design:* Bob Och
*Illustration Planning:* Wayne Hubbel
*Production:* Anne G. Seitz

Copyright © 1985
Williams & Wilkins
428 East Preston Street
Baltimore, MD 21202, U.S.A.

Accurate indications, adverse reactions, and dosage schedules for drugs are provided in this book, but it is possible that they may change. The reader is urged to review the package information data of the manufacturers of the medications mentioned.

*Made in the United States of America*

**Library of Congress Cataloging-in-Publication Data**

Main entry under title:

Lymphatic imaging.

   (Golden's diagnostic radiology series)
   Rev. ed. of: Clinical lymphography. 1977.
   Includes index.
   1. Lymphangiography. I. Clouse, Melvin E. II. Wallace, Sidney, 1929- · III. Series. [DNLM: 1. Lymphography. WH 700 L9847]
RC78.7.L9L87 1985     616.4′207572     84-13056
ISBN 0-683-01651-2

Composed and printed at the
Waverly Press, Inc.

85  86  87  88  89
10  9  8  7  6  5  4  3  2  1

# Series Editor's Foreword

The Golden's Diagnostic Radiology Series was conceived as a collection of current, inclusive, and authoritative reference sources for radiologists and nonradiologist specialists who have a primary interest in the individual text's subject. This newest volume of the Series, *Lymphatic Imaging*, more than fulfills that intent. The relevancy, the timeliness, and, consequently, the authoritativeness of this work are evidenced by its expanded scope, the reorganized format, and the emphasis which has been placed upon regional lymphatic systems and current imaging modalities.

The revised title of this edition, which was proposed by Dr. Clouse, much more appropriately bespeaks the scope and substance of this work than does *Clinical Lymphography*, the title of Dr. Clouse's first edition.

The Golden's Series authors are selected only after a rigorous review process and are then invited to prepare specific manuscripts. The stature of the authors of previous texts in this Series is testimony to the selectivity of this process. The authors of these editions dealing with the lymphatic system either have earned, or are destined to earn, that same level of recognition and acclaim. Those authors of the first edition who have contributed to the current volume have, where appropriate, significantly revised their material to reflect current concepts, clinical applications and imaging procedures relating to the lymphatic system. Several new authors, invited because of their special interest and knowledge, have contributed new material which greatly enhances the value and clinical relevancy of this edition. Included in this group are Thomas H. Adair, Ph.D., R. Thomas Bergeron, M.D., Arthur C. Guyton, M.D., Theresa C. McLoud, M.D., Jack E. Meyer, M.D., Deborah L. Reede, M.D., Marceau Servelle, M.D., and Jesus Zornoza, M.D.

Melvin E. Clouse, M.D., principal author and editor of this volume, has masterfully restructured and reorganized its format. He has been responsible for its expanded content and for coordinating those myriad details required to bring a multiauthored manuscript to completion.

On behalf of George S. Stamathis, Senior Editor, John Gardner, Vice President and Editor-in-Chief, and Sara Finnegan, President of the book publishing division of Williams & Wilkins, I extend heartiest congratulations and sincerest appreciation to Dr. Clouse and his contributing authors for the successful completion of this monumental task. This text is the single most comprehensive, authoritative treatise yet published dealing with the anatomy, physiology, pathology, and imaging of the lymphatic system.

This volume will make major contributions to physician knowledge and, consequently, have a direct and major impact upon patient care. Because of its scope and content, its relevance to both radiologists and attending physicians, this authoritative, yet concise and clearly written, volume is destined to earn its rightful place among the classics of medical literature.

JOHN H. HARRIS, JR., M.D., D.Sc.
Editor
June 1985

# Foreword

This volume greatly expands as well as updates the previous text, *Clinical Lymphography*. The important history, anatomy, and techniques are reviewed. A whole chapter is devoted to the physiology of lymph formation and reabsorption. The pathology of malignant lymphomas is presented separately and is a useful correlate to their images. The interpretation of both solid tumors and lymphomas is updated not only considering lymphographic images but their appearance using lymphographic scintigraphy and computed tomography as well. Specific chapters relate to proper imaging of the lymphatic system in the abdomen, thorax, and neck. These provide important guides to the clinician considering abnormalities in these areas. Percutaneous aspiration biopsy of lymph nodes has become an increasingly important medical tool and is well reviewed in the book. Finally, a specific chapter concerns the emerging imaging technique of lymphographic scintigraphy.

This volume affords the reader the opportunity of having in one place all of the materials pertinent to a clinical review of lymphatic imaging.

SAMUEL HELLMAN, M.D.
Physician-in-Chief
Memorial Sloan-Kettering
Cancer Center
January 21, 1985

# Preface to the Second Edition

During the past 30 years, diagnostic imaging techniques have undergone an incredible evolution from conventional radiographic imaging to sophisticated angiography, nuclear medicine, ultrasonography, computed tomography (CT), and, most recently, magnetic resonance imaging.

In 1945, Professor Marceau Servelle began studying the lymphatics of patients with lymphedema using Thorotrast, and in 1952 the clinical technique for the studies performed today was introduced in a publication written by Professor John B. Kinmonth, a British surgeon at St. Thomas Hospital in London. When the initial water-soluble contrast medium was replaced by Ethiodol, a large number of diseases of the lymphatic system could be studied.

Lymphography rapidly became the gold standard for imaging techniques used to study the lymphatic system because for the first time one could study the architecture of normal as well as abnormal lymph nodes. Lymphography had deficiencies, however, when imaging the cervical, axillary, and mediastinal lymph nodes and those nodes above the cisterna chyli (i.e., superior mesenteric, celiac, splenic, and hepatic areas). For this reason CT and ultrasound were rapidly incorporated into the staging of patients with lymphoma as well as solid tumors. In certain areas where lymphography is deficient, such as patients with head, neck, and lung cancer, CT has become the primary staging procedure. In other areas, such as the lymphomas, CT has largely replaced lymphography in the staging of patients with non-Hodgkin's lymphoma and in those patients with stage III or IV Hodgkin's disease. A combination of CT and lymphography is essential for the work-up and staging of patients with clinical stages I and II Hodgkin's disease. In the work-up of patients with genitourinary cancer, the examinations remain largely complementary.

This book was written primarily for radiologists in a busy department, practicing surgeons, residents, and oncologists involved in the care of patients with malignant disease. The format lends itself to easy and rapid reference beginning with a history of the discovery of the lymphatic system, normal anatomy, and the technique of lymphography and lymphographic scintigraphy and continuing with the physiology of lymph formation, control and flow, abnormal peripheral and mesenteric lymphatics, interpretation of lymphangiograms, benign lymph node disease, pathology of malignant lymphoma, lymphoma of the abdomen and retroperitoneum, lymphatic imaging of solid tumors of the abdomen and retroperitoneum, lymph node imaging of the thorax, head, and neck, percutaneous lymph node biopsy techniques, and complications of lymphography.

Each chapter is accompanied by a reference list that includes the major contributors to the subject. A detailed chapter on lymphatic anatomy of the abdomen, retroperitoneum, pelvis, and thorax emphasizes the appearances on lymphographic and computed tomographic images. Because of the difficulty of demonstrating normal lymph nodes by CT in the external, internal, and common iliac areas as well as the para-aortic, upper abdomen, and thorax, abnormal lymph nodes are used to illustrate the anatomy of these areas.

McKusick presents his extensive experience with radionuclide lymphography and deals with gallium-67 citrate, lymphoscintigraphy of the internal mammary chain, the iliopelvic area for genitourinary metastases to the internal iliac nodes, and the preoperative and postoperative mapping of lymph drainage of the skin before radical lymphadenectomy for melanoma metastases.

The technique of lymphography described in the text has proven over the years to be the least complicated and to use the lymphographer's time most efficiently without the need for special instruments. The more complicated techniques of cervical, testicular, and mammary lymphography have been omitted because they are time consuming and complicated and because the results have limited value. The general interpretation of lymphangiograms is important enough to merit a separate chapter.

The book would not be complete without the chapter on physiology by Thomas H. Adair and Arthur Guyton from Jackson, Mississippi. The dynamics of lymph formation and its function and factors that control its formation and flow are essential information for anyone working in the field. The chapters on abormal peripheral lymphatics by Dr. O'Donnell, a vascular surgeon, and abnormal mesenteric lymphatics by Professor M. Servelle, who performed lymphography on patients with lymphedema in 1945 using Thorotrast, are especially good, concise reviews of the lymphedemas, both congenital and acquired, describing the current clinical and surgical techniques for management. These chapters are up-to-date reviews of the subjects for surgical residents and practicing surgeons as well as radiologists.

Lymphography is not performed for benign disease of lymph nodes. However, this chapter has been included because of the importance of differentiating benign from malignant disease. Professor Robert J. Lukes has written an excellent review of the classification of lymphomas for the oncologist and radiologist. Although continually evolving, the functional approach based on immunological and cytochemical techniques has greatly increased our understanding of the non-Hodgkin's lymphomas by separating them into T, B, and U cell systems. Unquestionably, classification will change further, but this approach will accommodate further investigation of the basic biological mechanism of these disorders and ultimately a fundamental biological approach to therapy.

The chapter on lymphoma of the abdomen and retroperitoneum describes the advantages and disadvantages of lymphography and CT in the staging of patients with biopsy-proven lymphomas and an algorithm for the staging work-up.

Wallace and Jing present their vast experience with lymphatic imaging using lymphography and CT for the staging and management of solid tumors at the M. D. Anderson Hospital. Lymph node imaging of the thorax by Drs. McLoud and Meyer is an especially good concise review of lymphatic anatomy of the thorax and the use of CT in staging of patients with lung cancer. CT of cervical lymph nodes is a welcome addition to lymph node imaging because of the unreliability of lymphography in this area and the dramatic improvement in staging of head and neck tumors by high resolution CT. The approach by Drs. Reede and Bergeron is concise but comprehensive. Percutaneous lymph node biopsy is especially important to the radiologist, oncologist, and clinician staging patients with malignant disease. Routine use of aspiration biopsy of abdominal neoplasms and lymph nodes has shown it to be a safe and accurate method of establishing tissue diagnosis without surgery. Laparotomy can be avoided in incurable cases or in patients with recurrent disease, thus obviating the necessity for prolonged hospitalization. The chapter by Dr. Zornoza is, therefore, a must for one working in the field. The book concludes with a discussion of the real but infrequent complications of lymphography.

MELVIN E. CLOUSE, M.D.

# Preface to the First Edition

During the past 20 years diagnostic roentgenology has undergone an incredible evolution in techniques for imaging normal and abnormal anatomy. The evolution has progressed from the conventional techniques of body imaging to the use of sophisticated contrast media and shipment.

The development of lymphography is but one of the new techniques of diagnostic radiology. Study of the lymphatic system on a routine clinical basis was made possible with the starting publication by Dr. John B. Kinmonth, a British surgeon at St. Thomas Hospital, London, in 1952. The initial studies with water-soluble contrast media were of limited clinical use. The introduction of oily contrast media made lymphography applicable to the study of a large number of diseases of the lymphatic system and has produced an enormous amount of literature on the subject.

This book has been written primarily for those performing lymphography in a busy radiology department and for practicing surgeons, residents, and oncologists. The format lends itself to easy and rapid reference beginning with history, normal anatomy, technique, interpretation, abnormal lymphatics, benign lymph node disease, lymphoma, carcinoma, complications, radionuclide studies, and immunospecific lymphography. Each chapter is accompanied by a reference list that includes the major contributors on the subject material. Harrison has written a detailed anatomic and lymphographic chapter on anatomy of the lymphatic system. The technique of pedal lymphography described in the text has proven over the years to be the least complicated and makes the most efficient use of the lymphographer's time without the need of specialized instruments.

The technique of percutaneous lymph node aspiration biopsy is also described. The more complicated techniques of cervical, testicular, and mammary lymphography have been omitted because they are time consuming and complicated and because the diagnostic results have limited value. The importance of general interpretation of the lymphogram merits a separate chapter.

Chapter 3 is not intended as a complete reference text on the physiology of the lymphatic system but is a brief review of the formation, function, and circulation of lymph. The chapter on "Abnormal Lymphatics" by O'Donnell, a vascular surgeon, is an especially good, concise review of the lymphedemas, both congenital and acquired, describing the current clinical and surgical techniques of management. It is an up-to-date review of the subject for surgical residents and practicing surgeons as well as the radiologist.

The place of lymphography for benign diseases of the lymph node has not been clearly established, but the importance of differentiating benign from malignant disease is stressed. Lukes has written an excellent review of the classification of lymphomas for the clinician and radiologist. The chapter on "Lymphography in Lymphoma" by Hessel, Adams, and Abrams is especially clear and concise. Wallace and Jing present their vast experience with lymphography in carcinoma from the M. D. Anderson Hospital in Chapter 9, describing in detail its usefulness in staging and management of solid tumors especially in the genitourinary tract.

A review of the complications and method of management is presented in Chapter 10. Potsaid and McKusick in Chapter 11 review the use of radionuclide lymphography dealing extensively with gallium-67.

The chapter by Order on immunospecific radionuclide lymphography must be considered investigational. It has been included because of its exciting potential. Dr. Order presents a review of tumor antigenicity and possible uses of immunospecific reagents, the method of direct immunospecific lymphography—its diagnostic and therapeutic potential.

MELVIN E. CLOUSE, M.D.

# Acknowledgments

The problem of acknowledgment is always difficult because so many have contributed to the final product. The book could never have been completed without the editorial assistance of Sally Ann Edwards, who communicated with all of the authors as well as the publisher, collating and editing the chapters as well as completing the index. I would also like to thank Jeff Potter, the Research Assistant, for his help in literature research and review as well as Mr. Richard Wolfe, the rare book librarian at the Countway Library of Medicine at Harvard, for retrieving reference books and figures of the early anatomists used in preparing Chapters 1 and 2. The secretaries at the New England Deaconess Hospital, especially Ann Ryan, were most helpful in typing the revised edition. Stanley M. Bennett, Chief of Photography at the Massachusetts General Hospital, and Kathleen Grady, the Photographic Assistant, were very helpful in preparing the illustrative material. I am especially grateful and would like to thank each of the contributors for their work and diligence in preparing chapters of such high quality on schedule.

# Contributors

**Thomas H. Adair, Ph.D.**
Assistant Professor of Physiology and
Biophysics, The University of
Mississippi School of Medicine,
Jackson, Mississippi

**R. Thomas Bergeron, M.D.**
Professor of Radiology, New York
University Medical Center, New York,
New York

**Melvin E. Clouse, M.D.**
Associate Professor of Radiology,
Harvard Medical School, and
Chairman, Department of Radiology,
New England Deaconess Hospital,
Boston, Massachusetts

**Arthur C. Guyton, M.D.**
Professor of Physiology and Biophysics,
The University of Mississippi School of
Medicine, Jackson, Mississippi

**Dewey A. Harrison, M.D.**
Assistant Professor of Radiology, Stony
Brook Medical School and Nassau
County Medical Center, East Meadow,
New York

**Bao-Shan Jing, M.D.**
Professor of Radiology, University of
Texas, M. D. Anderson Hospital and
Tumor Institute, Houston, Texas

**Robert J. Lukes, M.D.**
Professor of Pathology, University of
Southern California School of
Medicine, Los Angeles, California

**Kenneth A. McKusick, M.D.**
Associate Professor of Radiology,
Harvard Medical School, and Clinical
Director of Nuclear Medicine,

Massachusetts General Hospital,
Boston, Massachusetts

**Theresa C. McLoud, M.D.**
Associate Professor of Radiology,
Harvard Medical School, and Chief of
Thoracic Radiology, Massachusetts
General Hospital, Boston,
Massachusetts

**Jack E. Meyer, M.D.**
Associate Professor of Radiology,
Harvard Medical School, and Director
of Oncologic Radiology, Massachusetts
General Hospital, Boston,
Massachusetts

**Thomas F. O'Donnell, Jr., M.D.**
Associate Professor of Surgery, Tufts
University School of Medicine, and
Chief of Vascular Surgery, New
England Medical Center, Boston,
Massachusetts

**Deborah L. Reede, M.D.**
Assistant Professor of Radiology, New
York University Medical Center, New
York, New York

**Marceau Servelle, M.D.**
Cardiovascular Section, Clinique
Ambroïse Paré, Neuilly-sur-Seine,
France

**Sidney Wallace, M.D.**
Professor of Radiology and Chief,
Section of Clinical Diagnostic
Radiology, University of Texas, M. D.
Anderson Hospital and Tumor
Institute, Houston, Texas

**Jesus Zornoza, M.D.**
Department of Radiology, Danbury
Hospital, Danbury, Connecticut

# Contents

Series Editor's Foreword. . . . . . . . . . . . . . . . . . . . . . . . . . . . .    v
Foreword. . . . . . . . . . . . . . . . . . . . . . . . . . . . . . . . . . . . . .    vii
Preface to the Second Edition  . . . . . . . . . . . . . . . . . . . .    ix
Preface to the First Edition  . . . . . . . . . . . . . . . . . . . . . .    xi
Acknowledgments . . . . . . . . . . . . . . . . . . . . . . . . . . . . .    xiii
Contributors . . . . . . . . . . . . . . . . . . . . . . . . . . . . . . . . .    xv

Chapter  1    **History**. . . . . . . . . . . . . . . . . . . . . . . . . . . . . . . . .    **1**
              *M. E. Clouse*
Chapter  2    **Normal Anatomy** . . . . . . . . . . . . . . . . . . . . . . . .    **15**
              *D. A. Harrison and M. E. Clouse*
Chapter  3    **Radionuclide Lymphography** . . . . . . . . . . . . . . .    **95**
              *K. A. McKusick*
Chapter  4    **Technique** . . . . . . . . . . . . . . . . . . . . . . . . . . . . .    **111**
              *M. E. Clouse*
Chapter  5    **Physiology—Lymph Formation,**
              **Its Control, and Lymph Flow** . . . . . . . . . . . . . . . .    **120**
              *T. H. Adair and A. C. Guyton*
Chapter  6    **Abnormal Peripheral Lymphatics** . . . . . . . . . . .    **142**
              *T. F. O'Donnell, Jr. and M. E. Clouse*
Chapter  7    **Malformations of the Mesenteric Lymphatics** . . . . . . . .    **180**
              *M. Servelle*
Chapter  8    **Interpretation** . . . . . . . . . . . . . . . . . . . . . . . . .    **203**
              *S. Wallace, B.-S. Jing, M. E. Clouse, and D. A. Harrison*
Chapter  9    **Benign Lymph Node Disease** . . . . . . . . . . . . . . .    **224**
              *M. E. Clouse*
Chapter 10    **Lymphoma—The Functional Approach to the**
              **Pathology of Malignant Lymphoma** . . . . . . . . . . . . .    **243**
              *R. J. Lukes*
Chapter 11    **Lymphoma of Abdomen and Retroperitoneum** . . . . . . . . .    **264**
              *M. E. Clouse*
Chapter 12    **Lymphatic Imaging of Solid Tumors** . . . . . . . . . .    **290**
              *B.-S. Jing and S. Wallace*
Chapter 13    **Lymph Node Imaging of the Thorax** . . . . . . . . . . .    **451**
              *T. C. McLoud and J. E. Meyer*
Chapter 14    **Computed Tomography of Cervical Lymph Nodes** . . . . . .    **472**
              *D. L. Reede and R. T. Bergeron*
Chapter 15    **Percutaneous Lymph Node Biopsy** . . . . . . . . . . . . .    **496**
              *J. Zornoza*
Chapter 16    **Complications** . . . . . . . . . . . . . . . . . . . . . . . . .    **511**
              *M. E. Clouse*

              **Index**. . . . . . . . . . . . . . . . . . . . . . . . . . . . . . . . .    **521**

# 1

# *History*

MELVIN E. CLOUSE, M.D.

Hippocrates' description of white blood and Aristotle's description of structures containing colorless fluid make it probable that lymph and lymph vessels were observed by the Alexandrian School in ancient times. These descriptions were lost with the decline in learning during the Middle Ages but were rediscovered in late Renaissance. According to Cruikshank (1786), a student of Hunter and the personal physician of Samuel Johnson, a Roman anatomist named Eustachius discovered the thoracic duct in a horse and described it in his treatis, *De Vena Fin Pari*, in 1563. He called the thoracic duct the vena Alba thoracica.

The glory of discovering the lymphatic vessels belongs to Gasparo Asellius, Professor of Anatomy and Surgery at Pavia, who on July 23, 1622, vivisected a well fed dog before members of the Order of Physicians to observe the recurrent nerve (Fig. 1.1). According to Drinker (1942), as an afterthought he decided to observe diaphragmatic motion. On opening the abdominal cavity and pulling the stomach aside, which he noted to be full, he was astonished by small white vessels in the mesentery along with the intestine. Asellius at first thought them to be nerves, but when real nerves were seen, he incised one and observed chyle rush out. He performed the same experiment on a dog whose stomach was empty and could not demonstrate these vessels. They were observed again when the experiment was repeated on another well fed dog. Asellius called them the vasa lactea and ascribed their function to absorbing chyle from the intestines and transporting it to the liver to be mixed into the blood stream.

Asellius' discovery was completely submerged for some time by Harvey's publication, *An Anatomical Disquisition on the Motion of the Heart and Blood in Animals*, in 1628. Even at the peak of his career, however, Harvey did not believe in the existence of Asellius' lymphatics or their function.

Asellius' book, *De Lactibus sine Lacteis Venis*, which contains his excellent diagrams of the mesenteric lymphatics and lymph nodes, was not only the first book on the lymphatic system but the first to have anatomic drawings in color.

In 1651 Pecquet described the thoracic duct and the cisterna chyli (Fig. 1.2). He found the cisterna chyli while performing an autopsy on a well fed dog and observed white fluid after removal of the heart. He first thought it was pus but after careful dissection found the thoracic duct. Almost simultaneously, van Horne, Professor of Anatomy at Leiden in 1652, also described the thoracic duct.

In 1652–1653 Thomas Bartholin and Olaf Rudbeck assembled the known parts of the lymphatic system and recognized them as a system (Fig. 1.3). Batholin was the first investigator to use the term lymphatic. The chyle vessels discovered by Asellius had been thought to convey food substances to the liver, but, when Bartholin ligated the portal tracts, he observed dilated lymphatics above the ligature and collapsed lymphatics below. At the same time he observed the thoracic duct, its inflow into the large veins, and the cisterna chyli. Immediately after his work was published, it became known that Rudbeck had presented essentially the same material before the Queen of Sweden at Uppsala prior to Bartholin's publication. Because of this, a violent argument erupted with each accusing the other of plagiarism. It is probable that each investigator working independently made the same discovery.

Anatomists until the time of Anton Nuck in 1685 considered the lymphatic vessels to have only one coat—the intima (Fig. 1.4). Nuck demonstrated a second fibrous coat in the thoracic duct of horses. Cruikshank in 1790 demonstrated a muscular coat as well as the intima in large lymphatics, but he could not demonstrate a muscular wall in smaller lymphatics.

According to Cruikshank the vasa vasorum in the lymphatic wall was described by William Hunter in 1762, who also noted contraction of the lymphatic vessels in response to irritation but could not demonstrate nerve innervation.

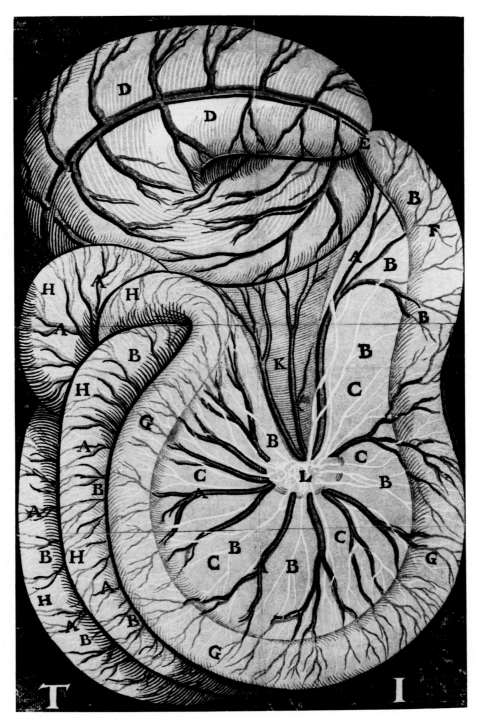

FIGURE 1.1. MESENTERIC LYMPHATIC VESSELS (B VENAE LACTEAE) (From Asellius, 1627.)

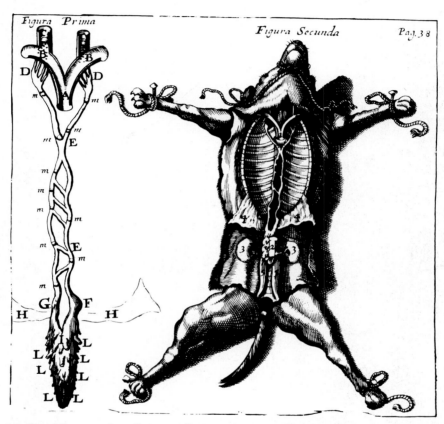

FIGURE 1.2. FROM BOOK BY JEAN PECQUET, DISCOVERER OF THE THORACIC DUCT AND CISTERNA CHYLI (From Pecquet, 1651, p 38.)

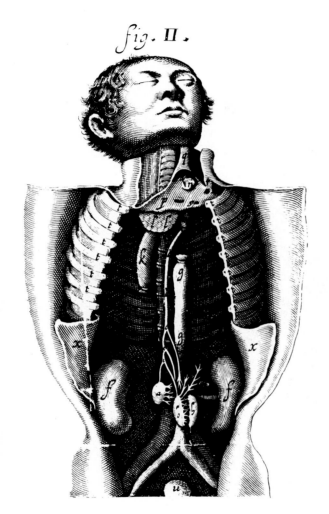

FIGURE 1.3. HUMAN CISTERNA CHYLI AND THORACIC
DUCTS
(From *The Anatomical History of Thomas Bartholinus of
the Lacteal Vein of the Thorax.* London, 1673.)

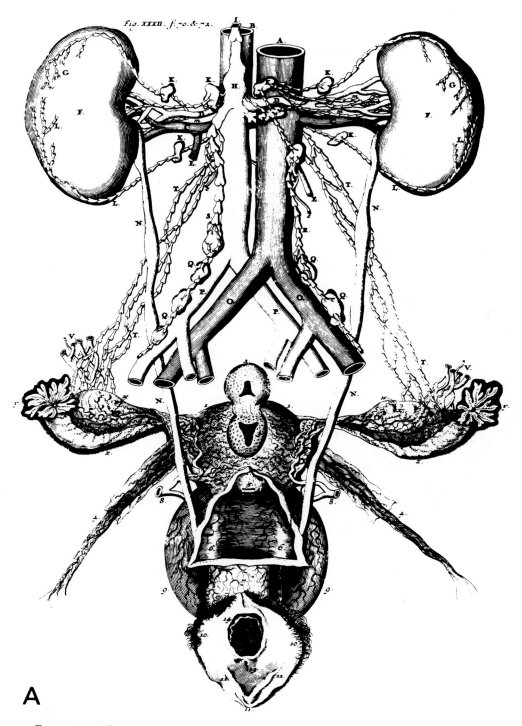

FIGURE 1.4*A*. LYMPHATICS OF THE RENAL AND REPRODUCTIVE SYSTEMS (From Nuck, 1692.)

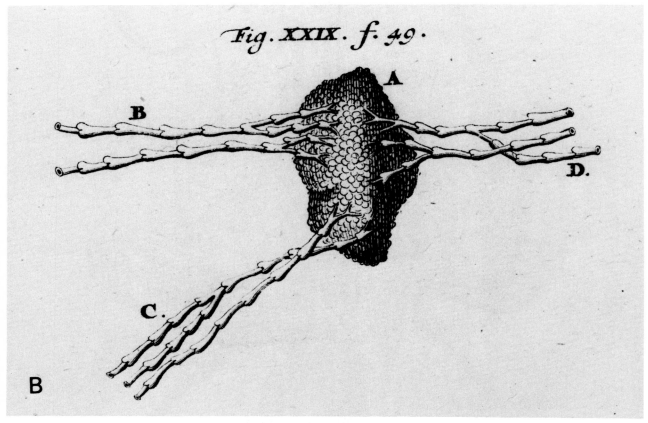

FIGURE 1.4*B*.  LYMPHATIC VESSELS AND NODES
An especially good drawing of valves. (From Nuck, 1692.)

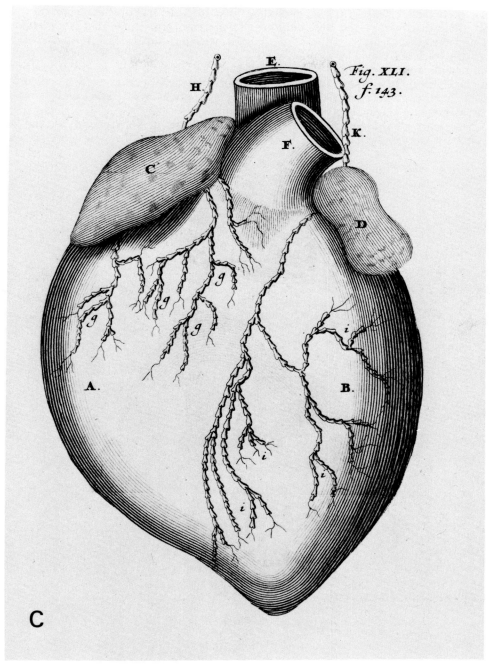

FIGURE 1.4C. HEART LYMPHATICS (From Nuck, 1692.)

Wrisberg in 1808 and Cruikshank in 1786 observed nerves in the vicinity of lymphatic vessels but could not demonstrate direct nerve innervation of the thoracic duct. It was not until 1925 that nervous innervation of the lymphatics was properly demonstrated by Lawrentjew. Dissecting cats and dogs, he described a periadventitial plexus of small ganglia surrounding the thoracic duct. Fibers from the intercostal and vagus nerves entered the thoracic duct. Branches from the lesser splanchnic nerve also supplied fibers to the lower thoracic duct and cisterna chyli.

Valves in the lymphatic vessels were almost certainly observed by Bartholin and Rudbeck, but Frederick Ruysch (1638–1731) is considered—if not their discoverer—the best demonstrator of the valves (Fig. 1.5).

Lymph nodes were seen by Herophilus, who noted certain veins in the mesentery that terminated in glandular bodies. These same glands were noted by Asellius, who thought them part of the pancreas because the lymph vessels were thought to pass through the pancreas on their way to the liver. For this reason they were labeled *pancreas Asellii* in *De Lactibus sine Lacteis Venis.* It was not until 1863 that His demonstrated them to be an integral part of the lymphatic system. In fact His' original description of the internal architecture and blood supply to the lymph nodes was so accurate that it has not changed.

Accurate demonstration of the course and

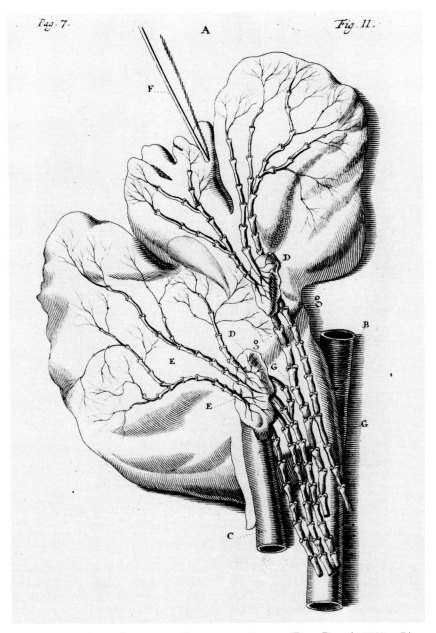

FIGURE 1.5. LIVER LYMPHATIC VESSELS AND VALVES (From Ruysch, 1665, p 7.)

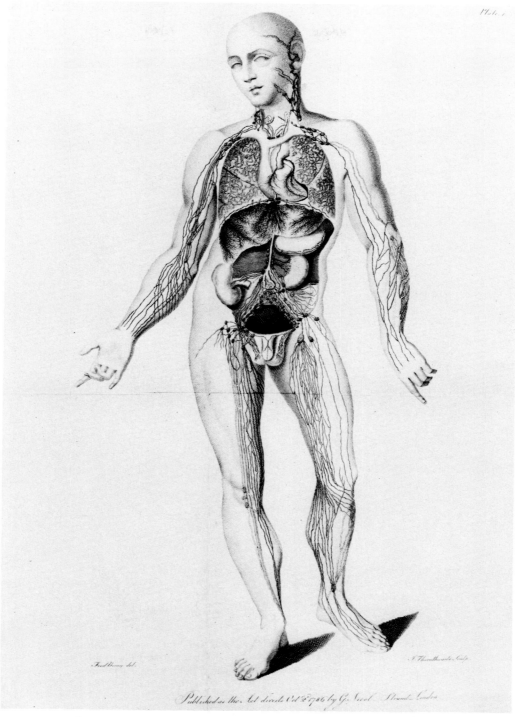

FIGURE 1.6. PERIPHERAL AND VISCERAL LYMPHATIC VESSELS AND NODES
(From Cruikshank, 1786, p 192.)

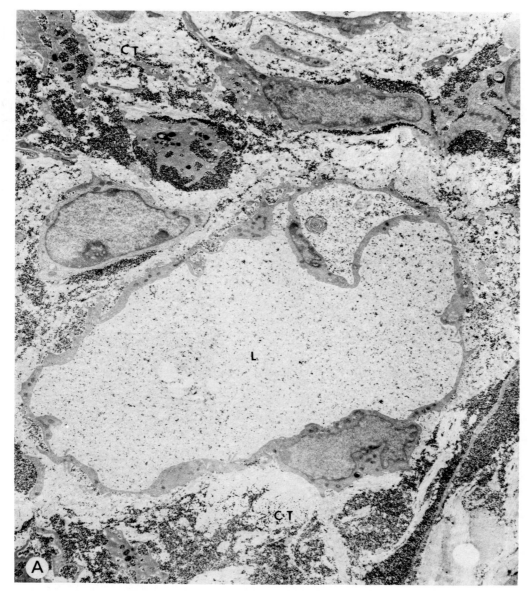

FIGURE 1.7A. ELECTRON MICROGRAPH OF THE LYMPHATIC CAPILLARY AND SURROUNDING CONNECTIVE TISSUE AFTER
THE INTERSTITIAL INJECTION OF COLLOIDAL THORIUM
Note the presence of tracer throughout the connective tissue (*CT*) and within the lymphatic lumen (*L*).

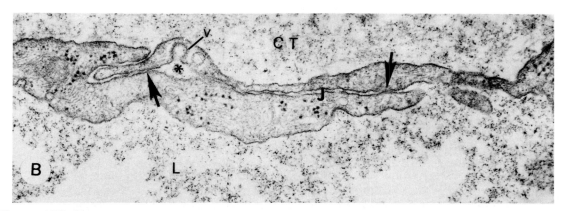

FIGURE 1.7*B*. Although the Adjacent Endothelial Cells Are Extensively Overlapped, the Width of the Intercellular Clefts (∗) is Extremely Varied over Its Length

In addition, points of close apposition are also observed (*arrows*). Colloidal ferritin occurs in the connective tissue (*CT*) and the lumen (*L*) of the vessel. Plasmalemmal vesicles (*v*) also contain ferritin. *J*, intercellular junction.

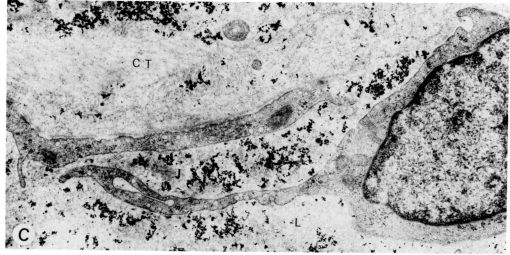

FIGURE 1.7*C*. Electron Micrograph of a Patent Intercellular Junction (*J*) Containing Colloidal Thorium
*L*, lumen; *CT*, connective tissue. (Courtesy of Dr. L. V. Leak and Dr. J. F. Burke.)

interconnection of lymphatic vessels was made possible by Anton Nuck in 1692. Using a time-consuming technique of injecting mercury into the lymphatics, he succeeded in visualizing practically the entire lymphatic system. It was from Nuck's technique that Mascagni in 1787 and Cruikshank in 1790 demonstrated the lymphatic topography in all parts of the body (Fig. 1.6). Gerota in 1896 introduced a new analytical technique using Prussian blue paint dissolved in turpentine and ether. On the basis of this improved technique, Jossifow in 1930 and Rouvièr in 1932 published books on the complete lymphatic system.

William Hunter was probably the first to appreciate the functional significance of the lymphatic system. He demonstrated absorption of chyle from the intestinal tract into the lymphatics. In a lecture published posthumously in 1784, he stated that lymphatic vessels all over the body (whether from the skin, lining of body cavities, or intestinal tracts) were the absorbing vessels and together with the thoracic duct transported chyle to the blood vascular system.

The mechanism of lymph formation was elusive. It was generally believed until 1850 that lymph passed from the blood stream into lymphatic vessels by direct communication through thin tubules—the vasa serosa. The chief architects of the vasa serosa theory were Boerhaave (1738, 1742) and Vieussens (1705), who demonstrated canaliculi between blood vessels and the lymphatics. These were later shown to be artifacts of their primitive histological techniques.

Virchow in 1858 contested the vasa serosa theory for lymph formation but believed there were communications through intercellular canaliculi. Von Recklinghausen in 1862 opposed the intercanalicular theory but thought the communication was direct through very small lymphatics and blood vessels. Ludwig's theory, more nearly correct, was based on simple filtration of fluid and molecular substances caused by intravascular pressure (blood pressure). Heidenhain criticized Ludwig's simple filtration theory because certain substances increased lymphatic flow. The vasa serosa theory was not abandoned, however, until after Schwann discovered the cell as the basic form of living substances within the body.

In 1894 Starling proved these theories incorrect. Starling's theory was that the blood capillary endothelium is a semipermeable membrane that is permeable to water and crystalloids but impermeable to proteins. Hydrostatic pressure in the arterial limb of the capillary induces filtration of water and crystalloids into the interstitial space. As the hydrostatic pressure in the venous limb diminishes, the plasma osmotic pressure becomes the driving force for resorption of crystalloids and water. The proteins cannot be absorbed into the blood through the semipermeable membrane (the capillary endothelium) but are absorbed by the lymphatics.

The anatomic basis for absorption of fluid and large molecules into the initial lymphatics (lymphatic capillaries) has been demonstrated by Leak and Burke (1966) and Casley-Smith (1972). Using electron microscopy these authors have demonstrated "open" junctions between the lymphatic endothelial cells for passage of fluid and large molecules. Smaller molecules may pass directly through the endothelial cell membrane into the lymphatic lumen (Figs. 1.7 and 1.8). The lymphatic endothelial cells are anchored by small fibrils to the surrounding connective tissues.

Although there have been many investigators in the field of lymphology, Cecil K. Drinker, Professor of Physiology at the Harvard School of Public Health, must be considered the father of modern lymphology because of his extensive observations and studies on the formation of lymph, its content, and changes in disease states (Drinker, 1942).

The concept of radiographic visualization of the lymphatics was published 35 yr after Roentgen's discovery of x-rays. In 1930 and 1931 Funaoka from Japan and Carvalho of Portugal performed lymphography by injecting Thorotrast into the lymph nodes and subcutaneous tissues of animals and cadavers. In 1932 Pfahler showed lymphatics in a live man using the indirect method of lymphography. The indirect method of visualizing the lymphatics relied on the absorption of contrast material into the lymphatics from the connective tissue, body cavities, and organs. One week after the injection of Lipiodol into the maxillary sinuses, the lymphatics leading from the region were observed. The contrast media used for indirect lymphography were Thorotrast, oily solutions (such as Lipiodol), and water-soluble compounds (such as Urografin, Biligrafin, Joduron, and Collargol). Numerous investigators attempted to visualize the lymphatics indirectly, but this method was impractical because lymphatic vessels do not absorb the contrast material rapidly enough to visualize the vessels and nodes adequately.

The direct method of lymphography involved direct injection of contrast material into the nodes and lymph vessels. Teneff and Stoppani in 1936 and Servelle in 1945 visualized the lym-

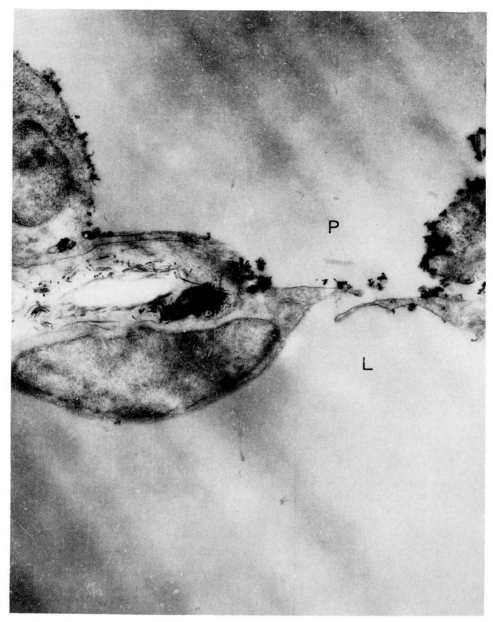

FIGURE 1.8. MOUSE DIAPHRAGM

There is a gap between two lymphatic endothelial cells. *L*, lymphatic lumen; *P*, peritoneal cavity for passage of large molecules. The overlapping nature of the junction implies that it can close on diaphragmatic contraction. Original magnification ×20,000. (From Casley-Smith, 1972.)

phatic channels and nodes in the pelvis by injecting Thorotrast into the inguinal nodes. In addition, Servelle performed lymphangiography in patients with lymphedema, using Thorotrast, and published a series of 12 patients in 1946.

It was not until 1952, when Kinmonth developed his revolutionary approach for identifying the pedal lymphatics by injecting patent blue violet dye (11%) into the subcutaneous tissues, that lymphography became a useful clinical tool. With this technique, the lymphatics are readily seen for direct cannulation because of the rapid absorption of the patent blue violet dye. Kinmonth then cannulated the vessel directly and injected water-soluble contrast material. Thus the procedure could be performed on patients with normal lymphatic vessels and used to study a wide spectrum of diseases of the lymphatic system.

It is interesting that Hudack and McMaster in 1933 at the Rockefeller Institute outlined the cutaneous lymphatics in humans using 11% patent blue violet dye and observed the network of dermal lymphatics draining into the subcutaneous chains with channels leading into the axilla. Presumably, they did not think of directly injecting contrast material into the lymphatic vessels—hence lymphography as a useful clinical tool did not arrive until 1952!

The first studies of Kinmonth were on the pathological changes of lymphedema using water-soluble contrast media, Biligrafin and Urografin. Thorotrast could not be used because of its now known toxicity. Water-soluble contrast material is excellent for examination of vessels but is unsatisfactory for studying nodes, and, in addition, it is diluted by the lymph in the lumbar area.

Hreschyshyn et al. (1961), Wallace et al. (1961), and Malek (1959), all almost simultaneously (1959–1961), modified the direct approach by using oil-soluble contrast material. This permits excellent visualization of the para-aortic lymph channels and nodes and the thoracic duct.

# REFERENCES

Asellius G: *De Lactibus sine Lacteis Venis*. Mediolani, apud Io B Bidellium, 1627.

Bartels P: Das lymph gefasssystem. In: *Handbuch d. Anatomie d. Menschen*. Jena, G. Fischer, 1909.

Bartholin T: *De Lacteis Thoracicis in Homine Brutisque*. Hafniae, M Martzan, 1652.

Boerhaave H: Oratio de Uso Rationii Mechanicii in Medicine, habita 24 Sept 1702. In *Opusc ommnia*. Hagaecomitis, 1738.

Boerhaave H: *Praelectiones Academiae in Proprias Institutiones Rei Medicae*. 1742.

Carvalho R, Rodriguez A, Pereina S: Lamise en evidence por la radiographie du system lymphatique chez la vivant. *Ann Anat Pathol (Paris)* 8:193, 1931.

Casley-Smith JR: The role of the endothelial intercellular junctions in the functioning of the initial lymphatics. *Angiologica* 9:106, 1972.

Cruikshank W: *The Anatomy of the Absorbing Vessels of the Human Body*. London, G Nicol, 1786.

Drinker CK: *The Lymphatic System: Its Part in Regulating Composition and Volume of Tissue Fluid*. Stanford, Stanford University Press, 1942.

Funaoka S, Tachikawa R, Yamaguchi O, Fijita S: Kurz Mitteilung über die Roentgenographie dies Lymphagefässsystem souie über den Mechanismes der symphstromung. *Ab Dritten Abst Inst Kaiserlich Univ Kyoto* 1:11, 1930.

Gerota D: Zur Technik der Lymph gefässinjektion. Eine nue Injektionsmasse der Lymphagefasse. Polychrome Injektion. *Anat Anz* 12:216; *Verh Anat Ges* 151–152, 1896.

Harvey W: An anatomical disquisition on the motion of the heart and blood in animals. In: *The Works of William Harvey, M.D.*, translated by R Willis from the Latin with a life of the author. London, Sydenham Society, 1847.

Heidenhain R: Versuche and Frozen zur Lehre von der Lymphbildung. *Pflügers Arch* 49:209, 1891.

His W: Uber das Epithel der Lymphagefasswurzeln und uber die von Recklinghausen's schen Saftcanalchen. *Z Wiss Zool* 13:455, 1863.

Hreschyshyn MM, Sheehan F, Holland JF: Visualization of retroperitoneal lymph nodes. Lymphangiography as an aid in the measurement of tumor growth. *Cancer* 14:205, 1961.

Hudack S, McMaster PD: The lymphatic participation in human cutaneous phenomenon. A study of the minute lympatics of the living skin. *J Exp Med* 57:751, 1933.

Jossifow GM: *Das Lymphgefässsystem der menschen*. Jena, 1930.

Kinmonth JB: Lymphangiography in man. *Clin Sci* 11:13, 1952.

Lawrentjew AP: Zur Lehre von der Innervation des Lymphsystems. Über die Nerven des Ductus Thoracicus beim Hunde. *Anat Anz* 60:475, 1925–1926.

Leak LV, Burke JF: Fine structure of the lymphatic capillary and the adjoining connective tissue area. *Am J Anat* 118:785, 1966.

Malek P: Physiologische, Pathologische und Anatomische Grundlagen der Lymphographie. IX International Congress of Radiology, Munchen, 1959.

Mascagni P: *Vasorum Lymphaticorum Corporis Humani Historia et Ichonographia*. Siena, 1787.

Nuck A: *Adenographia Curiosa et Uteri Foeminei Anatome Nova*. Lugd B, 1692.

Pecquet J: *Experimenta Nova Anatomica quibus Incognitum Chyli Receptaculum et ab eo per Thoracem in Ramos usque Subclavis Vasa Lactea Deteguntur*. Paris, 1651.

Pfahler GG: A demonstration of the lymphatic drainage of the maxillary sinuses. *AJR* 27:352, 1932.

Rouvièr H: *Anatomie des Lymphatiques des l'homme*. Paris, Masson, 1932.

Rudbeck O: *Nove Exercitatio Anatomica, Exhibens Ductus Hepaticos Aquosos, et Vasa Glandularum Serosa*. Arosiae, 1653.

Ruysch F: *Dilucidatio Valvularum in Vasis Lymphaticis et Lacteis*. Hagaecomitiae, 1665.

Servelle M: A propos de la lymphographie experimentale et clinique. *J Radiol Electro Med Nucl* 26:165, 1944–1945.

Servelle M: Lymphangiographic et elephantiasis. *Arch Mal Colur* 39:409–426, 1946.

Starling EH: The influence of mechanical factors on lymph production. *J Physiol (Lond)* 16:224, 1894.

Teneff S, Stoppani F: Apropos de la lymphographie. *J Radiol Electrol Med Nucl* 20:74, 1936.

van Horne J: Novus Ductus Chyliferus. Nunc Primum Delineatus, Descriptus Eruditorium Examini Expositas. Lugd Batav, 1652.

Vieussens R: *Novum Vasorum Corporis Humani Systema*. Amstelod, 1705.

Virchow R: *Die Cellular pathologie inihrer Begründung auf physiologische gewebelehre*. Berlin, 1858.

von Recklinghausen FD: *Die Lymphgefasse und ihre Beziehung zum Bindegewehe*. Berlin, A Hirschwald, 1862.

Wallace S, Jackson L, Schaffer B: Lymphangiograms: their diagnostic and therapeutic potential. *Radiology* 76:179, 1961.

Wrisberg H: *Observations Anatomical de Nervis Vescerum Abdominis*, part 3. Götting, 1808.

# 2

# *Normal Anatomy*

**DEWEY A. HARRISON, M.D., AND MELVIN E. CLOUSE, M.D.**

Immediately after its introduction by Professor John B. Kinmonth, lymphography became the gold standard for imaging the retroperitoneum in patients with biopsy-proven malignant disease. This was especially so for patients with Hodgkin's or non-Hodgkin's lymphoma. For the first time, radiologists, clinicians, and oncologists had a method for directly imaging diseased retroperitoneal nodes. For the lymphomas, accuracy of 81–95% has been reported (Takahashi and Abrams, 1967; Castellino and Marglin, 1974; Hessel et al., 1977; Castellino, 1982; Clouse et al., 1985). The patient's size and weight, presence or absence of bowel gas, and degree of body fat do not affect the quality of the images. In addition, a large number of nodes can be imaged, including isolated or generalized disease, and the presence of contrast material in the nodes provides a guide for node biopsy under fluoroscopy. An additional benefit includes the presence of contrast material remaining in nodes for long term follow-up.

Disadvantages of lymphography include its somewhat invasive nature and allergies to patent blue violet dye and contrast material. The main disadvantage, however, is that lymphography does not delineate those nodes above the cisterna chyli (including the celiac, mesenteric, hepatic and splenic nodes) nor the primary drainage nodes from the testes. For these reasons, computed tomography (CT) was enthusiastically embraced soon after it was introduced and became universally utilized as an imaging modality, especially for those areas that could not be probed by lymphography.

The advantages of CT are that accuracy figures near those of lymphography have been reported and that it yields excellent global anatomy of the celiac, mesenteric, hepatic and splenic hilar nodes as well as abdominal viscera and retroperitoneal organs and nodes. The method of CT is less operator dependent, results are reproducible for accurate follow-up, and it can be used to guide biopsy for bulk disease as well as for determining radiation treatment portals.

The disadvantages of CT, even under ideal circumstances, are its inability to delineate intranodal architecture and its reliance on size as the criterion for abnormality even though enlargement may not occur with displacement or obliteration of normal retroperitoneal architecture. Lymph nodes smaller than 1.5 cm in diameter were once considered normal and those above 1.5–2 cm abnormal. Now nodes 1–2 cm are considered suspicious, and those greater than 2 cm, definitely abnormal. One may find a group of nodes all less than 1 cm in diameter, but if the entire conglomeration of nodes is greater than 2.0 cm in diameter, the mass should be considered abnormal. In addition, enlargement to greater than 3 cm in diameter can occasionally be caused by reactive hyperplasia.

Guidelines must be followed for node clusters according to anatomic area and age of the patient. As a general rule, nodes are larger in younger patients than in older patients. The inguinal nodes are usually larger than the iliac nodes, and iliac nodes are larger than para-aortics. The low para-aortic nodes are also larger than the high para-aortic nodes near the cisterna. Nodes in the inguinal region may be near 2 cm in size after lymphography due to enlargement that occurs with filling and the inflammatory reaction to contrast material. The high para-aortic and retrocrural nodes normally are small aggregates of lymphatic tissue 1–3 mm in diameter. Lymph nodes in the retrocrural space are now considered abnormal if they exceed 6 mm in size (Callen et al., 1977).

CT identification of all lymph node areas requires adjacent soft tissue interfaces produced by the presence of fat. Contrasting fat planes must be adequate, and bowel, blood vessels, and ureters must be properly opacified and identified. In most adult patients the para-aortic and paracaval regions are endowed with adequate fat to delineate planes and structures. In the iliac region, however, a relative paucity of fat makes lymph node assessment somewhat difficult.

The CT technique used in imaging lymph

nodes varies, but precise attention to technical factors is crucial. Oral and intravenous contrast materials are widely used. Careful monitoring and imaging are also necessary. Nodes may enhance after intravenous contrast administration as well. This consideration becomes important when differentiating nodes from surrounding vessels. Also, on a single slice one may delineate all of the nodes in that slice, but intraslice nodes—those within the 2-cm slice thickness—could be missed. In lymphography, even though large numbers of nodes are opacified, all of the nodes in the retroperitoneal area generally do not fill.

One must weigh the advantages and disadvantages of each modality in determining which method should have priority. In this chapter, normal roentgen anatomy of the lymphatic system is presented for lymphangiography and CT. The anatomy of the lower extremity and retroperitoneum is illustrated as shown by dorsal pedal lymphography with CT after lymphography as a correlation for each nodal area. The lymphatic anatomy of areas not shown by dorsal pedal lymphography is illustrated using CT. In these areas, especially above the inguinal ligament, normal retroperitoneal, iliac, splenic, mesenteric, and hepatic hilar nodes are difficult to recognize so the anatomy is demonstrated using scans of diseased nodes.

## DEVELOPMENTAL CONSIDERATIONS

By injecting pig embryos, Florence Sabin in 1902 learned the first concepts of developmental anatomy of the lymphatics. At approximately the sixth week of embryonic life (10-mm state), paired jugular sacs become recognizable. The original concept postulated that lymphatic endothelium was a derivation of venous endothelium from a process of sprouting. Huntington and McClure (1906–1907) and Kampmeier (1912) subsequently postulated that lymphatic structures originated from fusion of mesenchymal clefts and that their connection with developing contiguous veins came secondarily. Still there is disagreement on the exact mechanism of initial derivation of the lymphatics, but otherwise the system's developmental anatomy is clearly established (Tondury, 1967).

As differentiation continues, the lymphatics rapidly separate and grow together, anastomosing into their own system. In spite of the development into a separate system, however, lymphatiocovenous communications have been demonstrated to persist, even in fully developed animals (Bron et al., 1963). Paired lymphatic sacs become evident in the inguinal region adjacent to the common iliac veins, and two other unpaired sacs develop along the posterior abdominal wall. One of these sacs gives rise to the cisterna chyli; the other develops into a retroperitoneal sac that extends into the lymphatic network of the mesentery, stomach, and retroperitoneal organs.

The thoracic duct can first be recognized in embryos of approximately 23–24 mm. The embryonic thoracic duct consists of two sacs which are bilaterally symmetrical. Their starting point is in the abdominal cavity at the level of the cisterna chyli. Dorsal to the aorta, the right duct crosses at about the level of the fourth thoracic vertebra to join the duct of the oppostie side. Thus, a single trunk forms on the left side and then merges with the jugular portion of the thoracic duct. The jugular portion of the thoracic duct is a caudal outgrowth of the jugular lymph sac on the left. In the embryo the two primitive ducts are connected by numerous cross anastomoses over the course of the aorta. Persistence and growth of a part of the embryonic duct system and involution of other parts result in the adult anatomic structure now accepted by most authorities on the anatomy of the thoracic duct. Although embryonic development of the thoracic duct can result in many variations, the usual adult form is a single duct passing into the thorax and opening into the venous system of the left side (Davis, 1915).

Lymph nodes do not appear until the vessels are well established. They are first recognizable as masses of lymphoid tissue in complex networks of developing vessels. Excepting the cisterna chyli, lymphoid masses destined to be nodes develop contiguously with the primitive sacs. The lymphoid masses divide into smaller portions. Then, penetration by vessels occurs and the tissue becomes enclosed in a connective tissue capsule. The original lymphoid tissue becomes the medullary cords and cortical nodules. Enclosing lymphatic capillaries form the sinusoidal system. All structures of the node are present and completely arranged at birth with the exception of differentiation of germinal centers (secondary nodules) within primary nodules.

## GENERAL ANATOMIC CHARACTERISTICS

The functions of the lymphatic system can be summarized as (a) production and transport of thymus-dependent small lymphocytes that operate mainly in the cellular immunity mechanism; (b) production of large lymphocytes and plasma cells, which in turn produce circulating antibodies; (c) return of interstitial proteins to blood; (d) filtration of body fluids through nodal sinuses; and (e) transfer of absorbed fats from intestinal lacteals to the thoracic duct (Drinker and Yoffey, 1941; Gowans, 1959; Rusznyak et al., 1967; Kuisk, 1971).

### Lymphatic Vessels

The normal lymphatic system is a closed network of vessels that commences with lymphatic capillaries in soft tissues, extends to larger vessels that pass through lymph nodes, and again collects in another network of closed vessels. Communication with the cardiovascular system predominantly is through anastomoses with neck veins by way of the thoracic duct (Davis, 1915; Clark, 1942; Brash, 1943). Lymphatic capillaries are the functional units of the system in its role of absorption and interchange of fluid substances and cells (Casley-Smith, 1967).

The capillaries are lined with endothelial cells and vary in shape throughout the body. The capillaries form anastomotic complexes with diameters ranging from a few microns to approximately 1 mm (Fig. 2.1). Electron microscopy can demonstrate overlapping endothelial cells that interlock with fine microfibrils. This complex is cemented to interstitial tissues. The microfibrils play a crucial role in maintaining patency of vital endothelial interconnections when pressure in the interstitium rises. Pappenheimer et al. (1951) elaborated on the significance of these interconnections (Pappenheimer pores) in a description of the "pore theory of molecular diffusion and filtration." This pathway appears to be the mechanism for movement of substances composed of large molecules. Smaller molecules pass directly through the endothelial cytoplasm.

Anatomically, larger lymphatic vessels (approximately 0.5–0.75 mm in diameter) are very similar to veins, containing three layers in their walls. The adventitia is composed of longitudinal and transverse bundles of smooth muscle and collagen fibers. Most of the medium-sized vessels possess a smooth muscle media of varying muscular configurations. The intima consists of endothelium and elastic fibers, the infolding of which forms valves to prevent backflow of lymph (Ham and Leeson, 1961; Bloom and Fawcett, 1962). Differing from veins, lymphatic vessels branch into divisions of similar diameters. Vessels are classed as afferent or efferent based on their functional relationship to the nodes. The thoracic duct is the largest of the vessels (4–6 mm in diameter) (Fig. 2.2).

Alternating bands of constriction and dilatation approximately 1 cm apart are characteristic of vessels filling in lymphography. The areas of constriction are lymphatic valves that become conspicuous as the viscous oily contrast material

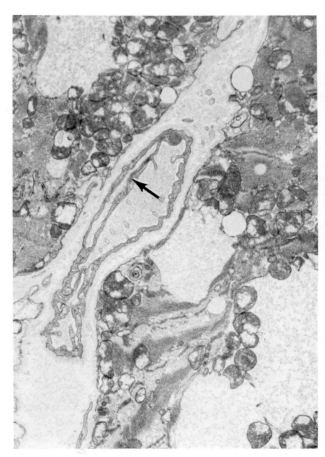

FIGURE 2.1. ELECTRON MICROGRAPH OF CROSS-SECTION OF LYMPHATIC CAPILLARY

The capillary consists of a single layer of endothelial cells blending into surrounding connective tissue. Note infolding that produces valves (*arrow*). Original magnification ×10,000. (Courtesy of Dr. Margaret Billingham, Department of Pathology, Stanford University Medical Center.)

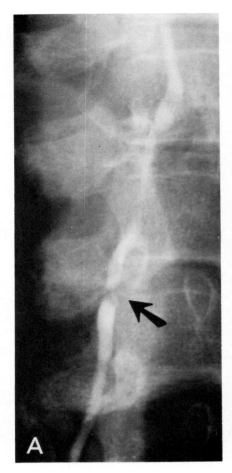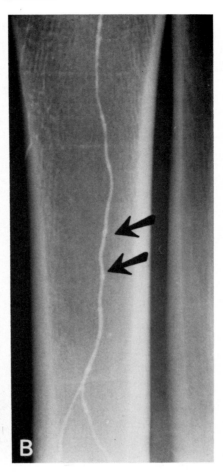

FIGURE 2.2. CONTRAST FILLING OF LYMPHATIC VESSELS

*A*: Segment of the thoracic duct. *B*: Lower extremity vessel filled with contrast material. *Arrows* indicate the areas of constriction and dilatation, which are characteristic of lymphatic valves during contrast infusion.

slightly distends the surrounding portion of the vessels (Fischer and Zimmerman, 1959; Jacobsson and Johansson, 1959; Fuchs, 1969; Jackson and Kinmonth, 1974b). Although the valves influence antegrade flow, movement of fluid along the vessel is determined primarily by external forces (Drinker and Yoffey, 1941).

## Lymph Nodes

The glandular structures (nodes of the lymphatic system) consist of groups of round lymphoid cells contained in a complex of reticulum fibers (Fig. 2.3). The thymus, spleen, tonsils, other collections of lymphoid tissue (Peyer's patches), and, to some extent, bone marrow contain cells that are similar in many respects to those cells of lymph nodes. Immunity is their common bond (Drinker and Yoffey, 1941).

Nodes vary extensively in size, shape, and

color and occur singly or in clusters. The specific characteristics of nodal groups depend to a large degree on their location and neighboring organs (Rouvière, 1938). Nodal parenchyma consists of a peripheral portion (cortex) and a more central core (medulla) (Fig. 2.3).

Nodes have four basic components: aggregates of lymphoid tissue (nodules), lymphatic capillaries, blood vessels, and supportive tissue framework (histological framework). Lymphoid elements predominate (Ham and Leeson, 1961; Bloom and Fawcett, 1962; Tjernberg, 1967). As noted in Figure 2.4, lymphoid nodules are encountered throughout the periphery of the node just within the capsule and subcapsular space (marginal sinus).

The supportive tissue framework of the node has considerable importance in lymphography (Tjernberg, 1967). Lymph nodes commonly lie in fatty tissue, but the node itself is surrounded

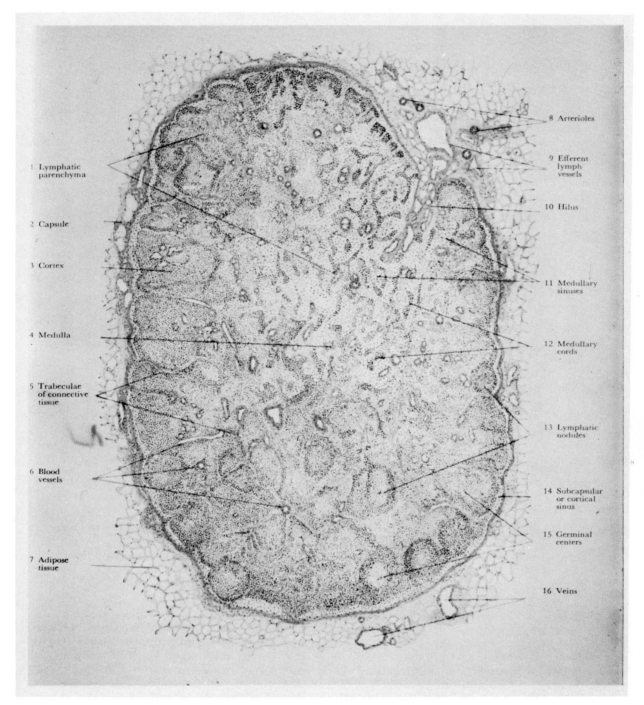

FIGURE 2.3. TYPICAL LYMPH NODE ARCHITECTURE

The parenchyma is predominant and is enclosed by a fibrous capsule. The capsule is interrupted by an indentation (hilus) where the arterioles enter and the venules and efferent lymph vessels emerge. As represented, nodes often are embedded in adipose tissue.

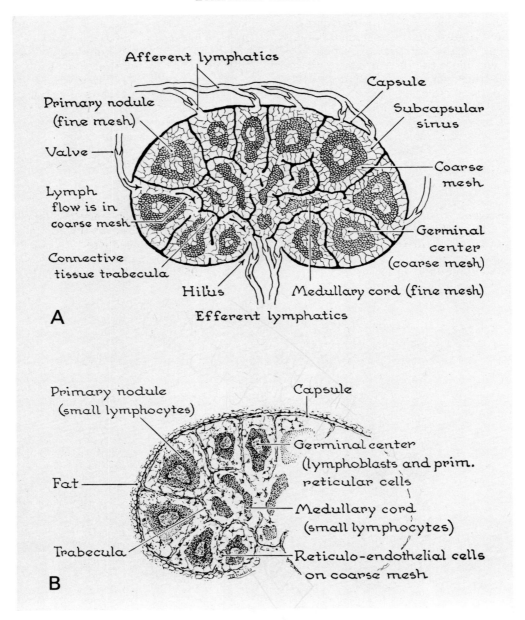

FIGURE 2.4. ARCHITECTURAL RELATIONSHIP OF FUNCTIONAL CONSTITUENTS OF LYMPHATIC SYSTEM
(EXCLUDING CAPILLARIES)

*A*: Afferent vessels penetrate the surface of the node through the capsule. During lymphographic injections, contrast material follows a course very similar to that of lymph flow. *B*: Note the difference in appearance of the primary follicles (densely stained homogeneously) and the secondary follicle (pale-stained central germinal center). Medullary cords branch and anastomose with each other and with cortical follicles. During lymphography these lymphoid elements produce the characteristic stippled radiolucencies observed in the nodes; their radiographic opacification is due to the surrounding contrast material, which settles in the supportive tissue framework. (Adapted from Ham and Leeson, 1961, p 390.)

by a capsule of dense collagenous fibers, fibroblasts, and some smooth muscle. Radiating from the capsule and hilus and extending into the substance of the node are connective tissue strands or trabeculae that provide nodal support and carry blood vessels. In addition to the trabeculae, an extensive network of reticular fibers projects from the capsule and trabeculae throughout the node. These fine reticular fibers form a lacy, interdigitating communication of minute spaces (sinus system). The portion beneath the capsule is the subcapsular or marginal sinus, while those segments found in the cortical and medullary regions are named respectively (Fig. 2.4A). Physiologically these sinuses serve as areas for permeation of fluid (Ham and Leeson, 1961; Rusznyak et al., 1967). During lymphography the oily contrast material in the si-

nuses opacifies the nodes (Fischer and Zimmerman, 1959; Fuchs, 1969) (Fig. 2.5).

Analysis of the lymphadenogram (nodal phase) has paramount significance during lymphography (Fig. 2.6). The roentgen appearance of the internal architecture of a node depends on the relative amounts of lymphatic tissue or other tissue of similar density (e.g., neoplasm) within the node and on the volume of contrast material deposited in the sinuses (Tjernberg, 1967).

## LOWER EXTREMITY LYMPHATICS

The roentgen appearance of the course and anatomic relationships of lymphatics of the extremities was first described by Kinmonth (1952). In subsequent years, the usual or normal pathways of lymphatic drainage of the lower

extremities and their relationships to various anatomic landmarks seen during lymphography have been well established (Kinmonth et al., 1955a, b; Jacobsson and Johansson, 1959; Malek et al., 1959, 1964; Fischer et al., 1962; Larson

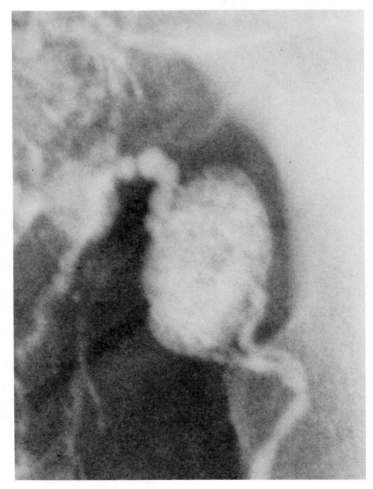

FIGURE 2.5. AFFERENT VESSELS DURING CONTRAST INJECTION

Note the afferent vessels transporting the oily substance to the node. After permeating the node through the sinuses, the material exits through a large efferent vessel.

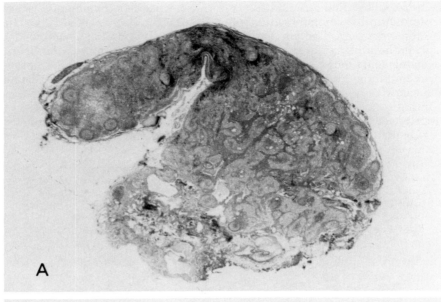

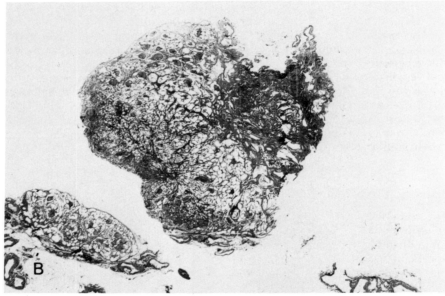

FIGURE 2.6. PHOTOMICROGRAPHS OF NODES

*A*: Mild reactive hyperplasia emphasizes the lymphoid elements in a node that has not undergone lymphography. Original magnification ×8. *B*: Sections of nodes with lymphographic contrast material entrapped in the reticular network. Original magnification ×9. (Courtesy of Dr. Margaret Billingham, Department of Pathology, Stanford University Medical Center.)

and Lewis, 1967; Kuisk, 1971; Browse, 1972a). A technically successful examination is imperative in order to obtain maximal diagnostic accuracy in assessing normal or abnormal lymphograms.

Vessels of the lower extremities consist of superficial (subcutaneous) prefascial and deep subfascial systems. Both systems accompany or are accompanied by corresponding blood vasculature. Dorsal pedal lymphatic injections (routine clinical lymphography) normally will not opacify the deep subfascial system. The superficial system is composed of anterior and posterior vessels. These vessels are usually opacified in routine clinical lymphography.

## Anterior Superficial System

If a lymphatic vessel on the medial aspect of the dorsum of the foot is injected more proximally, the opacified vessels course continuously anteriorly with the greater saphenous vein. Cannulation and injection of a vessel lateral on the dorsum will opacify vessels that predominantly course anteriorly and laterally below the knee.

From approximately the midcalf to the proximal third of the lower extremity, the lateral vessels cross in a gentle curve toward the medial side. As vessel filling continues, the lateral vessels become entirely medial just proximal to the knee, and their course continues along the greater saphenous vein as the medial chain vessels. Therefore, injection of any vessel on the dorsum results in opacification of the major portion of the superficial system, the origins (anteromedially and anterolaterally) of which ultimately accompany the greater saphenous vein and drain into the inguinal lymph nodes (Fig. 2.7).

The anteromedial chain tends to originate with slightly larger vessels on the dorsum but ascends with fewer vessels below the knee as compared to the anterolateral chain. Also, the anteromedial vessels are less variable in number and character in this region. Below the knee the anterolateral vessels are serpiginous and branch frequently as they begin to course medially. Usually anterolateral vessels deviate medially; anteromedial vessels seldom become lateral. Above the knee both groups are medially placed and display frequent bifurcations. Upon reaching their destination, the inguinal nodes, there are 10–20 vessels with similar characteristics (Fig. 2.8).

### Posterior Superficial System

The posterior component of the superficial prefascial lymphatics contributes far less to the system but can be opacified by cannulating and injecting a superficial vessel below the lateral malleolus. These vessels are smaller and more tortuous than the anterior component, and they contribute only one to three subcutaneous trunks. Posteriorly, these trunks accompany the lesser saphenous vein to the popliteal fossa. The afferents empty into one to three popliteal nodes. Efferent vessels then emerge, turn anteromedially, become deep subfascial vessels, and thereafter follow the deep blood vessels on the medial aspect of the thigh. Subsequent drainage is into deeper, more proximal inguinal nodes.

### Deep Subfascial System

Valves in lymphatics of the lower extremity direct flow from the deep to the superficial system, contrasting the flow pattern in the venous system. Techniques to perform lymphangiography on the deep subfascial system of the lower extremity have been devised, hence some knowledge of its roentgen appearance has been gained (Malek et al., 1959, 1964; Larson and Lewis, 1967).

The deep system of the lower leg and thigh collects lymph from the muscles, fascia, and joints. Some of the deep lymphatics of the thigh are demonstrated by opacification of the posterior superficial lymphatics. Once past the popliteal region, these vessels become subfascial as they continue in the thigh (see "Posterior Superficial System"). Lymphographically the ascending vessels of the superficial and deep systems do not seem to communicate extensively.

Ngu (1964) postulated an interesting concept pertaining to lymphatic drainage of the lower leg and thigh. His postulate suggests separate pathways of drainage for each of these regions. Evidence to support this theory was derived from the observation that there were separate nodes of drainage for each of these areas and that in the presence of postinflammatory edema below the knee, normal thigh lymphatics were maintained. Although the observations were accurate, the postulate was not proven. No attempts were made to opacify simultaneously the deep system of the lower leg and thigh for possible communication above the knee.

### Inguinal Lymphatics

Lymphographically, lymphatics of the inguinal region are strikingly variable. Contrast filling of the inguinal lymphatics shows wide variations in the number and course of the vessels with even more extensive variations in the number, size, and appearance of the nodes (Fischer et al., 1962). This significant variability of nonmalignant nodes can simulate malignancy in this region (Greening and Wallace, 1963; Wallace et al., 1962; Butler, 1969; Castellino et al., 1974). Therefore it is quite tenuous to interpret the inguinal nodes as containing primary or secondary malignant disease without substantial abnormality in higher regions (Wallace et al., 1961, 1962; Abrams et al., 1968; Kuisk, 1971; Browse, 1972a; Castellino, 1974) (Fig. 2.9).

Those nodes lymphographically considered as inguinal fall below the inguinal ligament and are divided into the superficial and deep groups. Specific distinction between these groups by lymphography can be difficult. The superficial group is further subdivided into superior and inferior groups. The superior nodes are more proximal than the inferior group and thus are closer to the femoral canal. Lymphographically, the inferior group is visualized far more fre-

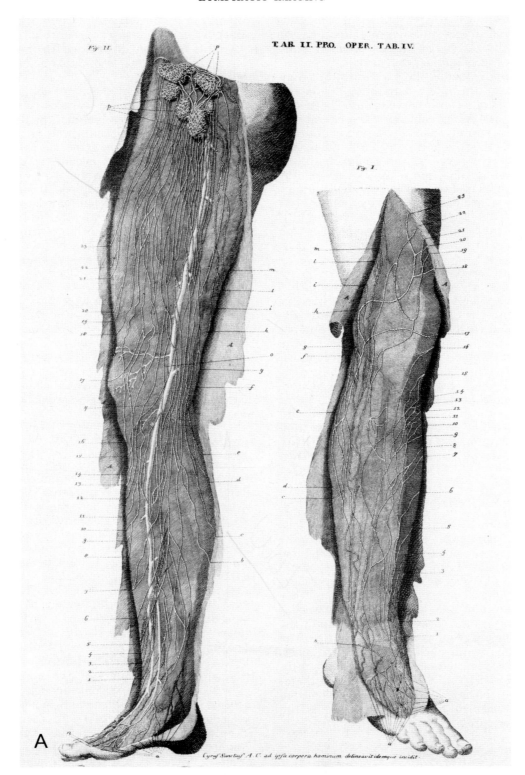

**FIGURE 2.7. LOWER EXTREMITY LYMPHATIC VESSELS**

*A*: (From Mascagni, 1787.) *B* and *C*: Vascular phase of lymphography shows course of injected contrast material. In *B* note that all channels have become medial.

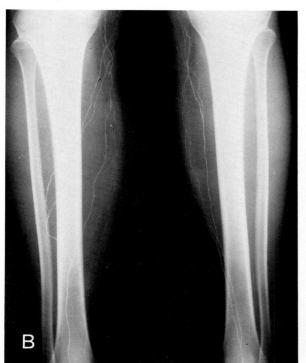
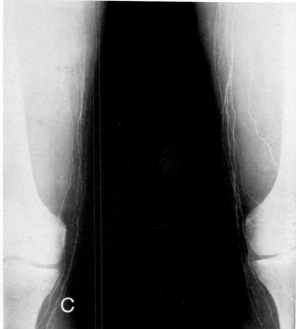

FIGURE 2.7*B* and *C.*

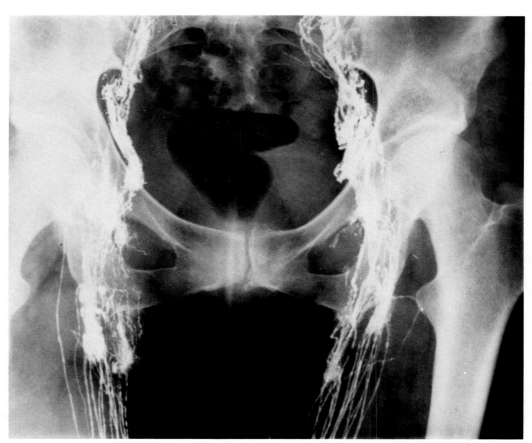

FIGURE 2.8. NUMEROUS LOWER EXTREMITY VESSELS TRAVERSING INGUINAL REGION
Note the similarity in appearance, particularly in size, even after frequent divisions distally.

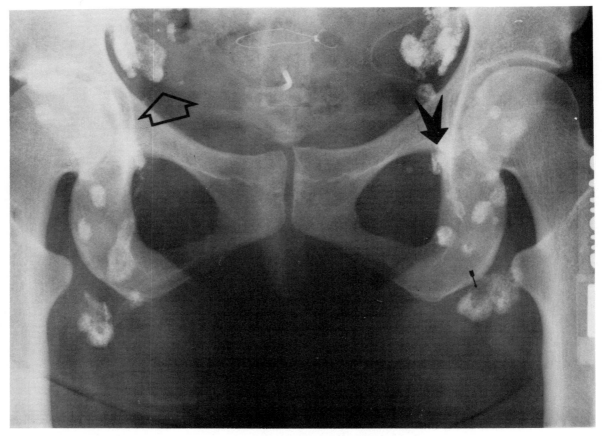

FIGURE 2.9. NORMAL INGUINAL NODES

The inguinal nodes are enlarged and characteristically foamy. Striking filling defects are also typical. Left inguinal node (*small arrow*) possesses sufficient characteristics to cause a false-positive diagnosis of nodal malignancy. The more cephalad low iliac nodes (*upper arrows*) appear less ominous but still can be easily misinterpreted.

quently than the superior group that drains the perineal structures (Fuchs, 1969, 1971b; Kuisk, 1971).

The deep inguinal group is also located more proximal and closer to the inguinal ligament than the superficial inferior group. The most proximal nodes of the deep inguinal group are larger, more constant, and occasionally seem continuous with the above external iliac group. In the inguinal fossa, medial to the femoral vein and immediately below the medial external iliac nodes, is a relatively large constant node (Fig. 2.10). This node has descriptively been called the *node of Rosenmüller, Pirogow,* and *Cloquet* (Kubik et al., 1967; Kuisk, 1971; Fuchs, 1971b).

Vessels from the lower nodes pass superiorly, sometimes bypassing a higher inguinal group on their way to the external iliac nodes. The efferents that emerge from the inguinals are larger and more tortuous than antecedent afferents,

and lymphographically the valves become more apparent and accentuated.

Lymph nodes in the inguinal region shown by CT can vary in size and exact location. These nodes are seen below the inguinal ligament at the level of the femoral heads (Fig. 2.11). On sections through the femoral neck, the sartorius, rectus, femoris, and iliofemoral vessels can be identified and should not be confused with lymph nodes. The nodes tend to be more medially positioned, and when normal, they are much smaller than the muscle bundles, varying in size from a few millimeters up to 1.5 cm. With 1- and 2-cm sections, these nodes may not be demonstrated.

To a greater extent, the clearly identifiable inguinal nodes are those anterior and medial to the femoral vessels. Nodes more posterior tend to rest adjacent to the muscle bundles and can be difficult to discern unless enlarged. The su-

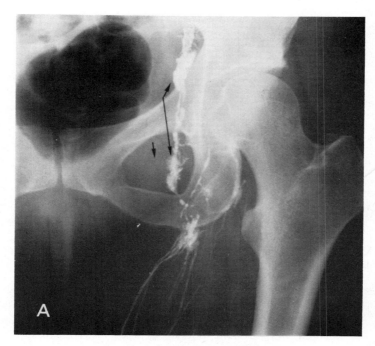

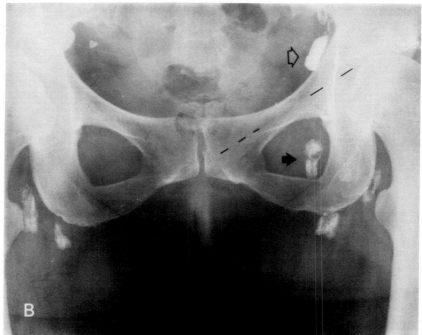

FIGURE 2.10. NODE OF ROSENMÜLLER, PIROGOW, OR CLOQUET

*A*: The node is shown communicating with the external iliac group (*arrows*). *B: Open arrow* shows opacified external iliac node; *broken line* delineates area of inguinal ligament; *solid arrow* points to node of Rosenmüller. Although the presence of this node is quite constant, its appearance is quite variable.

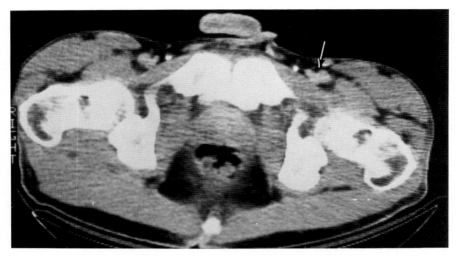

FIGURE 2.11. CT SECTION THROUGH SYMPHYSIS PUBIS
Note contrast material in the normal superficial inguinal nodes medial to the femoral artery and vein (*arrow*).

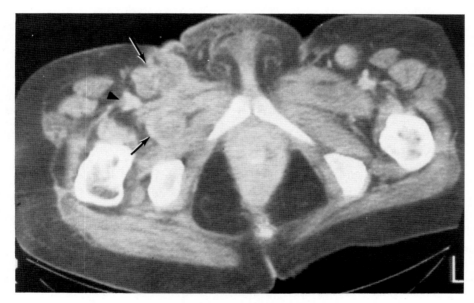

FIGURE 2.12. CT SECTION AT INFERIOR MARGIN OF SYMPHYSIS PUBIS
Note very large superficial and deep inguinal nodes (*arrows*) with necrotic centers in a patient with rectal carcinoma. *Arrowhead*, femoral artery and vein.

perior superficial group is closer to the inguinal ligament and can be seen as small, discrete soft tissue densities around the femoral vessels outlined by subcutaneous fat. CT generally reveals more nodes than are consistently seen by lymphography. Generally the three- to five-node mass in the inguinal region should be less than 1.5 cm in diameter all together. The node of Rosenmüller or Cloquet, the most medial node of the deep inguinal group, lies just below the inguinal ligament and may continue the internal chain of the external iliac group or course parallel to this chain and empty directly into the obturator node. Bulky adenopathy, when present, tends to destroy the interface between fat and soft tissue densities (Fig. 2.12).

# ILIAC LYMPHATICS

The next region visualized by lymphography is the pelvic (iliac) lymphatic bed. These nodes are located between the inguinal ligament inferiorly and the bifurcation of the common iliac blood vessels. Specific names for these lymphatics basically correspond to the adjacent iliac blood vessels.

## External Iliac Group

The external iliac lymphatics consist of three chains: lateral (external), intermediate (middle), and medial (internal) (Fig. 2.13). The lateral (external) chain is usually composed of one to three vessels that run along the lateral aspect of the external iliac artery. Lymphography usually demonstrates the most inferior node of this group. It is variously called the *lateral retrocrural node* (Herman et al., 1963) or the *lateral lacunar node* (Kubik et al., 1967) and is a rather constant, fairly large node (Fig. 2.10). Herman et al. (1963) describe one to three additional smaller nodes within this group.

The intermediate (middle) chain is less routinely demonstrated and is usually composed of fewer vessels than the lateral or medial chain (Herman et al., 1963; Kuisk, 1971). It is positioned between the artery and the vein, and anastomotic connections with the lateral and medial chains are common. The entire intermediate group usually comprises two to four nodes. Fuchs (1969) states that the middle retrocrural node is frequently absent.

The medial (internal) chain contains the greatest number of vessels (Herman et al., 1963). This chain is medial to the vein, superior to the obturator nerve, and more dorsal to the vein than the other external iliac chains. Herman et al. (1963) describe the dorsal location of this chain as being "prolapsed into the pelvis," and Fuchs (1969) specifically states that this group is situated close to the pelvic wall. Critical analysis of the lymphographic appearance of this group requires oblique and/or stereoscopic views of the region (Fig. 2.14). The most inferior node of this group is called the *internal retrocrural node* (Herman et al., 1963) or the *medial lacunar node* (Kubik et al., 1967; Fuchs, 1969). Although small additional nodes may be found in this chain, the middle node is the largest and most commonly opacified node of this group. This single node may represent the group in its entirety due to fusion with the node of Rosenmüller

or nodes of the intermediate chain (Herman et al., 1963; Fuchs, 1979; Kuisk, 1971).

Nevertheless, whether this node is seen on the lymphogram independently or tapered toward other nodes in an apparently inseparable cluster, thorough familiarity with the regional anatomy and internal architectural morphology of this node has high priority to the oncological lymphologist. This node is a most important lymphatic drainage site for the majority of male and female pelvic organs and is a common site for deposition of metastatic pelvic malignancies (Rouvière, 1938; Kuisk, 1971). Optimal visualization of this node frequently requires stereoscopy and occasionally laminagraphy.

The deep femoral lymphatics communicate with the middle node through the deep inguinal chain (Kuisk, 1971).

The term *obturator node* is lost in a myriad of confusion (Herman et al., 1963; Fuchs, 1969; Kuisk, 1971), and lymphologists who use the term must specify the anatomic location of the node to which they refer. In an attempt to correlate lymphographic anatomy with surgical and pathological anatomy, Herman et al. (1963) concluded that the lymphogram conforms more accurately with the anatomic description of Rouvière (1938) and therefore that lymphographic terminology is more precise than surgical terminology. Anatomic descriptions state that obturator nodes are part of the external iliac chain (Rouvière, 1938; Clark, 1942). The term *obturator node* tends to designate specifically the middle node of the internal chain of the external iliac group (Herman et al., 1963) (Figs. 2.14*D* and 2.15).

On CT scans, the three chains of the external iliac lymphatics accompany the external iliac artery to the aortic bifurcation. Separation of the nodes into each chain is difficult by CT because normal-sized nodes (i.e., 1 cm in diameter) overlap and surround the associated blood vessels and a lymph node is seldom differentiated from the accompanying blood vessel on a plain scan. For this reason, CT demonstrates the external iliac nodes only after contrast lymphography (Fig. 2.14*D*). Note also that nodes increase in size by approximately 20–30% after lymphography due to the presence of contrast material and the associated inflammatory reaction secondary to the oily contrast material (Steckel and Cameron, 1966).

As with bipedal lymphography, there is much

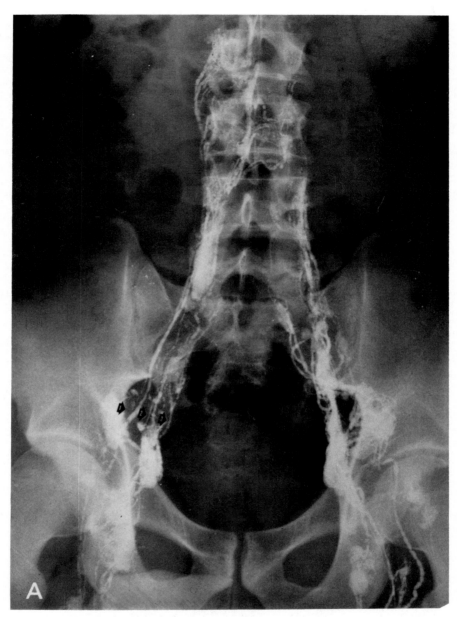

FIGURE 2.13. EXTERNAL ILIAC LYMPHATICS

*A*: Frontal projection during vascular phase of lymphogram. Three chains are demonstrated and indicated by *arrows: (1)* lateral, *(2)* intermediate, and *(3)* medial. Note the normal undulating vessel appearance; looping and crossover in the paralumbar region are also characteristic vessel-filling patterns. *B*: Better delineation of respective chains is obtained with a posterior oblique projection. *C*: Nodal retention phase depicting external iliac chains in frontal projection. *D*: Posterior oblique projection of the nodal retention phase. Note fusion of node of Rosenmüller with internal retrocrural node *(3)*.

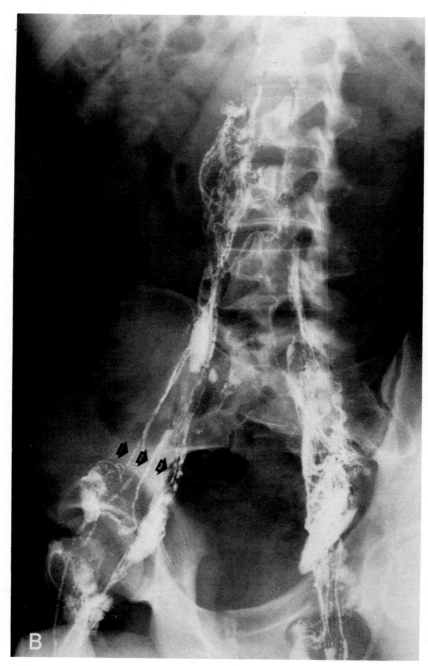

FIGURE 2.13*B*

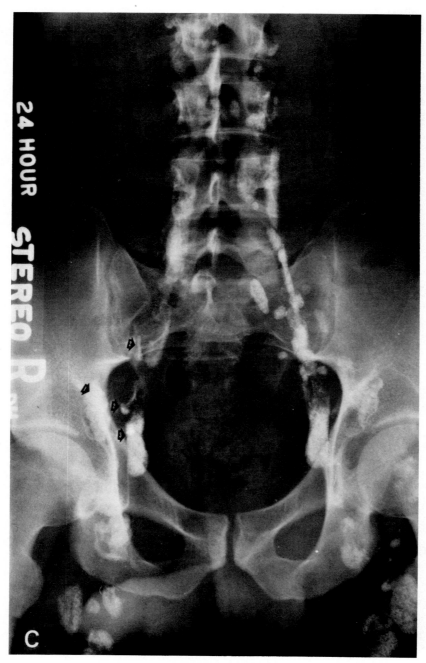

FIGURE 2.13*C*

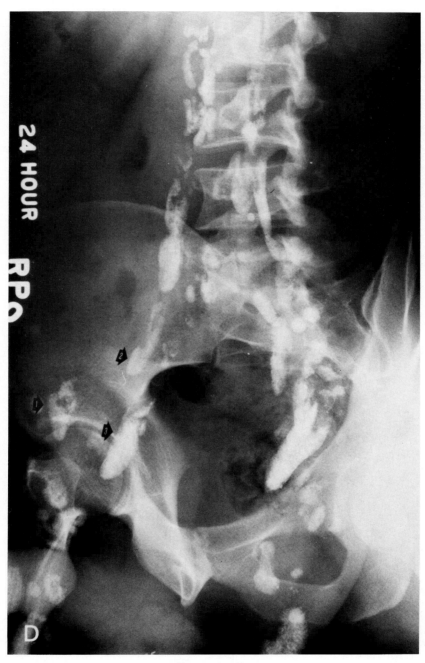

FIGURE 2.13D

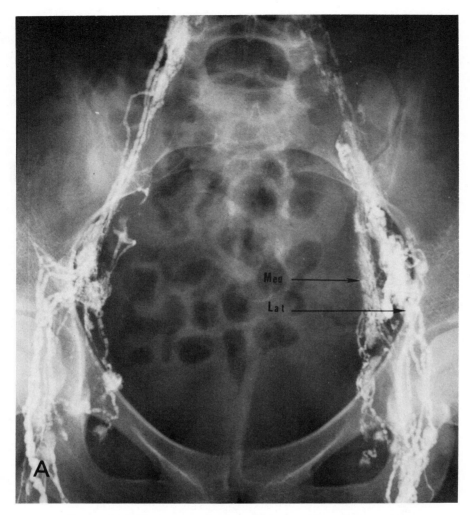

FIGURE 2.14. MEDIAL AND LATERAL EXTERNAL ILIAC LYMPHATICS

A: Frontal projection of vascular filling phase. In this projection the extensive superimposition of vessels and nodes is typical. B: Nodal retention phase in the frontal projection. Stereoscopic or oblique projections are imperative for adequate assessment. C: Left posterior oblique coned view delineates the respective nodal groups. The lateral and medial chains are endowed with more numerous, larger, and better opacified nodes. Commonly the intermediate group is the least endowed. The configuration of larger nodes is elongated and ovoid. Smaller nodes tend to be more nearly round. The medial (internal) chain is fused extensively into a single cluster. This cluster is fused with the middle node of the medial chain, which is the *obturator node* according to Rouvière (1938) and Herman et al. (1936). D: *Arrow*, contrast-filled obturator node; *OI*, obturator internus muscle; *RM*, rectus muscle.

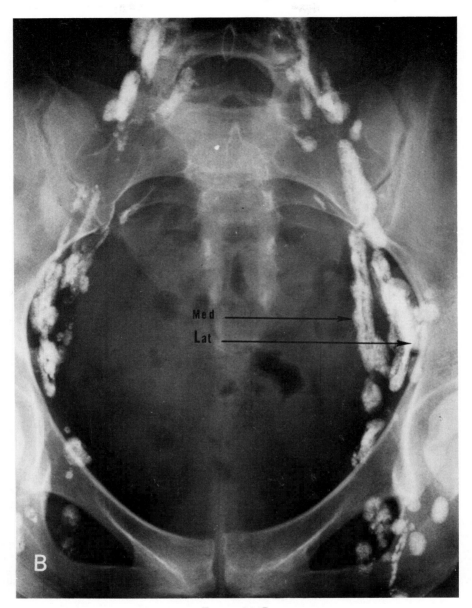

FIGURE 2.14B

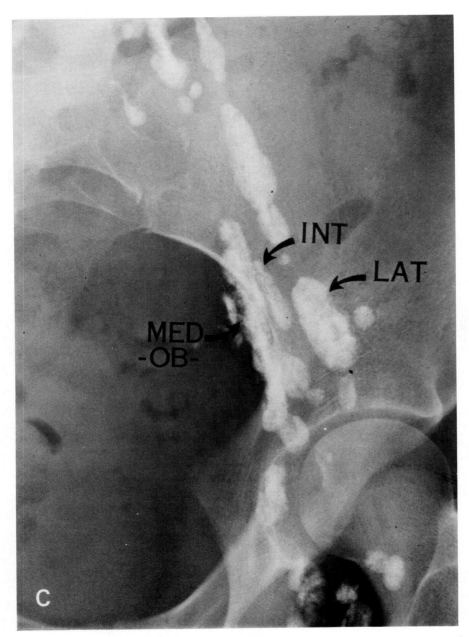

FIGURE 2.14C

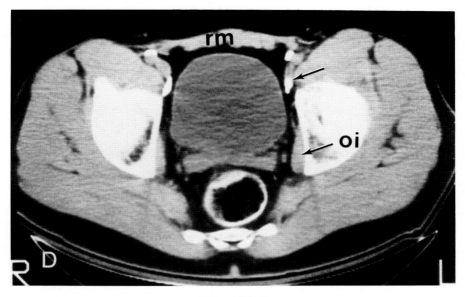

FIGURE 2.14*D*

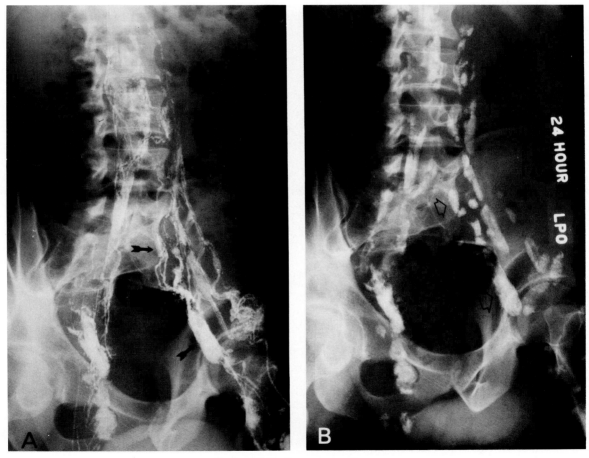

FIGURE 2.15. OBTURATOR NODE

*A*: Posterior oblique projection of the filling phase demonstrates a dominant medial chain (*upper arrow*). The middle node and Rosenmüller's node are fused (*lower arrow*). *B*: Subsequent nodal retention phase in the posterior oblique projection shows opacification of the large fused node. Continuation of the medial chain is shown by the more cephalad *arrows*.

controversy as to the precise location of the obturator node on CT scans. Anatomically and lymphographically, the obturator node is the middle node of the internal chain of the external iliac group. It lies above the inguinal ligament and falls deep in the pelvis to a position adjacent to the obturator internus muscle (Fig. 2.14D). It continues to be frequently confused with hypogastric nodes along the chain of the internal obturator artery (Cunéo and Marcille, 1901). The obturator node lies just superior to the inguinal ligament and receives drainage from the medial deep inguinal chain of nodes, specifically the node of Rosenmüller or Cloquet (Rouvière, 1938).

Even when sufficient pelvic fat is present, normal-sized external iliac nodes are almost impossible to differentiate from the external iliac artery and vein. Nodes 2 cm or greater in size are generally very easy to differentiate and more than an isolated large node—such as invasion of fat planes—is usually found to substantiate the presence of abnormality (Fig. 2.16).

## Internal Iliac (Hypogastric) Group

Internal iliac (hypogastric) nodes are usually four to eight in number and are located along the distribution of the internal iliac artery (Figs. 2.16B and 2.17) (Cunéo and Marcille, 1901). The anterior group is located along the hypogastric artery between the origins of the umbilical and obturator arteries. In addition, there are nodes in relation to the uterine artery, to the prostatic branches of the inferior vesicle and middle hemorrhoidal arteries, and to the inferior gluteal, internal pudendal, and superior gluteal arteries. Two or three nodes are also placed along the lateral sacral arteries opposite the second and third sacral foramina (i.e., the lateral sacral nodes). The hypogastric nodes include a few intercalated nodes along the course of the lymphatic trunks that accompany the middle hemorrhoidal artery. This group contributes to lymphatic drainage of the musculoskeletal structures of the pelvis as well as the organs intrinsic to the pelvic cavity. Most of these nodes are near their respective drainage sites (Rouvière, 1938; Brasch, 1943; Fuchs, 1969). Topographically these nodes can be further grouped into the nodes adjacent to the internal iliac blood vessels that drain the pelvic viscera and into the parietal nodes that drain the musculoskeletal portion of the pelvic wall.

The presence of specific nodes of the parietal and visceral subgroups is quite variable. At present, however, specific node clusters are named according to adjacent internal iliac blood vessel branches or tributaries. Pedal lymphography seldom reveals internal iliac nodes. Some data indicate wide anatomic variability of the internal iliac nodal groups (Reiffenstuhl, 1964; Howett and Greenberg, 1966). Thus, nonopacification or erratic minimal opacification of these nodes lymphographically is common. The most commonly opacified internal iliac group is the lateral sacral nodes of the parietal subgroup, and these are seen only in approximately 50% of normal lymphograms (Herman et al., 1963) (Figs. 2.17–2.19).

As the anatomic descriptions indicate and CT partially demonstrates, the hypogastric nodes are generally quite small and quite variable. Therefore, unless there are abnormal nodes (i.e., enlarged significantly in size), hypogastric nodes are difficult to demonstrate by CT on 1-cm slices through the pelvis. Frequently a very small cluster of densities (2–3 mm) outlined by pelvic fat near branches of the hypogastric artery and vein is compatible with lymph nodes. Since the primary drainage nodes from the pelvic viscera (i.e., bladder, uterus, prostate, cervix, and ovary) are largely the external iliac nodes, external iliac adenopathy is much easier to demonstrate by CT.

## Common Iliac Group

The common iliac arteries begin at the aortic bifurcation, usually in the vicinity of L4. External and internal iliac blood vessels communicate at approximately the level of the sacral promontory of S2. Between these two landmarks, the adjacent lymphatic vessels and nodes are termed the *common iliac group*.

The lateral chain of the external iliacs continues as the lateral chain of the common iliac group. It is lateral and slightly posterior to the artery. The intermediate chain can be found both anterior and posterior between the artery and the vein. The medial chain is dorsal and medial to the blood vessels. The three chains communicate extensively with each other. Communications between left and right common iliacs occurs with 50% frequency (Herman et al., 1963; Fuchs, 1969, 1971b) (Fig. 2.18).

The aortic bifurcation influences the anatomic relationships of the common iliac vessels and nodes. The connection of the medial common iliac chain is influenced far more by the aortic bifurcation than the intermediate or lateral chains. Influencing factors are (a) the precise lumbar vertebral level and acuteness of the angle of the bifurcation and (b) the distortion of the bifurcation by arterial atherosclerotic disease.

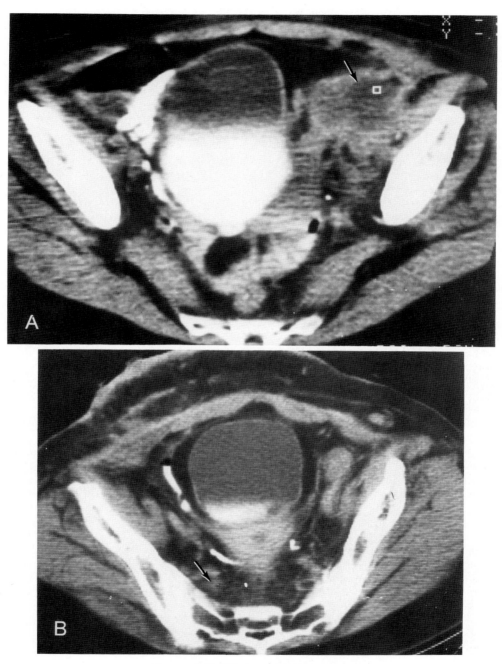

FIGURE 2.16. CT ABOVE ACETABULUM
*A*: Note the very large external iliac node with necrotic center in this patient with non-Hodgkin's lymphoma. *B*: CT through ilium showing a large left external iliac node. Multiple densities just anterior to the lateral margin of the sacrum are consistent with abnormal hypogastric nodes (*arrow*) in this patient with metastatic carcinoma of the rectum.

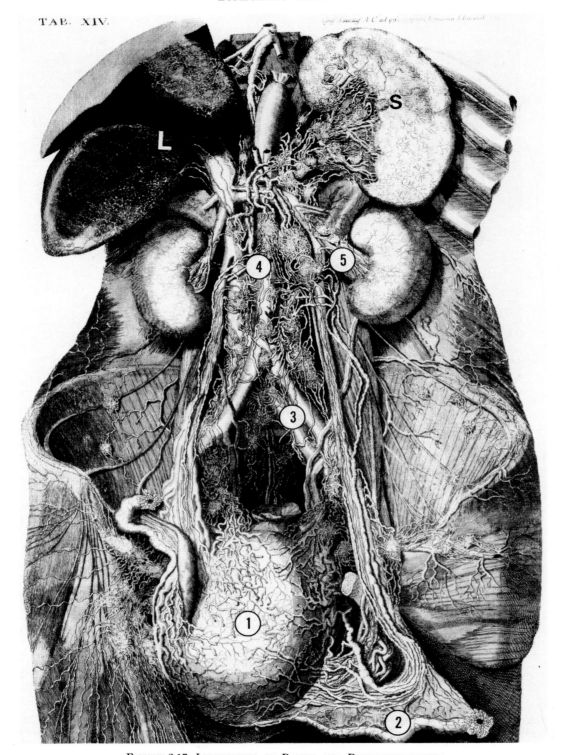

**FIGURE 2.17. LYMPHATICS OF PELVIS AND RETROPERITONEUM**
Uterus (*1*); fallopian tube and broad ligament (*2*); common iliac (*3*); para-aortic and paracaval (*4*); renal (*5*); splenic (*S*); and liver (*L*). (From Mascagni, 1787.)

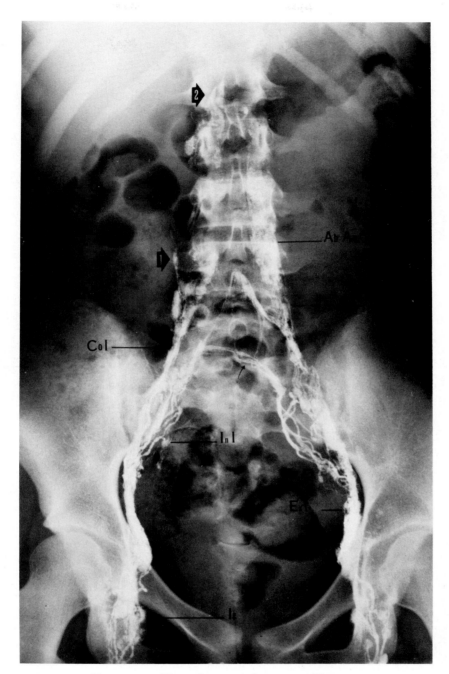

FIGURE 2.18. WELL OPACIFIED LYMPHATIC VESSELS

These vessels demonstrate with clarity the commonly described, characteristic vascular filling pattern. *Ig*, inguinals; *ExI*, external iliacs; *InI*, internal iliacs or hypogastrics; *CoI*, common iliacs; *small arrow*, extensive vessel communication between contralateral and ipsilateral. Also note the inverted "V" appearance of connecting right and left medial chains at the aortic bifurcation (*Ab Ao*, abdominal aortic or paralumbar). The left chain is the most richly endowed of the three. *Arrow 1*, right paralumbar "skip channel"; *arrow 2*, cisterna chyli.

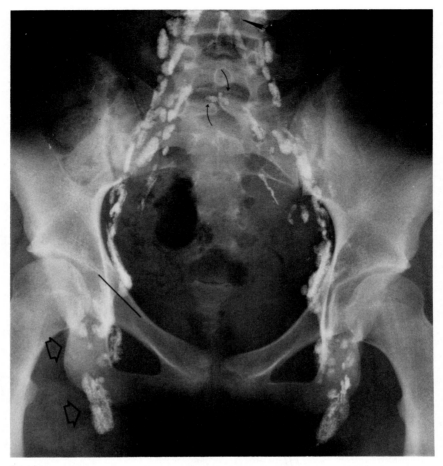

FIGURE 2.19. FRONTAL PROJECTION OF PATIENT IN FIGURE 2.18

External iliac nodes are above the line delineating the inguinal ligament. The lateral sacral nodes of the right internal iliac chain are opacified, but it is difficult to distinguish between these nodes and the nodes of the medial common iliac chain in this projection. Stereoscopic views and/or oblique projections assist greatly in this distinction. Vessel-filling patterns are helpful also. *Open arrow*, inguinal nodes; *small curved arrows*, nodes of the promontory; *top arrow*, aortic bifurcation.

The tendency is for the right and left medial chains to complete their course just inferior to the aortic bifurcation, forming an inverted "V" (Fig. 2.18).

The medial chain is important because it serves as one of the important pathways of communication between the pelvic visceral structures (e.g., ovary, fallopian tubes, uterus, bladder and prostate, and the abdominoaortic region (Fuchs, 1969; Browse, 1972a). From the pelvic viscera, efferents connect with the medial common iliac chain that connects with the abdominoaortic channels through intermediate chains that anastomose freely with each other.

Generally, a continuous series of vessels and nodes progresses up to the aortic bifurcation. The number of nodes along each chain is approximately three to six nodes with the medial chain of the left containing the fewest number (Fuchs, 1969). Few gaps are found, and lymphographically, coarse opacification and sharp delineation of nodes in this region should be expected (Browse, 1972a) (Fig. 2.19). These nodes are much less misleading in diagnostic oncology than nodes more caudally positioned (see Chapter 12 on neoplasms). Even in this area nebulous filling defects in a single node or few nodes can genuinely frustrate lymphographic attempts to confirm or negate the presence of metastatic neoplasms (Castellino et al., 1973; Parker et al., 1974a).

Most common iliac nodes, especially the lateral and intermediate groups, are oval (Fig. 2.20). The medial chain nodes usually are slightly smaller and more nearly round. On normal lymphograms with histological correlation, an elon-

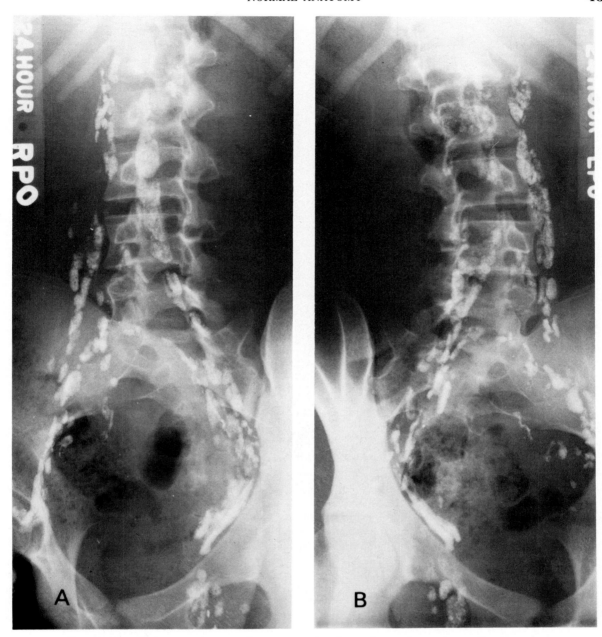

FIGURE 2.20. POSTERIOR OBLIQUE PROJECTIONS OF SAME LYMPHOGRAM AS IN FIGURE 2.19

Pelvic and paralumbar (abdominoaortic) nodes are shown far more discretely. The right posterior oblique view separates the more posterior right lateral sacral nodes from the medial chain nodes of the common iliac group.

gated transitional node in the right lateral chain has been observed frequently at the point of transition between the common iliacs and lumbar group (abdominoaortics) (D. A. Harrison, unpublished data). The normal internal architecture of this node is compact and homogeneous (Fig. 2.21*B*).

In patients less than 20 yr of age, the roentgen appearance of the internal architecture of common iliac nodes can differ slightly and falsely suggest lymphoma (Castellino et al., 1975). Nodes in these patients present a more reticulated or foamy pattern (relatively more lucent to opaque areas) than in adults. When normal, foaminess is not striking and tends to be generalized and uniform throughout the intra-abdom-

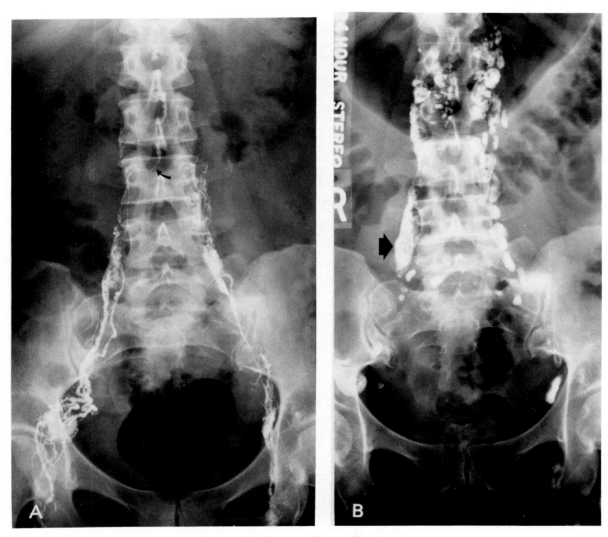

FIGURE 2.21. BENIGN NODAL HYPERPLASIA

*A*: Vascular filling of a lymphogram that shows asymmetry of the pelvic vessels. Paralumbar crossover is demonstrated superiorly (*arrow*). *B*: Nodal retention phase of the same lymphogram. *Arrow* illustrates the large, elongated, homogeneously opacified, right common iliac node (transitional node). More superior abdominoaortic nodes are slightly larger than usual and have relatively more lucencies than usual dispersed throughout their internal architecture (foaminess). Oblique projections (*C* and *D*) display this appearance distinctly. Postlaparotomy histological examination proved these nodes to contain benign follicular hyperplasia. This entity can simulate lymphomata and is the basis of most false lymphographic interpretations.

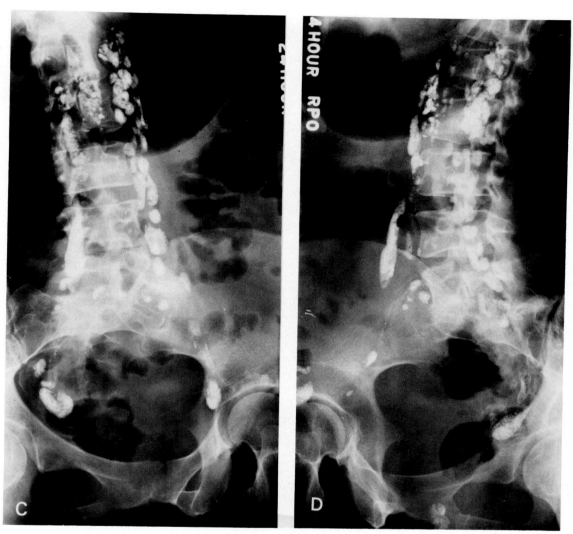

FIGURE 2.21C and D.

inal nodes (Figs. 2.21 and 2.22). Also, a significant increase in size of the nodes is not present with normal foaminess. Histologically, relatively more collections of lymphatic components to sinusoidal spaces can be found (Butler, 1969). Therefore, relatively less contrast material settles in the nodes.

Lateral chain nodes are positioned on the lateral aspect of the common iliac artery. Lymphography usually demonstrates three densely opacified nodes. The most superior node often represents the entire chain (elongated transitional nodes at the aortic bifurcation).

The intermediate chain becomes slightly more posterior to the artery and vein than its predecessors of the external iliac group. Having become more posterior, and therefore closer to the nodes of the medial chain, clear delineation and precise localization of individual intermediate nodes can be quite difficult. Some separation of these individual nodes for critical evaluation and interpretation can be accomplished with proper radiographic technique (see "External Iliac Group"). The intermediate chain averages two to four more nodes than the lateral or medial chains and thus produces a continuous sequence

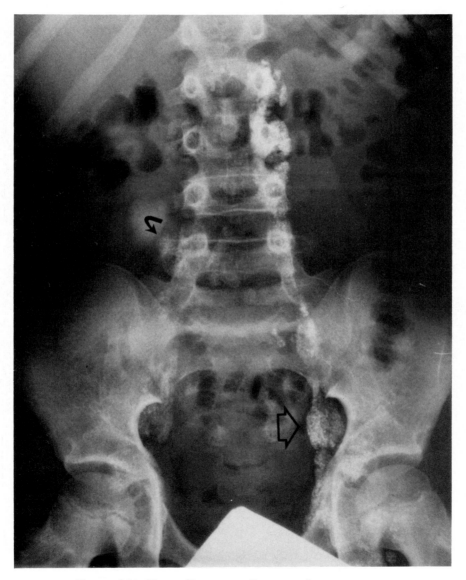

FIGURE 2.22. NODAL RETENTION PHASE OF LYMPHOGRAPHY
Frontal projection on a pediatric patient. *Arrows* show nodes that are extensively foamy but are without histological evidence of neoplasm.

of nodes devoid of a gap. The lymphographic appearance of a succession of nodes in an uninterrupted column may not represent simple continuity of a single chain, however, but actually may be the confluence and superimposition of intermediate and medial chains (Fuchs, 1969).

The medial common iliac chain is deep in the pelvis and medial to the artery and vein. Included in this chain are the subaortic or promontory nodes (Rouvière, 1938; Herman et al., 1963). Marked asymmetry between left and right medial common iliac nodes is characteristic. Predominantly this chain contains one to two chain nodes that are on the right. Other nodes superimposed over the lumbosacral area may have this appearance, and differentiation from incidentally filled nodes of the internal iliac group some-

times can be difficult. On frontal roentgenograms, medial nodes are frequently superimposed over the sacral promontory. Rouvière (1938) described these nodes as subaortic nodes or nodes of the promontory (Fig. 2.19).

Even with excellent bowel opacification and intravenous contrast administration, normal nodes in the common iliac area are difficult to delineate because the fat surrounding the blood vessels is insufficient. In addition, small nodes at the bifurcation of the aorta and inferior vena cava are difficult to demonstrate because of overlapping blood vessels in this region. Normal common iliac nodes are seldom demonstrated by CT; hence, anatomic demonstrations are created after intralymphatic injection of contrast material (Fig. 2.23).

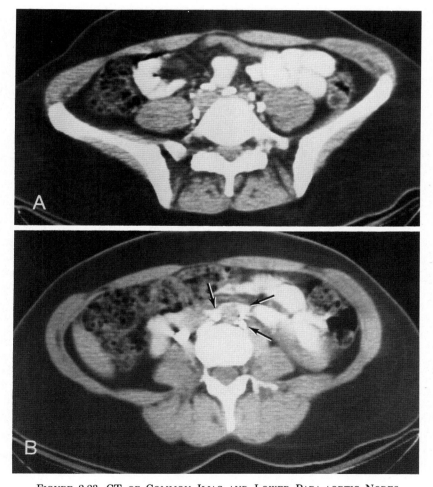

FIGURE 2.23. CT OF COMMON ILIAC AND LOWER PARA-AORTIC NODES

*A*: Contrast-filled, normal common iliac nodes at L4-5, just below aortic bifurcation. *B*: Lower para-aortic nodes (*arrow*) located just above the bifurcation at L3-4 surround the inferior vena cava and abdominal aorta.

## GENITOURINARY LYMPHATICS

### Pararenal Lymphatics

The lymphatics of the posterior pararenal space and capsule are composed of superficial and deep lymphatics. The superficial network first reported by Stahr (1899, 1900, 1903) and then explored by Kumita (1909) lies immediately below the peritoneum (Gerota's fascia). Lymphatics in the pararenal fascia exit only in regions where the capsules of the kidney and adrenal gland are in contact with the peritoneum. This area is more extensive on the right because the colon, adrenal gland, and stomach cover a large part of the anterior surface of the left kidney (Rouvière, 1938).

The deep lymphatic network is placed deep to the pararenal fascia (pararenal space) and receives lymphatics from the superficial network. The collecting trunks from the deep lymphatic network empty into nodes at the origin of the renal artery and vein. On the right the lymphatics empty into nodes between the inferior vena cava and aorta at the termination of the renal vein. On the left side, the trunks terminate in para-aortic nodes near the renal blood vessels and in front or on the left border of the aorta. Occasionally, lymphatics from both right and left sides empty into nodes near the origin of the inferior mesenteric artery.

The lymphatic network from Gerota's fascia communicates with lymphatics from the peritoneum, and on the right it empties into lymphatics on the visceral surface of the liver and diaphragm. The superficial network also communicates with lymphatics that drain the superficial network of the cecum, appendix, and colon. While on the left, they communicate with lymphatics which drain the transverse and descending colon. These communications explain the presence of metastases from cecal and right colon carcinoma in the hilum of the liver with biliary obstruction high in the portal area rather than low in the common duct. Occasionally, this network may communicate with juxta-aortic nodes on the diaphragmatic and lower intrathoracic and intercostal collecting trunks. Efferent trunks from the inferior part of the pararenal fascia frequently unite with testicular or ovarian lymphatics or lymphatics from the posterior abdominal wall (Ssysganow, 1930; Pellé and Pellé, 1931).

### Renal Lymphatics

Lymphatics of the kidney are composed of the network in the fibrous capsule (Stahr, 1900; Gabrielle, 1925; Nicolesco, 1930; Ssysganow, 1930)

as well as the renal parenchyma. Lymphatics from the cortex and medulla of the kidney run toward the base of the renal pyramids around the blood vessels. They unite at the corticomedullary junction and follow the blood vessels above the surface of the pyramid. Networks from the capsule and parenchyma emerge from the columns of Bertin and run in the renal sinus along the blood vessels on the surface of the calyces and intrarenal part of the pelvis to the hilum with other constituents of the renal pelvis. They are divided into anterior, middle, and posterior groups according to the position in front or behind the renal vessels or between the renal artery and vein.

On the right, the anterior collecting trunks drain chiefly the anterior half of the kidney and run along the anterior aspect of the renal artery and renal vein passing in front of or behind the inferior vena cava to terminate in the right lateral periaortic nodes between the renal and inferior mesenteric arteries. The middle collecting trunk also terminates in the right lateral periaortic nodes. The posterior collecting trunk from the posterior half of the kidney runs along the posterior surface of the main trunk of the renal artery and terminates in nodes situated on the right crus of the diaphragm behind the inferior vena cava and along the right border of the aorta between the renal artery and inferior mesenteric arteries.

On the left, the anterior trunks run in front of the renal vein and empty into lateral aortic nodes near the origin of the left renal vein. The highest trunk may terminate in a node situated at the junction of the left renal and adrenal veins, while the lowermost trunk may end in a node at the junction of the renal and left spermatic veins. The middle connecting trunk empties into lateral periaortic nodes near the junction of the renal and adrenal veins. The posterior collecting trunks empty into nodes in the periaortic chain near the origin of the renal artery (Mascagni, 1787; Stahr, 1900; Cunéo, 1902; Kumita, 1909; Hasumi, 1930; Nicolesco, 1930; Ssysganow, 1930) (Figs. 2.24, 2.25, and 2.29A).

Lymphatics of the calyces and renal pelvis drain from submucosal networks into collecting trunks that empty into the first order drainage node of the lateral periaortic nodes above and in the vicinity of the corresponding renal arteries.

### Ureteral Lymphatics

Lymphatics of the ureter drain from deep mucosal lymphatics into the adventitia. The col-

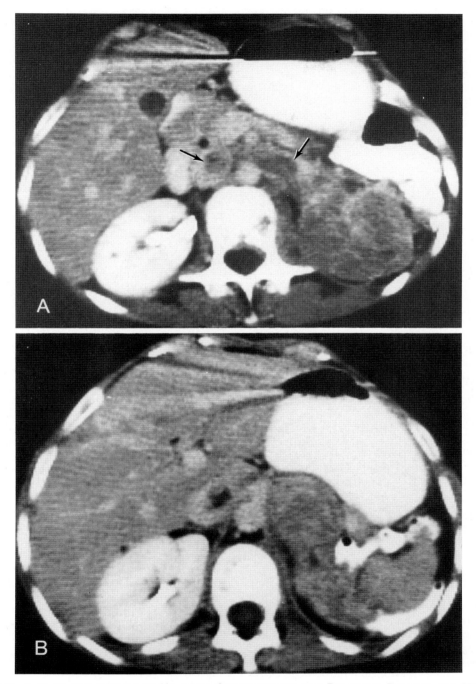

FIGURE 2.24. A 31-YR-OLD FEMALE 16 YR AFTER CHEMOTHERAPY AND RADIATION THERAPY FOR HODGKIN'S
DISEASE WITH HYPERNEPHROMA

*A*: Tumor thrombus in left renal vein and inferior vena cava (*arrows*). Note the direct extension into the retropancreatic
area with obliteration of the aorta. *B*: Massive enlargement of nodes adjacent to the celiac artery is evident.

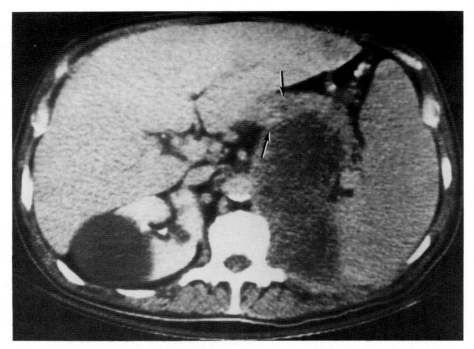

FIGURE 2.25. RECURRENT HYPERNEPHROMA WITH LARGE MASS FILLING LEFT GUTTER
Metastatic disease to retropancreatic area has displaced the pancreas and splenic vein (*arrows*) anteriorly.

lecting trunks are continuous with those of the urinary pelvis above and with those of the urinary bladder below. Superiorly, the trunks may empty into the para-aortic nodes near the origin of the spermatic artery or inferiorly into the common and external iliac nodes. The middle segment of the ureter drains to the lateral para-aortic nodes near the origin of the inferior mesenteric artery or into common iliac nodes. The inferior ureteral segment terminates in the common iliac, external iliac, and hypogastric nodes (Sakata, 1903; Nicolesco, 1929a, b).

## Bladder Lymphatics

The rich network of lymphatics from the mucosal and muscular coats of the bladder drain into collecting trunks of the trigone and the posterior and anterior walls of the bladder (Fig. 2.26). Trunks from the trigone area course laterally and posteriorly toward the inferior segment of the ureter, passing in front of it, accompanying the uterine artery in the female and the artery of the vas deferans in the male, and terminating in external iliac nodes (usually the medial and middle group of the chain; rarely the lateral group). Lymphatics from the posterior wall extend from the posterolateral angle of the

bladder, above and in front of the ureter, and across the umbilical artery from above and behind, to empty into the medial and middle group of external iliac nodes. Lymphatics from the inferior part of the posterior wall exit into collecting trunks of the trigone area. From the anterior wall, lymphatics exit from the middle part of the lateral border of the bladder near the region of the middle vesicle artery across the lateral border of the bladder and descend toward the origin of the middle vesicle and umbilical artery to converge with collecting trunks from the posterior wall before terminating in the middle group of the external iliac chain. Frequently a small intercalating node is present along the course of the bladder lymphatics, but for all practical purposes, the first order drainage nodes from the bladder are the external iliac nodes in the medial and middle group of the chain and occasionally in the hypogastric and common iliac nodes (Mascagni, 1787; Rouvière, 1938).

## Prostatic Lymphatics

The collecting trunks from the parenchyma and capsule of the prostate empty into the external iliac nodes from the base and upper part of the prostate, into the hypogastric nodes from the

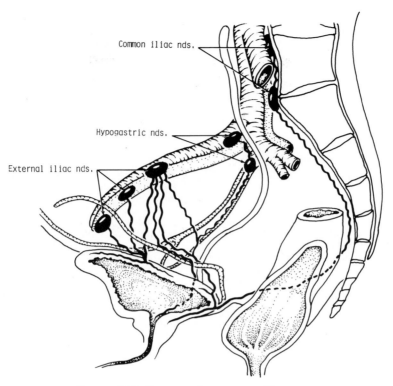

Common iliac nds.

Hypogastric nds.

External iliac nds.

FIGURE 2.26. BLADDER LYMPHATICS DRAINAGE
Note drainage to external iliac, hypogastric, and common iliac nodes via the sacral promontory.

inferior part of the prostate, into sacral promontory nodes from the posterior surface of the prostate, and into hypogastric nodes along the internal pudendal artery from the anterior-inferior segment of the prostate. Intercalated nodes, according to Marcille (1903), lie between the rectum and the prostate. If all of the small retroprostatic intercalating nodes are withdrawn from consideration, however, the first order drainage nodes from the prostate are the external iliac, hypogastric, and lymph nodes of the sacral promontory (Poirier and Cunéo, 1902; Marcille, 1903; Caminiti, 1905) (Fig. 2.27).

### Lymphatics of the Seminal Vesicles

The lymphatics of the seminal vesicles are intimately connected with lymphatics from the prostate, bladder, and rectum and empty into the middle chain of the external iliac nodes (Cordier, 1931).

### Ovarian Lymphatics

First studied by His (1865), the lymphatics exit from the ovary in the vicinity of the hilum and descend along the ovarian blood vessels to terminate in periaortic nodes (Poirier, 1889; Bruhns, 1898; Marcille, 1903). On the right, the trunks empty into precaval and lateral caval nodes adjacent to the inferior vena cava and below the origin of the renal artery. On the left, the lymphatic trunks ascend to a higher level and terminate in lateral aortic and para-aortic nodes above or below the left renal pedicle (Figs. 2.17 and 2.28). Accessory drainage from the ovary empties into the middle chain of the external iliac group near the junction of the common iliac nodes. The first order drainage nodes from the ovary, therefore, are to the periaortic and external iliac chains.

### Lymphatics of the Fallopian Tubes

Lymphatic drainage of the fallopian tubes is almost identical to that of the ovary. On the right, the efferent channels terminate in precaval nodes near the bifurcation of the aorta. On the left, the nodes may be situated slightly higher along the lateral periaortic nodes and adjacent to the left renal pedicle (Figs. 2.17 and 2.28).

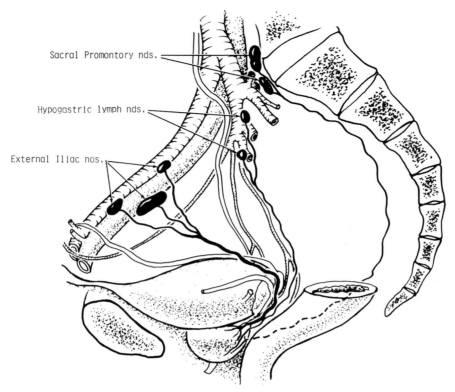

Sacral Promontory nds.

Hypogastric lymph nds.

External Iliac nds.

FIGURE 2.27. PROSTATIC LYMPHATIC DRAINAGE
Note drainage to the external iliac and hypogastric nodes and to the nodes of the sacral promontory.

Accessory pathways drain into the external iliac and hypogastric nodes (Poirier, 1889; Bruhns, 1898; Pellé and Pellé, 1931).

## Lymphatics of Uterus and Cervix

Collecting trunks from the body of the uterus may drain through the broad ligament and follow the drainage course of the fallopian tubes and ovaries to terminate on the right in the lateral periaortic nodes and the left in the lateral preaortic and periaortic nodes near the origin of the inferior mesenteric artery (Marcille, 1903). Vessels may also empty into the external iliac chain (Cunéo and Marcille, 1901), generally into the middle group of the external iliac chain near the bifurcation of the common iliac artery or along the course of the broad ligament through the inguinal canal into superficial inguinal nodes (Mascagni, 1787; Poirier, 1889; Bruhns, 1898; Marcille, 1903).

Lymphatic drainage from the uterine cervix may take one of three pathways: to the superior and middle nodes of the medial and middle group of external iliac nodes; to the hypogastric nodes near the origin of the uterine artery; or to the laterosacral nodes of the sacral promontory.

First order drainage, therefore, enters the medial middle group of the external iliac chain and the hypogastric nodes of the promontory. The fundus and body of the uterus terminate in the lateral para-aortic and preaortic nodes near the origin of the inferior mesenteric artery, in nodes of the middle group of the external iliac chain, and occasionally in superficial inguinal nodes (Figs. 2.17 and 2.28B).

## Vaginal Lymphatics

Lymphatic drainage from the vaginal area enters either the medial and middle groups of the external iliac nodes, the hypogastric nodes, or the nodes of the sacral promontory.

## Testicular Lymphatics

In males aged 20–35 yr, testicular malignancies rank first (Twito and Kennedy, 1975), but current methods of therapy effectively control a significant number of these neoplasms. With treatment, some forms have an overall 5-yr control rate of greater than 90%. Because these neoplasms are particularly prone to disseminate by the lymphatics, lymphography can be quite useful in efforts to stage lymphatic extension of the disease (Von Keiser, 1967; Fuchs, 1971a; Safer et al., 1975).

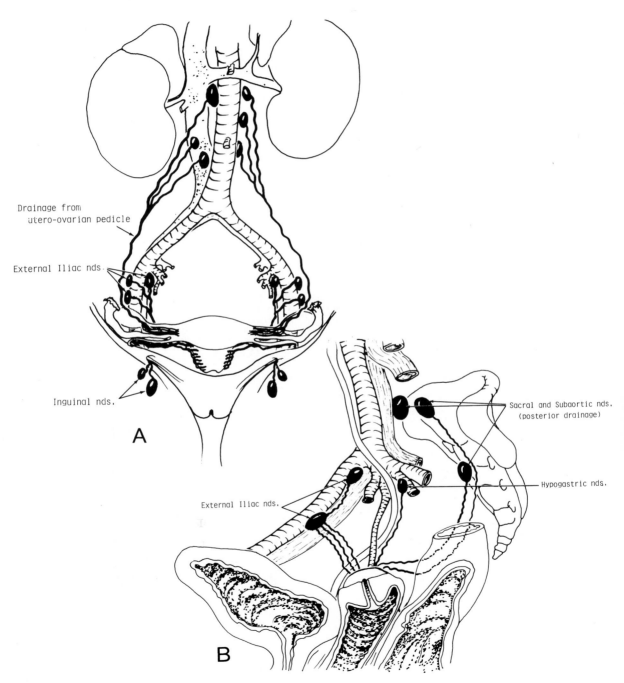

FIGURE 2.28. LYMPHATICS OF FEMALE REPRODUCTIVE ORGANS
*A*: Lymphatics of the uterus, ovaries, and fallopian tubes. *B*: Lymphatics of the cervix.

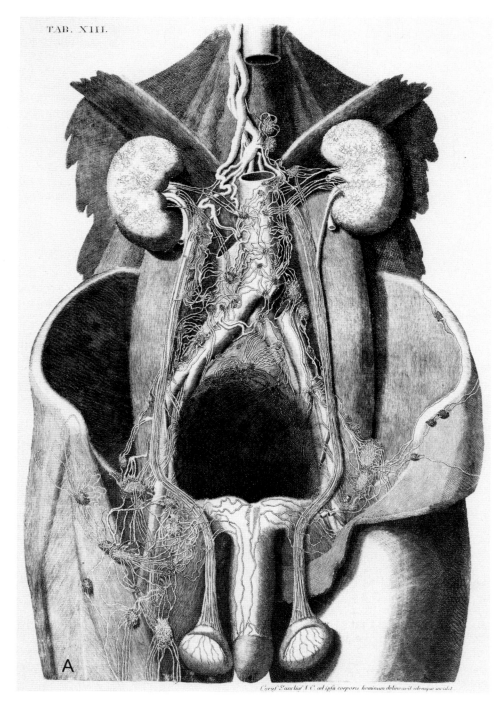

FIGURE 2.29. PRIMARY LYMPHATIC DRAINAGE VESSELS AND NODES OF GLANDULAR TISSUE OF TESTICLES
*A*: (From Mascagni, 1787.) *B*: Diagram according to descriptions by Rouvière (1938). Vessels emanate from the gland, bypassing the nodes usually demonstrated by clinical lymphography. Note the clusters of nodes in the region of the renal pedicles bilaterally. Also illustrated is cross-communication. The relationship of the gonadal center nodes to the paralumbar (paracaval/para-aortic) nodes as represented has been confirmed by simultaneous dorsal pedal and testicular lymphography (Chiappa et al., 1966).

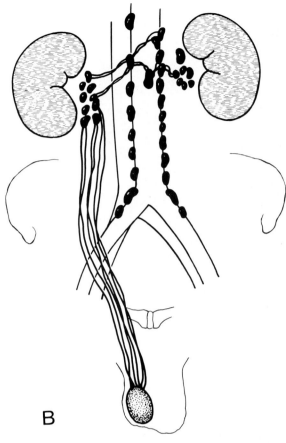

**B**

FIGURE 2.29B.

## Anatomy

Anatomic descriptions of testicular lymphatics have emphasized the character and course of the vessels (Rouvière, 1938; Clark, 1942; Brash, 1943). Two sets of efferent vessels emanate from each testicle; a superficial system drains the tunica vaginalis, and a deep system drains the epididymis and the body of the gland. The superficial and deep systems travel from each testicle as a unit of six to eight trunks that ascend in the spermatic cord, pass through the inguinal ring, and follow the testicular blood vessels along the psoas major muscle. These lymph vessels empty into the corresponding lumbar lymph nodes. Vessels that drain only the glandular portion of each testicle empty into the lateral aortic nodes adjacent to the renal bed (preaortic) nodes. Vessels that drain the ductal portion of the testicle (epididymis) preferentially terminate in the distal aortic or proximal common iliac nodes. Vessels draining the serosal covers and scrotum differ and usually terminate in the external iliac or inguinal nodes (Chavez, 1967).

Embryological development explains the range of terminal drainage sites of the testicular region (Lemeh, 1960). The glandular portion of the testicle originated as an organ high in the posterior abdominal cavity. The ductal system joined the organ in its descent into the pelvis. Hence, ductal drainage is comparable to that of organs of the pelvic region because these organs arise simultaneously and in the same position. Drainage of the more superficial enveloping tissue follows patterns of structures more in contiguity with the abdominal wall and scrotum (an outpouching of the abdominal wall) following the more superficial lymphatic vascular pathways (inguinals) (Fig. 2.29).

### Lymphographic Anatomy

Chiappa et al. (1966) elucidated the lymphographic anatomy of the entire testicle through sequential use of both injection techniques. Lymphographically, six to eight lymphatic vessels course from each testicle to their respective primary drainage sites. These vessels turn medially and empty into primary drainage sites located variously between T11-12 to L4-5 (Chiappa et al., 1966; Wahlqvist et al., 1966). Crossover is common. In some series at least 50% of testicular lymphograms demonstrated crossover (Wahlqvist et al., 1966). Right to left crossover is more common, but evidence for the reverse course has been well established. Regardless of the course, crossover is observed more frequently between L2 and L5.

Nodal opacification should demonstrate a primary testicular drainage center that is adjacent to the renal pedicle of either side. On the right, this is in the region of L1-3; on the left, it is in the L2 region. Although no constant pattern is observed, secondary testicular nodal drainage in the lumbar aortic region can be opacified by testicular injections. These are the nodes usually well opacified by dorsal pedal lymphography (Chiappa et al., 1966).

Retrograde opacification of pelvic nodes was not a finding of some authors (Busch and Sayegh, 1963), but evidence supporting retrograde flow has resulted from other studies (Wahlqvist et al., 1966). Definite statements implicating physiological flow patterns derived from lymphographic data should not be considered conclusive, however, because of the unphysiological nature of the procedure. Nevertheless, retrograde flow should be considered of clinical importance because there is inferential evidence of its occurrence. Opacification of mediastinal nodes is common (Busch et al., 1965; Wahlqvist et al., 1966), and thoracic duct filling with minimal aortic

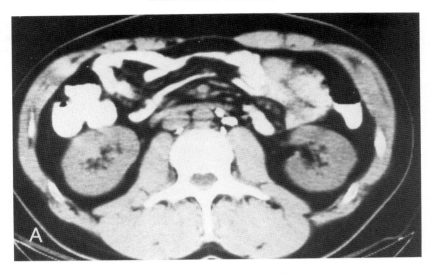

FIGURE 2.30. PRIMARY TESTICULAR DRAINAGE

*A*: Contrast-filled normal nodes at level of renal veins, primary drainage area for testes. *B*: A 30-year-old male with left seminoma. CT section at the lower pole of the kidneys (L3). Note enlarged left para-aortic nodes (*arrow*), the primary drainage area for the left testis. *C*: CT section through the renal vein shows two or three small para-aortic nodes obliterating the left lateral aortic shadow (*arrow*).

nodal filling also occurs (Wahlqvist et al., 1966). Opacification of supraclavicular nodes in the region of the termination of the thoracic duct is a common feature also.

Separate injections within a few days, using both techniques, outline with precision the extent of lymphatic dissemination of testicular neoplasms. Testicular injections visualize with far more definity the primary sites of drainage of the deeper testicular tissues than dorsal pedal injections. This method can delineate early lym-

phatic metastases of locally noninvasive neoplasms more efficiently. Dorsal pedal lymphography, the more comprehensive technique, better delineates more progressive testicular neoplasms. Testicular neoplasms that have disseminated distally can be demonstrated with greater precision by dorsal pedal lymphography than testicular injections (Chiappa et al., 1966; Kuisk, 1971). Figure 2.30 is a CT demonstration of normal node and metastatic disease to testicular drainage area.

## PARA-AORTIC LYMPHATICS

The abdominoaortic lymphatics are those vessels and nodes immediately above the common iliacs along the course of the lumbar vertebrae, inferior vena cava, and abdominal aorta. These lymphatics are also commonly termed *para-aortic, periaortics, lumbar,* and *paralumbar lymphatics.* The terms *right* and *left juxta-aortic groups* also have been used (Herman et al., 1963). Although location of these vessels and nodes is related to major regional blood vessels (i.e., inferior vena cava and aorta), radiographic visualization of the vertebral bodies enables the radiologist to use the vertebral column quite conveniently as a landmark. The functional anatomy of the abdominoaortic nodes and the architecture of their interconnections enable one to anticipate which nodes should be more routinely

demonstrated by clinical lymphography. Also, knowledge of actual anatomy enables one to better appreciate the potential for many lymphographic variations. Although the lymphographic flow patterns cannot be rigidly correlated with physiological flow patterns, analysis of sequentially visualized lymphatic vessels can be quite informative in attempts to anticipate routes of lymphatic dissemination of neoplasms (Busch et al., 1965; Wallace, 1968).

### Lymph Vessel Anatomy

According to Rouvière's (1938) anatomic descriptions, vessels in this region are continuations of the common iliacs that ascend the borders of the aorta. Para-aortic vessels also com-

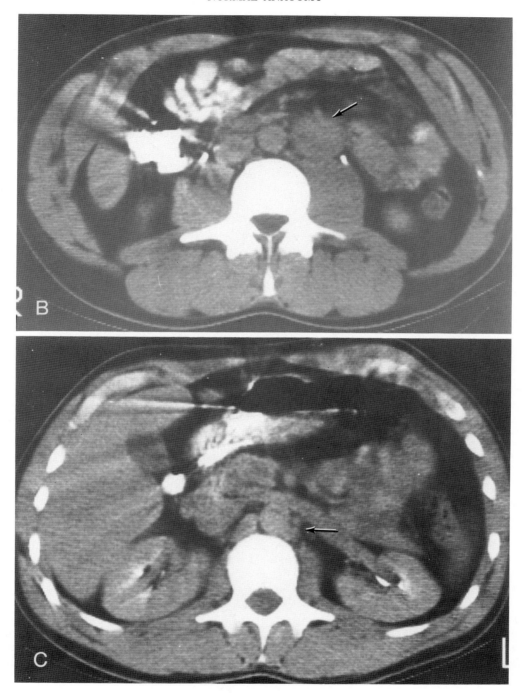

FIGURE 2.30*B* and *C*.

municate extensively, however, and receive drainage from other intra-abdominal sources. Organs that commonly drain directly into the para-aortic lymphatics are the testes, ovaries, fallopian tubes, corpus uteri, kidneys, adrenals, and abdominal wall lymphatics (Rouvière, 1938; Reiffenstuhl, 1964).

Coursing superiorly along the wall of the aorta, the para-aortic vessels empty into the cisterna chyli near the first to second lumbar vertebral bodies. More common clinical indications for lymphography emphasize nodal anatomy and function more than the highly variable structural arrangement of the lymphatic vessels (Rosen-

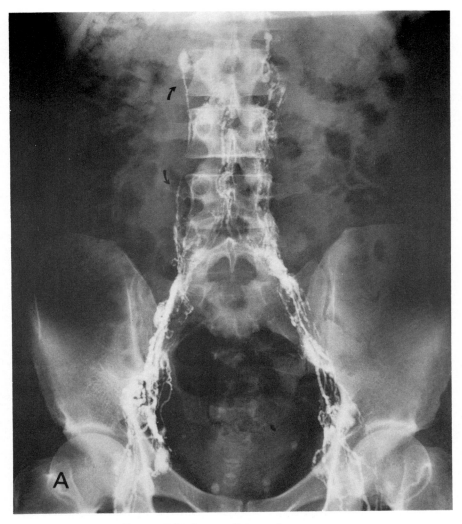

FIGURE 2.31. LYMPH VESSEL ABERRATION

*A*: Filling of a vessel with an atypical looping course along the right paralumbar region (*arrows*). Lateral (*B*) and frontal (*C*) projections of the same lymphogram in the nodal phase. The region traversed by looping vessel is devoid of opacified nodes. Laparotomy revealed no nodal abnormalities or other apparent reasons for this phenomenon. Histological examination of the opacified nodes was normal.

berg, 1968; Kaplan et al., 1973). Takahashi and Abrams (1967) were instrumental in developing lymphography as it is used currently in neoplastic disease and established criteria for distinguishing the normal from abnormal para-aortic lymphatic vessels and nodes. Their original criteria indicate the far greater significance of nodal characteristics in determining the presence of malignant disease. Vessel aberrations, including lymphaticovenous communications that indeed prove to be abnormal, rarely are the sole indicators of an abnormal lymphogram (Wallace and Jackson, 1968) (Fig. 2.31).

## Lymphographic Vascular Anatomy

In general, para-aortic vessels ascend along the sides of the aorta (Herman et al., 1963). A middle chain is filled occasionally from the right common iliac vessels but rarely contains as much contrast media as either lateral chain. The usual course of either chain is within 2–3 cm of the lateral edge of the vertebral body or within the confines of the transverse processes of the vertebral body (Abrams et al., 1968; Jackson and Kinmonth, 1974b).

Approximately 30% of confirmed normal lym-

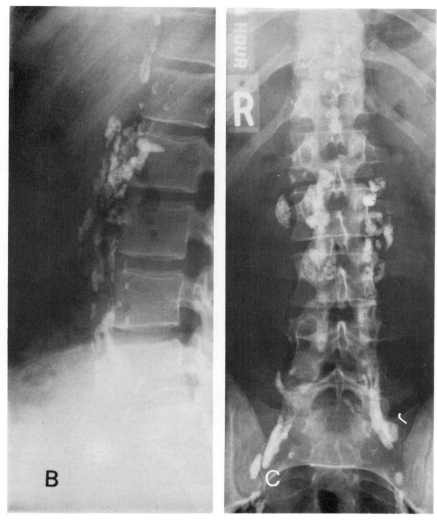

FIGURE 2.31*B* and *C*.

phograms exhibit right lower para-aortic skip channels (Jackson, 1972; Jackson and Kinmonth, 1974b) (see Fig. 2.18). Lymphographic-pathological correlations have produced convincing evidence that the position of these looping channels is unrelated to deviation either by normal or abnormal lymphatics or other structures. Reasonable explanations for these phenomena have been elusive thus far. On the lateral projection, most of the vessels and nodes are anterior to the anterior edge of the vertebral body but within 3–4 cm (Abrams et al., 1968) (Fig. 2.32).

Contralateral opacification of the para-aortic chains occurs in approximately half of normal lymphograms. Cross-filling is most often demonstrated in the L4-5 region (Fuchs, 1971b; Jackson and Kinmonth, 1974a). The para-aortic ves-

sels terminate at the level of L1-2. Two lumbar trunks and an intestinal trunk connect with the cisterna chyli, which fills with contrast media unpredictably.

## Lymph Node Anatomy

Approximately 25–30 abdominoaortic (lumbar) nodes surround and are in direct contiguity with the aorta and inferior vena cava (Rouvière, 1938; Clark, 1942; Brash, 1943; Gray, 1959). Anatomically, these nodes can be grouped according to their specific relationships to the adjacent major blood vessels: the right aortic, midaortic, and left aortic nodes. The right aortic nodes extensively encompass the inferior vena cava and can be subgrouped according to their specific

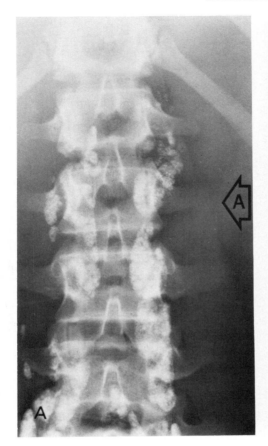
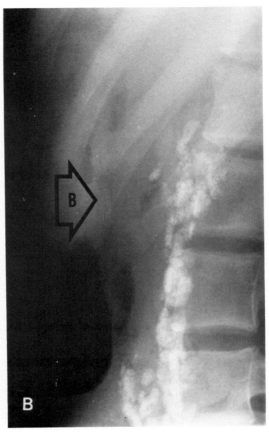

FIGURE 2.32. CONED VIEWS OF ABDOMINOAORTIC NODES IN FRONTAL, LATERAL, AND BOTH OBLIQUE POSITIONS

*A*: More opacified nodes can be observed in the left chain, and the height to which these nodes are visible exceeds that of the middle and right chains. Most of the midchain nodes are poorly shown because of superimposition over the vertebral column; therefore, differentiating between pre- and retroaortic nodes in this projection is virtually impossible. The right chain contains few opacified nodes between L2-4. Note that the nodal size and position concur with described criteria of normal lymphographic anatomy (*arrow A*). *B*: This projection demonstrates the paralumbar nodes to be within the confines of established criteria of normal position (less than 3 cm anterior to the vertebral bodies) (*arrow B*). *C* and *D*: Oblique projections separate the nodal chains giving a more three-dimensional picture of the abdominoaortic group. *E*: CT demonstration of normal contrast-filled para-aortic nodes at the lower border of L2.

relationships with the cava: precaval, interaortocaval, retrocaval, and laterocaval nodes. Preaortic and retroaortic (midaortic) nodes are located approximately at the midpoint of the diameter of the aorta, either anteriorly (pre-) or posteriorly (retro-). Left aortic nodes are situated more along the course of the left lateral aspect of the aorta (Fig. 2.32).

The lymphographic anatomy of the right aortic chain does not conform to classical descriptions. Anatomically, right aortic (paracaval) chain nodes are more numerous than the mid- or left aortic chains (Rouvière, 1938). The right aortic nodes that are anterior to the vena cava are situated near the termination of the renal vein. Posteriorly positioned nodes are concentrated at the origin of the psoas major muscle and on the right crus of the diaphragm.

Preaortic nodes of the midaortic group lie directly on the anterior surface of the abdominal aorta at levels that correspond to the celiac artery, renal arteries, and superior and inferior mesenteric arteries. Retroaortic nodes of the midaortic group lie on the dorsal aspect of the abdominal aorta, somewhat toward the left. Strict separation of some of the more lateral retroaortic nodes from left aortic nodes can be difficult.

Left aortic nodes form a continuous chain on the left lateral border of the aorta, anterior to the psoas major muscle and the left crus of the diaphragm. The two lateral chains receive drain-

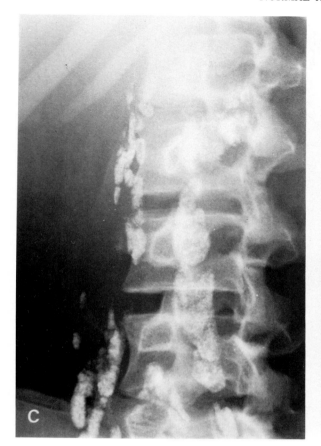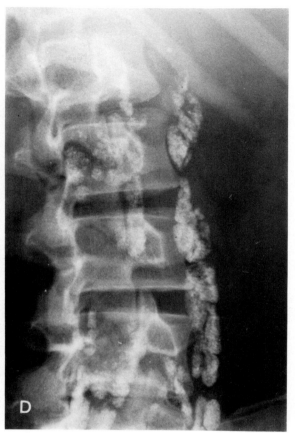

FIGURE 2.32C and D.

age from the following areas: (a) the common iliacs; (b) the testes or ovaries, fallopian tubes, and uterine corpus; (c) the kidneys and perirenal tissues; (d) the adrenals; and (e) the lymphatics that drain the abdominal wall. Afferents to the preaortic group of the midaortic chain emanate from the lymphatics of regions corresponding to the three major regional visceral arteries. Some communication with the two lateral nodal groups can be demonstrated, although it is seldom prominent. Retroaortic nodes of the midaortic group receive drainage from the intermediate chain of the common iliac lymphatics and the two lateral aortic groups.

A great deal of communication exists among the nodes of the lumbar group. Lumbar nodes, as functionally positioned, are the terminal abdominal lymphatic drainage areas of virtually all structures below the diaphragm. From this final common pathway, abdominal lymphatic flow enters the cisterna chyli and leaves the abdomen through the thoracic duct. These nodes have the same significance to lymphatic drainage as the

aorta has to arterial blood flow and the inferior vena cava has to venous return below the diaphragm.

In spite of their importance, however, paralumbar nodes are not the primary nodal drainage sites of all intra-abdominal groups.

## Lymphographic Nodal Anatomy

The lymphographic appearance of the lumbar nodes can produce diagnostically reliable data that are most contributory in the assessment of neoplastic disease of the retroperitoneal nodes (Baum et al., 1963; Viamonte et al., 1963; Fuchs, 1969; Kuisk, 1971; Castellino et al., 1974). Therefore, skilled analysis of the position, size, and appearance of each para-aortic/paracaval node and correlation with the total lymphographic pattern will produce the diagnostic accuracy of which the procedure is capable. Individually and as a group, these nodes are more constant than pelvic nodes; nevertheless, some variability is most often present as normal anatomy. Thor-

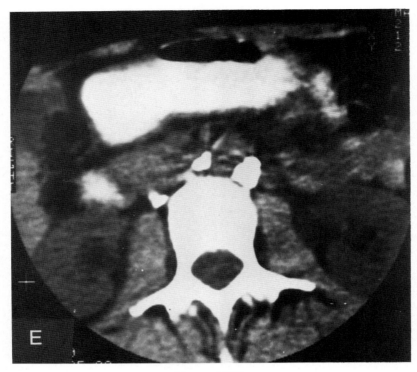

FIGURE 2.32*E*.

ough assessment of the nodes should include stereoscopic views, multiple projections, and, if necessary, laminagraphy.

Lymphographically, paralumbar nodes are usually oval and vertically oriented and have sharp margins around the vertical edges. Small nodes tend to be nearly round. Abrams et al. (1968) and Takahashi and Abrams (1967) established a limit for size in normal nodes. Normal para-aortic nodes proved seldom to be greater than 3 cm in their greatest diameter (Fig. 2.33). Prior to the work of Takahashi and Abrams, Wiljasalo (1965) devised what was termed a *projection difference index* as a measure of normal nodal size, but few lymphographers still consider it to have significant clinical value.

The internal lymphographic architecture of nodes is mostly determined by the amount of oily contrast material that permeates the subcapsular or marginal sinus, the intermediate sinus, and the medullary sinuses. Contrast material cannot permeate the follicular tissue; thus, minute lucencies are interspersed among contrast-filled sinuses. The node assumes a fine granular but homogeneous appearance with sharp, distinct margins. Of the patients with malignant lymphoma who undergo lymphography and in whom nodal opacification shows this

characteristic internal architecture, fewer than 1% will have occult retroperitoneal disease (Castellino et al., 1974). Presently, some data suggest that 20–25% of patients evaluated for metastatic malignancy who have normal internal nodal architecture by lymphography may have occult nodal metastases (Parker et al., 1974b; Castellino, 1975). Various stimuli unrelated to neoplasm can incite a variety of reactive responses within the node, however; hence, normal nodes can lymphographically appear somewhat reticular, can occasionally be described as foamy (relatively more lucencies), and still not contain lymphoma. Nodes that are reactive and without intrinsic malignancy tend to be uniform, individually and as a group (see Fig. 2.21). In spite of this, however, follicular hyperplastic responses of nodes have been shown to be the greatest source of diagnostic error when one attempts to determine the presence or absence of lymphoma (Hodgkin's or non-Hodgkin's) by lymphography (Castellino, 1974).

Similarly, complete contrast filling of the sinuses seldom occurs in every lymph node on the lymphogram. Although the para-aortic nodes have proved to be the most reliable group to show features of high diagnostic accuracy, even these nodes can be misleading. Incomplete con-

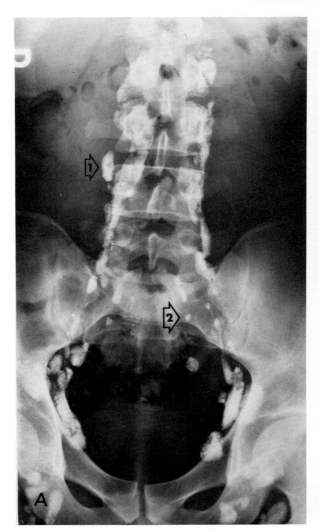
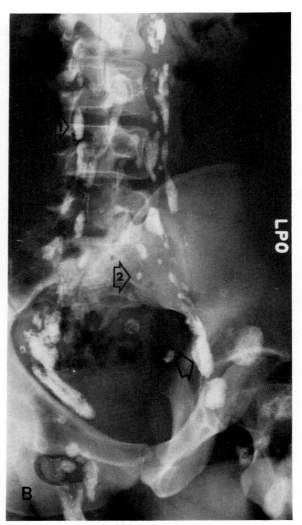

FIGURE 2.33. FRONTAL, LEFT, AND RIGHT POSTERIOR PROJECTIONS OF NODAL RETENTION PHASE OF NORMAL LYMPHOGRAPHIC ANATOMY

Note the larger, less uniform, more caudad nodes. The internal architecture is more reticular (foamy) and has multiple filling defects. The inguinal nodes display this pattern most floridly. The more inferior external iliacs have a similar character but become somewhat more uniform than the inguinal nodes. A: Note the marked superimposition of most of the nodes either over other nodes or osseous structures, thus limiting the delineation. B and C: These oblique views offer maximal visualization of all regional nodes. Fusion of the middle (obturator) node and the internal retrocrural nodes on the right is obvious (*open arrow* in C). The hilus of the middle nodes on the left becomes apparent (*open arrow* in B). Arrow 2 in A, B, and C identifies a small node in the medial chain of the common iliac group. Oblique views clearly differentiate this node from the larger, though less opacified, more caudad node (lateral sacral node of the internal iliac group (hypogastric)). Increased uniformity of these more cephalad nodes is apparent. The appearance of the three chains (dominant left chain) is strikingly typical. The position, size, and internal architecture of one of the paralumbar nodes are indicated (*arrow 1* in A, B, and C). All of the criteria for a normal paralumbar node are well emphasized by this node in the three projections.

trast filling of the sinuses can be unrelated to any disease entity. Benign processes, especially fibrolipomatous disease, frequently produce incomplete nodal filling, although not to the degree found in iliac and inguinal nodes. Also, small filling defects in the node can be produced by

normal nodal hilar vessels (Viamonte et al., 1963; Wallace and Jackson, 1968).

Densely opacified, homogeneous, sharply delineated lymphadenograms should not be expected routinely above the second lumbar vertebral body and rarely occur above the first ver-

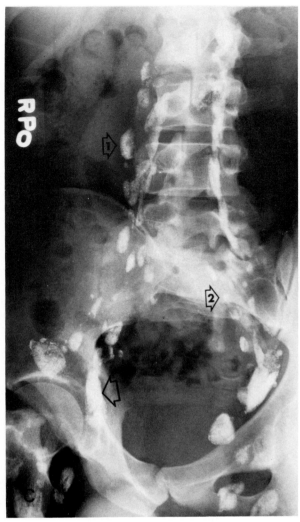

FIGURE 2.33C.

tebral body. Clusters of nodes near the first and second lumbar vertebrae most often will contain minute areas of incomplete filling.

### Right Aortic Chain

Left and midaortic chains have been shown lymphographically to contain many more nodes than the right aortic chain because many paracaval nodes are not in the pathway of the vessels transporting the greatest volume of contrast medium (Fuchs, 1971c; Jackson and Kinmonth, 1974b; D. A. Harrison, unpublished data). Contrast-bearing common iliac vessels continue superiorly along the aortic wall. The major chains generally do not extend beyond 2–3 cm of the lateral border of the vertebral column and thus ascend as para-aortic vessels.

This route of lymphatic transport of contrast media leads to opacification of nodes near the aorta. Although some filling of aberrant vessels is not rare, nodes along their routes seldom are optimally delineated. A large number of caval nodes are located more laterally and/or more anteriorly to the lymphatic vessels transporting the greatest volume of contrast medium (see Fig. 2.31). This mechanism of contrast transport accounts for nonvisualization of paracaval nodes known to exist, but it does not explain the skip channels in the L4-5 region. Evidence exists to confirm the absence of any nodes adjacent to these vessels (Jackson and Kinmonth, 1974b). The top of the column of the right chain reaches the level of L2 in approximately 30% of lymphograms (Fuchs, 1969, 1971b).

### Midaortic Chain

The midaortic chain (preaortic and retroaortic) is formed by a column of nodes that is superimposed over the vertebral column near the midline. Usually nodes are more opacified in this chain than in the right chain but less than in the left chain. The inferior nodes of this chain are found in the region of L3-4, often in clusters; the chain terminates at the L2 level in 35–40% of lymphograms (Fuchs, 1969; Kuisk, 1971; Jackson and Kinmonth, 1974b). Lymphographic differentiation of anterior from posterior nodes can be difficult. Whether positioned anteriorly or posteriorly on the aortic surface, these lymph nodes universally project over the spine. Stereoscopic views and laminagraphy are quite useful in delineating individual nodes, but in most clinical circumstances complete separation of each node of this column is not necessary.

The quality and quantity of nodes in this chain vary widely. Jackson and Kinmonth (1974b) have reported absence of the entire chain in 40% of lymphograms, but others report total absence as a rare occurrence (Fuchs, 1969; D. A. Harrison, unpublished data). The difficulty is precise localization of each individual node. Occasionally, nodes of both lateral chains are slightly more medially positioned; conversely, midchain nodes may be more laterally positioned, particularly toward the left. Since no criteria of lymphographic anatomy can infallibly localize each individual node in subtle situations, a conclusion of complete absence of this chain can become quite arbitrary.

### Left Aortic Chain

The left aortic chain is the most constant of the three chains and regularly contains more

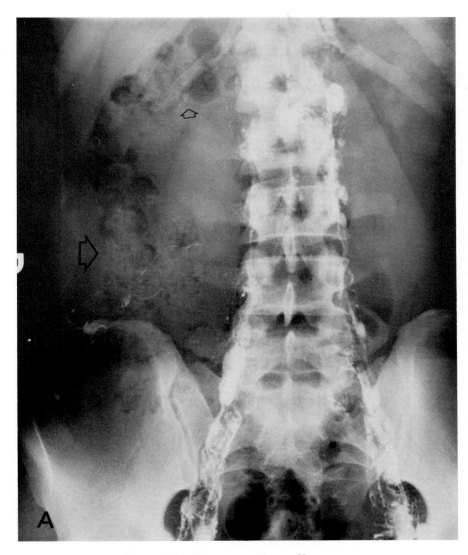

FIGURE 2.34. UNCOMMON NODAL VARIATION

*A*: Aberrant vessel filling during contrast injection. The large, inferior *arrow* indicates the multiple tortuous, serpiginous vessels widespread in the right hemiabdomen. Vessels are opacified above and below the right iliac crest. The smaller, superior *arrow* denotes filling of subcostal lymph vessels. *B*: Nodal retention phase shows opacification of nodes (*arrows*) that received contrast material from aberrantly filled vessels.

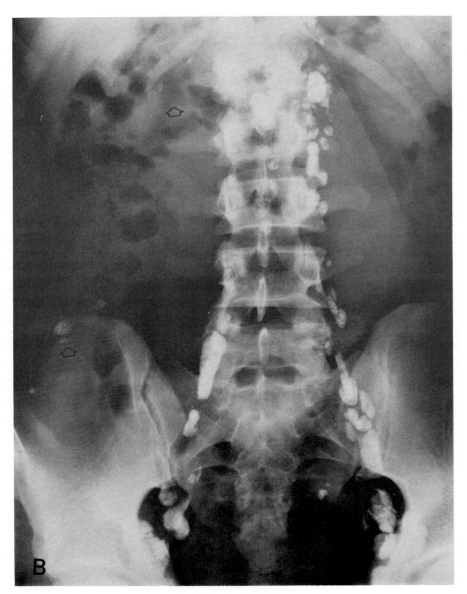

FIGURE 2.34*B*.

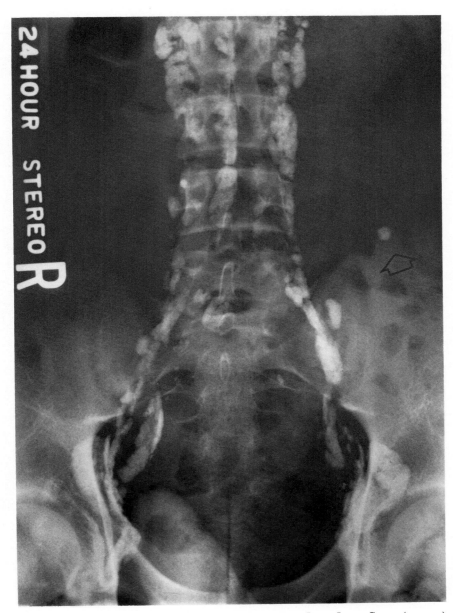

FIGURE 2.35. OPACIFICATION OF NODE OVER REGION OF LEFT ILIAC CREST (*ARROW*)

nodes considered characteristic of the abdominoaortic group. From their origin (immediately superior to the common iliac nodes) to their termination (seldom below L2), these homogeneous, well opacified nodes form an almost uninterrupted column along the left lateral border of the vertebrae. Lateral extension can be influenced by the state of the aorta, but the column is usually within 2 cm of the lateral edge of the vertebrae (Abrams et al., 1968; Fuchs, 1969; Jackson and Kinmonth, 1974b).

The nodes superior to the renal pedicle become fewer and less homogeneously opacified than the nodes in the caudal cluster. With few exceptions, the left chain is the most constant of the three abdominoaortic (paralumbar) chains. Nodes in this chain are visualized to L2 with frequencies up to 90% (Fuchs, 1969; D. A. Harrison, unpublished data). Some nodal opacification is demonstrated at the level of L1 in 30% of lymphograms (Fuchs, 1969). Nodes at this level in either chain become less densely opacified and form clusters that are almost inseparable. These clusters often simulate large nodes with filling defects that appear ominous.

*Para-aortic Nodes*

Although a large number of para-aortic nodes can vary from several millimeters to 1.5 cm in size, CT demonstration of significant numbers of normal para-aortic nodes is unusual. Occasionally one does see small bits of what appear to be nodal tissue adjacent to the aorta and cava when separation of the vascular and soft tissue planes by fat is excellent. For this reason, normal nodes in the para-aortic area are seen on CT scans after contrast lymphography. Although nodes are very apparent with contrast and many are 1.5 cm in size, they are enlarged because of the presence of Ethiodol and its associated inflammatory reaction.

*Uncommon Nodal Variations*

Those nodes that are visualized uncommonly are situated extrinsic to usual lymphographic regions. One such area is the pelvic–lower lumbar region. Opacification of these nodes occurs from vessels low in the pelvis that course superiorly and are quite lateral. These nodes are found over the region of the iliac crest (Figs. 2.34 and 2.35). Occasionally nodal opacification is observed beyond the terminal points of the abdominoaortic lymphatics (superior to the cisterna chyli) but still adjacent to the vertebral column (Fig. 2.36). Such nodes have been observed bilaterally and also superimposed over the vertebral column.

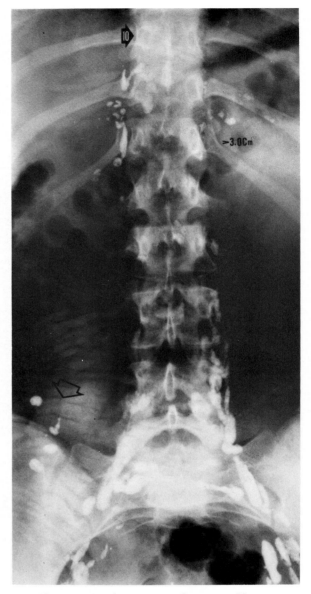

FIGURE 2.36. ABERRANTLY OPACIFIED NODES
These nodes are over the right iliac crest (*open arrow*) and adjacent to the thoracic vertebral column to T10 (*arrow 10*). Left parathoracic nodes extend 3 cm beyond the edge of the vertebral body.

Other nodes that occasionally fill are popliteal (Fig. 2.37), mediastinal, bilateral hilar, paratracheal, supraclavicular, and even axillary. Although an aberration from usual nodal filling, opacification of these nodes can be a normal variant. Therefore, interpretation of these nodes utilizing abdominoaortic criteria can produce dubious diagnostic conclusions. Concrete data on the spectrum of normal lymphographic anatomy

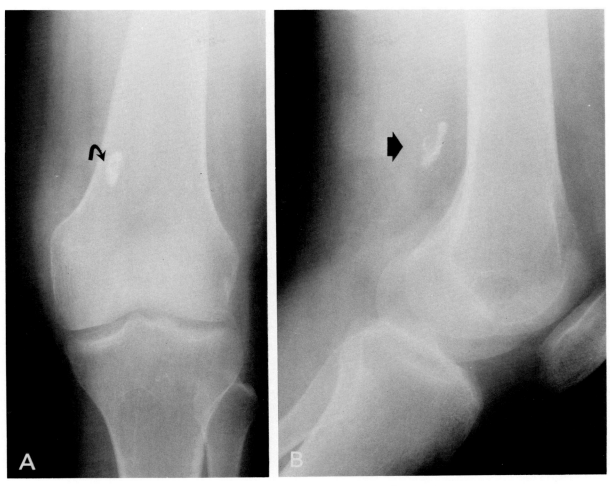

FIGURE 2.37. OPACIFIED POPLITEAL NODE (*ARROWS*)
Frontal (*A*) and lateral (*B*) projections.

of any of these nodes are not presently available (Baltaxe and Constable, 1968; Wallace and Jackson, 1968; Fuchs, 1969; Yee et al., 1969; Negus et al., 1970; Kuisk, 1971).

## VISCERAL ABDOMINAL LYMPHATICS

The lymphatics of the upper abdominal viscera drain primarily into the celiac, superior mesenteric, and inferior mesenteric nodes largely in relationship to their respective arteries.

### Hepatic Nodes

Superficial lymphatics from the superior surface of the right hepatic lobe pass through the diaphragm to the diaphragmatic nodes near the esophagus or inferior vena cava or course inferiorly to the celiac nodes along the phrenic artery. Vessels from the area of the falciform ligament drain into the anterior diaphragmatic nodes and from the anterior surface of the liver

to the hilum. Drainage from the visceral (inferior) surface passes to the hilum (Fig. 2.38). On the left, channels from the diaphragmatic surface drain to the left gastric nodes, to the left superior lumbar trunks along the inferior phrenic artery, or to the anterior diaphragmatic nodes. Lymphatics from the caudate and quadrate lobes drain to the hilum. Efferent vessels along the anterior border drain the gallbladder along the epiploic foramen to the hepatic nodes.

Lymphatic drainage from deep liver tissues begins at the terminal portion of the portal venous radicals and passes to the hilum by a large number of ducts. Efferents from the hepatic hilar node follow the hepatic artery to the celiac nodes,

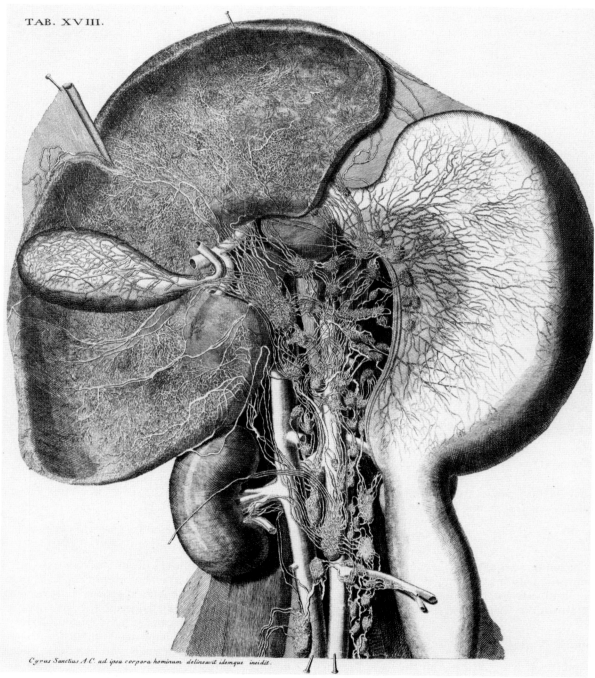

FIGURE 2.38. DRAINAGE FROM VISCERAL (INFERIOR) SURFACE OF LIVER
(From Mascagni, 1787.)

which empty into the left lumbar trunks (Figs. 2.39–2.41). Some minor lymphatics from the liver drain to the left gastric nodes through the gastrohepatic ligament. A small number of lymphatics located along the hepatic veins empty into inferior vena caval nodes just below or above the diaphragm. Efferents from this group drain into the retrosternal nodes or to the upper anterior mediastinal nodes along the phrenic nerve (Mascagni, 1787).

### Celiac and Gastric Nodes

These are the nodes in intimate contact with the celiac artery proper (Figs. 2.39, 2.40 and 2.42). According to Rouvière (1938), these nodes are placed along the left gastric, hepatic, and celiac arteries. The nodes are closely related to their respective arteries and for this reason are described with the left gastric and hepatic chains.

The left gastric chain is composed of three groups of nodes: the nodes in the left gastropancreatic fold, the nodes of the lesser curvature of the stomach, and the nodes of the cardiac area of the stomach circling the esophagogastric junction (Figs. 2.39, 2.40 and 2.43).

Nodes of the left gastropancreatic group follow the course of the left gastric artery from its origin and lie along the lesser curvature of the stomach. The nodes are found mainly above and behind the left gastric vessels in the substance of the left gastropancreatic fold. They frequently lie in intimate contact with the lesser curvature of the stomach, and it is difficult to determine whether they properly belong to the left gastropancreatic group or to the nodal group along the lesser curvature of the stomach. Nodes of the lesser curvature of the stomach commence at the point where the left gastric artery reaches the gastric wall and follow more accurately the path of this blood vessel and its terminal branches.

The parietal group and nodes of the cardiac area are located at the terminal branches of the left gastric artery and form a pericardiolymphoid ring at the esophagogastric junction (Figs. 2.39 and 2.43A). The cardia of the stomach as well as a portion of the fundus and the entire lesser curvature drain into the nodes around the cardia, the lesser curvature of the stomach, and the left gastropancreatic fold along the left gastric artery to the celiac nodes.

### Gastroduodenal Nodes

The inferior portion of the greater curvature of the stomach is drained by the right gastroepiploic nodes, which in turn drain into the nodes near the pyloric canal (infraduodenopyloric nodes). The infraduodenopyloric group drains into the retropyloric nodes that lie along the course of the gastroduodenal artery between the duodenopyloric wall and the pancreas and are called the *gastroduodenal group* (Fig. 2.39) (Jamieson and Dobson, 1907).

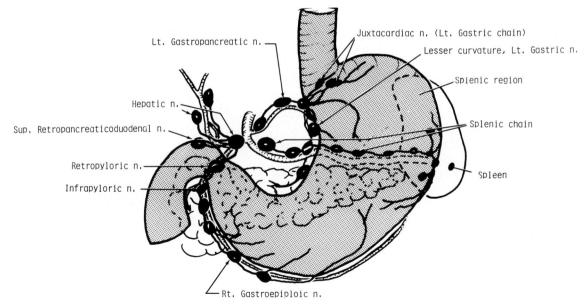

FIGURE 2.39. DIAGRAM OF CELIAC, GASTRIC, HEPATIC, AND SPLENIC NODES (From Rouvière, 1938.)

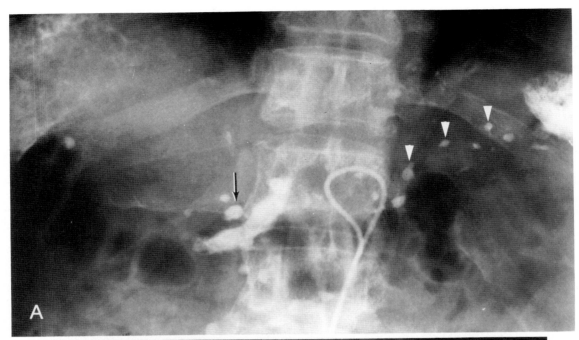

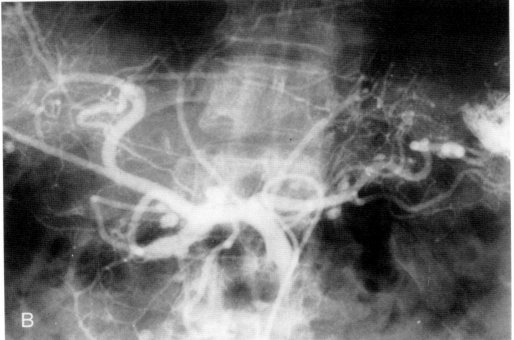

FIGURE 2.40. A 56-YR-OLD MALE 35 YR AFTER THOROTRAST ANGIOGRAPHY

*A*: Plain film prior to angiography. Note the dense, contracted spleen. There is Thorotrast in the splenic (*arrowheads*) and hepatic nodes (*arrow*). *B*: Film taken during the arterial injection shows the relationship of the splenic nodes to the splenic artery. *C* and *D*: CT scans in same patient—for comparison.

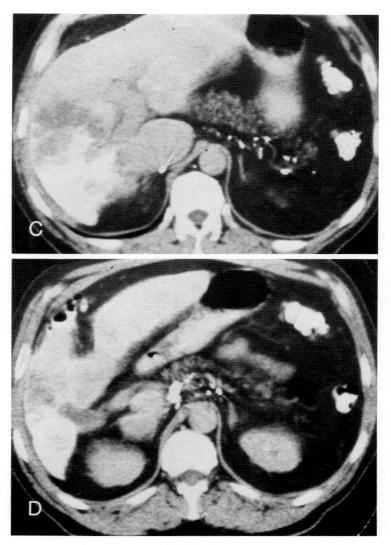

FIGURE 2.40C and D.

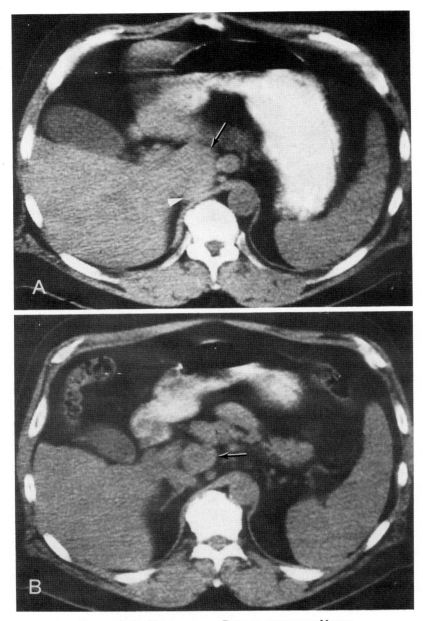

**FIGURE 2.41. HEPATIC AND RETROPANCREATIC NODES**

*A*: Hepatic adenopathy (*arrow*) obliterates edge of caudate lobe in this 65-yr-old male with hepatoma. The inferior vena cava is compressed (*arrowhead*). *B*: Section below *A* shows lower edge of caudate lobe and better demonstrates a large hepatic node (*arrow*). *C*: Massive retropancreatic adenopathy (splenic, celiac, hepatic, and retropyloric groups) is displacing the pancreas and splenic vein (*arrow*) anteriorly in this 66-yr-old female with non-Hodgkin's lymphoma.

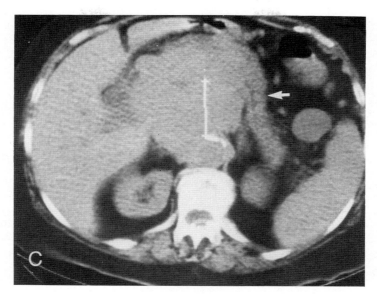

FIGURE 2.41C.

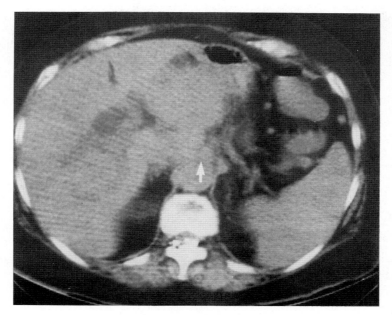

FIGURE 2.42. CELIAC AND HEPATIC HILAR NODES

Note enlarged mass of celiac nodes encasing the celiac artery (*arrow*) and hepatic hilar nodes in this 66-yr-old female with non-Hodgkin's lymphoma.

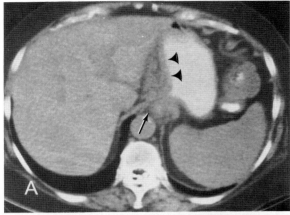

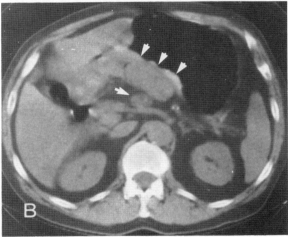

FIGURE 2.43. GASTRIC NODES

*A*: Note the enlarged left gastric nodes along the lesser curvature (*arrowheads*) and cardia of stomach (i.e., pericardiolymphoid ring in cardiac area of the stomach (*arrow*)) in this 77-yr-old female with histiocytic lymphoma. *B*: CT air-contrast study of the stomach in a patient with gastric carcinoma. Note the large nodes in left gastric chain (*arrowheads*) indenting the lesser curvature of the stomach and the enlarged node anterior to the hepatic artery.

## Splenic and Pancreatic Nodes

Lymphatic drainage of the pancreas is analogous to that of other organs in that the channels follow the course of the arterial blood supply (Figs. 2.39 and 2.40). The blood supply to the pancreas comes from numerous arteries, however, so there is a consequent confusion and overlap in terminology describing lymphatic drainage of this organ. A general term, *peripancreatic lymphatics,* may be more germane, but Rouvière classifies these lymph nodes as *suprapancreatic nodes* and *infrapancreatic nodes.*

The suprapancreatic nodes follow the course

of the splenic artery and lie along the upper and posterior borders of the pancreas. This chain continues into the phrenosplenic ligament to the hilum of the spleen. At this point it often continues in front of the hilum along the left gastroepiploic artery. The fundus and body of the stomach along the greater curvature are also drained by this chain of splenic nodes (Figs. 2.39, 2.44, and 2.45).

The infrapancreatic nodes are located along the lower border of the tail and body of the pancreas. The efferent trunks of the infrapancreatic nodes drain into the suprapancreatic nodes. All of the infrapancreatic nodes, however, do not belong to the splenic group. The most medial of these, near the duodenojejunal angle, belong to the superior mesenteric nodes, which lie along the course of the posteroinferior pancreaticoduodenal artery, a branch of the superior mesenteric artery and the terminal segments of the inferior mesenteric vein.

The nodes throughout the pancreas are further divided into anterior and posterior pancreaticoduodenal nodes that lie, respectively, anteriorly and posteriorly along the head of the pancreas and follow the course of the pancreaticoduodenal arteries. The superior portion of the head of the pancreas and upper duodenum drains to infrapyloric nodes and efferent trunks from the anterior pancreaticoduodenal nodes. The infrapyloric nodes, in turn, drain into the retropyloric nodes or into the nodes of the horizontal portion of the hepatic chain. The posterior pancreaticoduodenal nodes drain into the hepatic and celiac chains, into the right periaortic nodes, or into the superior mesenteric nodes.

The first order of drainage nodes from the pancreas is therefore (*a*) superiorly from the tail into the hilum of the spleen and from the body and head into the suprapancreatic (splenic chain) nodes of the left gastrohepatic fold and hepatic nodes; (*b*) inferiorly into the periaortic, mesenteric, and inferior pancreatic nodes; (*c*) posteriorly into the posterior pancreaticoduodenal and superior mesenteric nodes; and (*d*) anteriorly from the head and body into the infra- and retropyloric nodes, anterior pancreaticoduodenal nodes, and nodes at the root of the mesentery (Bartels, 1904; Rouvière, 1938).

The splenic chain is thus formed successively by nodes along the left gastroepiploic artery, the gastrosplenic ligament, the splenic hilum, and phrenosplenic ligament and by the suprapancreatic nodes. These nodes receive lymphatics from the gastric region of the splenic chain, the spleen, and the body and tail of the pancreas

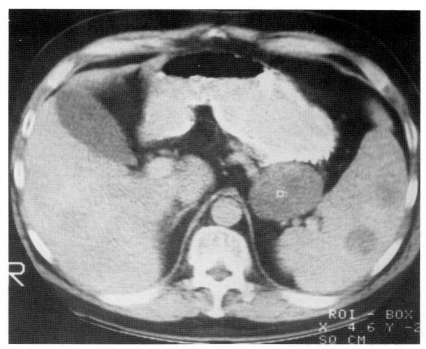

FIGURE 2.44. A 50-Yr-Old Male with Non-Hodgkin's Lymphoma
Note low-density area in the enlarged spleen and enlarged splenic node.

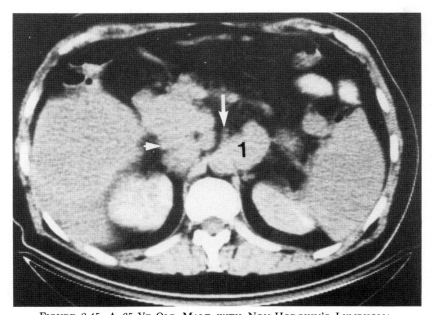

FIGURE 2.45. A 65-Yr-Old Male with Non-Hodgkin's Lymphoma
CT scan just above superior mesenteric artery (*arrow*) shows splenic nodes (*1*) and peripancreatic nodes about the head of the pancreas compressing the inferior vena cava (*arrowhead*).

with the exception of a few collecting trunks from the pancreas that empty into the inferior pancreaticoduodenal nodes. The splenic chain terminates in a group of nodes situated immedi- ately to the left of the celiac artery behind and above the initial segment of the splenic artery. This node also receives drainage from the left renal pedicle and the intestinal lymph trunk.

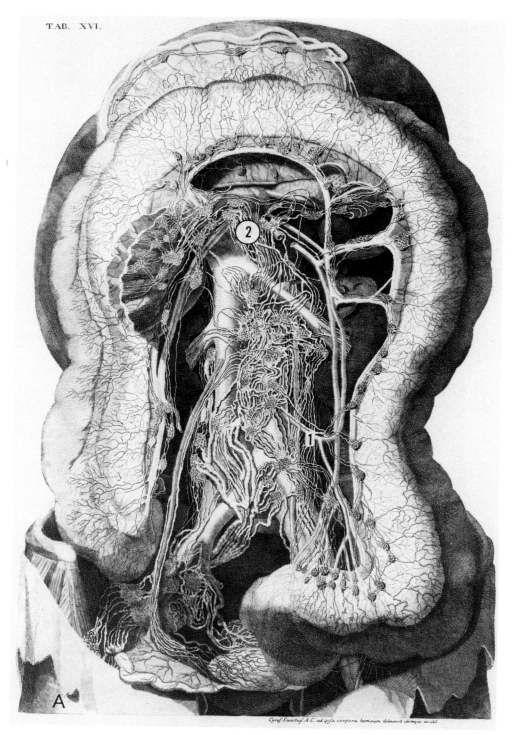

**FIGURE 2.46. MESENTERIC LYMPHATICS**

*A*: Note the inferior (*1*) and superior (*2*) mesenteric arteries. (From Mascagni, 1787.) *B*: (From Rouvière, 1938.)

## Mesenteric Nodes

The mesenteric vessels and lymph nodes accompany the mesenteric arteries and are divided into nodes of the mesentery (placed along the course of the superior mesenteric arteries) and the intestinal nodes (placed along branches of the arteries of the large intestine). Intestinal nodes occur along the middle right and ileocolic arteries (branches of the superior mesenteric artery), the left colic and sigmoid arteries (branches of the inferior mesenteric artery), as well as the inferior mesenteric trunks and its terminal branches.

The lymph nodes of the mesenteric group proper are as a group numerically the greatest number in the body (Cruikshank, 1790). Rouvière (1938) indicates their number to be 150–300. The superior mesenteric nodes are divided into three groups: the peripheral group is situated near the mesenteric border of the intestines; the middle group is placed near the midpoint of the mesenteric, along the terminal segment of the intestinal branches of the mesenteric arteries, and along the first series of arterial arcades;

and the central group lies at the root of the mesentery around the trunks of the superior mesenteric artery and vein. At the beginning of the jejunum, it is difficult to differentiate among the three nodal groups because the middle group is often fused with the central group. The peripheral and middle groups receive lymphatics directly from the small intestine. The middle group also receives lymph from the efferent trunks of the juxtaintestinal nodes (Fig. 2.46).

All efferents from the middle group end in the nodes of the central group. The central group also receives lymph from the ascending and transverse colon, the infrapancreatic lymph nodes (which are placed near the duodenojejunal angle), and the area juxtaposed to the terminal part of the inferior mesenteric vein. The efferent vessels from the central group of superior mesenteric nodes empty into the lumbar trunks, generally the left, or into the initial part of the thoracic duct. The left lumbar trunk frequently extends over the left lateral aspect of the aorta, above the renal artery and into the left lumbar trunk (Mascagni, 1787).

The nodes draining the left colon, sigmoid,

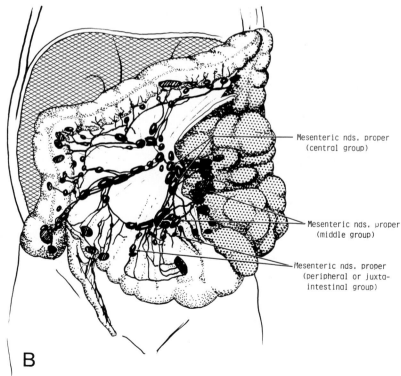

Mesenteric nds. proper (central group)

Mesenteric nds. proper (middle group)

Mesenteric nds. proper (peripheral or juxta-intestinal group)

B

FIGURE 2.46*B*.

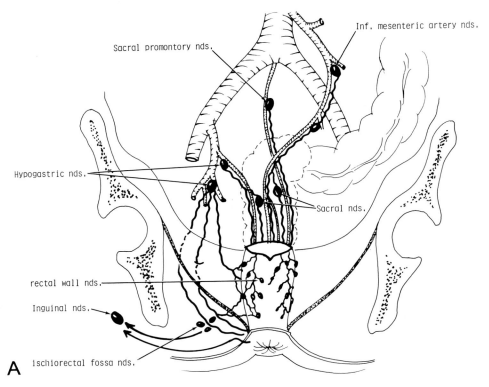

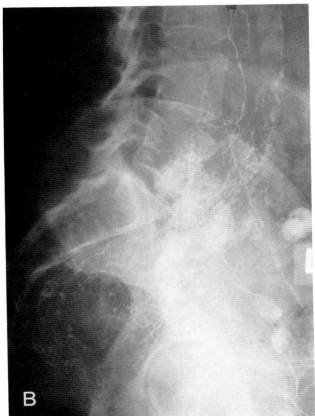

**FIGURE 2.47. RECTAL LYMPHATICS**

*A*: (From Ackerman, 1977.) *B*: Postlymphangiography film of patient with obstruction of para-aortic nodes (histiocytic lymphoma). Note retrograde filling of the lymphatics of the sigmoid and rectum

and rectal area send their efferent trunks to the nodes of the inferior mesenteric chain, which in turn drain into the preaortic and into the left lateral para-aortic nodes placed near the beginning of the inferior mesenteric artery. The nodes of the left colic artery are partially united with the superior mesenteric central group of nodes by means of lymph nodes and channels lining the terminal segment of the inferior mesenteric artery and vein.

With the exception of intercalated (pararectal) nodes, the first order drainage of the rectum enters the inferior mesenteric nodes, chiefly those near the bifurcation of the inferior mesenteric artery. The greater part of lymphatics of the anus drain to superficial inguinal nodes. Some trunks from the anal canal and inferior part of the rectum drain to the middle hemorrhoidal hypogastric nodes, the laterosacral nodes, or sacral promontory nodes (Rouvière, 1938) (Fig. 2.47).

## ADRENAL LYMPHATICS

In the retroperitoneal area, lymphatics from the adrenal gland are connected with those of the liver, diaphragm, and intrathoracic nodes. The first order drainage nodes from the adrenal glands are the right and left para-aortic nodes from the point of origin of the celiac artery to a point somewhat below the renal pedicles. A few renal collecting trunks may enter directly into the intrathoracic and posterior mediastinal lymph nodes (Fig. 2.48).

## THORACIC LYMPHATICS AND NODES

### Parietal Intrathoracic Lymphatics

The parietal intrathoracic lymphatics and nodes, according to Rouvière, are divided into three groups: the posterior parietal nodes, diaphragmatic nodes, and anterior parietal or internal mammary nodes.

The posterior parietal nodes are located pos-

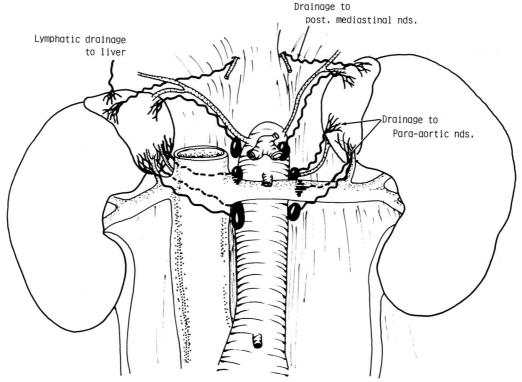

FIGURE 2.48. LYMPHATICS OF ADRENAL GLAND

(From Rouvière, 1938.)

teriorly near the costovertebral junction and lie in the intercostal spaces along the intercostal blood vessels and nerves. Each intercostal space contains one to six nodes just beneath the endothoracic fascia. The posterior parietal or intercostal nodes receive afferents from the parietal pleura, vertebrae, and spinal muscles. The efferent lymphatics of the first and second intercostal spaces terminate in inferior nodes of the internal jugular or transverse cervical chain, in the juxtasubclavian junction, or directly in one of the large collecting trunks at the base of the neck or thoracic duct. The efferent trunks from the third to sixth intercostal spaces empty directly into the thoracic duct, and those from the lower five or six intercostal spaces empty into the thoracic duct near the level of D12.

The juxtavertebral nodes are located in the efferent pathway of the intercostal nodes, lie adjacent or anterior to the vertebral bodies, and drain into the thoracic duct.

### Diaphragmatic Lymph Nodes

The diaphragmatic lymph nodes are divided into an interior pericardial group and a middle or lateral pericardial group (Rouvière, 1938). The anterior pericardial group is located in a median retroxyphoid position and consists of one to three nodes on the diaphragm. Nodes are normally present and placed to the right and left of the midline behind the anterior extremity of the seventh rib and the seventh costal cartilage. Each contains one to three nodes (Fig. 2.49A).

The middle or juxtaphrenic group is located on the right and left sides of the pericardium at the entrance of the phrenic nerve, hence the designation *juxtaphrenic nodes* (Fig. 2.49B). The group consists of two aggregations of lymph nodes, the left (frequently absent) and the more important right groups. The right group consists of one to three nodes, frequently located in front of the inferior vena cava at the entrance of the right phrenic nerve, between the inferior vena cava and the pericardium, or left of the inferior vena cava between the diaphragm and the pericardium (Sledziewski, 1930) (Fig. 2.49).

The anterior pericardial group receives efferent lymphatics from the greater part of the diaphragm, diaphragmatic pleura, anterior and superior surfaces of the liver, superior epigastric region, and anterior abdominal wall. The efferent lymphatics and the anterior group drain into the internal mammary nodes.

The middle or juxtaphrenic group receives lymphatics from the adjacent parts of the diaphragm, pleura, pericardium, and liver. The ef-

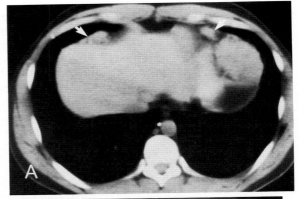

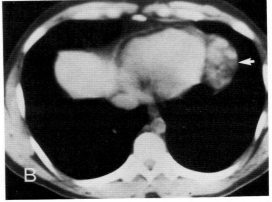

FIGURE 2.49. RECURRENT HODGKIN'S DISEASE
*A*: Note the right and left anterior pericardial nodes (*arrows*). *B*: The left juxtaphrenic pericardial nodes (*arrow*) are enlarged.

ferent lymphatics from the middle or juxtaphrenic group drain into lymphatics that follow the course of the phrenic nerve into anterior mediastinal nodes, pass posteriorly to terminate in the posterior mediastinal and juxtaesophageal nodes, or penetrate the diaphragm and empty into celiac nodes.

### Anterior Mediastinal (Internal Mammary) Nodes

The internal mammary nodes are located on either side of the sternum in front of the transverse thoracic muscle and follow the course of the internal mammary blood vessels. The nodes are generally more numerous at the superior segment of the sternocostal plate and are almost always found at the level of the first and second intercostal spaces but may extend as low as the third to fourth intercostal spaces and are usually absent between the fourth and sixth. The efferent vessels to the internal mammary lymphatics course from the abdominal wall, the anterior thoracic wall and intercostal muscles, and the pectoral muscles and mammary glands. They also receive lymphatic drainage from the anterior and middle pericardial nodes. The efferents drain into the thoracic duct on the left, the lymphatic ducts on the right, or the jugular and subclavian veins separately or together at the jugulosubclavian angle.

## Visceral Lymphatics of Thorax

Rouvière divides the visceral intrathoracic nodes into four principal groups: the anterior mediastinal or prevascular nodes, the posterior mediastinal nodes, the paratracheobronchial nodes, and the intrapulmonary nodes of the lung and pulmonary root (i.e., hilar nodes) (Figs. 2.50 and 2.51).

The *anterior mediastinal prevascular nodes* are located in the superior portion of the mediastinum in front of the large vessels that enter and exit from the heart. They consist of three chains of nodes to the right and left of the midline and a transverse group connecting two vertical chains.

The anterior mediastinal chain is located in front of the superior vena cava and right innominate vein and consists of two to five nodes, most often along the phrenic nerve near the right border of the thymus. The right anterior mediastinal chain is part of an ascending right anterior mediastinal path, which has its origin in the anterior part of the pulmonary root and sometimes drains nodes in the right juxtaphrenic aggregation of the diaphragm around the right phrenic nerve and inferior vena cava. It receives afferent lymphatics from the diaphragm, diaphragmatic and mediastinal pleura, heart, pericardium, right lung, and thymus and terminates in the right jugulosubclavian area.

The left anterior mediastinal chain is prearterial (i.e., preaortocarotid) (Fig. 2.51). It begins in the ductal node in the aortopulmonic window and descends along the phrenic nerve in front of and on the superior border of the aortic arch to ascend on the anterolateral surface of the common carotid artery. A few nodes are placed along its path near the lateral border of the thymus. These vessels form the left anterior mediastinal or preaortocarotid pathway. The efferents drain the pleura, pericardium, heart, thymus, and left lung. The left anterior mediastinal pathway terminates in the thoracic duct or directly in the jugulosubclavian angle.

The transverse anterior mediastinal group is located along the superior and inferior borders

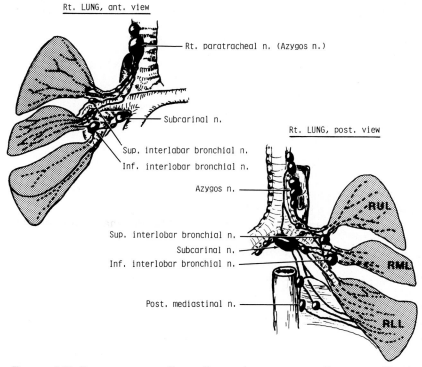

FIGURE 2.50. LYMPHATICS OF RIGHT LUNG, ANTERIOR AND POSTERIOR VIEWS
*RUL*, right upper lung; *RML*, right medial lung: *RLL*, right lower lung. (From Rouvière, 1938.)

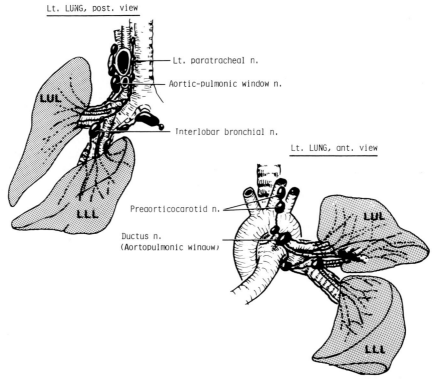

FIGURE 2.51. LYMPHATICS OF LEFT LUNG, ANTERIOR AND POSTERIOR VIEWS
*LUL*, left upper lung; *LLL*, left lower lung. (From Rouvière, 1938.)

of the left innominate vein and unites the right and left anterior mediastinal trunks.

The *posterior mediastinal nodes* are placed behind the esophagus and in front of the aorta, hence juxta-aortic, juxtaesophageal, or interaortoesophageal nodes. They are located in the lower part of the mediastinum below the level of the inferior pulmonary veins and extend to the diaphragm. The afferent drainage to the posterior mediastinal nodes is from the diaphragm, diaphragmatic pleura, esophagus, pericardium, and inferior lobes of the lung. Efferent vessels from the posterior mediastinal nodes empty into the subcarinal nodes and thoracic duct (Fig. 2.50).

The *paratracheobronchial nodes* can be further divided into the paratracheal nodes proper, the nodes at the bifurcation or subcarinal nodes, the intertracheal bronchial node, and the nodes of the pulmonary root (Figs. 2.50 and 2.51).

The paratracheal nodes consist of two chains on the right and left lateral aspects of the trachea. The right paratracheal chain consists of three to six nodes arranged in single file beginning at the arch of the azygos vein, hence the azygos node, and ending superiorly in a node

immediately below the right subclavian artery. Anteriorly, the chain is bounded by the superior vena cava and the right innominate vein; medially, by the trachea; and laterally, by the mediastinal pleura. The azygos node is generally the largest. The afferents drain directly from the right lung, bronchial nodes, and bifurcation as well as from the trachea, esophagus, and thymus. The right paratracheal nodes terminate in the right jugulosubclavian angle or the internal jugular vein.

The left paratracheal chain usually consists of four to five nodes along the anterior and medial aspect of the vertical segment of the recurrent nerve lateral to the left posterolateral border of the trachea and medial to the pleura and posterior arch of the aorta and left subclavian artery. Afferent drainage to the left paratracheal nodes is from a continuation of lymphatics from the left lung by means of the left suprabronchial node or ductal node in the aortopulmonic window. The left paratracheal lymph chain also receives drainage from the esophagus and trachea and terminates in the thoracic duct or near the left jugulosubclavian angle.

Because the drainage of the aortopulmonic

group is to the anterior mediastinal nodes, the nodes of the aortopulmonic window for practical clinical reasons are included in the anterior mediastinal group as in Chapter 13.

Subcarinal nodes of the tracheal bifurcation occupy the interval from the trachea, formed by its division into the right and left mainstem bronchi, to just above the pulmonary veins. The group usually consists of three to five nodes extending along the border of the right and left mainstem bronchi in contact with the inferior pulmonary vein immediately behind the pericardium and in front of the esophagus, azygos vein, and aorta. The subcarinal nodes form a crossroad drainage between the lymphatic vessels from the diaphragm, heart, pericardium, esophagus, inferior part of the trachea, bronchi, and lung. The efferent vessels most frequently drain into the right paratracheal chain but occasionally into the left, passing either in front of or behind the trachea and bronchus. CT scans have shown normal nodes in this region to be 6–10 mm in diameter (Genereux and Howie, 1984).

The intrapulmonary nodes located near the hilum, as well as those of the pulmonary root, are included as a single group, although anatomically and surgically they have been considered in separate categories. According to Rouvière, the nodes of the pulmonary root comprise those nodes from the origin of the bronchi to the mediastinal surface of the lung. Even in the early literature, however, there was confusion as to what comprised the intrapulmonary or pulmonary nodes proper (Barety, 1874; Sukiennikow, 1903; Poupardin, 1909; Engel, 1926; Steinert, 1928). The intrapulmonary nodes accompany the bronchial tree, others the pulmonary artery and veins, and still others are related to all three. They are generally placed in angles of division of the bronchi, arteries, or veins, are all near the hilum, and can be found by dissecting the bronchi and blood vessels that accompany the fissures. Thus Rouvière considered the intrapulmonary nodes to be lymphoid elements that were originally extrapulmonary (along the bronchoarterial tree at the root of each lobe) but that they became united into pulmonary tissue upon extension of the pulmonary parenchyma, which projected over the elements of the pulmonary root and enclosed the neighboring lobes. In this manner the nodes become either interlobar or lobar and drain the lymphatics of the lung. Because chest radiographs, hilar tomography and CT do not distinguish the nodes of the pulmonary root as described by Rouvière, the intrapulmonary nodes are considered under the general

category of hilar nodes with a description of lymphatic drainage as outlined by Rouvière.

## Pulmonary Lymphatics

Right upper lobe lymphatic drainage is divided into anteromedial and posterolateral regions. The anteromedial region drains the anterior portion of the upper lobe and empties into the lymphatics of the paratracheal chain via the azygos node. The posterolateral region drains into the paratracheal region as well as the subcarinal nodes through the superior interlobar bronchial nodes.

Lymphatics from the right middle lobe are connected on the anterior surface to the paratracheal nodes and to the superior as well as the inferior interlobar bronchial nodes. The interlobar bronchial nodes, in turn, empty into the subcarinal nodes. Drainage from the right lower lobe is divided into the superior and inferior regions. The superior region drains into the inferior interlobar bronchial and subcarinal nodes. Drainage from the inferior region drains into the inferior interlobar bronchial nodes, subcarinal nodes, or paratracheal nodes as well posterior mediastinal nodes through the inferior pulmonary ligament (Fig. 2.50).

Lymphatics from the left lung are divided into upper and lower lobe regions. The upper lobe region consists of anterior collecting vessels that are prevenous and prearterial and terminate in the ductus nodes or in other nodes of the left anterior mediastinal chain. The posterior collecting vessels are retroarterial and suprabronchial. They empty into left suprabronchial nodes and, by this communication, with the left paratracheal nodes, with ductal nodes to the preaortocarotid nodes (anterior mediastinal nodes), and with the subaortic node (node of the loop of the left recurrent nerve). The intermediate collecting trunks are prebronchial and supra-arterial and empty into the preaortocarotid chain, into the right paratracheal nodes through the subcarinal nodes, or into both. In the inferior region, drainage is to the superior region of the upper lobe, but the inferior region also drains into nodes of the tracheal bifurcation, interlobar bronchial nodes, and subcarinal nodes.

Drainage from the left lower lobe follows three routes. The upper region follows vessels that are retroarterial and suprabronchial. They empty into left suprabronchial nodes, which in turn are connected with the paratracheal and anterior mediastinal nodes as well as with subcarinal nodes from the posterior aspect of the lower lobe bronchus. The midregion of the left lower lobe drains to the same nodes as the upper region, but the course is interrupted by interlobar nodes as well as subcarinal nodes. The inferior region drains to subcarinal nodes as well as aortoesophageal (posterior mediastinal) nodes through the inferior pulmonary ligament (Fig. 2.50).

In summary, the superior lymphatic region of the right upper lobe (the anteromedial region) drains to right paratracheal nodes through the azygos node. Drainage from the mid region of the right lung includes the posterolateral region of the upper lobe, middle lobe, and superior segment of the lower lobe and empties into the right lateral paratracheal and subcarinal nodes. The inferior lymphatic drainage region includes

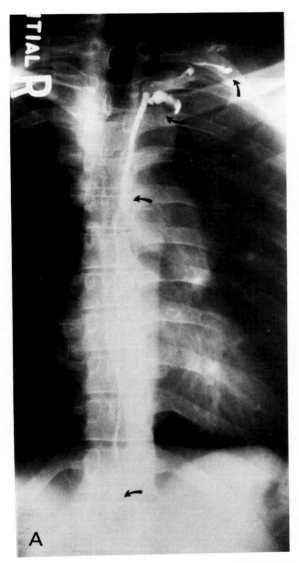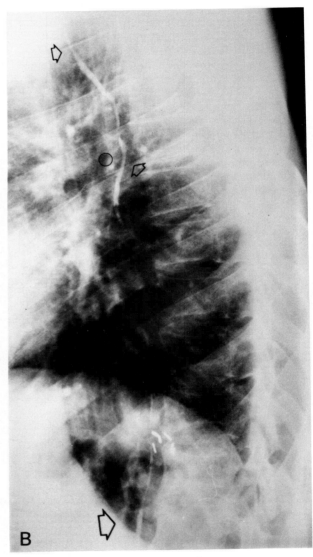

FIGURE 2.52. THORACIC DUCT

*A:* This frontal projection displays the morphology of the usual adult thoracic duct. From its origin (cisterna chyli) to its termination (venous system on the left), all segments are visible. *B:* The course of the thoracic duct on a lateral view. Note the posterior course taken until reaching the level of the bronchus (*circle*). Further ascent through the thorax is parallel with the trachea (*open arrow* at top). *C:* The most common thoracic duct anomaly is some form of duplication. One form of duplication (*arrow*) is illustrated. *D:* Segment of contrast-filled ducts from the cisterna. *E:* Contrast-filled thoracic duct at D5. Note the adenopathy in the aortic pulmonary window (*arrow*). *F:* Thoracic duct at D3-4. Note the contrast-filled thoracic duct just posterior to the esophagus at the apex of the aortic arch. *G:* Contrast-filled thoracic duct between and posterior to the esophagus and left subclavian artery. *H:* Thoracic duct at the jugulosubclavian confluens.

the basal segments of the lower lobe, and most of its lymphatics empty into the right paratracheal nodes through the superior and inferior interlobar bronchial nodes to the paratracheal nodes and subcarinal nodes. The inferior lymphatic region also drains into posterior mediastinal nodes through the inferior pulmonary ligament.

On the left the superior lymphatic region comprises the superior region of the upper lobe, and drainage is to the left paratracheal chain, the ductus node of the left anterior mediastinal chain, and the nodes of the aortopulmonic window. The middle lymphatic region includes the inferior portion of the upper lobe as well as the superior and middle regions of the lower lobe.

The collecting trunks empty superiorly into the anterior mediastinum and left paratracheal nodes and inferiorly into the subcarinal nodes. The inferior lymphatic region, represented by the inferior parts of the lower lobe, drains into the subcarinal nodes.

Drainage from the superior portion of the left lung in its entirety and the mid region of the left lung in part drain into the left anterior mediastinal and left paratracheal nodes and then into the jugulosubclavian angle. The remainder of the left lung (that is, the inferior and part of the middle region) and the entire right lung empty into tributaries of the right paratracheal region and of the right jugulosubclavian venous confluens. It thus becomes possible, by knowing the

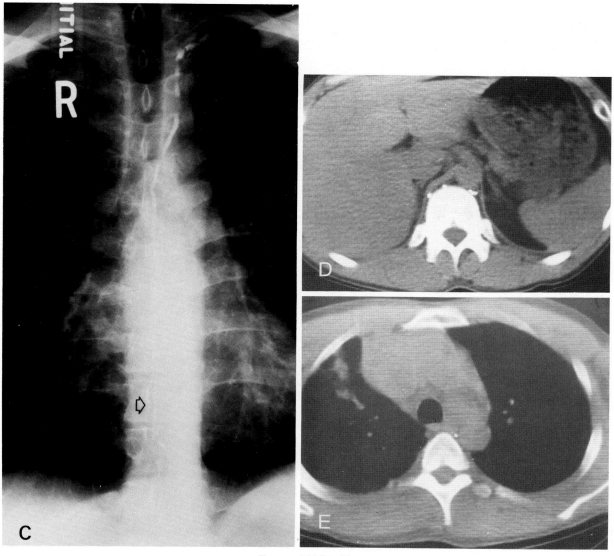

FIGURE 2.52C to E.

lymphatic anatomy, to predict the spread of metastasis from a primary lung lesion as demonstrated by McCort and Robbins (1951) and described by McCloud and Meyer in Chapter 13.

## Thoracic Duct

The thoracic duct is the principal lymphatic vessel in the body (Fig. 2.52). With the exception of the convex surface of the liver, lymphatic flow from all structures below the diaphragm is transmitted to the thoracic duct. Above the diaphragm it receives lymphatic flow from all of the structures on the left when joined by the left bronchial, mediastinal, subclavian, and jugular trunks. Lymph flow enters the blood system as the thoracic duct ends its course, usually anastomosing into the left subclavian vein. The significance of the thoracic duct to function of the lymphatic system in health and diseased states becomes readily apparent.

Although good opacification of the thoracic

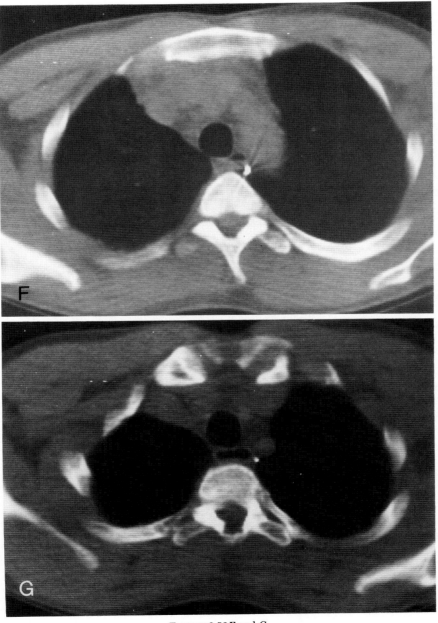

FIGURE 2.52*F* and *G*.

duct during lymphography would have enormous value in many clinical situations, routine satisfactory delineation without excess risk is not yet technically feasible. Various modifications of antegrade and retrograde techniques have been reported (Pomerantz et al., 1963; Nusbaum et al., 1964; Shieber, 1974; Cox and Kinmonth, 1975; Gothlin et al., 1975), but substantial evidence supporting their efficacy is not available presently. Since present methods do not routinely opacify the entire thoracic duct, the exact role of lymphography in evaluation of the thoracic duct is unclear.

Anatomic studies by Davis (1915) have depicted the usual adult structure and frequency of anatomic variations. In 14 of 22 dissections, the thoracic duct was single and traveled cephalad into and through the thorax on the right lateral aspect of the aorta. At the level of the fifth thoracic vertebra, it crossed to the left side and opened into and through the venous system of the left side. Lymphographic studies have corroborated these postmortem studies (Pomerantz et al., 1963; Wirth and Frommhold, 1970; Kinmonth, 1972).

Three subdivisions of the thoracic duct are based on embryological development (Fuchs, 1969; Wirth and Frommhold, 1970): the abdominal, thoracic, and cervical segments (Fig. 2.52D–G). Its abdominal segment begins as two lumbar trunks which combine to form the cisterna chyli. This relationship has been demonstrated in 50–72% of observed lymphograms (Fuchs, 1969; Wirth and Frommhold, 1970; Rosenberger and Abrams, 1971). Delineation of the cisterna chyli by these same authors occurred in 30–87% of lymphograms. The cisterna chyli occurs most often at the level of L1-2 with frequencies of 38–91% of lymphographic studies by Rosenberger

and Abrams (1971), Fuchs (1969), and Wirth and Frommhold (1970), respectively. The morphological character of the cisterna chyli also varies widely. Even within the same patient, the character of the cisterna chyli can vary when examined by consecutive filming (Rosenberger and Abrams, 1971). Usually, however, a saccular structure less than 5 cm in length but wider than the adjacent thoracic duct is characteristic. The configuration also can be round, oval, or linear (Fuchs, 1969; Wirth and Frommhold, 1970).

Leaving the cisterna chyli the thoracic duct continues into the thoracic segment, emerging through the aortic hiatus of the diaphragm. It then courses between the aorta and the azygos vein. Contrast filling of the entire thoracic segment of the duct occurs infrequently. The cephalad portion of the duct is visible more frequently than the caudad section because there are more valves above the sixth thoracic vertebra and at the termination of the duct as it enters the venous system (Nusbaum et al., 1964). These valves delay contrast emptying into the venous system by the cephalad portion. Simultaneously, the caudad portion permits uninhibited antegrade flow of contrast medium. Retrograde flow of contrast medium does not occur in the presence of intact valves (Nusbaum et al., 1964; Kinmonth, 1972). The flow of contrast medium (lymph) along the course of the thoracic duct does not appear to be assisted by active peristalsis (Pomerantz et al., 1963; Nusbaum et al., 1964; Dumont, 1967).

Although the aorta can greatly influence the course of the thoracic duct, the usual course observed roentgenographically correlates with classical anatomic descriptions. On the frontal projections the initial or caudad subsection is superimposed over the vertebral body, either at the midline or somewhat to the right of the spinous processes. This correlates with the right lateral aortic wall. On the lateral projection, it lies immediately anterior to the vertebrae.

From approximately T10-12, the thoracic duct deviates toward the left. At the level of the sixth thoracic vertebra, the duct crosses the left mainstem bronchus. It then courses anteriorly to travel just posterior and to the left but parallel with the trachea (Fig. 2.52E).

Continuation of the thoracic duct into the cervical segment is somewhat more dramatic. It rises 3–4 cm above the medial edge of the clavicle and then sharply arches anteriorly and inferiorly as it merges into the wall of the junction of the left internal jugular and subclavian veins as a bulbous structure. In this region, the valves are markedly accentuated (Fig. 2.52F–H).

The most common variation of the thoracic

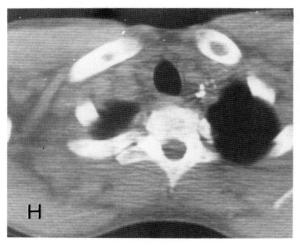

FIGURE 2.52H.

duct is some form of duplication (Davis, 1915; Fuchs, 1969; Wirth and Frommhold, 1970; Rosenberger and Abrams, 1971). Fortuitous filling of multiple intrathoracic, supraclavicular, cervi-

cal, and even axillary nodes occurs under normal circumstances. Knowledge of these variations has obvious significance in the management of patients with malignancies.

## UPPER EXTREMITY LYMPHATICS

Clinical indications for lymphography of the upper extremity and cervical lymphatics include confirmation of lymphedema, primary or secondary, or delineation of the extent of lymphedema in the upper extremity (Kuisk, 1971; Browse, 1972b) (see Chapter 7 on lymphedema). For oncological purposes the clinical rewards for overcoming the technical difficulties of performing upper extremity lymphography are insignificant. Malignancies that affect lymph nodes in the axillary, supraclavicular, or cervical regions are often accessible to palpation. Also, the natural history of malignant lymphomas, particularly Hodgkin's disease, is such that all of these nodal groups are included in treatment planning if either group has confirmed involvement. Additionally, interpretation of the lymphographic features of the majority of the nodes in these regions is extremely complex and often misleading (Fisch, 1968; Kuisk, 1971).

### Forearm and Arm

The anatomic and lymphographic description of this section is based primarily on the comprehensive work of Rouvière (1938) and Fisch (1968). As in the lower extremities, the upper extremity is drained by superficial and deep lymphatics. Multiple superficial plexuses drain the digits and the volar aspect of the palm. These plexuses drain into somewhat larger vessels that merge dorsally. These vessels eventually anastomose with the major superficial lymphatics of the forearm.

The lateral and medial lymphatics ascend the upper extremity. The lateral group courses the forearm laterally and accompanies the cephalic vein. The medial group courses medially and accompanies the basilic vein. Some of the ascending medial channels pass through the epitrochlear nodes at the elbow, but most continue superiorly to the lateral axillary nodes. Many of the lymphatics of the lateral group become medially directed at the elbow and continue superiorly with the medial group. Those channels that persist laterally with the cephalic vein pass through the deltoidopectoral nodes. From these nodes efferent vessels then course to the subclavicular axillary nodes or the inferior cervical nodes.

The vessels of the deep system ascend in juxtaposition to the arteries of the upper extremity. Some terminate in nodes along the brachial artery, but most continue to empty into the lateral group of axillary nodes. Fewer vessels are in the deep system than the superficial. Some communication exists between the superficial and deep systems.

### Axilla

Almost all of the hand, forearm, arm, and thoracic wall lymphatics drain into the axillary lymph nodes. Like the nodes in the inguinal region, these nodes vary in size and number. Generally they are somewhat larger than more centrally located nodes and range between 20 and 30 in number. Anatomically, these nodes are subgrouped into (a) lateral group, (b) anterior or pectoral group, (c) posterior or subscapular group, (d) central or intermediate group, and (e) medial or subclavicular group (apical). The nodes in the apex of the axilla (medial or subclavicular) are separated from the more inferiorly positioned subgroups by the pectoralis minor tendon.

The *lateral group* is composed of four to six nodes that lie medial and posterior to the axillary vein. Afferent vessels originate from the arm and efferent vessels empty into the central, subclavicular (apical), and inferior deep cervical nodes.

The *anterior group* consists of four to six nodes along the lower border of the pectoralis major muscle. Afferent vessels emanate from the anterior-lateral thoracic cage and the lateral and central portions of the mammary gland. Efferent vessels empty into the central and subclavicular (apical) nodes.

The *posterior nodes* are somewhat small. The group usually consists of six or seven nodes positioned on the inner wall of the axilla along the course of the dorsal thoracic artery. Afferent vessels drain the lateral thoracic wall, and efferent vessels drain into the nodes of the central group.

The *central group* has three to five nodes that are somewhat larger and are positioned more inferiorly along the axillary artery. Afferent vessels empty into the subclavicular (apical) nodes.

The *medial (subclavicular or apical) group* is positioned in the apex of the axillary fossa. The six to 12 nodes in this subgroup receive afferents from all other, more inferior axillary nodes. Efferent vessels unite to form the subclavian trunk, which empties directly into the junction of the internal jugular and subclavian vein or into the jugular trunk. The subclavian trunk may empty into the thoracic duct.

Lymphography demonstrates the axillary nodes unpredictably but most often very poorly. Complete contrast filling of these nodes is not achieved by usual clinical lymphographic methods (Fuchs, 1969; Kuisk, 1971).

## CERVICAL LYMPHATICS

Cervical lymphography has limited clinical utility. As with upper extremity and axillary lymphography, cervical lymphography is difficult to perform and currently is incapable of producing reliable information as to the true extent of malignant disease. Hence, the reward for overcoming the technical difficulties is insignificant (Fisch, 1968; Kuisk, 1971).

Cervical lymph nodes broadly include Waldeyer's tonsillar ring, lymph nodes at the transition between the head and neck regions, and the true cervical nodes (Rouvière, 1938; Fisch, 1968). Waldeyer's ring is formed by a circular arrangement of lymph nodes. In the pharynx, this arrangement consists of the posterior lingual, palatine, tubal, and pharyngeal tonsils. Nodes at the transition region of the head and neck are arranged in a circular configuration and include occipital, retroauricular, parotidean, submandib-

ular, submental, retropharyngeal, and sublingual lymph nodes. These nodes are both superficial and deep to the superficial fascia. Except for the retropharyngeal and sublingual groups, these nodal groups form a chain in the region of the transition between the head and neck.

The retropharyngeal and sublingual groups are incorporated in the chain as well, but they are also positioned in the vicinity of the pharyngeal wall and tongue, respectively. The nodes superficial to the superficial fascia drain the posterior aspect of the face, scalp, ears, posterior aspect of the head, and upper neck region. Efferent drainage is to the deep cervical nodes.

True cervical nodes are anatomically divided into the medial and lateral groups. These divisions are further subdivided into superficial and deep groups.

## REFERENCES

Abrams HL, Takahashi M, Adams DF: Usefulness and accuracy of lymphangiography in lymphoma. *Cancer Chemother Rep* 52:157, 1968.

Baltaxe HA, Constable WC: Mediastinal lymph node visualization in absence of intrathoracic disease. *Radiology* 90:94, 1968.

Barety: De l-adénopathie trachéo-bronchique en général et en particulier dans la scrofule et la phtisie pulmonaire, précédée de l'étude topographique des ganglions trachéo-bronchiques. Thèse, Université de Paris, 1874.

Bartels P: Ueber die Lymphgefässe des Pankreas. I. Ueber Lymphatische Verbindungen zwischen Duodenum and Pankreas beim Hunde. *Arch Anat Physiol Anat Abt* 299–330, 1904.

Baum S, Bron KM, Wexler L, Abrams HL: Lymphangiography, cavography, and urography. Comparative accuracy in the diagnosis of pelvic and abdominal metastases. *Radiology* 81:207, 1963.

Bloom W, Fawcett DW: The lymphatic system. In *A Textbook of Histology*. Philadelphia, WB Saunders, 1962, p 291.

Brash JC: Blood-vascular and lymphatic systems. In Brash JC, Jamieson EB (eds): *Cunningham's Textbook of Anatomy*, ed 8. New York, Oxford University Press, 1943, p 1177.

Bron KM, Baum S, Abrams HL: Oil embolism in lymphangiography. *Radiology* 80:194, 1963.

Browse NL: Normal lymphographic appearances: lower limb and pelvis. In Kinmonth JB (ed): *The Lymphatics: Diseases, Lymphography and Surgery*. Baltimore, Williams & Wilkins, 1972a, p 20.

Browse NL: Normal lymphographic appearances of the lower limb and axilla. In Kinmonth JB (ed): *The Lymphatics: Diseases, Lymphography and Surgery*. Baltimore, Williams & Wilkins, 1972b, p 70.

Bruhns C: Ueber die Lymphgefässe der weiblichen Genitalien nebst einigen Bemerkungen uber die Topographie der Leistendrusen. *Arch Anat Physiol Anat Abt* 57–80, 1898.

Busch F, Sayegh ES: Roentgenographic visualization of human testicular lymphatics: a preliminary report. *J Urol* 89:106, 1963.

Busch FM, Sayegh ES, Chenault OW Jr: Some uses of lymphangiography in the management of testicular tumors. *J Urol* 93:490, 1965.

Butler JJ: Non-neoplastic lesions of lymph nodes of man to be differentiated from lymphomas. *Natl Cancer Inst Monogr* 32:233, 1969.

Callen PW, Korobkin M, Isherwood I: Computed tomographic evaluation of the retrocrural prevertebral space. *AJR* 129:907, 1977.

Caminiti: Recherches sur les lymphatiques de la prostate humaine. *Ann Mal Organ Génito-urin* 23:1441–1460, 1905.

Casley-Smith JR: The functioning of the lymphatic system under normal and pathological conditions: its dependence on the fine structures and permeability of the vessels. In Rüttimann A (ed): *Progress in Lymphology*. New York, Hafner, 1967, p 348.

Castellino RA: Observations on "reactive (follicular) hyperplasia" as encountered in repeat lymphography in the lymphomas. *Cancer* 34:2042, 1974.

Castellino RA: The role of lymphography in apparently localized "prostatic" carcinoma. *Lymphology* 8:16, 1975.

Castellino RA: Imaging techniques for staging abdominal Hodgkin's disease. *Cancer Treat Rep* 66:697, 1982.

Castellino RA, Ray G, Blank N, Govan D, Bagshaw M: Lymphangiography in prostatic carcinoma. Preliminary observations. *JAMA* 223:877, 1973.

Castellino RA, Billingham M, Dorfman RF: Lymphographic accuracy in Hodgkin's disease and malignant lymphoma with a note on the "reactive" lymph node as a cause of most false-positive lymphograms. *Invest Radiol* 9:155, 1974.

Castellino RA, Bellani FF, Gasparini M, Terno G, Musumeci R: Lymphography in childhood: six years experience with 242 cases. *Lymphology* 8:74, 1975.

Chavez CM: Lymphatic drainage of the testicle. In Rüttimann A (ed): *Progress in Lymphology.* New York, Hafner, 1967, p 191.

Chiappa S, Uslenghi C, Bonadonna G, Marano P, Ravasi G: Combined testicular and foot lymphangiography in testicular carcinomas. *Surg Gynecol Obstet* 123:10, 1966.

Clark ER: The lymphatic system. In Schaeffer JP (ed): *Morris' Human Anatomy: A Complete Systematic Treatise,* ed 10. Philadelphia, Blakiston, 1942, sect VIII, p 786.

Cordier G: Note sur les lymphatiques de la vésicule séminale. *Ann Anat Pathol Anat Norm Méd-Chir* 8:293–294, 1931.

Cox SJ, Kinmonth JB: Lymphography of the thoracic duct. *J Cardiovasc Surg* 16:120, 1975.

Cruikshank W: *Anatomy of the Absorbing Vessels of the Human Body,* ed 2. London, G Nicol, 1790.

Cunéo B: Note sur les ganglions lymphatiques régionaux du rein. *Bull Mém Soc Anat Paris* 6e série, 4:235–236, 1902.

Cunéo B, Marcille M: Topographie des ganglions ilio-pelviens. *Bull Mém Soc Anat Paris* 6e série, 3:653–663, 1901.

Cutler SJ, Myers MH, Green SG: Trends in survival rates of patients with cancer. *N Engl J Med* 293:122, 1975.

Davis HK: A statistical study of the thoracic duct in man. *Am J Anat* 17:211, 1915.

Drinker CK, Yoffey JM: *Lymphatics, Lymph and Lymphoid Tissue: Their Physiological and Clinical Significance.* Cambridge, MA, Harvard University Press, 1941.

Dumont AE: Lymph flow in the regulation of circulatory congestion and pancreatic interstitial pressure. In Rüttimann A (ed): *Progress in Lymphology.* New York, Hafner, 1967, p 91.

Engel S: Die Topographie der bronchialen Lymphknoten. *Klin Wochenschr* 1:1136–1137, 1936.

Fisch U: *Lymphography of the Cervical Lymphatic System.* Philadelphia, WB Saunders, 1968.

Fischer HW, Lawrence MS, Thornbury JR: Lymphography of the normal adult male. *Radiology* 78:399, 1962.

Fischer HW, Zimmerman G: Roentgenographic visualization of lymph nodes and lymphatic channels. *AJR* 81:517, 1959.

Fuchs WA: Normal anatomy. In Fuchs WA, Davidson JW, Fischer HW (eds): *Lymphography in Cancer.* New York, Springer-Verlag, 1969, p 42.

Fuchs WA: Neoplasms of epithelial origin. In Abrams HL (ed): *Angiography,* ed 2. Boston, Little, Brown, 1971a, vol II, p 1369.

Fuchs WA: Normal anatomy of the lymphatics. In Abrams HL (ed): *Angiography,* ed 2. Boston, Little, Brown, 1971b, vol II, p 1337.

Fuchs WA: Technique and complications of lymphangiography. In Abrams HL (ed): *Angiography,* ed 2. Boston, Little, Brown, 1971c, vol II, p 1325.

Gabrielle H: *Le Canal Thoracique. Etude Anatomique et Expérimentale.* Imprimerie de Trévoux, G Patissier, 1925.

Genereux GP, Howie JL: Normal mediastinal lymph node size and number: CT and anatomic study. *AJR* 142:1095–1100, 1984.

Gothlin J, Dahlback O, Dencker H, Hakansson C-H, Lunderquist A: Retrograde angiography of the human thoracic duct. *AJR* 124:472, 1975.

Gowans JL: The recirculation of lymphocytes from blood to lymph in the rat. *J Physiol (Lond)* 146:54, 1959.

Gray H: The lymphatic system. In Goss CM (ed): *Anatomy of the Human Body,* ed 27. Philadelphia, Lea & Febiger, 1959, p 775.

Greening RR, Wallace S: Further observations in lymphangiography. *Radiol Clin North Am* 1:157, 1963.

Ham AW, Leeson TS: Hemopoietic tissue. In *Histology,* ed 4. Philadelphia, JB Lippincott, 1961, p 361.

Hasumi S: Anatomische Untersuchungen ueber das Lymphgefässystem des maennlichen Urogenitalsystems. *Jpn J Med Sci Anat* 2:159–186, 1930.

Hays DM: The staging of Hodgkin's disease in children reviewed. *Cancer* 35:973, 1975.

Herman PG, Benninghoff DL, Nelson JH, Mellins HZ: Roentgen anatomy of the ilio-pelvic-aortic lymphatic system. *Radiology* 80:182, 1963.

Hessel SJ, Adams DF, Abrams HL: Lymphography in lymphoma. In Clouse ME (ed): *Clinical Lymphography.* Baltimore, Williams & Wilkins, 1977.

His W: Beobachtungen ueber den Bau des Saeugethier-Eierstockes. *Arch Mikrosk Anat* (von Schultze) 1:151–202, 1865.

Howett M, Greenberg AJ: Direct lymphangioadenography of the uterine cervix. *Obstet Gynecol* 27:392, 1966.

Huntington GS, McClure CFW: The development of the main lymphatic system channels of the cat and their relation to the venous system. *Anat Rec* 1:36, 1906–1907.

Jackson BT: Normal lymphographic appearances: lumbar region. In Kinmonth JB (ed): *The Lymphatics: Diseases, Lymphography and Surgery.* Baltimore, Williams & Wilkins, 1972, p 44.

Jackson BT, Kinmonth JB: Lumbar lymphatic crossover. *Clin Radiol* 25:187, 1974a.

Jackson BT, Kinmonth JB: The normal lymphographic appearances of the lumbar lymphatics. *Clin Radiol* 25:175, 1974b.

Jacobsson S, Johansson S: Normal roentgen anatomy of the lymph vessels of upper and lower extremities. *Acta Radiol [Diagn] (Stockh)* 51:321, 1959.

Jamieson JK, Dobson JF: The lymphatic system of the stomach. *Lancet* 1:1061–1066, 1907.

Kampmeier OF: The development of the thoracic duct in the pig. *Am J Anat* 13:401, 1912.

Kaplan HS, Dorfman RF, Nelsen TS, Rosenberg SA: Staging laparotomy and splenectomy in Hodgkin's disease: analysis of indications and patterns of involvement in 285 consecutive, unselected patients. *Natl Cancer Inst Monogr* 36:291, 1973.

Kinmonth JB: Lymphangiography in man. A method of outlining lymphatic trunks at operation. *Clin Sci* 11:13, 1952.

Kinmonth JB, ed: *The Lymphatics: Diseases, Lymphography and Surgery.* Baltimore, Williams & Wilkins, 1972.

Kinmonth JB, Harper RK, Taylor GW: Lymphangiography by radiological methods. *Clin Radiol* 2:217, 1955a.

Kinmonth JB, Taylor GW, Harper RK: Lymphography: a technique for its clinical use in the lower limb. *Br Med J* 1:940, 1955b.

Kirschner RH, Abt AB, O'Connell MJ, Sklansky BD, Greene WH, Wiernik PH: Vascular invasion and hematogenous dissemination of Hodgkin's disease. *Cancer* 34:1159, 1974.

Kubik I, Tondury G, Rüttimann A, Wirth W: Nomenclature of the lymph nodes of the retroperitoneum, the pelvis, and the lower extremity. In Rüttimann A (ed): *Progress in Lymphology.* New York, Hafner, 1967, p 52.

Kuisk H: *Technique of Lymphography and Principles of Interpretation.* St Louis, Warren H Green, 1971.

Kumita: Über die parenchymatösen Lymphbahnen der Nebenniere. *Arch Anat Physiol Anat Abt* 321–327, 1909.

Larson DL, Lewis SR: Deep lymphatic system of the lower extremity. *Am J Surg* 113:217, 1967.

Lemeh CN: A study of the development and structural relationship of the testis and gubernaculum. *Surg Gynecol Obstet* 110:164, 1960.

Malek P, Kolc J, Belan A: Lymphography of the deep lymphatic system of the thigh. *Acta Radiol [Diagn] (Stockh)* 51:422, 1959.

Malek P, Belan A, Kocandrle VL: The superficial and deep lymphatic system of the lower extremities and their mutual relationship under physiological and pathological conditions. *J Cardiovasc Surg* 5:686, 1964.

Marcille M: Lymphatiques et ganglions ilio-pelviens. Thèse, Université de Paris, 1902; and *Tribune Medicale,* 1903, pp 165–170.

Mascagni: *Vasorum Lymphaticorum Corporis Humani. Historia et Iconographia.* Senis, P Carli, 1787.

McCort JJ, Robbins LL: Roentgen diagnosis of intrathoracic lymph node metastases in carcinoma of the lung. *Radiology* 57:339–359, 1951.

Negus D, Edwards JM, Kinmonth JB: Filling of cervical and mediastinal nodes from the thoracic duct and the physiology of Virchow's node. Studies by lymphography. *Br J Surg* 57:267, 1970.

Ngu VA: The lymphatic drainage of the leg and its implications. *Clin Radiol* 15:197, 1964.

Nicolesco J: Sur les vaisseaux et les ganglions lymphatiques regionaux de l'uretere. *Ann Anat Pathol Anat Norm Méd-Chir* 6:331–333, 1929a.

Nicolesco J: Sur les vaisseaux et les ganglions lymphatiques régionaux de l'uretère. (Segment inferieur.) *Ann Anat Pathol Anat Norm Méd-Chir* 6:847–848, 1929b.

Nicolesco J: Sur les lymphatiques du rein. *Ann Anat Pathol Anat Norm Méd-Chir* 7:503–508, 1930.

Nusbaum M, Baum S, Hedges RC, Blakemore WS: Roentgenographic and direct visualization of the thoracic duct. *Arch Surg* 88:105, 1964.

Pappenheimer JR, Renkin EM, Borrero LM: Filtration, diffusion and molecular sieving through peripheral capillary membranes. A contribution to the pore theory of capillary permeability. *Am J Physiol* 167:13, 1951.

Parker BR, Blank N, Castellino RA: Lymphographic appearance of benign conditions simulating lymphoma. *Radiology* 111:267, 1974a.

Parker BR, Castellino RA, Fuks ZY, Bagshaw MA: The role of lymphography in patients with ovarian cancer. *Cancer* 34:100, 1974b.

Pellé A, Pellé A: Lymphatiques de la trompe. *Ann Anat Pathol Anat Norm Med-Chir* 8:509–510, 605–610, 1931.

Poirier P: Lymphatiques des organes génitaux de la femme. *Prog Med* 10:491–493, 509–511, 527–529, 568–569, 590–592, 1889.

Poirier P, Cunéo B: Les lymphatiques. In Poirier P, Charpy A (eds): *Traité d'Anatomie Humaine.* Paris, 1902.

Pomerantz M, Herdt JRL, Rockoff SD, Ketcham AS: Evaluation of the functional anatomy of the thoracic duct by lymphangiography. *J Thorac Cardiovasc Surg* 46:568, 1963.

Poupardin: De quelques éléments du pedicle pulmonaire. *Thèse, Université de Paris,* 1909.

Reiffenstuhl G: *The Lymphatics of the Female Genital Organs,* translated by LD Ekvall. Philadelphia, JB Lippincott, 1964.

Rosenberg SA: Contribution of lymphangiography to our understanding of lymphoma. *Cancer Chemother Rep* 52:213, 1968.

Rosenberg SA, Kaplan HS: Clinical trials in the non-Hodgkin's lymphomata at Stanford University. Experimental design and preliminary results. *Br J Cancer* 31:456, 1975.

Rosenberger A, Abrams HL: The thoracic duct. In Abrams HL (ed): *Angiography,* ed 2. Boston, Little, Brown, 1971, vol II, p 1351.

Rouvière H: *Anatomy of the Human Lymphatic System,* translated by MJ Tobias. Ann Arbor, MI, Edwards Brothers, 1938.

Rusznyak I, Földi M, Szabo G: *Lymphatics and Lymph Circulation, Physiology and Pathology,* ed 2. New York, Pergamon Press, 1967.

Rüttimann A (ed): Panel discussion IV. In *Progress in Lymphology.* New York, Hafner, 1967.

Safer ML, Green JP, Crews QE Jr, Hill DR: Lymphangiographic accuracy in the staging of testicular tumors. *Cancer* 35:1603, 1975.

Sakata K: Ueber den Lymphapparat des Harnleiters. *Arch Anat Physiol Anat Abt* 1–12, 1903.

Shieber W: The demonstration of thoracic duct abnormalities by lymphangiography. *Angiology* 25:73, 1974.

Sledziewski H: Note sur les voies efférentes des ganglions lymphatiques infrapéricardiques. *C R Assoc Anat* 3e Cong Fed Internat et 25e Reunion, Amsterdam, 1930, pp 374–377.

Ssysganow AN: Ueber das Lymphsystem der Nieren und Nierenhuellen beim Menschen. *Z Anat Entwicklungsgesch* 91:770–831, 1930.

Stahr H: Bemerkungen über die Verbindungen der Lymphgefässe der Prostata mit denen der Blase. *Anat Anz* 16:27–29, 1899.

Stahr H: Der Lymphapparat der Nieren. *Arch Anat Physiol Anat Abt* 41–80, 1900

Stahr H: In Bergmann E, Bruns P, Mikulicz J (eds): *Handbuch der Praktisschen Chirurgie. 3. Chirurgie des Unterleibes.* Stuttgart, Enke, 1903, pp 320–321.

Steckel RJ, Cameron TP: Changes in lymph node size induced by lymphangiography. *Radiology* 87:753–755, 1966.

Steinert R: Untersuchungen über das Lymphsystem der Lunge. Zugleich ein Beitrag zur Frage der Topographie der bronchialen Lymphknoten. *Beitr Klin Tuberk* 68:497–510, 1928.

Sukiennikow: Topographische Anatomie der bronchialen und trachealen Lymphdrüsen. *Diss Berlin,* 1903; and *Klin Wochenschr* 40:316–318, 347, 369–372, 1903.

Takahashi M, Abrams HL: The accuracy of lymphangiographic diagnosis in malignant lymphoma. *Radiology* 89:448, 1967.

Tjernberg B: The histology of the lymph node. In Rüttimann A (ed): *Progress in Lymphology.* New York, Hafner, 1967, p 71.

Tondury G: Embryology and topographic anatomy of the lymphatic system. In Rüttimann A (ed): *Progress in Lymphology.* New York, Hafner, 1967, p 10.

Twito DI, Kennedy BJ: Treatment of testicular cancer. *Annu Rev Med* 26:235, 1975.

Viamonte M Jr, Altman D, Parks R, Blum E, Bevilacqua M, Recher L: Radiographic-pathologic correlation in the interpretation of lymphangioadenograms. *Radiology* 80:903, 1963.

Von Keiser D: Testicular tumors. In Rüttimann A (ed): *Progress in Lymphology.* New York, Hafner, 1967, p 190.

Wahlqvist L, Hulten L, Rosencrantz M: Normal lymphatic drainage of the testis studied by funicular lymphography. *Acta Chir Scand* 132:454, 1966.

Wallace S: Dynamics of normal and abnormal lymphatic systems as studied with contrast media. *Cancer Chemo-*

*ther Rep* 52:31, 1968.

Wallace S, Jackson L: Diagnostic criteria for lymphangiographic interpretation of malignant neoplasia. *Cancer Chemother Rep* 52:125, 1968.

Wallace S, Jackson L, Schaffer B, Gould J, Greening RR, Weiss A, Kramer S: Lymphangiograms: their diagnostic and therapeutic potential. *Radiology* 76:179, 1961.

Wallace S, Jackson L, Greening RR: Clinical applications of lymphangiography. *AJR* 88:97, 1962.

Wiljasalo M: Lymphographic differential diagnosis of neoplastic disease. *Acta Radiol Suppl* 247, 1965.

Wirth W, Frommhold H: Lymphography. The normal thoracic duct and its variations: comparative anatomical-lymphographic study. In Viamonte M, Koehler PR, Witte M, Witte C (eds): *Progress in Lymphology II.* Stuttgart, Georg Thieme Verlag, 1970, p 1860.

Yee L, Llewellyn GA, Williams PA, May IA, Dugan DJ: Scalene lymph node dissection. A study of 354 consecutive dissections. *Am J Surg* 118:596, 1969.

# 3

# *Radionuclide Lymphography*

**KENNETH A. McKUSICK, M.D.**

The lymphatic system may be imaged using radiolabeled agents by one of two fundamental techniques: by injecting a radiocolloid that will drain into the lymphatic chain, or intravenously injecting a radiopharmaceutical that has a predilection for tumor in lymph nodes. The most commonly used, intravenously injected tumor agent is gallium-67.

It is a curious historical sidelight that there were nearly two decades elapsed between observation and clinical application of radiolabeled gallium uptake by soft tissue tumors. Originally discovered in 1875 as a class III metal with a high boiling point, pharmacological data were needed in the late 1940s when gallium was considered as a coolant in nuclear-powered naval vessels. In 1952, Dudley and Marrer at Oak Ridge reported high concentrations of radiogallium (reactor-produced $^{72}$Ga) deposited in sites of osteogenic activity. They noted that the tissue distribution of cyclotron-produced (and carrier-free) $^{67}$Ga differed from $^{72}$Ga with less bone uptake, longer blood residence time, higher soft tissue uptake, and different excretion patterns. Shortly, nonosseous tumor accumulation of $^{67}$Ga was observed in a metastasis from the breast to lung and was thought to represent uptake in tumor calcium (years later, analysis of the tissue showed no excessive calcium). As so entertainingly recounted by Raymond Hayes, Ph.D.

(1978) in "The Medical Use of Gallium Radionuclides: A Brief History with Some Comments," the true cause for the $^{67}$Ga uptake in that patient was not appreciated, although the Oak Ridge investigators had recognized that gallium pharmacokinetics could be altered from that of a bone-seeking agent by making it carrier-free.

The advent of improved imaging instruments renewed interest in the use of $^{67}$Ga as a bone agent and in the effect of carrier gallium on $^{67}$Ga distribution. "To our amazement," wrote Hayes, recounting the Oak Ridge workers' experience, "in one of the first few studies with carrier-free $^{67}$Ga, we observed a completely unexpected, intense localization of $^{67}$Ga in the afflicted lymph nodes of a patient with Hodgkin's disease."

The clinical usefulness and the biological mechanisms of $^{67}$Ga uptake in Hodgkin's and non-Hodgkin's lymphoma have been extensively investigated over the past 15 yr. It has been shown that $^{67}$Ga uptake is related to tumor cell type and that detection is related to tumor size, location, dose, and instrument used. $^{67}$Ga incorporation into tumor cells may be facilitated by transferrin, and because of the similarity of gallium to the ferric ion, its transportation may be linked to lactoferrin and siderophore tumor activity, shown to be increased in some $^{67}$Ga-avid tumors (Hoffer, 1978).

## DIRECT TUMOR LOCALIZATION WITH $^{67}$Ga

In vivo radionuclide studies are performed most frequently for tumor detection in the brain, bones, and liver. Although there is a definite lack of nonspecificity, the studies are safe, noninvasive, painless, and relatively inexpensive with a high sensitivity. Gallium-67 citrate is a widely used tumor-avid radionuclide that is taken up most commonly by neoplasms arising from the liver, lung, or lymphatic system (Higasi and Nakayama, 1972; Langhammer et al., 1972; Littenberg et al., 1973a; Johnston et al., 1977; Andrews et al., 1978). $^{67}$Ga has been used for primary

detection of occult tumor, as a complementary method for tumor staging, for noninvasive reassessment of patients during the course of their disease, and for measurements of the response of tumor to therapy (Andrews and Edwards, 1975).

Clinical experience since 1969 has defined the role of gallium-67 in the management of lymphoma patients (Edwards and Hayes, 1969; Kay and McCready, 1972; Turner et al., 1972; Bakshi and Bender, 1973; Silberstein et al., 1974; Johnston et al., 1977; Anderson et al., 1983). Concurrently, there has been improvement in the prognosis of patients with lymphoma. This improvement may be attributed to improved diagnosis and therapy and to use of laparotomy and bone marrow biopsy, which have led to a better understanding of both the spread of this disease and a more useful histological classification (Lukes, 1972). Prognosis in lymphoma depends on both the extent of disease when first diagnosed and upon the histological type (Smithers, 1972; Jones et al., 1973; Hellman, 1974).

Hodgkin's lymphoma commonly presents as a swollen but painless peripheral node, although any organ can be involved (Rosenberg and Kaplan, 1966). The predominant histological feature of the tumor at the time of diagnosis (Lukes et al., 1966) determines its classification (Rye Conference Classification (Carbone, 1971)). The cell type may reflect the immunological state of the host and is characterized by an inverse relationship between the number of lymphocytes and Reed-Sternberg cells (Lukes, 1972). The disease is usually chronic when the Reed-Sternberg cells are infrequent and is more virulent when there is a paucity of lymphocytes (Lukes, 1972). Prognosis is also related to the histological characteristics in non-Hodgkin's lymphoma as classified by Rappaport (Jones et al., 1973). For example, nodular non-Hodgkin's lymphoma has a more favorable prognosis than diffuse lymphoma with a similar cell type.

It is probable that Hodgkin's lymphoma spreads in a nonrandom contiguous manner along lymphatic channels (Rosenberg and Kaplan, 1966). A pathway between the left lower cervical/supraclavicular nodes and the upper para-aortic nodes provides a mode of entry for tumor into the blood stream via the thoracic duct. Bone marrow and gastrointestinal tract involvement are more common in non-Hodgkin's lymphoma and are also more likely to be widespread on initial presentation than in Hodgkin's lymphoma. The extent of disease is a major determinant in the plan of therapy. The most widely used staging classification is the Ann Arbor Clinical Staging Classification (Carbone, 1971). In establishing the stage of disease, the intra-abdominal region is relatively inaccessible to clinical examination. Manual palpation may detect lymphadenopathy or organomegaly, but the mere presence of splenomegaly or hepatomegaly has variable significance.

Hellman (1974) has noted that radionuclide colloid scanning of the spleen is unreliable (false positive 20% and false negative 23%). The most significant findings on radiocolloid spleen scanning are splenomegaly (greater than 15 cm on the posterior view) and focal splenic defects (Miller et al., 1973). Using those strict criteria, the scan was only 43% sensitive in detection of intrasplenic tumor. Nonoperative clinical assessment of the liver in Hodgkin's disease is also unreliable (Rosenberg, 1972; Miller et al., 1973) but hepatic lymphomatous involvement is exceedingly rare without concomitant splenic involvement (Rosenberg, 1972; Ferguson et al., 1973). When lymphoma does extend below the diaphragm, the spleen has been shown to contain tumor in greater than 80% of patients (Rosenberg, 1972).

Extralymphatic abdominal disease may be detected by endoscopy, gastrointestinal contrast studies, arteriography, venography, and urography or $^{67}$Ga scintigraphy. Intra-abdominal lymph node tumor may be detected by bipedal lymphangiography, which does entail some risk of reaction to contrast agent and has a wide range in reported sensitivity from 54% (Alcorn et al., 1977) to 95% (Castellino and Marglin, 1981; Castellino, 1982; Clouse et al., 1985).

Because of the need for accurate staging, exploratory laparotomy may be undertaken if the patient's medical condition will allow it and if it might alter the plan of therapy. On the basis of findings at laparotomy, some modification of treatment was made in 40 of 114 patients in one series (Hellman, 1974). In addition, splenectomy permitted a reduction in the size of the radiation field, reducing radiation damage to the base of the left lung and the kidney, and in some patients splenectomy allowed more aggressive chemotherapy because of the increased total white cell and platelet count (Pannettiere and Coltman, 1973). There is some concern about serious postoperative infections in splenectomized children (Eraklis et al., 1967).

There would be a role for a noninvasive test that could accurately define the extent of lymphoma, especially if it could be performed repeatedly. Like $^{99m}$Tc bone scanning in breast and prostate cancer, $^{67}$Ga has been evaluated for staging lymphoma. After the initial report by Edwards and Hayes (1969) of the accumulation of gallium-67 citrate in cervical lymph nodes in a Hodgkin's disease patient, Langhammer et al. (1972) observed positive gallium-67 scans in 17 of 50 patients with non-Hodgkin's lymphoma. Gallium uptake was abnormal in 14 of 24 non-Hodgkin's lymphoma patients and 19 of 27 Hodgkin's patients in a follow-up study by Edwards and Hayes (1971). Kay and McCready (1972) studied 50 Hodgkin's lymphoma patients, and 76 of 96 sites of active tumor were gallium-positive; Turner et al. (1972) were able to identify 23 of 29 Hodgkin's sites using [67]Ga citrate.

Data from the Cooperative Group Study for Localization of Radiopharmaceuticals (Johnston et al., 1977; Andrews et al., 1978), based on observations from 668 Hodgkin's and non-Hodgkin's lymphoma studies (Table 3.1), indicate that gallium-67 scanning may be sensitive in the detection of *patients* with lymphoma, but it is less sensitive in the detection of individual histologically proven *sites* of disease. [67]Ga studies were positive in 88% and 76% of the untreated Hodgkin's and non-Hodgkin's patients, respectively, but identified fewer than 67% and 71% of proven sites in the same two diseases.

The incidence of false-positive [67]Ga uptake is 5% (Alder et al., 1975; Johnston et al., 1977; Andrews et al., 1978). Other than retained fecal activity, the most common reason for false-positive results is unsuspected infection. Numerous inflammations and infections have been noted to accumulate gallium (Lavender et al., 1971), and, in fact, gallium-67 citrate scanning is used in patients with sepsis or fever of undetermined origin (Littenberg et al., 1973b; Silva and Harvey, 1974; Teates and Hunter, 1975). Unusual pulmonary [67]Ga uptake may occur in patients who have undergone previous contrast lymphangiography secondary to contrast embolization; [67]Ga lung activity was present in 14 of 28 patients who had undergone contrast lymphangiography within 1 month prior to the radionuclide study (Lentle et al., 1974). Thymic uptake has been noted in a child with pneumonia (Johnson et al., 1978) and in 11–15% of children with no apparent disease (Donahue et al., 1981). [67]Ga thyroid uptake was increased in pediatric patients with acute lymphocytic leukemia and malignant lymphoma undergoing chemotherapy (Donahue et al., 1981).

TABLE 3.1.
SCANNING RESULTS IN UNTREATED TUMOR*

| | No. | Positive | Negative |
|---|---|---|---|
| | | (%) | (%) |
| Hodgkin's lymphoma | | | |
| Patients | 248 | 88 | 12 |
| Sites—all | 1308 | 56 | 44 |
| Sites—proven | 224 | 63 | 37 |
| Non-Hodgkin's lymphoma | | | |
| Patients | 296 | 76 | 24 |
| Sites—all | 1305 | 53 | 47 |
| Sites—proven | 396 | 55 | 45 |

*Based on Cooperative Study (Johnston et al., 1977; Andrews et al., 1978).

[67]Ga scanning appears to be most sensitive in the detection of lymphoma in the neck or chest, and least sensitive when the disease is in the abdomen or inguinal-femoral regions (McCready et al., 1972; Greenlaw et al., 1974; Alder et al., 1975; Andrews et al., 1978). In the Cooperative Group Study, the percentage of detected lesions in untreated Hodgkin's was the following: neck 80%, thorax 90%, abdomen 48%, inguinal-femoral 47%, and axilla 36% (Johnston et al., 1977).

[67]Ga accumulates in normal spleen and normal liver. Only if [67]Ga concentrates in a focal defect that is present on a [99m]Tc-sulfur colloid liver scan should it be considered abnormal and indicative of pathology (Suzuki et al., 1971; Lomas et al., 1972). If [67]Ga activity in the spleen is absent or considerably reduced, it is unlikely that the spleen contains lymphoma (Turner et al., 1972; Greenlaw et al., 1974; Alder et al., 1975).

[67]Ga concentration in lymphoma is related to the differentiation of the cell, to the ratio of viable to necrotic tumor (Edwards and Hayes, 1970), and to cell type. In the Cooperative Study, 89% of histiocytic lymphomas were [67]Ga-positive, whereas only 58% of sites of poorly differentiated lymphocytic lymphoma were gallium-positive. In Hodgkin's disease, the greatest number of positive [67]Ga sites were in patients with nodular sclerotic and lymphocyte-depleted disease, whereas in lymphocyte-predominant Hodgkin's only 42% of sites were [67]Ga-positive.

Direct intralymphatic injection of gallium-67 citrate has been attempted in the hope that [67]Ga would accumulate in any malignant lymph nodes in that lymphatic chain. No augmented lymph node uptake resulted, however, and the [67]Ga injected intralymphatically shortly became distributed the same as an intravenous injection (Edwards et al., 1971). Ito and co-workers (1982) found good correlation between positive [67]Ga uptake in metastatic lymph nodes after subcutaneous injection and cold lesions on lymphoscintigraphy with [99m]Tc-rhenium colloid.

The mechanisms by which [67]Ga accumulates in tumor are partially understood. Subcellular lysosomal localization of [67]Ga has been demonstrated in both murine lymphoma and Buffalo rat hepatomas (Hayes et al., 1971; Swartzendruber et al., 1971). There is rapid plasma membrane association of [67]Ga on lymphocytes in culture and an increase in uptake when those lymphocytes are stimulated with phytohemagglutinin (Merz et al., 1974). Membrane association was also observed on mouse fetal membrane and decidua (Otten et al., 1973). [67]Ga uptake is not necessarily related to proliferation by all cells. There is no increased uptake on proliferating intestinal crypt cells, which do accumulate labeled thymidine (Otten et al., 1973), nor is blood flow a major determinant of $^{67}$Ga concentration in tumor. $^{67}$Ga uptake was unrelated to blood flow in colon tumors but was in highest concentration at the invasive edge of the tumors (Nash et al., 1972).

In the periodic table, gallium is in group IIIA, which also includes aluminum and indium. Most salts of gallium are hydrolyzed in aqueous media and are insoluble at physiological pH. Citrate produces a soluble salt of gallium and therefore is usually used as the radiopharmaceutical, which is injected intravenously because it is absorbed poorly from the intestine. Approximately one-third of the injected dose combines with plasma proteins, especially transferrin, haptoglobin, and albumin in that order (Hartman and Hayes, 1969). The soluble remainder diffuses throughout the extracellular space or is excreted by the kidneys. Within the first 24 hr, 12% of the dose is excreted in the urine. Overall, 26% is renally excreted in the first week in patients with neoplasia (Nelson et al., 1972). An additional 10% is excreted via the gastrointestinal tract (Edwards and Hayes, 1970). Tissue distribution varies even in normal individuals. The highest initial uptake is in the liver and kidney (Table 3.2) but later shifts to the liver and spleen (Lavender et al., 1971). Splenic uptake is within phagocytic cells, whereas liver uptake is in both the RES Kupffer cells and hepatocytes (Nelson et al., 1972). The large intestine, kidney, liver, and spleen receive the highest radiation dose (Table 3.3). Whole body radiation dose is 0.26 rad/mCi; the critical organ is the large intestine 0.9 rad/mCi (MIRD/Dose Estimate, 1973).

In order to maximize the target-to-nontarget ratio, imaging is usually performed at least 48 hr after an intravenous injection of 50–100 μCi/kg of $^{67}$Ga citrate. Effective bowel cleansing may be necessary to remove excreted gallium. It is some-

**TABLE 3.2.**
**CONCENTRATION OF GA-67 IN VARIOUS TISSUES\*†**

| Tissue | % Administered Activity/Kg Mean |
|---|---|
| Spleen | 4.1 |
| Kidney cortex | 3.8 |
| Adrenal | 3.8 |
| Marrow | 3.6 |
| Liver | 2.8 |
| Bone | 2.6 |

\* Data from MIRD/Dose Estimate, 1973.

† Radioassay of autopsy tissue corrected for radioactive decay and normalized to a body weight of 70 kg.

**TABLE 3.3.**
**SUMMARY OF ESTIMATED ABSORBED DOSE PER UNIT OF ADMINISTERED ACTIVITY FROM A SINGLE INTRAVENOUS ADMINISTRATION OF RADIOACTIVE GA-67 CITRATE\***

| Tissue | Rads/mCi Injected |
|---|---|
| Gastrointestinal tract | |
| Upper large intestine | 0.56 |
| Lower large intestine | 0.90 |
| Gonads | |
| Ovaries | 0.28 |
| Testes | 0.24 |
| Kidneys | 0.41 |
| Liver | 0.46 |
| Marrow | 0.58 |
| Skeleton | 0.44 |
| Spleen | 0.53 |
| Total body | 0.26 |

\*Data from MIRD/Dose Estimate, 1973.

**TABLE 3.4.**
**PHYSICAL CHARACTERISTICS OF $^{67}$GA\***

| | | |
|---|---|---|
| Physical half-life | 7.80 hr | |
| Decay constant | 0.00885 hr$^{-1}$ | |
| Mode of decay | Electron capture | |
| Equilibrium dose constant for nonpenetrating radiation (g-rad/μCi-hr) | 0.0873 | |
| | $E_i$ (MeV) | $n_i$ |
| Principal photons: | 0.0933 | 0.380 |
| $E_i$, energy | 0.1845 | 0.239 |
| $n_i$, mean number/disintegration† | 0.3002 | 0.161 |
| | 0.3936 | 0.043 |

\*Data from MIRD/Dose Estimate, 1973.

† Photons whose mean number per disintegration is 0.05 or greater.

times necessary for the patient to receive additional cathartics and return an additional day for repeated imaging. After the first 48 hr following injection, there is minimal additional intestinal excretion. Blood clearance of gallium and tumor uptake may be accelerated by saturation of serum iron binding sites. Imaging earlier than 72 hr may be possible after an intramuscular injection of iron, which results in lower soft tissue and colonic background activity (Sephton and Martin, 1980; Smith and Dendy, 1981). It is thought that the effect is secondary to saturation of plasma transferrin with iron, enhancing tumor uptake and lesion to background ratios.

The physical characteristics of $^{67}$Ga are listed in Table 3.4. The 184-keV and 300-keV photopeaks may be utilized for imaging. The procedure requires 60–90 min to complete.

It is imperative that any physician, in interpreting a [67]Ga scan, become thoroughly familiar with the normal gallium scan and be aware of the benign processes that may concentrate the radiopharmaceutical. There is usually definition of the bony structures of the head, spine, and pelvis with accentuation of activity in the region of the epiphyses, especially in children (Larson et al., 1973). Although long bones are not usually apparent, regions of osteoblastic activity secondary to fracture, infection, or tumor and areas of very active bone marrow will concentrate the radiopharmaceutical. In the face, some gallium activity is seen in the region of the nose, lacrimal glands, and salivary glands. Parotid gland uptake may increase after radiation therapy to the neck and may lead to misinterpretation (Kashima et al., 1974). Sternal activity can be pronounced but may be separated from abnormal mediastinal concentration by utilizing a lateral projection. The numerous benign processes within the lung that may concentrate gallium include pneumoconiosis, pneumonia, and sarcoidosis (McKusick et al., 1973; Heshiki et al., 1974; Kinoshita et al., 1974; Siemsen et al., 1974). Breast tissue under the stimulation of cyclic estrogen or progestational agents or during lactation or menarche may show a marked concentration (Fogh, 1971; Larson and Schall, 1971). The liver and spleen normally accumulate gallium in a pattern similar to that seen on a [99m]Tc-sulfur colloid scan. During the first 24 hr, the kidneys may be apparent. Renal activity at 48 hr or later suggests the presence of pathology such as pyelonephritis, urinary obstruction, or tumor. Retained fecal radioactivity is often visible at 48 hr. Normally the fecal activity will decrease with time and change position within the abdomen, whereas a fixed concentration in pathological tissue will become more apparent with the passage of time. Re-examination of the patient for as long as a week may be necessary.

What is the role of [67]Ga in the management of patients with lymphomas? The variable sensitivity for detection of sites of disease precludes its use as a single test for staging. Negative findings at any site have less significance than positive uptake. It is unlikely that a patient's staging will be changed by [67]Ga imaging. Only 1 of 122 non-Hodgkin's lymphoma patients was upgraded by [67]Ga (Longo et al., 1980). However, initial therapy may be altered by discovery of unsuspected sites, especially in the lung, upper mediastinum, or bone (King et al., 1980). Unsuspected tumor was found in 23% of non-Hodgkin's and 26% of Hodgkin's sites in the Cooperative Study.

[67]Ga-positive sites of tumor have been shown to revert to a [67]Ga-negative state after therapy (Edwards and Hayes, 1970; Higasi and Nakayama, 1972; Bakshi and Bender, 1973; Henkin et al., 1974; Andrews and Edwards, 1975). Thus, [67]Ga can be used as one marker of response to therapy. In patients with known lymphoma who have undergone treatment, [67]Ga provides a relatively simple and noninvasive assessment of new symptoms that may arise in relatively inaccessible areas. For example, gallium scanning detected active mediastinal disease in six reported patients whose chest radiography changes were thought to have been secondary to previous radiation therapy (Kay and McCready, 1972).

[67]Ga has been useful as an adjunct to lymphangiography, computed tomography (CT), and ultrasound in treated patients. The Cooperative Group found lymphangiography to be somewhat more accurate than [67]Ga at proven sites in the pelvis and abdomen, but it also found a significant incidence of [67]Ga true-positive lesions where lymphangiography was negative. In a restaging study, Herman and Jones (1978) found that [67]Ga chest radiography and lymphangiography were the most helpful procedures for detection of active residual disease in 13% of 72 patients thought to be disease-free. In a separate study of non-Hodgkin's lymphoma, Fuks and co-workers (1982) compared the efficacy and accuracy of clinical examination, ultrasound, CT, lymphangiography, and [67]Ga for restaging. They found by laparotomy that lymphography was 17% and [67]Ga 50% accurate and recommended second-look operations for accurate appraisal of response to therapy. Because of the known false-negative rates in [67]Ga imaging, Anderson and co-workers (1983) advocate the use of higher doses in patients with proven disease. Using 7–10 mCi of [67]Ga citrate and careful imaging technique incorporating a triple-peak Anger camera, they studied 51 patients with non-Hodgkin's and 21 patients with Hodgkin's lymphoma. Overall, accuracy was 96% by site with a specificity of 90%. The data were insufficient to compare gallium to lymphangiography, but there was sufficient information to conclude that "a gallium scan is usually correct in differentiating active disease in the abdomen from bulky nodal fibrosis, that latter frequently delineated on computed tomographic scanning or ultrasound."

At the current time, [67]Ga imaging remains a useful test in the care of patients with lymphoma because of the correlation between a positive site and active disease. With the best imaging techniques, gallium should be considered in these patients for detection of unsuspected sites of tumor, for investigation of pain or fever, and for determining the significance of abnormal findings found on chest radiograph, ultrasound scan, CT scan, or lymphangiogram.

## LYMPHOSCINTIGRAPHY

Shortly after World War II, several investigators showed that radiocolloids (such as gold-198) concentrated in normally functioning reticuloendothelial cells after parenteral administration of the radiopharmaceutical and especially in regional lymph nodes after a subcutaneous injection (Hahn and Sheppard, 1946; Sheppard et al., 1947; Walker, 1950). Colloidal gold-198 was investigated as a possible radiotherapeutic agent (Hahn and Carothers, 1951, 1953; Sherman and Ter-Pogossian, 1953), but this approach was abandoned because the concentration of radionuclide was too often the highest in normal nodes and the lowest in nodes most heavily involved with tumor (Seaman and Powers, 1955).

As radiogold was being investigated for therapy, it became obvious that diagnostic information was being derived from the distribution patterns of radioactivity in normal versus abnormal lymph nodes. It was fortuitous that gold-198 also emits a 412-keV peak photon that can be detected easily by external probes, and it was a relatively simple matter to obtain useful images of the distribution of radioactivity in lymph nodes.

Colloidal gold-198, as a therapeutic agent, was found useful for the control of pleural and peritoneal effusions resulting from malignant tumors. After intraperitoneal administration of the agent for the treatment of malignant ascites, accumulations of radiogold were noted in the mediastinum of some patients, indicating passage of colloid from the abdominal cavity to the lymph nodes in the chest (Muller, 1956). This finding indicated another manner in which radiocolloid could be used diagnostically.

Diagnostic radionuclide lymphoscintigraphy using a colloid gold-198 was a relatively simple procedure to perform, but it had significant limitations stemming from the use of gold-198. This radionuclide has to be restricted in amount because of the high radiation dose that can result from beta radiation. As a consequence, the low photon flux and poor statistics made production of quality images difficult.

It was logical that several $^{99m}$Tc-radiocolloids were subsequently evaluated for lymphoscintigraphy. The current radiocolloid of choice is $^{99m}$Tc-antimony sulfide, which has a size (4–50 nm) and surface characteristics favorable for good clearance after an interstitial injection. A resurgence of interest in radionuclide interstitial lymphoscintigraphy has occurred since Ege (1976, 1977) reported on her extensive experience with internal mammary lymphoscintigraphy using $^{99m}$Tc-antimony sulfide injected into the posterior sheath of the rectus muscle in patients with carcinoma of the breast.

After an intravenous injection of $^{99m}$Tc-antimony sulfide, there is rapid clearance from the blood and uptake in the reticuloendothelial system of the liver, spleen, bone marrow, and lung. Upon injection into interstitial tissue (subcutaneous, intradermal, muscular), there is slower clearance from the site, with flow into the local lymphatic channels and passive retention in the sinusoids of the lymph nodes. The radiocolloid that does not go directly through the lymph node will undergo phagocytosis by the lymph node reticuloendothelial cells (Ege, 1982a, b). The dynamics of clearance from the interstitium, pathways of clearance, rate of accumulation, and discharge from lymph nodes allow quantitative and anatomic assessment of the lymphatic system.

Is lymphoscintigraphy just an interesting research tool, or is it essential to good medical practice today? The answer is not unequivocal either way. Nevertheless, the work of the past several decades with both gold-198 and $^{99m}$Tc-radiocolloids has been enlightening and has afforded images of some lymphatic systems in the extremities, chest, and pelvis not easily examined otherwise. Lymphoscintigraphy has furthered our understanding of the extent of disease in the lymphatic system and of its role in effective management of patients with carcinoma. It may be that this has been a prelude to development of interstitial and intralymphatic injections of receptor-specific substances for detection of micrometastatic lymph node disease or for therapy. At the very least, the techniques used for radiocolloid lymphoscintigraphy permit improved understanding of lymphatic system function.

Radiocolloid can be injected intratumor, intradigital, subcostal, subareolar, intradermal, subcutaneous, or intramuscular. Depending upon the size of the particle and the tissue in which it is injected, there is variable clearance from the injection site into the regional lymphatic channels. The path taken by the radiocolloid has been used to define the ports of radiotherapy in carcinoma of the breast (Siddon et al., 1982) and to plan surgery in patients with malignant melanoma (Bennett and Lago, 1983). Obstructed or replaced lymph nodes will not accumulate interstitially injected radiocolloid; there may be increased or no apparent abnormal uptake in nodes with micrometastases (Matsuo, 1974; Peyton et al., 1981; Bennett and Lago, 1983). Since unilaterally decreased or absent nodal uptake highly suggests tumor involvement in patients with carcinoma of the breast, pelvis, or testicles, lymphoscintigraphy can be used to gauge the extent of disease in internal mammary nodes as well as sacral, pelvic, hypogastric and internal iliac chains not normally identified on contrast lymphangiography. Interstitial lymphoscintigraphy appears to be highly reproducible. Ege (1977) found that injection of $^{99m}$Tc-antimony sulfide into the posterior rectus sheath offered consistent reproducibility of the internal mammary lymphatic structures in 96% of injections.

Consistency of imaging depends somewhat upon techniques of injection and imaging, but primarily it depends upon the preparation of the radiocolloid itself.

## $^{99m}$Tc-RADIOLABELED COMPOUNDS FOR INTERSTITIAL LYMPHOSCINTIGRAPHY

Because of the short half-life of $^{99m}$Tc (6.1 hr), an interstitially injected $^{99m}$Tc-radiocolloid must pass into the lymphatic channels with speed sufficient to permit imaging within 3–6 hr. The kinetics of radiocolloid particles was found to be strongly dependent upon particle size (Bergquist et al., 1983). Particles with diameters of less than 4–5 nm were exchanged through blood capillaries, whereas particles were found to remain in place at the interstitial site if they were greater than several hundredths of a nanometer. Particles in the 10–50 nm range were readily passed into the lymphatic capillaries. Bergquist and co-workers characterized the several $^{99m}$Tc-radiocolloids available from manufacturers and found that the outflow of small particle colloids around 40 nm was 20% by 5 hr, whereas the larger particle colloids (greater than 100 nm) cleared less than 10% by 5 hr. Lymph node uptake of the larger particles was a third that of the particles in the 10–40 nm range.

The same group (Strand and Persson, 1979) had compared parasternal nodal uptake after interstitial injections of $^{198}$Au-colloid, $^{99m}$Tc-antimony sulfide colloid, $^{99m}$Tc-tin colloid, $^{99m}$Tc-phytate and $^{99m}$Tc-sulfur colloid. Again the most rapid uptake was with the smaller particles in the range of 5–15 nm and included the $^{198}$Au and $^{99m}$Tc-antimony sulfide. A limited dual study in patients has been performed, demonstrating more nodes and offering better delineation of the internal mammary lymphatic chains. There is a more certain uptake in supraclavicular nodes after posterior rectus sheath injection using $^{99m}$Tc-antimony sulfide than with $^{99m}$Tc-phytate (Ege and Warbick, 1979; Kaplan et al., 1979).

Another compound, $^{99m}$Tc-dextran, has a molecular weight of 110,000 and has been shown to have rapid clearance and good lymph node uptake in experimental animals (Henze et al., 1982). This compound cleared from the interstitial space with a half-life of 30 min compared to a reported clearance of $^{99m}$Tc-antimony sulfide of 20.5 hr by Bergquist and co-workers (1983). Dextran is water soluble and will reflect lymphatic flow, although the reason for its uptake in lymph nodes is not known. In view of its rapid clearance after interstitial injection, this agent could permit more physiological assessment of lymphatic flow than is obtainable with intralymphatic injection of contrast agents and may play a role in the assessment of patients with lymphedema.

$^{99m}$Tc-antimony sulfide colloid remains an investigational phase III drug (Cadema Medical Products, Inc.). It is the agent most widely used for lymphoscintigraphy at this time in North America. The absorbed dose with $^{99m}$Tc-antimony sulfide is considerably less to the site of injection than that from gold-198 colloid. The dose to the injection site is 50–100 rad/$\mu$Ci with gold-198 (Strand and Persson, 1979), whereas Bronskill (1983) calculated the absorbed dose at the injection site to be 45.6 rad to the center of the rectus sheath and 21 rad to individual internal mammary lymph nodes using 450 $\mu$Ci of $^{99m}$Tc-antimony sulfide. In patients with malignant melanomas (Bergquist et al., 1982), the dose to the injection site has been calculated to be 30–35 rad/mCi. Although an apparently high dose to the injection site is delivered by these agents, the absorbed dose is considerably less than that from a fractionated radiotherapy dose and well within the tolerance dose of skin. A higher skin radiation dose may occur after inadvertent extravasation of routinely administered radionuclide liver or bone agents. The whole body burden from $^{99m}$Tc-antimony sulfide is calculated to be 10 mrem/Ci.

# CLINICAL APPLICATION

## Breast

Parasternal lymphoscintigraphy using gold-198 was introduced in 1966 (Schenk et al., 1966) as a test for imaging the internal mammary lymphatic system. Following up on this work, Ege (1976) first reported on the uptake and patterns of distribution of $^{99m}$Tc-antimony sulfide in internal mammary chain in 848 patients.

Two lymphatic systems that are clinically important to the management of patients with breast carcinoma can be examined by interstitial lymphoscintigraphy: the internal mammary and axillary. Lymphoscintigraphy has been used to detect previously unsuspected tumor involvement of lymph nodes, to plan the ports for radiation therapy (Dufresne et al., 1980), and to assess postoperative lymphedema (W. D. Kaplan, S. A. Slavin, H. D. Royal, R. Gelman, S. M. Laffin, J. A. Markisz, and I. C. Henderson, personal communication, 1984). The test may be performed repeatedly and without admitting the patient to the hospital.

Internal mammary scintigraphy as performed by Ege involves injection of 0.3 ml of 500 $\mu$Ci of $^{99m}$Tc-antimony sulfide into the posterior rectus sheath at the insertion of the diaphragm in the subcostal site. The point of injection is 3 cm inferior to the xiphoid process and medial to the midclavicular line. If the needle pierces the rectus sheath, an intraperitoneal injection may occur and result in inadequate uptake of $^{99m}$Tc-antimony sulfide in the parasternal chain. Similarly, a superficial injection may demonstrate axillary but not internal mammary chains. The test should not be performed within 3 weeks after breast surgery because postsurgical debris blocking the lymphatic chains would invalidate the results.

In order to allow sufficient time to elapse for transit of the radiocolloid from the injection site to the internal mammary chains, imaging is performed with a large-field-of-view camera 3 hr after injection, and 100,000 count images of the chest are usually obtained with the injection site excluded. The use of cobalt-57 markers of the supraclavicular notch and midline of the sternum and lateral views (Dufresne et al., 1980) is necessary for more precise localization and possible measurements of the depths and positions of the nodes identified. Initially, a single injection is performed on the same side as the carcinoma of the breast to detect any crossover of the parasternal lymphatic system. Crossover and communication between the parasternal and the axillary or superficial nodal groups is common and may have significance because of the possibility of spread to the contralateral nodes or chest. This was observed in 17% of one series (Dionne et al., 1983). The mean number of nodes identified is 7.8. Since there is considerable variation in the number and position of the internal mammary nodes and since normal crossover can occur at the subxiphoid, submanubrial, or substernal locations, injections in the contralateral side are necessary for complete internal lymphoscintigraphy. At least one node must be seen to be certain that the injection was properly placed, and if the diaphragmatic nodes are not seen, inadequate injection technique is assumed and no conclusions can be made about possible obstruction to the internal mammary system.

Nonvisualization of the proximal internal mammary chain may occur in normal individuals with congenital unilateral (12%) or fused substernal internal mammary systems. However, unilateral complete absence or nonvisualization of nodes proximal to the diaphragmatic node may indicate tumor involvement.

The first change that occurs in a node harboring metastasis is not known, but if the tumor expands in a node, there is decreased radiocolloid uptake (Ege, 1983). Changes in uptake indicating increasing certainty of tumor involvement are "relatively increased node uptake" (least likely), "decreased radiocolloid uptake," "interruption in sequence of lymphatics," "no hepatic uptake or other evidence of lymphatic patency," "alternate pathways of flow," and "localized radiocolloid blush" (Ege, 1983). Gold-198 colloid internal mammary scintigraphy predicted the absence of tumor in 10% and the presence of tumor in 90% of patients who underwent exploration and in whom a histological examination of the specimens was obtainable (Matsuo, 1974).

Does the internal mammary lymphoscintigram predict outcome? When internal mammary lymphoscintigraphy was normal, there was a 34% incidence of recurrence, whereas an abnormal lymphoscintigram was associated with 67%

recurrence in 243 patients (Ege and Clark, 1980). Dionne and co-workers (1983) advocate internal mammary lymphoscintigraphy for staging breast carcinoma. They emphasize that it is commonly thought that only primary breast tumors located in the medial portion of the breast tend to spread to the internal mammary chain, and yet they found that internal mammary lymphoscintigraphic involvement was present in 48% of patients who had superior and inferior quadrant disease, 57% if the disease was in the outer quadrant, and 33% if it was central. Thus, metastases to the internal mammary lymphatic system occur from anywhere in the breast. Internal mammary metastases may be present even if the axillary lymph nodes are negative. Both Dionne et al. (1983) and Ege (1977) reported that 17–18% of internal mammary lymphoscintigrams were abnormal in separate populations of breast carcinoma patients who had histologically negative axilla.

Axillary lymph nodes have been studied after subcutaneous injection of a radiocolloid in the medial surface of the arm and after interdigital or periareolar injections (Agwunobi and Boak, 1978; Black et al., 1980, 1981; Peyton et al., 1981). All investigators concluded that on the basis of histological studies lymphoscintigraphy could not rule out the presence of metastatic carcinoma in lymph nodes. Nonetheless, they suggested that axillary lymphoscintigraphy might be useful in postoperative management of patients who had undergone radical mastectomy and axillary resection. In another study, no lymphatic flow was evident in only 36% of patients; the appearance of flow in the remaining patients suggested incomplete resection and was a forewarning of postoperative lymphedema (Bourgeois et al., 1983).

Quantitative and qualitative studies of upper extremity lymphedema may be performed following interstitial injection of radiocolloid (W. D. Kaplan, S. A. Slavin, H. D. Royal, R. Gelman, S. M. Laffin, J. A. Markisz, and I. C. Henderson, personal communication, 1984). Using injections in interdigital subcutaneous space (two between the second and third digits) and intradermal injection on the ulnar styloid process, normal flow (that is no superficial channels and prompt axillary uptake) was differentiated from abnormal flow in which collateral and superficial channels were visible and radial and ulnar lymphatic uptake was poor. Quantitative objective measurements were used to assess lymphatic channels in patients considered for surgical anastomosis for the lymphedema, and the results were used to locate the lymphatic channels.

Interstitial lymphoscintigraphy is used as a noninvasive technique for localizing the internal mammary chains in carcinomas of breast patients for whom radiation therapy is planned (Ege, 1976; Rose et al., 1979; Dufresne et al., 1980; Siddon et al., 1982; Collier et al., 1983). To ensure adequate therapy using tangential or en face radiation beams, precise information about location and depth of nodes is helpful. Generally, the internal mammary nodes lie in the intercostal spaces lateral to the sternum. The variability of position and depth, the common findings of crossover, and the absence of tumor involvement have been shown (Ege, 1976, 1977; Rose et al., 1979; Collier et al., 1983; Dionne et al., 1983). CT, which can detect enlarged lymph nodes, is also being used to plan radiation therapy. Meyer and Munzenrider (1981) reported alteration of radiation therapy protocols in 7 of 18 patients with locally recurrent disease based on the detection of enlarged (over 6 mm) parasternal nodes suspected of containing tumor, which otherwise would not have been adequately treated. Poor correlation between CT and lymphoscintigraphy was found in 20 patients with stage I or II carcinoma of the breast in whom CT identified only 29% of functionally normal nodes as seen on $^{99m}$Tc-antimony sulfide examinations (Collier et al., 1983). Internal mammary lymphoscintigraphy correlated to CT in 20% of 243 possibly normal nodes. CT could not reliably distinguish between lymph nodes and vessels on the posterior surface of the anterior chest wall, and contrast did not increase CT specificity for vessels less than 2 mm in size. Lymphoscintigraphy resulted in modification of radiation therapy in 60% of the patients. Because nodes replaced by tumor will not take up $^{99m}$Tc-antimony sulfide, CT plays a complementary role by identifying enlarged nodes, which are probable sites of tumor involvement. At the same time lymphoscintigraphy was found to be a more specific test for location of functioning lymphatic systems.

External markers using cobalt-57 placed on the midline of the sternum provide points of reference so that one may calculate the lateral excursion and depth of functioning nodes seen on the lymphoscintigram (Rose et al., 1979; Dufresne et al., 1980). In 68 patients, an average of 8 nodes were found per patient, and an average of 4.3 lymph nodes were lateralized using both anterior and lateral views (some of the nodes were subxiphoid and beyond the fifth intercostal space, and others could not be seen on the lateral view). The mean distance of the nodes from the anterior surface of the sternum was 2.4 cm lateral (a range of 0–4.7 cm) and 1.8 cm deep (0.3–5.3 cm). Using a conventional radiation portal of 3 cm lateral to the midline and 3 cm deep, 29 of the 230 nodes would have been missed. Assuming that for effective radiation therapy the node must lie within 3 mm of the 100% isodense line, 6 of 15 of their patients were judged retrospectively to have had inadequate therapy; in 53 consecutive prospective therapy patients, 16 had a 1–3 cm increase in the tangential spread between medial and lateral beams and 15 more patients had a decrease in the volume of irradiated tissue.

Thus, internal mammary lymphoscintigraphy offers increased certainty that the internal mammary lymphatic chain is within the effective field of radiation therapy (as opposed to using an arbitrary reference) and also may lead to reduction in radiation of contiguous normal lung and heart tissue. Lymphoscintigraphic measurements of the distance of the nodes deep to the sternum may be made using tomographic scintigraphic techniques such as with a slant hole collimator or emission CT (Siddon et al., 1982). By imaging the patient in a manner similar to the position planned for radiation therapy, alignment of the three-dimensional lymphoscintigraphic data to the tangential field radiographs during radiotherapy simulation may be done to ensure an even more effective radiation dose to the lymph nodes.

## Malignant Melanoma

Spread of malignant melanoma occurs early by lymphatic channels to regional lymph groups. Lymphatic drainage of the skin, however, becomes less certain the more central the lesion on the body. Since an en bloc resection and lymphadenectomy are considered as means for surgical cure, knowing which nodal groups are at risk is imperative. It has been recognized that there are variable pathways of damage when melanoma is in the scalp or near the watershed area in the midline or Sappy's line (Sugarbaker and McBride, 1976). Sappy's line, a region 5 cm wide extending from above the umbilicus to the L2 vertebra, was described in the 19th century as an area drained by lymphatic channels to both the axilla and inguinal nodal systems (Sappy, 1874). Lymphoscintigraphic techniques may be used to ascertain which nodal groups are at most risk to harbor metastatic tumor from cutaneous melanoma, assuming the injection around the lesion will accurately describe the lymphatic pathways.

Similar to internal mammary lymphoscintig-

raphy, cutaneous lymphoscintigraphy should not be performed in recently operated patients because of the probability of blocked lymphatic channels or reactive lymph nodes. Preferably the study should be performed prior to initial removal of the lesion, although that opportunity is uncommon in our experience. Three weeks appears to be an adequate interval for performance of internal mammary lymphoscintigraphy after surgery (Ege, 1977), and the same guidelines are appropriate in cutaneous lymphoscintigraphy. One millicurie of $^{99m}$Tc-antimony sulfide is injected intradermally in two proximal sites near the edge of the lesion if it is on an extremity and surrounding the lesion in four sites if it is a truncal or scalp lesion (Sullivan et al., 1981). Immediate images of the injection site frequently demonstrate lymphatic channels, but images must be taken at 2–4 hr to detect regional lymph nodes reliably. To ensure that as wide an area as possible is imaged, a large-field-of-view camera is recommended. Specifically, each inguinal, axillary, and supraclavicular region bilaterally must be imaged. We have found that timed (10-min) images collected on a computer are preferable to preset count analog data.

Published data on lymphoscintigraphy in malignant melanoma patients are similar whether the radiopharmaceutical is $^{99m}$Tc-sulfur colloid (Meyer et al., 1979), gold-198 colloid (Robinson et al., 1977; Fee et al., 1978; Bennett and Lago, 1983), or $^{99m}$Tc-antimony sulfide (Sullivan et al., 1981; Munz et al., 1982a). All found that lymphatic drainage does not follow classical pathways. In truncal lesions, the lymphatics drained to more than one regional system in 11 of 28 patients examined after injection of $^{99m}$Tc-antimony sulfide (Munz et al., 1982a). These investigators also found that 96% of patients with truncal melanoma studied preoperatively showed uptake in one or both axilla either solely or in combination with inguinal, supraclavicular, posterior cervical, or parasternal nodes (Munz et al., 1982b). Sullivan and co-workers (1981) similarly found that in 11 of 11 truncal lesions there was uptake in one or both axilla including three lesions that were originally at Sappy's line. Generally, extremity lesions drain to the appropriate proximal lymphatic nodes. Drainage from the scalp lesions is variable, and in Sullivan's experience (1981) two of the three patients had drainage to one posterior from the cervical group and the other had bilateral drainage to both posterior triangles.

The drainage paths shown by lymphoscintigraphy predicted location of metastases. In 32 patients with stage I deeply penetrating melanoma followed for 15–30 months, 9 of 27 had metastatic nodal disease and all 9 had had radiocolloid uptake in the same region (Fee et al., 1978). Although it is logical to predict that lymphatic metastatic disease will occur in those nodal groups shown to drain a cutaneous lesion, no other long term study has been done to confirm this likelihood.

No conclusion can be drawn from uptake in nodes as to the presence or absence of tumor (Boak and Agwunobi, 1978; Fee et al., 1978; Sullivan et al., 1981). There was "no statistically significant correlation between the presence or absence of $^{99m}$Tc activity and the presence or absence of tumor" (Sullivan et al., 1981). Nodes that were replaced by tumor were cold.

Published data support the use of cutaneous lymphoscintigraphy in the management of patients with malignant melanoma if it is used as a guide to the surgeon contemplating regional lymphadenectomy. Any regional nodal system shown to have lymphatic channels from the original cutaneous lesions should be carefully followed subsequently for clinical evidence of metastatic disease.

## Ileopelvic Lymphoscintigraphy

Malignancies arising in the pelvis may metastasize to internal, external, and common iliac lymphatic channels. Unfortunately, contrast bipedal lymphangiography does not reliably fill the internal iliac node systems. Since these are often involved in lymphatic spread of pelvic tumor, noninvasive means to stage disease accurately would be useful. Contrast lymphangiography has been shown to be inaccurate for this purpose in carcinoma of the bladder, prostate, and cervix (Kolbenstvedt, 1975; Catalona and Scott, 1978). In part, this is because those tumors frequently spread to the internal iliac lymphatic group. Ultrasound and CT examinations suffer from being unable to separate tumor from nontumor nodal enlargement and are limited in resolution of small nodes and micrometastatic disease in those nodes (Levine et al., 1981).

The optimal site for injection of radiocolloid for ileopelvic lymphoscintigraphy appears to be the ischiorectal fossa via para-anal injections (Ege and Cummings, 1980). This may be augmented by bipedal radiocolloid injections in order to fill the distal lymphatic chains (Ege, 1982a, b). Using 1 mCi of $^{99m}$Tc-antimony sulfide each, in volumes of 0.2 ml, bilateral para-anal injections were made with the unanesthetized patient in the lithotomy position. Using a 22-gauge needle, 1.5 inches long, the radiolabel was

deposited through the levator muscles. Imaging was obtained 3 hr later using preset timed images (9 min) or preset count images (100,000 counts) (Kaplan, 1983). Normal findings are symmetrical and uniform delineation of the common iliac and para-aortic nodal systems to the level of the kidneys; consistent with obstruction of a lymphatic channel or tumor involvement of a node is the finding of asymmetric uptake, mottled uptake, or absent uptake. Unfortunately, tumor involvement of a node may be characterized by normal, absent, mottled, or even increased radiocolloid uptake (Whitmore et al., 1980; Iverson and Aas, 1982; Kaplan, 1983). Thus, the accuracy for nodal metastatic detection in individual nodes is low. Histological examination of pelvic nodes in 14 patients showed a sensitivity of 70% and a specificity of 48% for ileopelvic lymphoscintigraphy (Ege, 1982a, b). In another series of 15 patients with nonseminomatous testicular carcinoma, lymphoscintigraphy was 89% sensitive and 83% specific. These patients had retroperitoneal resection, and the tumor tended to spread to the para-aortic and preaortic nodes, which were systems more easily examined by contrast lymphography. Because of the level of nodal involvement, however, variable filling by bipedal contrast lymphography may adversely affect its accuracy. Limited clinical experience in patients with carcinoma of the prostate (Gardiner et al., 1979; Stone et al., 1979; Whitmore et al., 1980) indicates that the technique, lymphoscintigraphy, lacks precision for use in staging patients with that carcinoma.

Since ovarian carcinoma can metastasize by a transperitoneal route and lead to involvement of diaphragmatic lymphatics, internal mammary lymphoscintigraphy has been used as a prognostic marker. Performing internal mammary lymphoscintigraphy in 364 patients postoperatively, one group found that the test did not predict probability of relapse adequately (Dembro et al., 1982). Sensitivity was 51% and specificity was 71% compared to clinical data. A novel approach was taken by another group (Kaplan et al., 1981) based on the assumption that intraperitoneally injected particulates would migrate into the internal mammary lymphatic chains unless there were obstruction of the diaphragmatic lymphatics. Using a small injection of $^{99m}$Tc-labeled autologous red cells, data were collected in 15 patients with ovarian carcinoma in whom laparoscopic peritoneal examinations were done. The 5 patients with diaphragmatic metastases had no uptake in the internal mammary lymphatic chains following instillation of the injected red cells, and 9 of the 10 patients without diaphragmatic tumor had uptake in the internal mammary lymphatics. They concluded that intraperitoneal $^{99m}$Tc red cell internal mammary lymphoscintigraphy may play a role in the management of patients with ovarian carcinoma.

## Miscellaneous Applications

Interstitially injected radiocolloids are physiologically cleared into regional lymphatic chains; using appropriate imaging techniques, investigation of normal lymphatic dynamics, such as tissue of the heart and lungs, has been possible. The lymphoscintigraphic pattern of the lymphatics of the head and neck was studied in 45 patients after submucous injection in the mouth (Thommesen et al., 1981). No symmetry was found, there was marked variation in nodal uptake, and no typical pattern of drainage could be described to use as a diagnostic baseline. In patients with squamous cell carcinoma of the oral cavity, decreased flow to the ipsilateral lymph nodes after paratumor $^{99m}$Tc-sulfur colloid injection correctly identified metastases in a smaller number of patients (Parell et al., 1981). Lymphatic drainage from the larynx was studied by injection of radiocolloid in 36 patients (Jackson et al., 1981). Twenty-three of the 36 had evidence of regional lymphatic drainage, and it was noted that mediastinal and axillary nodal uptake was found in none. Lymphoscintigraphic assessment of mediastinal drainage was assessed in nine patients with esophageal carcinoma in whom lymphatic nodes were then dissected at surgery and examined histologically (Terui et al., 1982). Twenty-six of 106 examined nodes could be detected on imaging; among the visualized nodes 35% contained tumor, and of the nonvisualized nodes 4% harbored metastases. This is similar to histological correlative studies of the axillary, internal mammary, and pelvic lymph nodes and indicates that one cannot reliably assume the absence of tumor in a lymph node seen on lymphoscintigraphy. Tracheal and bronchial lymphatic drainage was studied by injection at bronchoscopy, using several different radiocolloids (Bethune et al., 1978). The technique was unaccompanied by complication, and patterns of drainage to local and regional nodes as well as cervical and celiac lymphatic systems were identified.

Lymphatic drainage of the heart has been characterized using intraoperative, percutaneous, and transcatheter intramural injections (Osbakken et al., 1982). In the dog, a lymph node superior to the aortic arch and between the superior vena cava and innominate artery consistently drains the anterior wall of the heart (Clark et al., 1980). Alterations in lymphatic drainage secondary to ischemic and idiopathic myopathic heart disease have been described (Miller et al., 1964). Lymphatic drainage from vessels as well as the heart was described in the rabbit after the injection of $^{99m}$Tc-antimony sulfide (Castronuovo et al., 1983). The investigators concluded that lymphoscintigraphy offered a useful tool for investigation of lymphatic drainage of the cardiovascular system.

Intravenous injection of monoclonal antibodies is under active investigation in the diagnosis of cancer (Sfakiamakis and Deland, 1982). When injected interstitially, monoclonal antibodies will migrate to regional lymph nodes and bind to target cells (Deland and Goldenberg, 1982; Weinstein et al., 1983). Ipsilateral uptake of $^{131}$I-labeled antibodies to carcinoembryonic antigen was found in regional lymph nodes after interstitial injection in 7 patients with carcinoma of the breast and 43 patients with various malignancies (Kolbenstvedt, 1975; Deland et al., 1979, 1980). All of the axillary metastases were detected. There was uptake in inguinal nodes free of disease, an observation which was speculated to be secondary to sequestration of antibody. The significance of lymphatic system exposure to tumor antigen remains conjectural (Weinstein et al., 1983). Interstitial delivery of labeled monoclonal antibodies to the lymphatic system has several advantages compared to intravenous injection: Lower doses may be used for diagnosis and therapy, there is a distinct possibility of detection of micrometastases, there is a shortened interval between injection and imaging, and there is no binding to circulating shed antigen. Although limited to studies of regional drained lymph nodes, the technique may become useful in the many malignancies already studied by conventional lymphoscintigraphy, including lymphoma and carcinoma of the breast, lung, pelvis, or colon.

## REFERENCES

Agwunobi TC, Boak JL: Diagnosis of malignant breast disease by axillary lymphoscintigraphy: preliminary report. *Br J Surg* 65:379, 1978.

Alcorn FS, Mategrano VC, Petasnick JP, Clark JW: Contributions of computed tomography in the staging and management of malignant lymphoma. *Radiology* 125:717, 1977.

Alder S, Parthasarathy KL, Bakshi SP, Stutzman L: Gallium-67 citrate scanning for the localization and staging of lymphomas. *J Nucl Med* 16:255, 1975.

Anderson KC, Leonard RCF, Cannellos CP, Skarin AT, Kaplan WD: High dose gallium imaging in lymphoma. *Am J Med* 75:327, 1983.

Andrews GA, Edwards CL: Tumor scanning with gallium-67. *JAMA* 233:1100–1103, 1975.

Andrews GA, Hubner KF, Greenlaw RH: [67]Ga citrate imaging in malignant lymphoma: final report of cooperative group. *J Nucl Med* 19:1013–1019, 1978.

Bakshi S, Bender MA: Use of gallium-67 scanning in the management of lymphoma. *J Surg Oncol* 5:539, 1973.

Bennett CR, Lago G: Cutaneous lymphoscintigraphy in malignant melanoma. *Semin Nucl Med* 13:61–69, 1983.

Bergquist L, Strand SE, Persson BR, Hafstrom L, Jonsson PE: Dosimetry in lymphoscintigraphy of Tc-99m antimony sulfide colloid. *J Nucl Med* 23:698, 1982.

Bergquist L, Strand SE, Persson BR: Particle sizing and biokinetics of metastatic lymphoscintigraphic agents. *Semin Nucl Med* 13:9–19, 1983.

Bethune DC, Mulder DS, Chiu RC: Endobronchial lymphoscintigraphy (EBLS). New diagnostic modality. *J Thorac Cardiovasc Surg* 76:446, 1978.

Black RB, Merrick MV, Taylor TV, Forrest APM: Prediction of axillary metastases in breast cancer by lymphoscintigraphy. *Lancet* 2:15, 1980.

Black RB, Merrick MV, Taylor TV, Forrest APM: Lymphoscintigraphy cannot diagnose breast cancer. *Br J Surg* 68:145, 1981.

Boak JL, Agwunobi TC: A study of technetium labeled sulfide colloid uptake by regional lymph nodes drainage a tumor bearing area. *Br J Surg* 65:374–378, 1978.

Bourgeois P, Fruhling J, Henry J: Postoperative axillary lymphoscintigraphy in the management of breast carcinoma. *Int J Radiat Oncol Biol Phys* 9:29–32, 1983.

Bronskill MJ: Radiation dose estimates for interstitial radiocolloid lymphoscintigraphy. *Semin Nucl Med* 13:20–25, 1983.

Carbone PP: Report of the committee on Hodgkin's disease staging classification. *Cancer Res* 31:1860–1861, 1971.

Castellino RA: Imaging techniques for staging abnormal Hodgkin's disease. *Cancer Treat Rep* 66:697, 1982.

Castellino RA, Marglin SD: Lymphographic accuracy in 599 consecutive, previously untreated patients with Hodgkin's disease and non-Hodgkin's lymphoma. In Weissleder H, Bartos V, Clodius L, Malek R (eds): *Progress in Lymphology*. Prague, Avicenum, Czechoslovak Medical Press, 1981, p 317.

Castronuovo JJ Jr, Lopez-Majano V, Flanigan P, Schuler JJ, Jonasson O: Cardiovascular lymphoscintigraphy. *Surgery* 94:351, 1983.

Catalona WJ, Scott WW: Carcinoma of the prostate: a review. *J Urol* 119:1–8, 1978.

Clark GL, Siegal BA, Sobel BE: External evaluation of regional cardiac lymph drainage in intact dogs. *J Invest Radiol* 15:134–139, 1980.

Clouse ME, Harrison D, Grassi CJ, Costello PC, Edwards SA, Wheeler HG: Lymphangiography, ultrasonography, and computed tomography in Hodgkin's disease and non-Hodgkin's lymphoma. *J Compt Tomogr* 9:1–8, 1985.

Collier BD, Palmer DW, Wilson JF, Greenberg MH, Komaki R, Cox JD, Lawson TL, Lawlor PM: Internal mammary lymphoscintigraphy in patients with breast cancer. *Radiology* 147:845, 1983.

Deland FH, Goldenberg DM: In vivo radioimmunological lymphoscintigraphy in cancer: the implications of positive findings. *J Can Assoc Radiol* 33:4–9, 1982.

Deland FH, Kim EE, Corgan RL, Casper S, Primus FJ, Spremulli E, McDowell E, Goldenberg DM: Axillary lymphoscintigraphy by radioimmunodetection of carcinoembryonic antigen in breast cancer. *J Nucl Med* 20:1243, 1979.

Deland FH, Kim EE, Goldenberg DM: Lymphoscintigraphy with radionuclide labeled antibodies to carcinoembryonic antigen. *Cancer Res* 40:2997–3000, 1980.

Dembro AJ, Ege GN, Busch RS: Internal mammary lymphoscintigraphy in the assessment of patients with ovarian carcinoma. *Int J Radiat Oncol Biol Phys* 8:1177–1183, 1982.

Dionne L, Freide J, Blais R: Internal mammary lymphoscintigraphy in breast carcinoma. A surgeon's perspective. *Semin Nucl Med* 13:35–41, 1983.

Donahue DM, Leonard JC, Basmadjian GP, Nitschke RM, Hinkle GH, Ice RD, Wilson DA, Tunell WP: Thymic gallium-67 localization in pediatric patients on chemotherapy: concise communication. *J Nucl Med* 22:1043, 1981.

Dudley HC, Marrer HH: Studies of the metabolism of gallium. III. Deposition in and clearance from bone. *J Pharmacol Exp Ther* 106:129–132, 1952.

Dufresne EN, Kaplan WD, Zimmerman RE, Rose CM: The application of internal mammary lymphoscintigraphy to planning of radiation therapy. *J Nucl Med* 21:697, 1980.

Edwards CL, Hayes RL: Tumor scanning with [67]Ga citrate. *J Nucl Med* 10:103–105, 1969.

Edwards CL, Hayes RL: Scanning malignant neoplasms with gallium 67. *JAMA* 212:1182, 1970.

Edwards CL, Hayes RL: Localization of tumors with radioisotope. In: *Clinical Use of Radionuclides; Critical Comparison with Other Techniques*. Oak Ridge USAEC Conf-71101, 1971.

Edwards CL, Hayes RL, Ominsky S, Byrd BL, Rafter JJ: Intralymphatic injection of [67]Ga for visualizing intraabdominal lymph nodes. *J Nucl Med* 12:431, 1971.

Ege GN: Internal mammary lymphoscintigraphy in breast carcinoma—the rationale, technique, interpretation and clinical application. A review based on 848 cases. *Radiology* 118:101–107, 1976.

Ege GN: Internal mammary lymphoscintigraphy in breast carcinoma—a study of 1071 patients. *Int J Radiat Oncol Biol Phys* 2:755–761, 1977.

Ege GN: Augmented ileopelvic lymphoscintigraphy: applications in the management of genitourinary malignancy. *J Urol* 127:265–269, 1982a.

Ege GN: Whether lymphoscintigraphy? *J Can Assoc Radiol* 33:66–67, 1982b.

Ege GN: Lymphoscintigraphy—techniques and applications in the management of breast carcinoma. *Semin Nucl Med* 13:26–41, 1983.

Ege GN, Clark R: IML in conservative management of breast carcinoma. *Clin Radiol* 31:55–63, 1980.

Ege GN, Cummings BJ: Interstitial radiocolloid ileopelvic lymphoscintigraphy: technique, anatomy and clinical application. *Int J Radiat Oncol Biol Phys* 6:1483–1490, 1980.

Ege GN, Warbick A: Lymphoscintigraphy: a comparison of 99Tc(m) antimony sulfide colloid and 99Tc(m) stannous phytate. *Br J Radiol* 52:124, 1979.

Eraklis AJ, Kevy SV, Diamond LK, Gross RE: Hazard of overwhelming infection after splenectomy in childhood. *N Engl J Med* 276:1225, 1967.

Fee HJ, Robinson DS, Sample WF, Graham LS, Holmes EC, Morton DL: The determination of lymph shed by colloidal gold scanning in patients with malignant melanoma: a preliminary study. *Surgery* 84:626, 1978.

Ferguson DJ, Allen LW, Griem ML, Moran ME, Rappaport HE, Ultmann JE: Surgical experience with staging laparotomy in 125 patients with lymphoma. *Arch Intern*

*Med* 131:356, 1973.

Fogh J: [67]Ga accumulation in malignant tumors and in pre-lactating or lactating breast. *Prog Soc Exp Biol Med* 138:1086–1090, 1971.

Fuks J, Aisner J, Wiernik P: Restaging laparotomy in the management of the non-Hodgkin's hepatomas. *Med Pediatr Oncol* 10:429–438, 1982.

Gardiner RA, Fitzpatrick JM, Constable AR, Cranage RW, O'Donoghue EPN, Wickham JEA: Improved techniques in radionuclide imaging of prostatic lymph nodes. *Br J Urol* 51:561, 1979.

Greenlaw RH, Weinstein MB, Brill AB, McBain JK, Murphy L, Kniseley RM: [67]Ga-citrate imaging in untreated lymphoma; preliminary report of Cooperative Group. *J Nucl Med* 15:404, 1974.

Hahn PF, Carothers EL: Radioactive metallic gold colloids coated with silver and their distribution in the lung and its lymphatics following intra-pulmonary administration: therapeutic implication in primary lung and bronchiogenic tumors. *Br J Cancer* 5:400–404, 1951.

Hahn PF, Carothers EL: Lymphatic draining following intrabronchial instillation of siliver-coated radioactive gold colloids in therapeutic quantities. *J Thorac Cardiovasc Surg* 25:265–279, 1953.

Hahn PF, Sheppard CW: Selective radiation obtained by the intravenous administration of colloidal radioactive isotopes in diseases of the lymphoid system. *South Med J* 39:559–562, 1946.

Hartman RE, Hayes RL: The binding of gallium by blood serum. *J Pharmacol Exp Ther* 168:193–198, 1969.

Hayes RL: The medical use of gallium radionuclides: a brief history with some comments. *Semin Nucl Med* 8:183–191, 1978.

Hayes RL, Nelson B, Swartzendruber DC, Brown DH, Carlton JE, Byrd BL: Studies in the intracellular deposition of [67]Ga. *J Nucl Med* 12:364, 1971.

Hellman S: Current studies in Hodgkin's disease. *N Engl J Med* 290:894–897, 1974.

Henkin RE, Polcyn RE, Quinn JL III: Scanning treated Hodgkin's disease in [67]Ga citrate. *Radiology* 110:151–154, 1974.

Henze E, Schelbert HR, Collins JD, Najafi A, Barrio JR, Bennett LR: Lymphoscintigraphy with Tc-99m labeled dextran. *J Nucl Med* 23:923, 1982.

Herman T, Jones S: Systemic restaging in patients with Hodgkin's disease: a Southwest Oncology Group study. *Cancer* 42:1976–1982, 1978.

Heshiki A, Schatz SL, McKusick KA, Bowersox DW, Soin JS, Wagner HN Jr: Gallium-67 citrate scanning in patients with pulmonary sarcoidosis. *AJR* 122:744, 1974.

Higasi T, Nakayama Y: Clinical evaluation of [67]gallium-citrate scanning. *J Nucl Med* 13:196–201, 1972.

Hoffer PB: The utility of gallium-67 in tumor imaging: a comment on the final report of the Cooperative Study Group. *J Nucl Med* 19:1082–1083, 1978.

Ito Y, Otsuka N, Nagai K, Muranaka A, Yoneda M: Lymphoscintigraphy by SC injection of [67]Ga-citrate. *Eur J Nucl Med* 7:260, 1982.

Iverson T, Aas M: Pelvic lymphoscintigraphy with [99m]Tc-colloid in lymph node metastases. *Eur J Nucl Med* 7:445–457, 1982.

Jackson BS, Rosenthal L, Attia E: Laryngeal lymphoscintigraphy. *Laryngoscope* 91:2085–2091, 1981.

Johnson PM, Berdon WE, Baker DH, Fawwaz RA: Thymic uptake of gallium-67 citrate in a healthy 4 year old boy. *Pediatr Radiol* 7:243–244, 1978.

Johnston GS, Go MF, Benua RS, Larson SM, Andrews GA, Hubner KF: Gallium-67 citrate imaging in Hodgkin's

disease: final report of cooperative group. *J Nucl Med* 18:692, 1977.

Jones SE, Fuks Z, Bull M, Kadin ME, Dorfman RF, Kaplan HS, Rosenberg SA: Non-Hodgkin's lymphoma. IV. Clinicopathological correlation in 405 cases. *Cancer* 31:806, 1973.

Kaplan WD: Ileo-pelvic lymphoscintigraphy. *Semin Nucl Med* 13:42–53, 1983.

Kaplan WD, Davis MA, Rose CM: A comparison of two technetium-99m labeled radiopharmaceuticals for lymphoscintigraphy. *J Nucl Med* 20:933–937, 1979.

Kaplan WD, Bloomer WD, Jones AG, Federschneider J, Knapp RC: Mediastinal lymphoscintigraphy in ovarian cancer using intraperitoneal autologous technetium-99m labeled erythrocytes. *Br J Radiol* 54:126, 1981.

Kaplan WD, Garnick MB, Richie JP: Ileopelvic radionuclide lymphoscintigraphy in patients with testicular cancer. *Radiology* 147:231–235, 1983.

Kashima HK, McKusick KA, Malmud LS, Wagner HN Jr: Gallium-67 Scanning in patients with head and neck cancer. *Laryngoscope* 84:1078–1089, 1974.

Kay DN, McCready VR: Clinical isotope scanning using [67]Ga citrate in the management of Hodgkin's disease. *Br J Radiol* 45:437–443, 1972.

King D, Dawson A, McDonald A: Gallium scanning in lymphoma. *Clin Radiol* 31:729–732, 1980.

Kinoshita F, Ushio T, Maekawa A, Ariwa R, Kubo A: Scintiscanning of pulmonary disease with [67]Ga citrate. *J Nucl Med* 15:227, 1974.

Kolbenstvedt A: Lymphography in the diagnosis of metastases from carcinoma of the uterine cervix. Stage I and II. *Acta Radiol [Diagn] (Stockh)* 16:81–97, 1975.

Langhammer H, Glaubitt G, Grebe SF, Hampe JF, Haubold U, Hor G, Kaul A, Koeppe P, Koppenhagen J, Roedler HD, Va der Schoot JB: [67]Ga for tumor scanning. *J Nucl Med* 13:25, 1972.

Larson SM, Milder MS, Johnston GS: Interpretation of the [67]Ga photoscan. *J Nucl Med* 14:208–214, 1973.

Larson SM, Schall GL: Gallium-67 concentration in human breast milk. *JAMA* 218:257, 1971.

Lavender JP, Lowe J, Barker JR, Burn JI, Chaudhri MA: Gallium-67 citrate scanning in neoplastic and inflammatory lesions. *Br J Radiol* 44:361, 1971.

Lentle BC, Castor WR, Khaliqi A, Dieuch H: The effect of contrast lymphangiography on localization of [67]Ga citrate. *J Nucl Med* 15:374, 1974.

Levine MS, Arger DH, Coleman BE, Mulhern CB Jr, Pollack HM, Wein AJ: Detecting lymphatic metastases from prostatic carcinoma. Superiority of CT. *AJR* 137:207, 1981.

Littenberg RL, Alazraki NP, Taketa RM, Reit R, Halpern SE, Ashburn WL: A clinical evaluation of gallium-67 citrate scanning. *Surg Gynecol Obstet* 137:424, 1973a.

Littenberg RL, Taketa RM, Alazraki NP, Halpern SE, Ashburn WL: Gallium-67 for localization of septic lesions. *Ann Intern Med* 79:403, 1973b.

Lomas F, DiBos P, Wagner HN Jr: Increased specificity of liver scanning with the use of [67]Ga citrate. *N Engl J Med* 286:1323–1329, 1972.

Longo D, Schilsky R, Blei L, Cano R, Johnston GS, Young RC: Gallium-67 scanning: limited usefulness in staging patients with non-Hodgkin's lymphoma. *Am J Med* 68:695, 1980.

Lukes RJ: Prognosis and relationship of histological features to clinical stage. *JAMA* 222:1294–1296, 1972.

Lukes RJ, Craver LF, Hall TC, Rappaport H, Ruben P: Report of the Nomenclature Committee. *Cancer Res* 26:1311, 1966.

Matsuo S: Studies on the metastases of breast cancer to lymph nodes. II. Diagnosis of metastasis to internal mammary nodes using radiocolloid. *Acta Med Okayama* 28:361–371, 1974.

McCready RV, Dance DR, Hammersley P, Morley R: Clinical and experimental observation on 67-Ga citrate uptake in tumors and other lesions. In: *Symposium on Medical Radioisotope Scintigraphy*, Monte Carlo, Principality of Monaco, October 23–28, 1972. I.A.E.A./SM-164/42.

McKusick Ka, Ghiladi A, Wagner HN Jr: Gallium-67 in pulmonary sarcoidosis. *JAMA* 223:688, 1973.

Merz T, Malmud LS, McKusick KA, Wagner HN Jr: The mechanism of [67]Ga association with lymphocytes. *Cancer Res* 34:2495, 1974.

Meyer CM, Lecklitner ML, Logic JR, Balch CE, Bessey PQ, Tauxe WN: Technetium-99m sulfur colloid cutaneous lymphoscintigraphy in the management of truncal melanoma. *Radiology* 131:205, 1979.

Meyer JE, Munzenrider JE: Computed tomographic demonstration of internal mammary lymph node metastasis in patients with locally recurrent breast carcinoma. *Radiology* 139:661, 1981.

Miller AJ, Peck R, Katz LN: The importance of the lymphatics of mammalian heart: experimental observations and some speculations. *Circulation* 29:485–489, 1964.

MIRD/Dose Estimate. Report No. 2. Summary of current radiation dose estimates to humans from [66]Ga-, [67]Ga-, [68]Ga-, and [72]Ga-citrate. *J Nucl Med* 14:755–756, 1973.

Muller JH: Intraperitoneal application of radioactive colloids. In Hahn PF (ed): *Therapeutic Use of Artificial Radioisotopes*. New York, John Wiley & Sons, 1956, p 269.

Munz DL, Altmeyer P, Holzmann A, Encke A, Hör G: Der Stellenwert der Lymphoszintigraphie in der Behandlung maligner Melanome der Haut. *Dtsch Med Wochenschr* 107:86, 1982a.

Munz DL, Altmeyer P, Sessler MJ, Hor G: Axillary lymph node groups. The center in lymphatic drainage from the truncal skin in man. Clinical significance for management of malignant melanoma. *Lymphology* 15:143, 1982b.

Nash AG, Dance DR, McCready VR, Griffiths JD: Uptake of [67]gallium in colonic and rectal tumors. *Br Med J* 3:508, 1972.

Osbakken MD, Kopiwoda SY, Swan A, Castronovo FP, Stauss HW: Cardiac lymphoscintigraphy following closed chest catheter injection of radiolabeled colloid into the myocardium of dogs: concise communication. *J Nucl Med* 23:883, 1982.

Otten J, Johnston GS, Pasten I: Cyclic AMP levels in fibroblasts: relationship to growth rate and contact inhibition of growth. *Proc Soc Exp Biol Med* 142:92–95, 1973.

Pannettiere F, Coltman CA: Splenectomy effects on chemotherapy in Hodgkin's disease. *Arch Intern Med* 131:362, 1973.

Parell GJ, Becker GD, Surpin GT: Prediction of lymph node metastasis by lymphoscintigraphy of the neck after pericancer injection of a radiocolloid. *Otolaryngol Head Neck Surg* 89:67, 1981.

Peyton JWR, Crosbie J, Bell TK, Roy AD, Odling-Smee W: High colloidal uptake in axillary nodes with metastatic disease. *Br J Surg* 68:507, 1981.

Robinson DS, Sample WF, Fee HJ, Holmes EC, Morton DL: Regional lymphatic drainage in primary malignant melanoma of the trunk determined by colloid gold scanning. *Surg Forum* 28:147, 1977.

Rose CM, Kaplan WD, Marck A: Parasternal lymphoscintigraphy: implication for the treatment planning of internal mammary lymph nodes in breast CA. *Int J Radiat Oncol Biol Phys* 5:1849–1853, 1979.

Rosenberg SA: Updated Hodgkin's disease; place of splenectomy in evaluation of management. *JAMA* 222:1296–1298, 1972.

Rosenberg SA, Kaplan HS: Evidence of an orderly progression in spread of Hodgkin's disease. *Cancer Res* 26:1225–1231, 1966.

Sappy C: *Anatomic physiology pathologic der vaisseaux lymphahquis considering chez l'homme et les virtebras*. Paris, A Delehaye, 1874.

Schenk P, Zumwonkle K, Becker G: Die szintigraphic der Para Stermalen Lymphsystems. *Nucl Med* 5:388–396, 1966.

Seaman WB, Powers WE: Studies on the distribution of radioactive colloidal gold in regional lymph nodes containing cancer. *Cancer* 8:1044–1046, 1955.

Sephton R, Martin J: Modification of distribution of gallium-67 in man by administration of iron. *Br J Radiol* 53:572–575, 1980.

Sfakiamakis GN, Deland FH: Radioimmunodiagnosis and radioimmunotherapy. *J Nucl Med* 23:840–850, 1982.

Sheppard CW, Goodell JPB, Hahn PF: Colloidal gold containing the radioactive isotope Au-198 in the selective internal radiation therapy of diseases of the lymphatic system. *J Lab Clin Med* 32:1437–1441, 1947.

Sherman AI, Ter-Pogossian M: Lymph node concentration of radioactive colloidal gold following interstitial injection. *Cancer* 6:1238–1240, 1953.

Siddon RL, Chin LM, Zimmerman RE, Mendel JB, Kaplan WD: Utilization of parasternal lymphoscintigraphy in radiation therapy of breast carcinoma. *Int J Radiat Oncol Biol Phys* 8:1059, 1982.

Siemsen JK, Sargent EN, Grebe SF, Winsor DW, Wnetz D, Jacobson G: Pulmonary concentration of [67]Ga pneumoconiosis. *AJR* 120:815, 1974.

Silberstein EB, Kornblut A, Shumrick DA, Saenger EL: [67]Ga as a diagnostic agent for the detection of head and neck tumors and lymphoma. *Radiology* 110:605, 1974.

Silva J Jr, Harvey WC: Detection of infections with gallium-67 and scintigraphic imaging. *J Infect Dis* 130:125–131, 1974.

Smith F, Dendy P: Modification of gallium-67 citrate distribution in man following administration of iron. *Br J Radiol* 54:398–402, 1981.

Smithers DW: Updated Hodgkin's disease; patterns of spread. *JAMA* 222:1298–1299, 1972.

Stone AR, Merrick MV, Chisholm GD: Prostatic lymphoscintigraphy. *Br J Urol* 51:556–560, 1979.

Strand SE, Persson BR: Quantitative lymphoscintigraphy. I. Basic concepts for optimal uptake of radiocolloids in parasternal lymph nodes of rabbits. *J Nucl Med* 20:1038, 1979.

Sugarbaker EV, McBride CM: Melanoma of the trunk: the results of surgical excision and anatomic guidelines for predicting nodal metastasis. *Surgery* 80:22–30, 1976.

Sullivan DC, Crocker BP, Harris C, Deery P, Seigler HF: Lymphoscintigraphy in malignant melanoma: [99m]Tc antimony sulfur colloid. *AJR* 137:847, 1981.

Suzuki T, Honjo I, Hamaoto K, Kousaka T, Torizuka K: Positive scintiphotography of cancer of the liver with [67]Ga citrate. *AJR* 113:92, 1971.

Swartzendruber DC, Nelson B, Hayes RL: [67]Gallium localization in lysosomal-like granules of leukemic and nonleukemic murine tissues. *J Natl Cancer Inst* 46:941–952, 1971.

Teates CD, Hunter JG: Gallium scanning as a test for inflammatory lesions. *Radiology* 116:383–387, 1975.

Terui S, Kato H, Hirashima T, Iizuka T, Oyamada H: An evaluation of the mediastinal lymphoscintigram for carcinoma of the esophagus studied with $^{99m}$Tc rhenium sulfur colloid. *Eur J Nucl Med* 7:99–101, 1982.

Thommesen P, Buhl J, Jansen K, Funch-Jensen P: Lymphoscintigraphy in the head and neck in normal diagnostic value. *ROFO* 134:80, 1981.

Turner DA, Pinsky SM, Gottschalk A, Hoffer PB, Ultmann JE, Harper PV: The use of $^{67}$Ga scanning in the staging of Hodgkin's disease. *Radiology* 104:97, 1972.

Walker LA: Localization of radioactive colloids in lymph nodes. *J Lab Clin Med* 36:440–449, 1950.

Weinstein JN, Steller MA, Keenan AM, Covell DG, Key ME, Sreber SM, Oldham RK, Hwang KM, Parker RJ: Monoclonal antibodies in the lymphatics: selective delivery to lymph node metastasis of a solid tumor. *Science* 222:423, 1983.

Whitmore WF III, Blute RD Jr, Kaplan WD, Gittes RF: Radiocolloid scintigraphic mapping of the lymphatic drainage of the prostate. *J Urol* 124:62, 1980.

# 4

# *Technique*

MELVIN E. CLOUSE, M.D.

The steps in lymphography are visualization of the lymphatics by vital dyes, surgical exposure of the vessel, direct cannulation, injection of contrast material, and roentgenographic imaging of the vessels immediately after completion of the injection and 24 hr later for lymph node detail.

## PEDAL LYMPHOGRAPHY

The technique generally used was developed by the British surgeon J. B. Kinmonth (1952). Kinmonth extended the technique of Hudack and McMaster (1933), who used patent blue violet dye to study the dermal lymphatics. In the United States, the only dye with Food and Drug Administration approval is isosulfan blue.

### Preparation of the Patient

The first step in the procedure is examination of the patient and review of the chart to be certain that the procedure is indicated and that there are no contraindications. The major contraindications are cardiovascular or pulmonary disease (i.e., heart failure, angina, interstitial fibrosis, emphysema, or previous radiotherapy to the lung).

Age, per se, is not a contraindication to lymphography. If lymphangiography is done judiciously, even patients with advanced age can be examined without significant risks. In a study by Sokol et al. (1977), patients with severe cardiac risk factors—such as previous myocardial infarction, heart failure, arrhythmias, and severe hypertension (greater than 180 over 100)—did not experience significantly more complications than those without such risks.

Previous radiotherapy to the lung is a significant contraindication because radiation therapy opens arteriovenous shunts, which predispose to systemic emboli (Davidson, 1969). The patient must also be quizzed about allergies to local anesthesia, vital dyes, and contrast material.

Lymphography may be performed on an outpatient basis, but it is better to observe the patient in the hospital for 24 hr. This may be accomplished through an observation unit or receiving ward.

The procedure is explained to the patient with special attention to local blue skin discoloration at the injection site that may persist for several weeks. Generalized light blue staining of the skin does not occur with isosulfan blue possibly because of its much lower concentration (30 mg of a 1% solution). According to the manufacturers, 34% of isosulfan blue is absorbed from the injection site in approximately 30 min with 69% and 100% absorption at 1 hr and 24 hr, respectively. However, care should be taken in administering even this dye to patients with chronic renal disease or obstructive uropathy.

Premedication is adjusted according to the patient's weight and age. For an average 70-kg patient a combined injection of atropine (0.4 mg), meperidine (Demerol, 75 mg), and pentobarbital (Nembutal, 100 mg) is given intramuscularly 30 min before the procedure is begun. For small patients or those over 60 yr of age, adequate premedication can be achieved with atropine (0.4 mg) alone or in combination with meperidine (75 mg).

The feet are shaved in the radiology department, prepared with an antiseptic surgical scrub, cleansed with alcohol, and then draped with sterile sheets. A lymphangiogram tray is used (Fig. 4.1).

### Vital Dyes

Various indicator dyes, such as direct sky blue, trypan blue, niagara sky blue, and methylene blue have been used for lymphangiography (Threefoot, 1960; Hreschyshyn et al., 1961; Riveros et al., 1967). The vital dyes are large molecular compounds that facilitate their absorption into the initial lymphatics rather than small molecular crystalloids that are absorbed into the

6 towels
16 4 × 3 sponges
1 swab
1 20-cc vial of lidocaine 1% plain
1 medicine glass
1 6-inch basin
2 smooth sponge forceps
1 Adson smoothed forceps
1 Miltex 3-C (or any small, sharp, pointed forceps)
1 suture scissors
1 small needle holder
3 curved mosquitoes
1 no. 3 knife handle with no. 15 blade
2 straight mosquitoes
1 10-cc ring Luer-loc syringe (for lidocaine)
2 10-cc Luer-loc syringes
3 no. 26 disposable needles
Available:
    4-0 silk suture
    sterile sheets
    1% isosulfan blue dye
    Harvard Apparatus injector
    proper surgical light
    Steri-Strip tape
    Ethiodol 2 10-ml vials

FIGURE 4.1. LYMPHANGIOGRAPHY TRAY CONTENTS

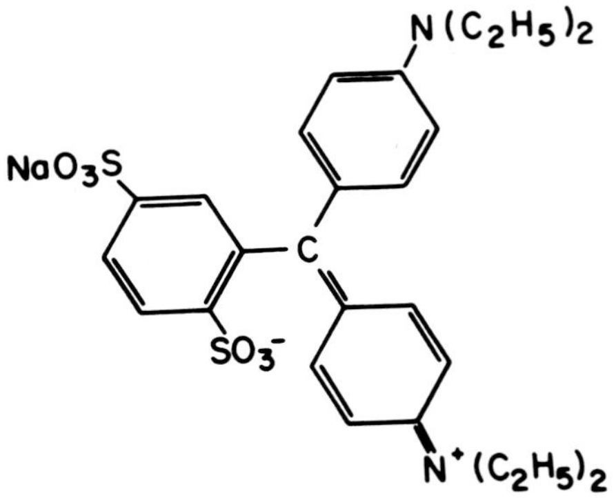

FIGURE 4.2. STRUCTURAL FORMULA OF ISOSULFAN BLUE
(From Hirsh et al., 1982, p 1062.)

blood vascular capillaries. Patent blue violet 11%, a triphenylmethane dye selected by Hudack and McMaster (1933) for outlining the skin lymphatics, was widely used for many years. It is rapidly absorbed into the lymphatics, slowly diffuses into the adventitia, and is rapidly excreted because it does not bind to plasma protein (Threefoot, 1960). Although it was used experimentally by Hudack and McMaster and in clinical studies for 25 yr, the dye was never approved by the Food and Drug Administration. No major problems were reported, but Gangolli and others (1967) found sarcomatous changes after repeated injections of the dye into subcutaneous tissues of Wistar albino rats. Because of the possible liability to radiologists, its use was discontinued.

Through the efforts of J. I. Hirsh at the Medical College of Virginia, extensive trials with isosulfan blue, the 2,5-disulfonic acid isomer of patent blue, was finally approved for lymphangiography (Hirsh et al., 1982) (Fig. 4.2). It is marketed under the trade name of Lymphazurin 1% in 5-ml single dose vials. The appropriate dose is 0.5 ml injected into the web spaces between the toes of each lower extremity. The maximum dose is 3 ml (30 mg). Within 24 hr, 10% is excreted unchanged in the urine. Approximately 90% is excreted through the bile.

When examination of the deep lymphatics of the leg is desired, the vital dye is injected into the tissues below the lateral malleolus. For examinations of the arm and axillary lymphatics, the vital dye is injected on the dorsal aspect between the fingers of the hand. For the cervical lymphatics, the posterior auricular area is used. A single dose of isosulfan blue is sufficient to fill a lymphatic, enabling it to be localized with a bright light at the cutdown site.

It is easier to expose and cannulate the lymphatic before the dye has extravasated into the surrounding tissue and stained the skin. It is, therefore, imperative to identify the lymphatic immediately after it has filled with dye. This can be accomplished by focusing a bright light on the dorsum of the foot after injecting the dye. The blood can be compressed from the small veins by stretching and compressing the skin and making it taut. The lymphatics can then be seen as light blue streaks underneath the skin. The lymphatics cannot be visualized in this manner in dark-skinned patients.

Sigurjonsson (1974) localized pedal lymphatics without aid of indicator dyes because of the considerable incidence of allergic reactions reported by Mortazavi and Burrows (1971). He reported no difference in failure rate or required operation time with or without indicator dyes. More recently, Kapdi (1979) reported a 96% success rate for performing lymphography without vital dye. The success was attributed to the fact that the author performed all examinations himself. Doss et al. (1980) have used fluorescein and ultraviolet light to identify and cannulate lymphatics. Their procedure is complicated by the fact that fluorescein is mixed with the patient's serum and injected subcutaneously. Approximately 60 to 90 min are required for lymphatic visualization—a long time in an active clinical department.

## Exposure of the Lymphatics

The site on the foot chosen to expose and cannulate a lymphatic is very important. The vessels near the toes are very small, and the

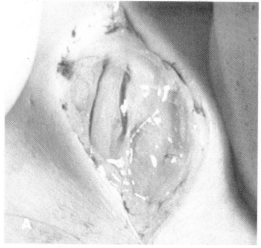

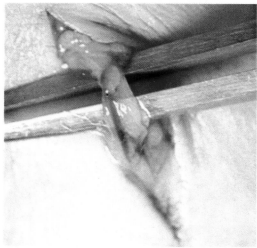
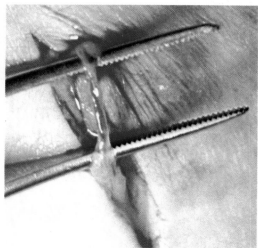

FIGURE 4.3. EXPOSURE OF LYMPHATIC VESSEL

*A*: Longitudinal incision over lymphatic. *B*: Lymphatic elevated by probing under it with the 3-C Miltex forcep. *C*: Exposed lymphatic before the soft tissue has been removed.

patient may dislodge the needle from this site by slight movement of his foot or toes. It is best to select a vessel on the lateral aspect of the dorsum of the foot or just lateral to the base of the first metatarsal. It is much easier to expose and cannulate a single lymphatic. Occasionally there may be two very small lymphatics parallel to each other, or the examiner may make the original incision at a bifurcation. The incision must then be extended in the direction of the largest trunk. If the first attempt is unsuccessful, a vessel higher up near the ankle may be chosen.

Lidocaine 1% is injected into the dermal and subcutaneous tissues on either side of the lymphatic. Injecting into the subcutaneous tissues helps the physician to dissect and free the lymphatic vessel from the surrounding tissues, elevates the skin, and reduces the chance of laceration of the lymphatic when the initial incision is made. A longitudinal incision is made over the lymphatic. When the vessel is exposed under direct vision, the incision is carried down into the subcutaneous tissues on either side of the vessel. The vessel is elevated by probing underneath it with a sharp pointed fine 3-C, Miltex forcep (Miltex Instrument Co., 300 Park Avenue South, New York, NY 10010) (Fig. 4.3) and held exposed by passing a smooth Adson forcep (Codman Instrument Co., Randolph, MA 02054) underneath the lymph vessel with the opposite hand. Fat and loose areolar tissue are stripped off the lymphatic for a distance of 1–2 cm with the fine Miltex forcep (Fig. 4.4).

Although it is usually easy to differentiate lymphatics from veins, it may at times be difficult. For this reason the foot is fluoroscoped immediately after the injection has begun. The walls of the small veins are usually thicker and denser when compressed, while the lymphatic vessel is clear and more transparent when it is collapsed and the vital dye is milked from the vessel.

## Cannulation

Various modifications of the Kinmonth technique have been described. Jing (1966), Iriarte et al. (1964), Lee et al. (1969), Kropholler et al. (1968), and Tong (1969) have described techniques of directly inserting a fine polyethylene catheter into the lymph vessel. There have also been a proliferation of instruments designed to make cannulation easier and to secure the needle in the vessel once it has been cannulated. Damascelli et al. (1969) described a special forcep for removing loose connective tissue around the vessel. Special cannulas have been designed by Viamonte and Stevens (1966), Howland (1972), DeRoo (1966), and Tegtmeyer (1974). In addition, Turner (1966), Youker (1966), and DeRoo (1966) have each described special clamps for holding the needle in place once the vessel has been cannulated.

Over the years we have found that the easiest method of cannulation is one that avoids the need for special equipment. As an example we do not use ligatures to obstruct and distend the vessel temporarily for cannulation. This is best accomplished with the smooth Adson forcep. The proximal portion of the lymph vessel is temporarily obstructed (Fig. 4.5). The vessel is distended by massaging the tissues and milking

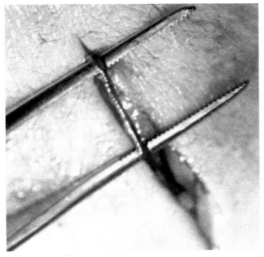

FIGURE 4.4. EXPOSED LYMPHATIC AFTER THE SOFT TISSUE HAS BEEN REMOVED READY FOR CANNULATION

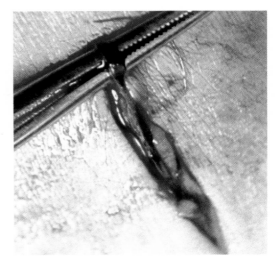

FIGURE 4.5. EXPOSED LYMPHATIC TEMPORARILY OBSTRUCTED BY ADSON FORCEP

the lymph up from the toes. The forcep is spread to make the vessel taut and semidistended (Fig. 4.6A). The lymphatic set (Randall Faichney Co., Avon, MA 02322) with a 27 or 30 gauge needle is grasped with a large sponge forcep, and the lymphatic vessel is punctured. In making the approach into the lymphatic vessel, the needle must be on a plane parallel to and just above the vessel so that the posterior wall of the lymphatic is not punctured (Fig. 4.6B).

A small amount of contrast material is injected manually by the assistant from a 10-ml syringe attached to the lymphatic set to distend the vessel further. The needle is then advanced 2–3 mm into the lumen. It is much easier to see small air bubbles alternating with the column of contrast material, indicating free passage into the lymphatic lumen, than to see a solid column of contrast material. For this reason small air bubbles are trapped in the lymphography set tubing near the needle before cannulation is attempted.

The lymphatic needle is stabilized with the index finger. The catheter and needle are secured with strips of ½-inch Steri-Strip (Minnesota Mining and Manufacturing Co., St. Paul, MN) tape that have previously been peeled from the heavy paper backing and taped to the surrounding drapes (Fig. 4.7). The heavy paper backing should remain on the corner to prevent the tape from sticking to the examiner's glove. As the lymphographer gains experience and anticipates the procedure, assistance is only needed for contrast injection to distend the lymph vessel at the initial puncture.

Occasionally contrast material may leak from the puncture site even when the needle is se-

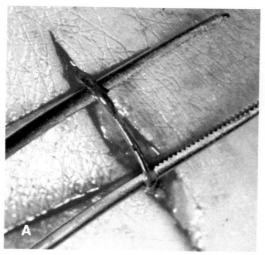 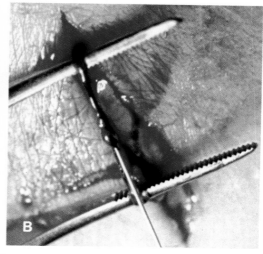

FIGURE 4.6. LYMPHATIC CANNULATION TECHNIQUE

*A*: Taut, semidistended lymphatic ready for cannulation. *B*: Lymphatic immediately after needle has punctured lymphatic; needle is on a plane parallel to the lymphatic. When the lymphatic has been punctured, a small amount of contrast material is injected to distend the vessel further, and the needle is advanced 2–3 mm.

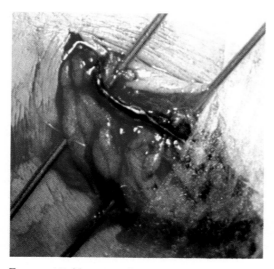

FIGURE 4.7. NEEDLE IN LYMPHATIC SECURED WITH
STERI-STRIP TAPE

The lymphatic is distended because the injection has begun. The needles in the subcutaneous tissue beneath the lymphatic elevate it to the skin surface.

curely in the vessel. In these instances a 4-0 silk ligature may be placed around the vessel distal to the needle tip but proximal to the puncture site by passing a fine Miltex forcep underneath the needle and vessel, grasping the suture, and pulling it underneath without disturbing the needle.

It is preferable to use a different vessel when a second puncture must be made because leakage of lymph and dye prevents vessel distention, thus making the second puncture more difficult. If this is not possible, the second puncture must be made proximal to the first to prevent leakage of contrast material during the injection.

The tubing is securely taped to the patient's foot. The patient remains supine during the procedure but may be given fluids and additional medication if necessary. The patient must never be left unobserved during the procedure.

## Contrast Material

The standard contrast material used for lymphography is Ethiodol (Savage Laboratories, Inc., Missouri City, TX 77459), an iodinated ethyl ester of the fatty acids of poppy seed oil. Ethiodol is obtained by transesterification of Lipiodol. It is mainly composed of ethyl diiodostereate, monoiodostereate, and moniodinated ethyl stereate (Guerbet Laboratories, 16-24 rue Jean-Chaptal, 93 Aulnaysouse, Boise, France). Ethiodol has completely replaced other oily contrast materials, such as Iodopin used by Bruun and Engeset (1956) and Lipiodol used by Zheutlin and Shanbrom (1958).

Zheutlin and Shanbrom found that Ethiodol produced good opacification of the nodes and was easier than Lipiodol to inject because it is less viscous. Ethiodol also provides excellent opacification of the lymph vessels and nodes because it does not diffuse through the vessel wall like water-soluble contrast media. It remains in the nodes for months and sometimes years, allowing one to evaluate the effects of treatment or progression of disease. The single disadvantage of Ethiodol is that it is not completely inert. It produces an inflammatory reaction in the lymph nodes and lungs that does not cause permanent damage and is not clinically significant.

The viscosity of Ethiodol at 15°C is 0.5–1.0 poise compared to 20.0 poise for Lipiodol. Ethiodol is a clear, light amber, oily fluid. If exposed to oxygen or sunlight, it will decompose (liberating iodine) and turn a dark brown color. It should not be used in this condition.

The biological fate of Ethiodol has been reported by Fischer (1959a, b), Koehler et al. (1964), and Threefoot (1968). The contrast material that is not held within the nodes enters the venous system via the thoracic duct of lymphovenous communication. When normal doses of Ethiodol (7 ml in each extremity) are used, the excess is largely filtered by the lungs. If excessive doses are given, there is spillover from the lungs into other organs.

Koehler et al. (1964) have shown that after 3 days an average of 23% of radioactively tagged [131]I Ethiodol (30 $\mu$Ci/g) remained in the lymph nodes of the dog, while an average of 50% was concentrated in the lungs. The remainder of an injected dose of 0.16 g/kg was distributed fairly evenly throughout the remaining body organs. The amount of contrast material entering the systemic circulation in humans should be considerably less because the usual dose is lower (0.2 ml/kg) and there are more iliac and para-aortic nodes to retain contrast material. The fate of the lipid molecule is unknown, but presumably it is degraded by $\beta$ oxidation (Koehler, 1968).

Iodine is stripped from the lipid molecule by esterases. Threefoot (1968) has shown that the lipid form of [131]I-labeled Ethiodol gradually decreases to insignificant amounts. By 9 days nearly all of the iodine is in the aqueous phase and is excreted by the kidneys in the iodide form.

## Dosage

To evaluate the inguinal, iliac, and para-aortic nodes and the thoracic duct by pedal lymphography in a 70-kg patient, 6–7 ml of Ethiodol are injected into the lymphatics of each extremity. The rate of injection is 0.0618–0.153 ml/min depending upon the size of the lymphatic. Too rapid a rate of injection will rupture the lymphatic.

For lymphography in the upper arm, 2–5 ml of Ethiodol are used. The injection is discontinued when the axillary nodes fill. The injection rate is 0.0618 ml/min.

## Injectors

The various types of injectors described for lymphography all offer a slow steady rate of injection. Wallace et al. (1961) described a manually operated C-clamp. Gilchrist (1965), Jing (1966), Arts (1967), and Cusick and Panning (1967) use gravity types of injectors. Various automatic injectors have been used by DeRoo (1966), Clementz and Olin (1961), and Viamonte (1964).

We use a Harvard Apparatus, model 941 automatic injector (Harvard Apparatus Co. Inc., Millis, MA 02054) (Fig. 4.8). The Harvard Apparatus injector is similar to that described by Clementz and Olin (1961). It operates on a screw-driven mechanism with a gear box, is simple to operate, and is very accurate at all rates of injection.

## Roentgenographic Technique

The foot and lower leg are fluoroscoped after the injection has begun to be certain that the needle is in the lymphatic and there are no peripheral lymphovenous communications. After approximately 4 ml have been injected, an anteroposterior film of the pelvis is taken to check for obstruction or lymphovenous communications in the pelvis.

A supine film of the abdomen is taken after 6–7 ml of Ethiodol have been injected. If the injection rate has been 0.153 ml/min, the total injection time will be just over 45 min. The cisterna chyli may not have filled, and it will be necessary to delay the complete film series for 15–30 min to allow for complete filling of the para-aortic vessels and cisterna chyli.

Seven views are routinely taken after the injection has been terminated and repeated 24 hr later for lymph node detail: an anteroposterior view of the abdomen; an anteroposterior view of the pelvis; right and left posterior oblique views of the abdomen, including the iliac and inguinal areas; lateral view of abdomen using lumbar spine technique; and posteroanterior and lateral views of the chest and thoracic duct to evaluate the presence of drainage into paratracheal nodes and the amount of embolized oil.

High quality films and short exposure times to prevent motion unsharpness are most important. High or low kilovoltage may be used for filming depending upon the preference of the examiner.

The technical factors are 40-inch target-to-film distance, Kodak X-omatic cassettes, and Kodak TML film (Table 4.1). Multiple views and, on occasion, ×2 magnification are more helpful than stereoscopy (Mannila and Wilja-

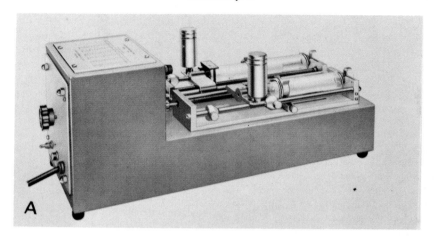

HARVARD APPARATUS

Infusion/Withdrawal Pump

Rates in ml/minute per Syringe

| SERIES 900, 930, 940, 950, 954 Syringe Sizes | | | | | |
|---|---|---|---|---|---|
| 50 ml. | 30 ml. | 20 ml. | 10 ml. | 5 ml. | 2 ml. |
| 114.0 | 74.1 | 58.2 | 30.9 | 20.4 | 11.8 |
| 45.9 | 29.7 | 23.3 | 12.4 | 8.16 | 4.71 |
| 22.9 | 14.8 | 11.6 | 6.18 | 4.08 | 2.36 |
| 11.5 | 7.41 | 5.82 | 3.09 | 2.04 | 1.18 |
| 5.73 | 3.69 | 2.91 | 1.53 | 1.02 | 0.591 |
| 2.29 | 1.48 | 1.16 | 0.618 | 0.408 | 0.237 |
| 1.15 | 0.741 | 0.582 | 0.309 | 0.204 | 0.118 |
| 0.573 | 0.369 | 0.291 | 0.153 | 0.102 | 0.0591 |
| 0.229 | 0.148 | 0.116 | 0.0518 | 0.0408 | 0.0237 |
| 0.115 | 0.0741 | 0.0582 | 0.0309 | 0.0204 | 0.0118 |
| 0.057 | 0.0369 | 0.0291 | 0.0153 | 0.0102 | 0.00591 |
| 0.0229 | 0.0148 | 0.0116 | 0.00618 | 0.00408 | 0.00237 |

B

FIGURE 4.8. INJECTORS
A: Harvard Apparatus injector pump. B: Injection rates (milliliters per minute per syringe).

salo, 1965) and tomography (DeRoo et al., 1965). The vessel phase must be compared to the node films to determine whether filling defects represent metastases or lymph node hila.

In addition, localized obstruction of one or more vessels by a node completely replaced by tumor may be demonstrated only in the vessel phase. Significant amounts of contrast material

TABLE 4.1.

| View | Milliamperes | Kilovolts |
|---|---|---|
| Chest | | |
| Posteroanterior | 3 | 110 |
| Lateral | 10 | 120 |
| Abdomen | | |
| Anteroposterior | 70 | 70 |
| Right posterior oblique-<br>left posterior oblique | 100 | 70 |
| Lateral | 160 | 70 |
| Pelvis | | |
| Anteroposterior | 60 | 70 |

remaining in the vessels after 24 hr and collateral circulation indicate obstruction.

Direct ×2 magnification is especially helpful for evaluating a conglomerate of nodes high in the para-aortic and iliac areas. The presence of multiple small superimposed nodes prevents one from clearly determining the boundary of each node. In addition to enlargement, magnification changes the spatial relationship of the node images to each other and thereby sharply delineates the node boundaries and the intranodal architecture. Questionable nodes at first examination will become clearly normal or abnormal with magnification. Magnification is least helpful when there is no node superimposition.

Direct magnification has been used by Ditchek and Scanlon (1967). In order to use direct ×2 magnification, a focal spot of 0.3 mm is needed. The advertised 0.3-mm focal spot may actually increase to 0.5 mm or become distorted at conventional milliamperage and kilovoltage. Special nonbiased tubes for 0.3-mm and under focal spots may be purchased, but they are expensive and not absolutely essential for lymphography.

### Follow-up

The needles are removed after the injection has been terminated. The wound is thoroughly cleansed with a saline scrub, sutured with 4-0 silk, and covered with Band-aids. The sutures are removed after 12 days by the patient's physician or radiologist.

Follow-up films of the abdomen are made to evaluate progress of treatment or recurrent disease until the node contains insufficient amounts of contrast material for evaluation.

## BREAST LYMPHOGRAPHY

Kett et al. (1970) performed direct lymphography of the breast on 88 patients by injecting 0.2 ml of an equal mixture of 11% patent blue dye and 1% lidocaine into the region of the mammary areola. The exposure is similar to pedal lymphography, but cannulation is much more difficult because of deep small fragile lymphatics and chest movement. After cannulation, 2 ml of Ethiodol are injected. The authors find direct lymphography useful for differentiating lymph node metastases from breast cancer. Because the procedure is time consuming and somewhat difficult, it has not gained wide acceptance.

## THYROID LYMPHOGRAPHY

Gruart et al. (1967) attempted to outline the cervical lymph nodes by injecting 8 ml of Ethiodol into the muscles at the base of the tongue and having the patient chew. Matoba and Kikuchi (1969) described a method of injecting Lipiodol ultrafluid directly into the thyroid gland. This outlines the gland and its nodules by spreading throughout the periacinar tissues. Later the external thyroid lymphatics and nodes fill. Many have found this method to be successful (Beales et al., 1971; Compana et al., 1974; Pelu et al., 1974; Sachdeva et al., 1974).

Although the method offers information about thyroid disease and is safe and trouble free, little physiological information is gained. Small parts scanning with the 10-MHz ultrasound units have completely obviated any clinical need for thyroid lymphography.

## REFERENCES

Arts V: An injection apparatus for lymphangiography. *AJR* 100:466, 1967.

Beales JS, Nundy S, Taylor S: Thyroid lymphography. *Br J Surg* 58:168, 1971.

Bruun S, Engeset A: Lymphadenography. *Acta Radiol* 45:389, 1956.

Clementz B, Olin T: Apparatus for controlled infusion of saline in angiography and contrast medium in lymphography. *Acta Radiol* 55:109, 1961.

Compana FP, DeAntoni E, Cordone MN, DiMatteo G: Thyrolymphadenography and thyroid scintigraphy. A diagnostic comparison. *Minerva Chir* 29:335, 1974.

Cusick H, Panning WP: A simple practical technique of lymphography. *Radiology* 88:576, 1967.

Damascelli B, Musumeci R, Uslenghi C: Instruments for lymphography. *Lymphology* 2:166, 1969.

Davidson JW: Lipid embolism to the brain following lymphography. *AJR* 105:763, 1969.

DeRoo T: An improved, simple technique of lymphography. *AJR* 98:948, 1966.

DeRoo T, Thomas P, Kropholler RW: The importance of tomography for the interpretation of lymphographic picture of lymph node metastases. *AJR* 94:924, 1965.

Ditchek T, Scanlon GT: Direct magnification lymphography. *JAMA* 199:654, 1967.

Doss LL, Alyea JL, Waggoner CM, Schroeder TT: Fluorescein-aided isolation of lymphatic vessels for lymphangiography. *AJR* 134:603, 1980.

Fischer HW: Lymphangiography and lymphadenography with various contrast agents. *Ann NY Acad Sci* 78:799, 1959a.

Fischer HW: A critique of experimental lymphography. *Acta Radiol* 52:448, 1959b.

Gangolli SD, Grasso P, Goldberg L: Physical factors determining the early local tissue reactions produced by food colourings and other compounds injected subcutaneously. *Food Cosmet Toxicol* 5:601, 1967.

Gilchrist MR: Lymphangiography. A local evaluation. *Minn Med* 48:1000, 1965.

Gruart FJ, Yoel J, Wagner AM: Value of perilingual lymphography in cancer of the head and neck. A means of exploration of the lymphatic system of the neck. *Am J Surg* 114:520, 1967.

Hirsh JI, Tisnado J, Cho SR, Beachley MC: Use of isofulfan blue for identification of lymphatic vessels: experimental and clinical evaluation. *AJR* 139:1061, 1982.

Howland WJ: A cannula method for lymphography. *AJR* 114:830, 1972.

Hreschyshyn MM, Sheehan F, Holland JF: Visualization of retroperitoneal lymph nodes. Lymphangiography as an aid in the measurement of tumor growth. *Cancer* 14:205, 1961.

Hudak S, McMaster PD: The lymphatic participation in human cutaneous phenomenon. A study of the minute lymphatics of the living skin. *J Exp Med* 57:751, 1933.

Iriarte P, Jagasia H, Thurman WG: Lymphangiography for malignant disease in children. *JAMA* 188:501, 1964.

Jing BS: Improved technique of lymphangiography. *AJR* 98:952, 1966.

Kapdi CC: Lymphography without the use of vital dyes. *Radiology* 133:795, 1979.

Kett K, Varga G, Lukac S: Direct lymphography of the breast. *Lymphology* 1:3, 1970.

Kinmonth JB: Lymphangiography in man: a method of outlining lymphatic trunks at operation. *Clin Sci* 11:13, 1952.

Koehler RP: Discussion: pulmonary hazards of lymphography (Threefoot SA). *Cancer Chemother Rep* 52:110, 1968.

Koehler RP, Meyers WA, Skelley JF, Schaffer B: Body distribution of Ethiodol following lymphangiography. *Radiology* 82:866, 1964.

Kropholler RW, Blom JMH, Irto I: Lymfografie met behulp van een polyeencatheter. *Ned Tijdschr Geneeskd* 112:696, 1968.

Lee KF, Roy WM, Hodes PJ: Improved techniques of lymphography: reliable isolation and cannulation method. *J Can Assoc Radiol* 20:48, 1969.

Mannila T, Wiljasalo M: Stereolymphography. *Ann Med Intern Fenn* 54:139, 1965.

Matoba N, Kikuchi T: Thyroidolymphography. *Radiology* 92:239, 1969.

Mortazavi SH, Burrows BD: Allergic reactions to patent blue dye in lymphangiography. *Clin Radiol* 22:389, 1971.

Pelu T, Modigliani V, Dal Pozzo G, Carini L: Thyroid adenolymphography. *Minerva Chir* 29:261, 1974.

Riveros M, Garcia R, Cabanas R: Lymphadenography of the dorsal lymphatics of the penis. Technique and results. *Cancer* 20:2026, 1967.

Sachdeva HS, Chowdhary GC, Bose SM, Gupta BB, Wig JD: Thyroid lymphography. *Arch Surg* 109:385, 1974.

Sigurjonsson K: Lymphography without the aid of vital dyes. *Lymphology* 7:121, 1974.

Sokol GH, Clouse ME, Kotner LM, Sewell JB: Complications of lymphangiography in patients of advanced age. *AJR* 128:43, 1977.

Tegtmeyer CJ: A new technique for cannulating lymphatic vessels: experience in 140 extremities. *Lymphology* 7:116, 1974.

Threefoot SA: Some chemical, physical and biological characteristics of dyes used to visualize lymphatics. *J Appl Physiol* 15:925, 1960.

Threefoot SA: Pulmonary hazards of lymphography. *Cancer Chemother Rep* 52:107, 1968.

Tong ECK: Improved technique of lymphatic cannulation for lymphography. Experience with 300 cases. *AJR* 107:877, 1969.

Turner AF: Lymphangiographic needle clamp. *AJR* 96:1053, 1966.

Viamonte M: Advances in lymphangioadenography. *Acta Radiol (Diagn) (Stockh)* 2:394, 1964.

Viamonte M, Stevens RC: A new tracer for lymphatic cannulation. *Radiology* 86:934, 1966.

Wallace S, Jackson L, Schaffer B, Gould J, Greening R, Weiss A, Kramer S: Lymphangiograms: their diagnostic and therapeutic potential. *Radiology* 76:179, 1961.

Youker JE: A clamp to facilitate lymphangiography. *Br J Radiol* 39:556, 1966.

Zheutlin N, Shanbrom E: Contrast visualization of lymph nodes. *Radiology* 71:702, 1958.

# 5

# *Physiology—Lymph Formation, Its Control, and Lymph Flow*

THOMAS H. ADAIR, Ph.D., AND ARTHUR C. GUYTON, M.D.

The lymphatic system is a drainage system through which fluid is actively pumped from the interstitial spaces to the blood vascular system. Most tissues of the body have lymphatic vessels. Exceptions are the superficial portions of the skin, the central nervous system, the deeper portion of peripheral nerves, the endomysium of muscles, and bones (Rusznyák et al., 1960; Yoffey and Courtice, 1970; Guyton, 1981), although even these tissues often have small interstitial channels called *prelymphatics* through which interstitial fluid can flow into nearby lymphatic vessels. The lymphatic system begins with very small *lymphatic capillaries* that are similar to blood capillaries but much larger (about 5-fold), thinner-walled, and infinitely more permeable (Casley-Smith and Florey, 1961; Leak and Burke, 1968a, b; Leak, 1970). The lymphatic capillaries coalesce to form *collecting lymphatics*, and these join to form large *lymphatic trunks*.

Small amounts of fluid containing plasma proteins continually leak from blood capillaries into the interstitium. The most important physiological function of the lymphatic system is to return this extravasated fluid and plasma protein to the blood vascular system (Mayerson, 1963; Guyton et al., 1975). This is especially true for protein because there is no other pathway through which this can return to the blood.

The lymphatic system also removes particulate matter, such as bits of degenerating tissue, particles of dirt, and bacteria from the interstitium (Rusznyák et al., 1960; Mayerson, 1963; Yoffey and Courtice, 1970), but this aspect of lymphatic function is not considered in this chapter. Instead, the emphasis of this chapter is on how the lymphatic system functions physiologically to help maintain a constant interstitial fluid volume by continuously returning extravasated protein and fluid to the blood vascular system. To understand how this system performs this function, it is first necessary to study the physical characteristics of the interstitium and, especially, how interstitial fluid is formed.

## INTERSTITIUM AND INTERSTITIAL FLUID

### Anatomy

The average 70-kg man has approximately 11 liters of fluid occupying the spaces between cells (Aukland and Nicolaysen, 1981; Guyton, 1981). Collectively, the spaces are called the *interstitium*, and fluid in these spaces is *interstitial fluid*. Within the interstitium are two major types of solid structures, called *collagen fibers* and *proteoglycan filaments* (Fig. 5.1). The collagen fibers have tensile strengths approaching one-sixth that of mild steel (Chapil, 1967) and provide most of the tensional strength of the tissues. Between the collagen bundles is a so-called ground substance containing billions of proteoglycan filaments that entrap the interstitial fluid. Weak cross-links among the proteoglycan filaments, collagen fibers, and protein molecules give the ground substance a gel-like consistency (Guyton et al., 1975; Granger, 1981).

Although perhaps 99.9% of interstitial fluid is normally trapped within the proteoglycan gel, small isolated vesicles and rivulets containing *free interstitial fluid* are also present (Gersh and Catchpole, 1960; Wiederhielm, 1972; Guyton et al., 1975). When tracer molecules are injected into circulating blood, they can be found flowing through the interstitium in small rivulets (Casley-Smith, 1981). On the other hand, interstitial fluid within vesicles is normally immobilized because vesicles are physically isolated and cannot move throughout the ground substance. In edematous states, clusters of vesicles become larger and more numerous, and they eventually coalesce, forming large spaces containing freely mobile interstitial fluid (Dennis, 1959).

gradient ($\pi c$-$\pi i$) is 23.5 mm Hg. Therefore, the net driving pressure is 30.2 − 23.5 or 6.7 mm Hg and is directed toward the interstitium, causing fluid to be filtered into the interstitium as indicated by the *arrows*. At the venous end of the capillary, the transcapillary hydrostatic pressure gradient is only 16.4 mm Hg, whereas the transcapillary colloid osmotic pressure gradient is 22.5 mm Hg. Therefore, at the venous end of the capillary the net driving pressure is 16.4 − 22.5 or −6.1 mm Hg and is directed back toward the capillary, causing fluid to be absorbed from the interstitium into the venous end of the capillary. The figure also shows the net driving pressure in the middle of the capillary to be +0.3 mm Hg, which causes a small but continuous filtration of fluid into the interstitium. Therefore, in the average capillary the rate of filtration of fluid into the interstitium slightly exceeds the rate of absorption of fluid from the interstitium.

In the entire human body about 20–40 liters of fluid are filtered into the interstitium each day. Most of this fluid is then absorbed by the capillaries, but about 2–4 liters of fluid containing approximately 100 g of plasma protein are not absorbed and must be carried away by the lymphatic system (Landis and Pappenheimer, 1963; Yoffey and Courtice, 1970; Guyton et al., 1975). The most vital physiological function of the lymphatic system is to remove continuously this excess protein from the tissue spaces and to return it to the systemic circulation. If the net rate of protein movement into the interstitium exceeds the capacity of the lymphatic system to remove protein, edema fluid will accumulate and the tissues will expand.

## FORMATION OF LYMPH

Lymph is simply the fluid in the lymphatic system. Near the end of the last century, the mechanism of lymph formation was critically debated. At the present time, essentially all investigators agree that perhaps 99.9% of lymph is simply interstitial fluid that has entered lymphatics from the interstitium through very large gaps in the lymphatic capillaries. In other words, lymph is formed in exactly the same way that interstitial fluid is formed, by filtration of fluid first through the blood capillary membrane, then passive flow of this fluid through the interstitium into the lymphatic capillaries. During its course through the interstitial spaces, the composition of interstitial fluid may be changed very slightly as nutrients are removed and metabolites are added, but this modification is usually so small it may be neglected. For all practical purposes, the fluid entering lymphatic capillaries is exactly the same as the free interstitial fluid (Yoffey and Courtice, 1970; Taylor et al., 1973). Lymph can probably be modified after it enters the lymphatic system by filtration or absorption of fluid through the lymphatic endothelium.

### Permeability of Lymphatic Capillaries

Interstitial fluid flows freely into lymphatic capillaries through large gaps between the lymphatic endothelial cells. These gaps offer little or no resistance to flow of interstitial fluid into lymphatic capillaries. Electron microscopic studies have shown the gaps to be sufficiently large to allow a variety of substances to pass through them, such as ferritin molecules, latex spheres, carbon particles, bacteria, and even red blood cells (Casley-Smith, 1964a, b, 1967; Allen, 1967). Because the gaps are not fixed in the anatomic sense, any given gap can intermittently open and close. A closed gap may cause fluid and particles to dam up temporarily in adjacent tissue, but, as fluid begins to accumulate and the tissue begins to expand, gaps seem to open up, allowing fluid and particles to enter the lymphatic capillary freely. Therefore, lymphatic capillaries are sufficiently permeable to accommodate passage of essentially all particulate matter that normally finds its way into interstitial spaces.

The ultrastructure of a typical lymphatic capillary is shown in Figure 5.3, which shows some of the various types of junctions between endothelial cells (Leak, 1970). The structural features of lymphatic capillaries that cause them to be more permeable than blood capillaries may be summarized as follows:

1. Unlike blood capillaries, lymphatic capillaries have a discontinuous basement membrane that exposes a large part of the endothelial cell surface to interstitial fluid.

2. As shown in Figure 5.3, lymphatic endothelium is very thin except in the perinuclear region.

3. Junctions between adjacent endothelial cells are completely open in some areas, whereas in other areas the cells are firmly attached. The open junctions form gaps that offer essentially no resistance to passage of fluid, protein, and even large particulate material.

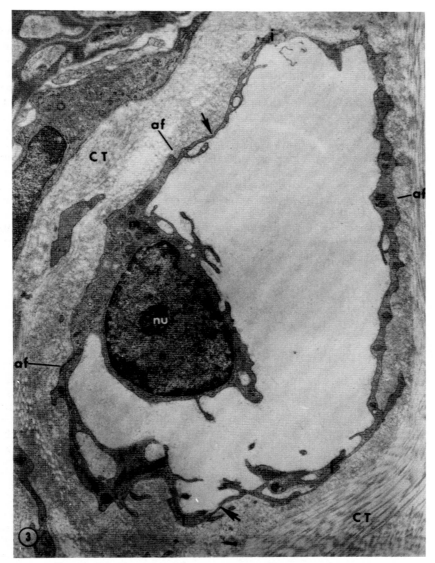

**FIGURE 5.3. ELECTRON MICROGRAPH OF A LYMPHATIC CAPILLARY**
Note the areas of overlap of endothelial cells and other points, at the *arrows*, where the cells are beginning to pull apart at their junctions. *af*, anchoring filaments; *CT*, connective tissue; *m*, mitochondria, *n*, nucleus; *nu*, nucleolus; *i*, intercellular junction. (From Leak, 1970.)

## Permeability of Larger Lymphatic Vessels

In contrast to lymphatic capillaries, larger lymphatic vessels are thought to have permeability characteristics similar to those of blood vessels. A number of studies have shown larger lymphatic vessels to be almost totally impermeable to plasma proteins and other macromolecules (Patterson et al., 1958; Mayerson et al., 1962; Renkin, 1979). In fact, studies indicate that they are capable of retaining solutes with molecular weights as low as 10,000. Therefore, once the proteins of interstitial fluid have entered the

lymphatic system through lymphatic capillaries, they seem to be trapped until they are eventually emptied into the systemic venous circulation.

## Lymph as Measure of Interstitial Fluid

Even though larger lymphatic vessels are normally almost totally impermeable to proteins and other macromolecules, there is little doubt that the lymphatics are freely permeable to water and most electrolytes. This means that imbalances in hydrostatic and osmotic pressure gradients across the lymphatic endothelium will cause fluid to be absorbed from the lymph or filtered into the lymph, according to the Starling hypothesis discussed previously (Guyton et al., 1979). Yet, for nearly a century many investigators have considered the protein concentration and colloid osmotic pressure of free interstitial fluid and lymph from the tissues to be identical. The reason for using lymph as a measure of free interstitial fluid is that lymph can be collected relatively easily, whereas interstitial fluid is still almost impossible to collect from nonedematous tissues.

Whether this assumption is valid is important for many reasons, but primarily because the colloid pressure of free interstitial fluid is one of the four Starling forces governing fluid balance in normal capillaries. At the present time, the majority of evidence suggesting that interstitial fluid and lymph from a tissue have identical protein concentrations and, therefore, identical colloid osmotic pressures has been derived from statistical studies. However, a growing belief among some physiologists is that protein-free fluid is continuously filtered out of the lymphatics. By continually filtering protein-free fluid from lymph into the tissues, proteins would become concentrated in the lymph. Therefore, the concentration of protein measured in lymph could be higher than the concentration of protein in interstitial fluid from which lymph is formed. Recent studies from our laboratories have demonstrated that lymph nodes can concentrate lymph proteins as much as 3-fold by continuously absorbing protein-free fluid from the lymph as it passes through the node (Adair et al., 1982a, b).

## INTERSTITIAL FLUID PROTEIN

By far the most important physiological function of the lymphatic system is to remove excess plasma protein from the interstitium. Even though most capillaries are almost totally impermeable to plasma proteins, this is never an absolute impermeability. Therefore, capillaries continually leak at least some protein into the interstitium, and over a 24-hr period the total amount of protein leaked equals about one-half the total amount of protein in all of the plasma. Yet, only a small portion of the protein can diffuse backward into the capillaries because the concentration of protein in the capillaries is greater than the concentration of protein in the interstitial fluid. As a result, nearly all protein that enters the interstitium must be returned to the systemic circulation by the lymphatic system. Without the lymphatic system, protein concentration and colloid osmotic pressure of the interstitial fluid would become so high within a few hours to a few days that capillary filtration dynamics would become very abnormal.

### Normal Concentration

The fluid that filters into the interstitium through arterial ends of capillaries has an average protein concentration of about 0.2 g/100 ml in subcutaneous tissue (Landis and Pappenheimer, 1963; Guyton, 1981). Approximately 90% of the fluid portion of this ultrafiltrate is then absorbed by the venous ends of capillaries; however, the absorbed fluid contains very little protein because there can be little diffusion of protein into the blood against the protein concentration gradient at the capillary wall. The result is that one-tenth of the fluid in the original capillary ultrafiltrate (containing essentially all of the filtered protein) remains unabsorbed and becomes interstitial fluid. Therefore, protein concentration of the ultrafiltrate has increased 10-fold, and the result is an average concentration of 2.0 g/100 ml in subcutaneous tissues. Thus, this mechanism continually concentrates proteins in the interstitial fluid even before the fluid flows into the lymphatic capillaries.

### Effect of Lymph Flow

Figure 5.4 schematically illustrates the relationship between lymph flow and interstitial fluid protein concentration. Lymph flow is equal to net filtration rate in this figure because in a steady state, when a tissue is neither gaining nor losing weight, lymph flow is equal to the rate of fluid filtration into the interstitium minus the rate of fluid absorption from the interstitium. The *solid curve* in the figure shows how the protein concentration of interstitial fluid changes when lymph flow (or net filtration) increases from zero to very high levels.

Because interstitial fluid is an ultrafiltrate of plasma, the protein concentration of interstitial fluid cannot become greater than the protein concentration of plasma (Guyton et al., 1975). The figure shows that when lymph flow is zero— that is, capillary filtration = capillary absorption—the protein concentration of interstitial fluid becomes exactly the same as the protein concentration of plasma. The reason for this is simply that the plasma proteins that do filter or diffuse into the interstitium become mainly trapped in the interstitium because fewer of them can diffuse backward into the capillary than in the forward direction because of their forward concentration gradient. Once the protein concentration of interstitial fluid becomes equal to the protein concentration of plasma, the proteins do then diffuse into the capillary as easily as out of the capillary. Therefore, when lymph flow is zero (capillary filtration = capillary absorption), the protein concentration of interstitial fluid will eventually become equal to the protein concentration of the plasma.

Figure 5.4 also shows that as lymph flow increases, protein concentration of interstitial fluid decreases. At very high rates of lymph flow, the protein concentration of interstitial fluid decreases maximally and becomes nearly equal to the protein concentration of capillary filtrate (Guyton et al., 1975; Taylor, 1981). This inverse relationship between lymph flow and interstitial fluid protein concentration has been demonstrated experimentally in lung, hindpaw, intestine, and other tissues by simply raising capillary pressure, measuring lymph flow and lymph protein concentration, and assuming that the protein concentration of lymph is equal to the protein concentration of free interstitial fluid (Taylor, 1981). The relationship can be explained by the following mechanism.

### Dissipation of Protein Concentration

Proteins are normally concentrated in the interstitial fluid for the reasons explained above, but the degree to which they are concentrated depends on the fraction of fluid in the capillary filtrate that is absorbed. If none of the fluid is absorbed, the protein concentration of interstitial fluid will become equal to the protein concentration of capillary filtrate. Conversely, if all of the fluid in the capillary filtrate is absorbed, the protein concentration of the interstitial fluid will become extremely high. As lymph flow increases, a smaller fraction of the capillary filtrate is absorbed because lymph flow is equal to the amount of fluid filtered out of the capillaries minus the amount of fluid absorbed by the capillaries. Therefore, as lymph flow increases, the proteins are concentrated to a lesser extent in the interstitium. If lymph flow were infinitely high, an infinitely small fraction of capillary filtrate would be absorbed so that the protein concentration of interstitial fluid would become equal to the protein concentration of capillary filtrate. Although it is impossible to achieve in-

finite lymph flow in physiological systems, lymph flow can be increased as much as 20- to 50-fold. Under such conditions the protein concentration of interstitial fluid can approach the protein concentration of capillary filtrate.

### Lymph Flow Effect during Increased Capillary Permeability

The *dashed curve* in Figure 5.4 illustrates that increasing lymph flow during increased capillary protein permeability causes the interstitial fluid protein concentration to decrease but not to the same low level as achieved in normal tissue (Taylor, 1981). Increased capillary protein permeability simply means that the size of pores in the capillary membrane is increased. The protein concentration of interstitial fluid is greater at any given lymph flow when protein permeability is increased because the protein concentration of capillary filtrate is then greater than normal due to easier movement of protein molecules through the capillary membrane. Therefore, the relationship between lymph flow and interstitial fluid protein concentration during increased capillary permeability can be explained in exactly the same manner as in normal tissues. The reason that the increased permeability curve of Figure 5.4 is shifted upward is simply that the protein concentration of the capillary filtrate is greater than in normal tissues.

In the liver, increased lymph flow is often associated with an increase in protein concentration of interstitial fluid, a phenomenon exactly opposite to that observed in most other tissues. The reason for this difference has been explained in the following way. Capillaries in the liver are normally so permeable to proteins that protein molecules are not sieved by the capillary wall to an appreciable extent. Instead, most of the protein sieving is believed to occur beyond the capillary membrane by the solid structures of the interstitial matrix. When excess capillary filtration occurs in the liver, the liver begins to swell, and the rate of liver lymph flow also increases. Because of the swelling, solid structures of the interstitium begin to separate, allowing proteins to move more freely through the interstitium (Granger et al., 1979; Laine et al., 1979). In this situation interstitial fluid that reaches a lymphatic capillary now has a protein concentration approaching the concentration in the plasma. In effect, then, factors that increase liver lymph flow cause an apparent increase in capillary permeability at the same time, thereby causing the protein concentration of the interstitial fluid to increase rather than to decrease.

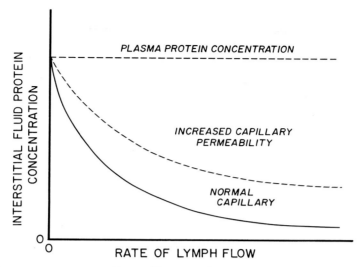

FIGURE 5.4. RELATIONSHIP BETWEEN LYMPH FLOW AND INTERSTITIAL FLUID PROTEIN CONCENTRATION

## Feedback Control

We have already seen that plasma protein is continually concentrated in the interstitial fluid by the capillary filtration-absorption phenomenon. As protein molecules accumulate in interstitial fluid, the protein concentration and colloid osmotic pressure of interstitial fluid increase. The increase in osmotic pressure in turn automatically increases the rate of fluid filtration out of the capillary and decreases the rate of fluid absorption into the capillary. This causes lymph flow to increase, thereby decreasing the protein concentration and colloid osmotic pressure (Fig. 5.4). In other words, a high colloid osmotic pressure produces increased lymph flow, and the increased lymph flow in turn decreases the colloid osmotic pressure of the interstitial fluid back toward normal; thus, the excess colloid osmotic pressure is corrected. To summarize, an increase in interstitial fluid protein increases the rate of lymph flow, and this washes the excess proteins out of the interstitium, automatically returning the protein concentration to its normal low level.

## Importance of Protein Control

The lymphatic system provides the only means by which interstitial fluid protein can be removed from the tissues. This is the most important physiological function of the lymphatic system because without the lymphatic system the interstitial fluid protein concentration would progressively increase and eventually approach the protein concentration of the plasma, at which point normal capillary filtration dynamics would no longer occur, and life would no longer continue. No other function of the lymphatic system can even approach this in importance.

## LYMPHATIC PUMP

The lymphatic system is endowed with millions of tiny pumps that actively propel lymph from the tissues to the venous circulation. Each pump consists of a short segment of lymphatic vessel between two bicuspid valves. Because the one-way valves can withstand back pressures of over 70 mm Hg in some cases (Ohhashi et al., 1980a), the lymph almost never flows backward through the valves toward the tissues of origin. Therefore, any force that intermittently compresses a lymphatic will automatically send the lymph flowing toward the openings into the venous circulation.

### Pumping by Extrinsic Lymphatic Compression

Compression of lymphatics by extrinsic tissue forces will cause the lymph to flow forward along the lymphatics. Such extrinsic pumping forces are generated by respiratory movements, muscle contractions, arterial pulsations, and simple passive movements.

#### Respiratory Movements

Rhythmic movements associated with breathing are thought to be especially important for pumping lymph in the thoracic duct, cisterna chyli, and other larger lymphatics in the chest and abdomen (Yoffey and Courtice, 1970). Respiratory motion of the diaphragm is particularly important for removing fluid and other substances from the peritoneal cavity (Allen, 1967). The peritoneal surface of the diaphragm has many large pores that connect with an extensive system of diaphragmatic lymphatics. As the surface of the diaphragm enlarges during expiration, the pores and lymphatics are pulled open. This creates a negative pressure or vacuum in the lymphatics that literally sucks fluid, cells, and other substances from the peritoneal cavity through the pores and into the diaphragmatic lymphatics. During inspiration the pores are closed tight and the lymphatics are compressed by the contracting diaphragm, forcing lymph to flow forward toward the thoracic duct (Allen, 1967; Bettendorf, 1978). This pumping mechanism provides the major pathway for absorption of blood from the abdominal cavity following peritoneal blood transfusions in infants (Allen, 1967).

*Muscle Contraction*

Rhythmic contraction and relaxation of skeletal muscle during brief periods of walking or running increases lymph flow up to 20-fold in dogs (White et al., 1933). Similarly, dye injected intradermally in human forearms enters the lymphatics sooner and moves along the lymphatics faster when the arm is briefly exercised (McMaster, 1937). On the other hand, recent studies have indicated that prolonged periods of mild exercise do not sustain the increase in lymph flow from superficial leg lymphatics in humans (Olszewski and Engeset, 1980). For the extrinsic muscle pump to produce a sustained increase in lymph flow, the rate of formation of lymph must be increased as well. Moderate or severe exercise would probably increase the rate of lymph formation (Hall et al., 1965; Yoffey and Courtice, 1970), perhaps by increasing capillary pressure in the exercising tissues. Under this situation the extrinsic muscle pump would most likely produce a sustained increase in lymph flow.

*Arterial Pulsation*

Many of the larger lymphatics lie close to arteries, and arterial pulsations have actually been recorded from the thoracic duct and cisterna chyli (Cressman and Blalock, 1939; Webb and Starzl, 1953). Presumably, such variations in lymphatic hydrostatic pressure can produce

some degree of lymphatic pumping. In isolated perfused rabbit ears the rate of lymph flow, as estimated from the rate of dye movement along the lymphatics, was found to be nearly zero when the ear was perfused at constant pressure. When the same ear was perfused using pulsatile pressure, however, lymph flow increased 15- to 20-fold (Parsons and McMaster, 1938). The authors concluded that arterial pulsations increase lymphatic pumping as well as the rate of lymph formation.

**Intrinsic Pumping by Lymphatics**

Most lymphatic vessels, except the lymphatic capillaries, contain smooth muscle cells in their walls. These vessels have been shown to undergo rhythmic contractions in almost all mammals studied, including man, horse, sheep, mouse, rat, guinea pig, rabbit, squirrel, bat, and dog (Rusznyák et al., 1960; Yoffey and Courtice, 1970; Guyton et al., 1975; Aukland and Nicolaysen, 1981). In a few studies in which intrinsic lymphatic contractions were not observed, anesthesia or tissue trauma may have obscured the normal contractile activity (Guyton et al., 1975; Aukland and Nicolaysen, 1981). Therefore, it is very likely that intrinsic contractions of lymphatics, with the possible exception of the lymphatic capillaries, are a universal feature of the mammalian lymphatic system.

The quantitative physiological significance of the intrinsic pumping mechanism has not been adequately determined. In recent years much information has accumulated describing the physical characteristics of lymphatic contractions: how individual contractile units, consisting of a segment of lymphatic with its two valves, work in concert to propel lymph effectively; and how the nervous system and local physical factors might regulate the frequency and strength of lymphatic contractions to handle larger volumes of lymph automatically during excessive lymph formation.

*Strength and Frequency*

The ability of the intrinsic lymphatic pump to propel lymph can be better appreciated by looking at the frequency of lymphatic contractions and especially the tremendous pressures that can be generated by the contracting lymphatics. Pulsatile side pressures recorded from various lymphatics in awake sheep were found to range from 1–25 mm Hg, with pulse frequencies of 1–30/min (Hall et al., 1965). Systolic pressures recorded from freely flowing superficial leg lymphatics in human beings have reached 30 mm Hg even during complete rest (Olszewski et al., 1980). Furthermore, pulsatile end pressures recorded from obstructed lymphatics in resting human beings reached values greater than 100 mg Hg, with pulse frequencies up to 35/min (Olszewski et al., 1980). In some cases, therefore, the intrinsic lymphatic pump is sufficiently powerful to propel lymph against pressures approaching those generated by the heart.

### Contraction Cycle

When a lymphatic vessel contracts, a very rapid wave of constriction can often be seen moving along the lymphatic in the direction of lymph flow. In other cases an entire lymphatic may appear to contract all at once. Smith (1949) described how trypan blue dye entering lymphatics after intradermal injection flowed rapidly through several valved segments of a lymphatic with each wave of contraction. The dye front, pausing as the lymphatic relaxed, swiftly proceeded during the next wave of contraction, illustrating the ability of lymphatic contractions to propel lymph.

The contraction cycle of lymphatics has many features common to the cardiac cycle (McHale and Roddie, 1976). By continuously recording lymphatic pressures and flow and calculating lymphatic volume, McHale and Roddie (1976) were able to show that the contraction cycle of lymphatics consists of a systole and a diastole. Systole includes a phase of isovolumetric contraction followed by a phase of rapid ejection of lymph. Diastole begins with a phase of isovolumetric relaxation and ends with a prolonged filling phase during which lymphatic pressure and volume slowly increase until the next systole is initiated.

To understand how a chain of individual contractile units can work together to propel lymph effectively, it is first necessary to understand that stretching the walls of a contractile unit will automatically cause that unit to contract. One can then imagine that when a single unit contracts it forces lymph into the next adjacent unit. Then, as the walls of that unit stretch to accommodate the incoming lymph, it too contracts, forcing lymph on to the next unit and so on. The velocity of a wave of such contractions along the length of a lymphatic vessel is about 4–5 mm/sec in a bovine mesenteric lymphatic (Ohhashi et al., 1980a). Thus, one can understand why long stretches of a lymphatic might appear to contract almost all at once.

### Regulation

Perhaps the most important factor regulating the rate and strength of lymphatic contractions is the degree of stretch in the lymphatic wall (Mawhinney and Roddie, 1973; McHale and Roddie, 1976; Hargens and Zweifach, 1977; Ohhashi et al., 1980a). When lymphatic hydrostatic pressure increases, the wall of a lymphatic vessel stretches, increasing the frequency and strength of the individual lymphatic contractions. Yet, if pressure in the lymphatic becomes too great and the lymphatic becomes overstretched, in time the vessel will stop contracting and will relax in a state of marked dilatation. Smith (1949) demonstrated some of these principles by simply occluding lymph flow in a contracting lymphatic. Immediately following occlusion, lymph rapidly accumulated upstream from the occlusion. As the lymphatic walls began to stretch, both the rate and strength of the contractions increased for a time, until the lymphatic eventually became overstretched and quiescent.

Figure 5.5 shows results from actual experiments illustrating the response of isolated segments of contracting bovine mesenteric lym-

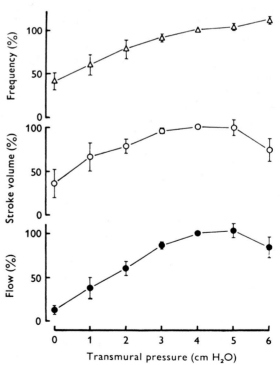

FIGURE 5.5. EFFECT OF TRANSMURAL PRESSURE ON FLOW, STROKE VOLUME, AND FREQUENCY OF CONTRACTION IN A LYMPHATIC
(From McHale and Roddie, 1976.)

phatics to increases in transmural pressure (McHale and Roddie, 1976). At first, as the transmural pressure of the isolated lymphatic was increased in 1-cm $H_2O$ steps, so too did the frequency, stroke volume, and rate of lymph flow increase. At the higher transmural pressures (greater than 5 cm $H_2O$), however, the vessel became overdistended, causing both the stroke volume and lymph flow to decrease.

Studies of mesenteric microlymphatics have shown that initiation of a lymphatic contraction partly depends on development of a threshold pressure (Hargens and Zweifach, 1977). For a given lymphatic, the authors could accurately predict a contraction by following the lymphatic hydrostatic pressure (or the lymphatic diameter) to a certain threshold level. Larger lymphatics were shown to have higher threshold pressures than smaller lymphatics. However, it is important to note that the lymphatics would continue to contract at lower frequencies when the lymphatic hydrostatic pressure was zero or even subatmospheric (Hargens and Zweifach, 1977). Such unstimulated contraction may reflect an inherent instability of lymphatic smooth muscle cells and suggests the existence of lymphatic pacemaker cells, thought to reside just downstream from a lymphatic valve (Ohhashi et al., 1980a). This type of unstimulated contraction could literally suck fluid from the tissues, helping to maintain a subatmospheric tissue fluid hydrostatic pressure (Guyton et al., 1971).

The lymphatic contractile mechanism appears to have a myogenic rather than neurogenic origin. That is, initiation of a lymphatic contraction does not require nervous stimuli; rather, it is mainly dependent on the degree of stretch of the vessel wall. A number of observations support this concept. First, lymphatics contract more rapidly and with greater force when the lymphatic wall is stretched. Second, lymphatics continue to contract in vitro when all nerves to the lymphatic are obviously severed (Mawhinney and Roddie, 1973; Ohhashi et al., 1980a). Third, lymphatics continue to contract in vivo for up to 1 hr after death (Campbell and Heath, 1973; Hargens and Zweifach, 1977). This phenomenon may explain why lymph continues to flow after death when the extrinsic pumping mechanism is obviously not operative.

Even though denervated lymphatics appear to be capable of pumping lymph, it is probable that in some instances nervous stimuli do play a role in regulating the strength and frequency of contractions, at least of larger lymphatics. The walls of lymphatics contain $\alpha$-adrenergic receptors

that are innervated by the autonomic nervous system (Acevedo, 1943; Russell et al., 1980). Electrical field stimulation or topical application of norepinephrine increases the rate of lymphatic contractions and decreases the amplitude of each individual contraction in a dose-related manner (Mawhinney and Roddie, 1973; Ohhashi et al., 1980b; Russell et al., 1980). Yet, exactly how a contracting lymphatic responds to normal levels of adrenergic stimulation is not entirely clear.

In summary, the intrinsic lymphatic pumping mechanism is primarily regulated myogenically. As lymph enters a segment of lymphatic, the lymphatic wall is stretched to some threshold level, whereupon a contraction is initiated. Greater stretching of the lymphatic wall produces stronger contractions of greater frequency. Yet, even without stretch, lymphatics continue to contract periodically, illustrating the possible presence of pacemaker cells in the lymphatic wall. The adrenergic nervous system may help to regulate the intrinsic lymphatic pump as suggested by the presence of adrenergic innervation of lymphatic vessels.

## Lymphatic Capillary Pump

Electron microscopy studies of the lymphatic capillary ultrastructure have provided strong evidence supporting the concept that lymphatic capillaries can also actively pump lymph.

### Structure

Figure 5.6 shows two structural features of the lymphatic capillary essential for pumping lymph: the valve-like slits between adjacent endothelial cells, and the anchoring filaments (Leak and Burke, 1968b). The anchoring filaments are hollow tubules with diameters of approximately 100 Å. They attach to the outer surface of endothelial cells and extend approximately 10 $\mu$m into the surrounding tissue where they are embedded in bundles of collagen fibers and in the ground substance of the tissues. In other words, the anchoring filaments tie the endothelial cells to the surrounding tissues. As fluid accumulates in the tissues and the structural elements in the tissues are pushed apart by the fluid, the lymphatic capillaries are automatically pulled open (Fig. 5.6) (Leak and Burke, 1968b). As the capillaries open, they automatically fill with interstitial fluid.

Figure 5.6 also shows that adjacent endothelial cells overlap. Because the anchoring filaments attach only to the outer flaps of endothelial cells,

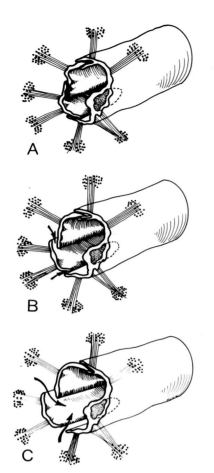

FIGURE 5.6. DRAWINGS OF A LYMPHATIC CAPILLARY
Note the progressive opening of valve-like slits between the endothelial cells (*arrows*) caused by expansion of the tissues with edema fluid. (From Leak, 1970.)

open the lymphatic capillaries and creating suction inside the capillaries. This suction pulls fluid from the surrounding tissue through the pores in the lymphatic capillary as the one-way flap valves are forced inward by the flowing fluid. Once the lymphatic capillary is completely filled and the lymph attempts to flow backward through the valves, the one-way valves automatically close, thus trapping the fluid in the capillary (Casley-Smith, 1967).

The fluid will then remain in the lymphatic capillary until the vessel is compressed by passive movements of the tissue, by contraction of a surrounding skeletal muscle, or even by contraction of the lymphatic endothelial cells themselves. The compressed lymphatic capillary will force the fluid forward into the collecting lymphatic and beyond the first bicuspid valve of this lymphatic; thus, the lymph is pumped forward by the lymphatic capillary and is trapped by the collecting lymphatic valve. Electron microscopy studies indicate that little if any fluid flows backward through the one-way flap valves when they are in a closed position.

In summary, the one-way flap valves of the lymphatic capillaries provide a unidirectional path for fluid to flow from the tissues into the lymphatic capillaries. Compression of the lymphatic capillaries forces the fluid on into the collecting lymphatics where the lymph is further pumped by the larger lymphatic pumping mechanism.

the inner flaps are free to open inward but cannot open outward. Fluid from outside the lymphatic capillary can push the inner flap open and flow into the capillary lumen. Once the fluid has entered the capillary, however, it cannot push the flaps outward to return to the surrounding tissue.

### Pumping Mechanism

Based on the ultrastructure of the lymphatic capillary, a mechanism has been proposed whereby the lymphatic capillary could pump lymph from the tissues (Allen, 1967; Casley-Smith, 1967; Leak and Burke, 1968a). The lymphatic capillary pump seems to operate in the following way. Fluid collects in the tissue, causing it to expand. As the tissue expands, the anchoring filaments act as guy wires, pulling

### Contraction of Capillary Endothelial Cells

Unlike the larger lymphatics, the lymphatic capillaries are not surrounded by smooth muscle cells, but the capillary endothelial cells do contain large numbers of filaments, which are thought to be actin or actomyosin filaments (Leak, 1970). Similar filaments have been identified in the endothelial cells of systemic blood capillaries as well and have been shown to cause the entire endothelial cell to contract when appropriately stimulated (Majno and Leventhal, 1967; Majno et al., 1969).

Lymphatic capillaries themselves have been observed to contract rhythmically in the bat's wing. Simultaneous measurements of hydrostatic pressure in both the lymphatic capillary and surrounding tissue spaces of the bat's wing have shown that immediately after a lymphatic capillary contraction is over, a subatmospheric pressure is recorded within the capillary lumen, which in turn provides a gradient for fluid to flow from the tissue into the capillary (Nicoll and Hogan, 1978; Hogan, 1981). Thus, it is probable that at least some lymphatic capillaries possess their own active pumping mechanism, even in the absence of outside compressive forces.

## DETERMINANTS OF LYMPH FLOW

Lymph flow has been measured in a variety of different organs and tissues by simply cannulating a lymphatic and measuring flow with calibrated pipettes or weighing techniques. In most organs, increases in lymph flow can be produced experimentally by increasing capillary hydrostatic pressure, decreasing plasma colloid osmotic pressure, or increasing capillary permeability. In other words, any factor that increases the net rate of fluid filtration from the capillaries also increases the lymph flow because lymph flow is equal to capillary filtration minus capillary absorption. Lymph flow increases almost linearly with increases in capillary filtration until capillary filtration becomes extremely high, at which point further increases in capillary filtration will cause lymph flow to respond in one of two ways: lymph flow may reach a plateau beyond which it will not rise further, or lymph flow may actually decrease (Guyton et al., 1975; Taylor, 1981).

### Interstitial Fluid Hydrostatic Pressure

Recent studies have demonstrated that increasing interstitial fluid pressure from normally negative values to positive values produces the nonlinear effect on lymph flow illustrated in Figure 5.7 (Taylor et al., 1973; Guyton et al., 1975). This experiment was performed in the dog hindlimb by measuring interstitial fluid pressure in perforated capsules permanently implanted subcutaneously and by measuring lymph flow from an adjacent subcutaneous lymph vessel during the development of edema. Qualitatively, the same relationship between interstitial fluid pressure and lymph flow was achieved whether the edema was created by obstructing venous outflow from the leg or by intravenously infusing large quantities of balanced electrolyte solution.

The figure shows that at the normal interstitial fluid pressure of about −6 mm Hg lymph flow was almost zero. As fluid began to collect in the tissues and the interstitial fluid pressure began to increase, lymph flow increased dramatically (about 20-fold) until the interstitial fluid pressure reached 0–2 mm Hg. Further increases in interstitial fluid pressure did not produce further increases in lymph flow. In effect, therefore, up to an interstitial fluid pressure of 2 mm Hg,

lymph flow is roughly related to the product of interstitial fluid pressure and the ability of the lymphatic pump to pull fluid out of the interstitium (Guyton, 1981).

One of the most important aspects of the relationship shown in Figure 5.7 is that lymph flow increases greatly as interstitial fluid pressure increases from normally negative values up to about zero but does not increase further when the interstitial fluid pressure increases much above zero (that is, much above atmospheric pressure). This means that the ability of the lymphatic system to oppose increases in the interstitial fluid volume (edema) occurs to its maximum extent before the interstitial fluid pressure rises much above zero. Because edema fluid does not significantly accumulate in the tissues until the interstitial fluid pressure becomes positive, the lymphatic compensatory mechanism against edema manifests itself before the edema actually occurs. That is, by the time a tissue has become edematous, the lymph flow has probably already increased to its maximum extent.

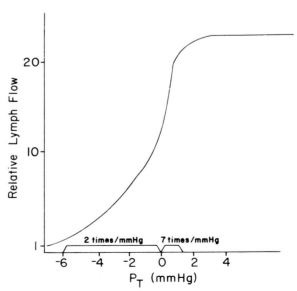

FIGURE 5.7. RELATIONSHIP BETWEEN INTERSTITIAL FLUID PRESSURE AND LYMPH FLOW

The graph illustrates the maximum level of lymph flow that is attained when the interstitial fluid pressure rises to positive values. (From Taylor et al., 1973.)

## Capillary Filtration

Lymph flow increases almost linearly with increases in capillary filtration until a point is reached where further increases in capillary filtration produce a variable effect on lymph flow, depending on the tissue. As Figure 5.8 illustrates, lymph flow may respond in one of two ways when capillary filtration is raised to very high levels. In subcutaneous tissue and muscle, lymph flow reaches a plateau at high filtration rates beyond which further increases in capillary filtration do not produce further increases in lymph flow (Guyton et al., 1975; Taylor, 1981). In intestine and lung, lymph flow may actually decrease even though capillary filtration continues to increase (Granger et al., 1977; Parker et al., 1979).

## Plateau in Lymph Flow

The reasons why lymph flow reaches an upper limit even though capillary filtration continues to increase are not known, but three possibilities have been offered to explain this effect.

### Failure of Lymphatic Capillary Pump

At high filtration rates the tissues become edematous. As edema fluid collects and solid structures of the tissue begin to separate, junctions between endothelial cells of lymphatic capillaries also begin to separate because they are tethered to solid structures of the tissue by anchoring filaments. Once spaces between endothelial cells are pulled open, endothelial cell flap valves become incompetent, allowing fluid to flow out of the lymphatic capillary as easily as into the lymphatic capillary. Therefore, when capillary filtration increases to the point that interstitial fluid pressure becomes positive and frank edema begins to develop, the lymphatic capillary pump is likely to become completely incompetent and unable to cause lymph flow to increase further (Guyton et al., 1975).

Even without the lymphatic capillary pump, however, the larger lymphatic pumping mechanism should still be able to pump fluid from the tissues when the interstitial fluid pressure is high. Therefore, it is likely that the plateau in lymph flow must also be related to failure of the lymphatic pumping mechanism of the larger lymphatics. The following two possibilities explain how the larger lymphatic pumping mechanisms could fail.

### Maximum Capacity of Larger Lymphatic Pump

The plateau in lymph flow observed at high rates of capillary filtration may be simply due to the fact that the lymphatic pump can pump so much and no more. Just as the heart has a maximum limit as to the amount of blood it can pump, the larger lymphatic pump must have an upper limit as well. The *bottom graph* in Figure 5.5 shows that the amount of fluid pumped by an isolated bovine mesenteric lymphatic increased progressively as transmural pressure increased until an upper limit of pumping was reached. Further increases in transmural pressure caused less lymph to be pumped, suggesting that the lymphatic pump was beginning to fail. Therefore, the upper limit of lymph flow may simply express maximum pumping capacity of the lymphatic pump.

### Lymphatic Compression by Positive Interstitial Pressure

As interstitial fluid pressure becomes positive and tissues become edematous, interstitial fluid presses on the outsides of larger lymphatics, which tends to flatten them for they are not tethered to solid structures of tissue as are lymphatic capillaries. If interstitial fluid pressure causes lymphatics to collapse, then further increases in lymph flow would not be possible (Guyton et al., 1975).

## Volume Overflow

The lymphatic system provides the major pathway for removing excess fluid and protein

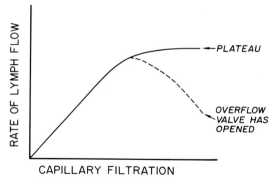

FIGURE 5.8. EFFECT OF INCREASING CAPILLARY FILTRATION ON LYMPH FLOW

In subcutaneous tissue and muscle, lymph flow reaches a plateau even though capillary filtration continues to increase. Lung and intestine often exhibit the relationship illustrated by the *dashed curve*, however, indicating that an overflow valve opens to cause lymph flow to decrease. (From Taylor, 1981, by permission of the American Heart Association, Inc.)

from the tissues; however, in several organs an-other type of system provides an alternative route through which interstitial fluid can leave the tissue when edema becomes severe. Such a system is called a *volume overflow system*; it actually means loss of the fluid into a cavity, such as the peritoneal cavity, alveoli, or intes-tinal lumen. Thus, when lymph flow has in-creased to its maximum extent in the liver, lung, or intestines and edema begins to develop, some of the edema fluid enters the volume overflow system (Taylor, 1981).

Two organs with volume overflow systems (lung and intestine) have been shown experimen-tally to exhibit the relationship between lymph flow and capillary filtration illustrated in Figure 5.8 by the *dashed curve*. When edema becomes progressively more severe in these organs, the amount of edema fluid that enters the volume overflow system also becomes progressively greater (Taylor, 1981), thus decreasing the amount of fluid that drains into the lymph. The mechanism for this is not well understood, but valves or gates to the volume overflow system may open wider and wider as more fluid goes through.

## INTERSTITIAL FLUID PRESSURE

### Measurement Techniques

Prior to 1960, it had been universally believed that the interstitial fluid pressure was almost always slightly above 0 (that is, slightly above atmospheric pressure). At that time we con-cluded on the basis of measurements made in our laboratories using permanently implanted perforated capsules that the interstitial fluid pressure was negative, averaging 5–7 mm Hg below atmospheric pressure (Guyton et al., 1960, 1971). During the past 20 yr a number of phys-iologists have supported the negative interstitial fluid pressure concept using our techniques as well as various other methods of measurement (Aukland and Nicolaysen, 1981; Brace, 1981). Yet, some techniques measure pressures that are more negative than others. The three most pop-ular methods for measuring interstitial fluid pressures are the following.

### Perforated Capsule Technique

Free interstitial fluid is normally confined to very small rivulets and vesicles, and it is difficult, if not impossible, to measure accurately the pres-sure in these pockets of free fluid simply because of their small size. By implanting a plastic cap-sule perforated with several hundred small holes into a tissue, the interstitial fluid can move into the capsule, creating a much larger pocket of free interstitial fluid, the pressure of which can be measured by inserting a needle into the lumen of the capsule through one of the many perfora-tions. In practice, the capsule is surgically im-planted, and the wound is allowed to heal for several weeks. By 4–5 weeks, the pressure is −5 to −7 mm Hg, and it remains at this level for the next several months. One week after implanta-tion, however, the capsule is surrounded by in-flammation and edema fluid, and the pressure at this time measures 2–5 mm Hg. Therefore, the true interstitial fluid pressure can only be accu-rately measured in a tissue free from inflamma-tion and edema fluid (Guyton et al., 1971, 1975).

### Wick Technique

Another method of measuring interstitial fluid pressure is with the wick technique (Scholander et al., 1968). The measuring apparatus consists of a small Teflon tube into which a wick com-posed of several cotton fibers is inserted. The wick is inserted into the tissues through a hollow needle. When the needle is withdrawn, the wick is left in contact with the tissue elements. Be-cause the cotton fibers are microtubules with large numbers of lateral pores, the interstitial fluid can enter these pores and make direct con-tact with a fluid-filled catheter and low compli-ance pressure transducer.

The pressure measured by the wick technique is usually about one-half to two-thirds as nega-tive as the pressure measured by the capsule technique. This difference in pressure could be caused by acute hemorrhage, acute inflamma-tion, and local destruction of lymphatics and small blood capillaries when inserting the wick. On the other hand, some investigators have sug-gested various reasons why the capsule technique might measure pressures that are too negative.

### Micropuncture Technique

This method of measuring interstitial fluid pressure involves insertion of small glass pipettes into pockets of free interstitial fluid. To identify these pockets, it is necessary to study thin struc-tures through which light can be transmitted. In the bat's wing, the interstitial fluid pressure has been found by some investigators to range from −1 to −4 mm Hg (Hogan and Nicoll, 1978, 1979), but Wiederhielm and Weston (1973) have measured slightly positive pressures. The reason that micropuncture methods measure pressures that are less negative than those measured using the capsule or wick techniques is not known but could be related to the necessity either of injecting small amounts of fluid into the tissue to make the pipette tip patent or of finding a pocket of fluid already present in the tissue.

## Evaluation of Measurement Techniques

Although the perforated capsule technique requires several weeks before accurate measurements can be made, there are a number of reasons for believing that the measurements that are made using this technique reflect more closely true free interstitial fluid pressure. First, factors which create inflammation, local edema, or local hemorrhage theoretically should cause interstitial fluid pressure to be higher (that is, less negative). Both the wick technique and the micropuncture technique are acute and invasive and are known to cause some degree of tissue disturbance; on the other hand, the perforated capsule technique measures interstitial fluid pressure 4 weeks after implantation of the capsule, and by this time the tissues have mainly healed, having already gone through a temporary high pressure phase.

Second, the perforated capsule technique has been used to measure changes in interstitial fluid pressure caused by various physiological interventions, and these changes have been very close to those predicted by the Starling concept of pressure equilibria (Guyton et al., 1971, 1975). For example, if concentrated solutions of dextran are perfused through the vasculature of a tissue, fluid is absorbed from the tissue into the vessels by osmosis; in turn, the interstitial fluid pressure becomes more negative. On the other hand, venous obstruction causes the interstitial fluid pressure to become higher (that is, less negative) because fluid is filtered into the tissues, and the tissues then become edematous. This type of validation has also been attempted with the wick technique, but changes in the observed pressures have been much smaller than simultaneously measured capsule pressures (Prather et al., 1971). Yet, although the wick technique probably does not measure the true interstitial fluid pressure, it has become very popular in recent years simply because the interstitial fluid pressure can be recorded almost immediately after insertion of the wick, whereas the capsule technique requires several weeks before measurements can be made.

In summary, the three most popular techniques for measuring interstitial fluid pressure are the perforated capsule technique, the wick technique, and the micropuncture technique. The pressures measured using the perforated capsule technique are almost always more negative than those measured using the other two.

## INTERSTITIAL EDEMA

Edema is defined as the presence of abnormally large amounts of fluid in the tissues, and interstitial edema is excessive amounts of fluid in the interstitial spaces. Any factor that increases the volume of interstitial fluid can cause interstitial edema, especially increases in capillary pressure, increases in interstitial fluid colloid osmotic pressure, decreases in plasma colloid osmotic pressure, and decreases in lymph flow. Each of these possible causes of edema is considered in this section, but first is a discussion of the relationship between interstitial fluid volume and interstitial free fluid pressure.

## Pressure-Volume Curve

One of the most important aspects of tissue fluid dynamics that has come from studying the relationship between interstitial fluid pressure and volume is the following. In the soft tissues of the body, edema will not occur as long as the interstitial fluid pressure is negative (that is, subatmospheric). Once the interstitial fluid pressure becomes positive, edema fluid rapidly collects in the tissues. In several hundred experiments we have never observed edema in the presence of negative interstitial fluid pressure (Guyton et al., 1971, 1975).

Figure 5.9 shows the relationship between interstitial fluid volume and interstitial fluid pressure in human beings as extrapolated from measurements made in dogs. The *solid curve* was generated in the following way. Four weeks prior to the experiments, perforated capsules were implanted subcutaneously in the hindlimbs of dogs. Interstitial fluid pressure could then be measured

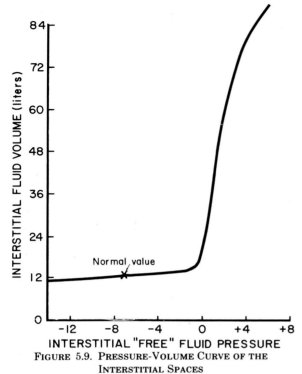

FIGURE 5.9. PRESSURE-VOLUME CURVE OF THE
INTERSTITIAL SPACES

These data on humans were extrapolated from data obtained in dogs. (From Guyton, 1981.)

at the time of the experiment by inserting a needle through the skin and through a perforation into a capsule. The legs were then removed from the dogs and perfused by an artificial perfusion system. By manipulating the colloid osmotic pressure of the perfusion fluid and the hydrostatic pressure of the perfusion system, interstitial fluid volumes of the legs were first decreased below normal and then increased progressively to far above normal while capsule pressures were measured at each stage of increased volume. The curve of Figure 5.9 (as extrapolated from these dog studies) was thus determined. Note the following two significant features of the curve: As long as interstitial free fluid pressure remained in the negative range, interstitial fluid volume changed only slightly. In other words, edema fluid did not begin to collect in the tissues as long as interstitial free fluid pressure was negative. Furthermore, once interstitial free fluid pressure had risen above zero, the slope of the pressure-volume curve suddenly changed, and interstitial fluid volume increased tremendously with much less increase in pressure. At the very top of the curve, the skin began to stretch, causing interstitial fluid volume to increase less rapidly.

In summary, the relationship between interstitial fluid volume and interstitial free fluid pressure indicates that as long as the interstitial fluid pressure is in the negative range, edema will not occur. Therefore, the physical cause of subcutaneous edema is usually positive pressure in the interstitial fluid spaces.

## Causes of Edema

Because the physical cause of edema is an increase in interstitial fluid pressure, any factor that causes interstitial fluid pressure to increase can, therefore, cause edema. The various specific causes of edema are listed below.

### Increased Capillary Pressure

When mean capillary pressure becomes abnormally high, increased amounts of fluid are filtered out of the capillaries. This causes interstitial fluid pressure to rise and tissues to become edematous. Factors that can cause capillary pressure to increase to such high levels include increased venous pressure, increased arterial pressure, arteriolar vasodilation, venous constriction or occlusion, and multiple plugging of venules, which increases flow and pressure in remaining capillaries. Perhaps most frequently, capillary pressure is increased by venous obstruction due to cardiac failure combined with simultaneous retention of fluid by the kidneys.

### Decreased Plasma Colloid Osmotic Pressure

Decreases in colloid osmotic pressure of plasma are caused by decreases in protein concentration of plasma. The following clinical conditions can cause plasma protein concentration to decrease to low enough levels to cause edema: nephrosis, poor nutrition or starvation, loss of protein from denuded surfaces of the body (severe burns), malabsorption syndromes, dilution of plasma proteins by infused fluids, and loss of plasma proteins from capillaries into interstitial spaces due to factors that increase capillary protein permeability.

### Increased Interstitial Colloid Osmotic Pressure and Decreased Lymph Flow

Interstitial colloid osmotic pressure increases when excessive amounts of protein build up in the interstitium. There are two major causes for this: obstruction of lymphatics and increased protein permeability of the capillary membrane. Because the lymphatic system provides the only means through which extravasated proteins can be removed from interstitial spaces and returned to the blood vascular system, obstruction of lymphatics increases the protein concentration and, therefore, increases the colloid osmotic pressure of the interstitial fluid. Theoretically, total obstruction of all lymphatics in a tissue would cause the protein concentration of the interstitial fluid to rise until it eventually would become equal to the protein concentration of the plasma, as described in detail elsewhere in this chapter. Increases in capillary protein permeability will also cause the protein concentration of interstitial fluid to increase because proteins then move more freely through capillary membranes and into interstitial spaces.

## SAFETY FACTOR AGAINST EDEMA

For many years clinicians have noted that edema will not occur until tissue fluid dynamics become severely abnormal. The ability of tissues to buffer imbalances in Starling forces allows them to maintain an almost normal degree of hydration with an initial Starling force imbalance of up to 18 mm Hg (Krogh et al., 1932; Guyton et al., 1975). That is, capillary pressure can often increase by 18 mm Hg or plasma colloid osmotic pressure can decrease by 18 mm Hg without causing edema. Thus, there is a safety factor against edema. This factor results from three physiological mechanisms.

### Negative Interstitial Pressure

We have already seen that the interstitial fluid pressure of subcutaneous tissues must increase from the normally negative value of −6 mm Hg up to atmospheric pressure (that is, up to 0 mm Hg) before edema will occur (Guyton, 1963). Therefore, the normal negativity of interstitial fluid pressure provides a safety factor of 6 mm Hg against edema.

### Removal of Interstitial Fluid by Lymphatics

When a transcapillary pressure disequilibrium causes interstitial fluid pressure to increase up toward atmospheric pressure, this in turn causes lymph flow to increase. This increase in lymph flow helps to prevent development of edema because it carries fluid away from the tissues. Maximally increased lymph flow constitutes an estimated safety factor of about 7 mm Hg because the lymphatics can remove an amount of fluid from the tissues approximately equal to the amount that is formed by a 7 mm Hg increase in capillary pressure (Taylor et al., 1973; Guyton et al., 1975).

### Decreased Interstitial Colloid Osmotic Pressure

As shown in Figure 5.4, increases in lymph flow result in decreases in interstitial fluid colloid osmotic pressure. When lymph flow increases, protein is literally washed from the interstitium; in turn, the protein concentration of interstitial fluid decreases (Rusznyák et al., 1960; Yoffey and Courtice, 1970; Guyton et al., 1975). If the initial interstitial fluid colloid osmotic pressure were 7 mm Hg and increased lymph flow reduced this to 2 mm Hg, the safety factor caused by decreasing the colloid osmotic pressure would be 5 mm Hg.

In summary, these three physiological components of the safety factor against edema, when added together, equal the total safety factor against edema of up to 18 mm Hg, which has been measured experimentally and observed clinically. Although the three physiological components of the safety factor are qualitatively similar in all tissues of the body, the total amount of safety factor against edema and the quantitative importance of each of the three physiological components of the safety factor may differ from tissue to tissue.

## Lymphatic Proliferation

When capillary filtration is elevated chronically and the tissues become chronically edematous, the lymphatic vessels draining the tissues proliferate, which increases their capacity for carrying fluid away from tissue spaces. Figure 5.10 demonstrates the effects of elevated left atrial pressure on pulmonary lymph flow in dogs (Uhley et al., 1962). The single point in the *bottom right-hand corner* of the figure illustrates the average lymph flow recorded in a previous study when left atrial pressure was acutely increased to about 40 cm $H_2O$ (Leeds et al., 1959); this point indicates that lymph flow had increased only to about 10 ml/hr despite the high left atrial pressure. Other points in the figure illustrate the relationship between pulmonary lymph flow and left atrial pressure after several weeks of moderate pulmonary congestion. The

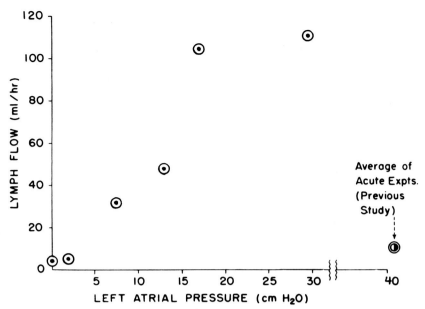

FIGURE 5.10. EFFECT OF LEFT ATRIAL PRESSURE ON LYMPH FLOW FROM THE RIGHT LYMPHATIC DUCT OF DOGS
The single point in the *bottom right corner* represents the average lymph flow in an earlier series of dogs (Leeds et al., 1959) when the left atrial pressure was elevated acutely. The other points, representing lymph flows recorded after several weeks of pulmonary congestion, illustrate a 25-fold increase in lymph flow caused by proliferation or enlargement of lymphatic vessels. (From Uhley et al., 1962, by permission of the American Heart Association, Inc.)

congestion was achieved by creating an aortico-caval anastomosis and administering desoxycorticosterone trimethylacetate and a salt-rich diet, which caused elevated left atrial pressure over a period of several weeks. The dogs were then anesthetized, and pulmonary lymph flow was measured as left atrial pressure was increased in steps up to about 30 cm $H_2O$. As shown in the figure, lung lymph flow was about 25 times higher in the animals that had been subjected to chronic pulmonary congestion than in the normal animals. Gross observation of the pulmonary lymphatics indicated that they had undergone

tremendous enlargement during the period of pulmonary congestion.

These studies indicate that the pulmonary lymphatic system can undergo proliferation or enlargement and that such enlargement may be a chronic safety factor for prevention of overt pulmonary edema. The studies may also explain how a patient with chronic mitral stenosis can have a pulmonary capillary pressure as great as 40–45 mm Hg without having significant pulmonary edema. Therefore, the lymphatic system appears to be able to restructure itself when lymph flow is chronically elevated by edema.

## SUMMARY

The most important physiological function of the lymphatic system is to remove extravasated fluid and plasma protein from interstitial spaces and to return these to the blood vascular system. This function is especially critical for plasma protein because there is no other pathway by which protein can be removed from interstitial spaces. Plasma proteins are continually concentrated in interstitial spaces because fluid containing protein continually leaks from blood capillaries into interstitial spaces, but fluid which is

absorbed into the blood capillary contains little protein.

The concentration of protein in interstitial spaces depends on the rate of lymph flow. Because lymph flow is equal to capillary filtration minus capillary absorption, a smaller fraction of capillary filtrate is absorbed as lymph flow increases. In turn, the interstitial fluid protein-concentrating mechanism is partially dissipated, and the protein concentration of the interstitial fluid decreases. In other words, when lymph flow increases, interstitial fluid protein concentration decreases. This mechanism functions as a negative feedback system to help keep the interstitial fluid protein concentration constant. For example, as protein molecules accumulate in interstitial fluid, the colloid osmotic pressure of interstitial fluid increases. This automatically increases the rate of fluid filtration out of the capillary and decreases the rate of fluid absorption into the capillary. Therefore, lymph flow increases. As lymph flow increases, proteins are washed from the interstitium, and the excess colloid osmotic pressure is corrected.

The lymphatic system actively removes fluid and protein from the interstitium because every segment of the lymphatic system is able to pump lymph actively. The energy required to pump lymph is generated by extrinsic tissue compressive forces and intrinsic lymphatic contractions. The ability of lymphatics to contract automatically when they fill with lymph and their walls are stretched is a universal feature of the mammalian lymphatic system with the possible exception of the lymphatic capillaries. In addition, the lymphatics will continue to contract periodically even without being stretched; this indicates that there may be pacemaker cells in the lymphatic wall.

Although the primary function of the lymphatic pump is to remove fluid and protein continuously from the interstitial spaces, in doing so, the lymphatic pump is also thought to generate negative interstitial fluid pressure. In normal subcutaneous tissues, interstitial fluid pressure averages about −6 mm Hg, but in various abnormal states, interstitial fluid pressure often becomes positive. When positive pressure occurs, tremendous amounts of fluid collect in interstitial spaces, causing typical extracellular edema. In several hundred experiments we have not observed subcutaneous edema in the presence of negative interstitial fluid pressure. Among factors that can increase interstitial fluid pressure to positive values and thereby cause edema are increased capillary pressure, decreased plasma colloid osmotic pressure, increased interstitial fluid colloid osmotic pressure, and decreased lymph flow. Because most tissues of the body can withstand an initial Starling force imbalance of up to 18 mm Hg without becoming edematous, there is a safety factor against edema of up to 18 mm Hg. Negative interstitial fluid pressure provides about 6 mm Hg of the safety factor, removal of interstitial fluid by lymphatics provides about 7 mm Hg, and the decrease in interstitial fluid colloid osmotic pressure that occurs when lymph flow increases provides about 5 mm Hg of the safety factor. There probably exists yet another safety factor against edema that is slower to develop but possibly has great importance in chronic states of edema. This is the ability of the lymphatic system to grow when lymph flow is chronically increased and thereby to increase its capacity for carrying fluid away from the tissue spaces.

# REFERENCES

Acevedo D: Motor control of the thoracic duct. *Am J Physiol* 139:600–603, 1943.

Adair TH, Drake RE, Guyton AC: Fluid ultrafiltration across the intranodal blood-lymph barrier modifies lymph flow and protein concentration. In Bartos V, Davidson JW (eds): *Advances in Lymphology.* Prague, Avicenium, Czechoslovak Medical Press, 1982a, pp 100–114.

Adair TH, Moffatt DS, Paulsen AW, Guyton AC: Quantitation of changes in lymph protein concentration during lymph node transit. *Am J Physiol* 243:H351–H359, 1982b.

Allen L: Lymphatics and lymphoid tissues. *Annu Rev Physiol* 29:197–224, 1967.

Aukland K, Nicolaysen G: Interstitial fluid volume: local regulatory mechanisms. *Physiol Rev* 61:556–643, 1981.

Bettendorf U: Lymph flow mechanism of the subperitoneal diaphragmatic lymphatics. *Lymphology* 11:111–116, 1978.

Brace RA: Progress toward resolving the controversy of positive vs. negative interstitial fluid pressure. *Circ Res* 49:281–297, 1981.

Campbell T, Heath R: Intrinsic contractility of lymphatics in sheep and in dogs. *Q J Exp Physiol* 58:207–217, 1973.

Casley-Smith JR: An electron microscopic study of injured and subnormally permeable lymphatics. *Ann NY Acad Sci* 116:803–830, 1964a.

Casley-Smith JR: Endothelial permeability—the passage of particles into and out of diaphragmatic lymphatics. *Q J Exp Physiol* 49:365–383, 1964b.

Casley-Smith JR: The function of the lymphatic system under normal and pathological conditions: its dependence on the fine structure and permeability of the vessels. In Rüttimann A (ed): *Progress in Lymphology.* New York, Hafner, 1967, pp 348–359.

Casley-Smith JR: The fine structure of tissues and tissue channels. In Hargens AR (ed): *Tissue Fluid Pressure and Composition.* Baltimore, Williams & Wilkins, 1981.

Casley-Smith JR, Florey HW: The structure of normal lymphatics. *Q J Exp Physiol* 46:101–106, 1961.

Chapil M: *Physiology of Connective Tissue.* London, Butterworth, 1967, p 14.

Cressman RD, Blalock A: The effect of the pulse upon the flow of lymph. *Proc Soc Exp Biol Med* 41:140–144, 1939.

Dennis JB: Effects of various factors on the distribution of ferrocyanide in ground substance. *Arch Pathol* 67:533, 1959.

Florey H: Observations on the contractility of lacteals. Part II. *J Physiol (Lond)* 63:1–18, 1927.

Földi M: The lymphatic system. A review. *Z Lymphol (J Lymphol)* 1:16–19, 44–56, 1977.

Gersh I, Catchpole HR: The nature of ground substance of connective tissue. *Perspect Biol Med* 3:282, 1960.

Granger DN, Mortillaro NA, Taylor AE: Interaction of intestinal lymph flow and secretion. *Am J Physiol* 232:E13–E18, 1977.

Granger DN, Miller T, Allen R, Parker RE, Parker JC, Taylor AE: Permselectivity of cat liver blood-lymph barrier to endogenous macromolecules. *Gastroenterology* 77:103–109, 1979.

Granger HJ: Physicochemical properties of the extracellular matrix. In Hargens AR (ed): *Tissue Fluid Pressure and Composition*. Baltimore, Williams & Wilkins, 1981.

Guyton AC: A concept of negative interstitial pressure based on pressures in implanted perforated capsules. *Circ Res* 12:399–414, 1963.

Guyton AC: *Textbook of Medical Physiology*. Philadelphia, WB Saunders, 1981.

Guyton AC, Armstrong GG, Crowell JW: Negative pressure in interstitial spaces. *Physiologist* 3:70, 1960.

Guyton AC, Granger HJ, Taylor AE: Interstitial fluid pressure. *Physiol Rev* 51:527–563, 1971.

Guyton AC, Taylor AE, Granger HJ: *Circulatory Physiology II: Dynamics and Control of the Body Fluids*. Philadelphia, WB Saunders, 1975.

Guyton AC, Parker JC, Taylor AE, Jackson TE, Moffatt DS: Forces governing water movement in the lung. In Fishman AP, Renkin EM (eds): *Pulmonary Edema*. Bethesda, MD, American Physiological Society, 1979.

Hall JG, Morris B, Woolley G: Intrinsic rhythmic propulsion of lymph in the unanaesthetized sheep. *J Physiol (Lond)* 180:336–349, 1965.

Hargens AR, Zweifach BW: Contractile stimuli in collecting lymph vessels. *Am J Physiol* 223:H57–H65, 1977.

Hogan RD: The initial lymphatics and interstitial fluid pressure. In Hargens AR (ed): *Tissue Fluid Pressure and Composition*. Baltimore, Williams & Wilkins, 1981.

Hogan R, Nicoll PA: Initial lymphatic activity role in regulating interstitial fluid. *Physiologist* 21:55, 1978.

Hogan R, Nicoll PA: Quantitation of convective forces active in lymph formation. *Microvasc Res* 17 (pt 2):S145, 1979.

Kedem O, Katchalsky A: Thermodynamic analysis of the permeability of biological membranes to non-electrolytes. *Biochim Biophys Acta* 27:229–246, 1958.

Krogh A, Landis EM, Turner AH: The movement of fluid through the human capillary wall in relation to venous pressure and to the colloid osmotic pressure of the blood. *J Clin Invest* 11:63–95, 1932.

Laine GA, Hall JT, Laine SH, Granger HJ: Transsinusoidal fluid dynamics in canine liver during venous hypertension. *Circ Res* 45:317–323, 1979.

Landis EM, Pappenheimer JR: Exchange of substances through the capillary walls. In Hamilton WF, Dow P (eds): *Handbook of Physiology*. Sect 2: Bethesda, MD, American Physiological Society, 1963, vol II, pp 961–1034.

Leak LV: Electron microscopic observations on lymphatic capillaries and the structural components of the connective tissue-lymph interface. *Microvasc Res* 2:361–391, 1970.

Leak LV, Burke JF: Electron microscopic study of lymphatic capillaries in the removal of connective tissue fluids and particulate substances. *Lymphology* 1:39–52, 1968a.

Leak LV, Burke JF: Ultrastructural studies on the lymphatic anchoring filaments. *J Cell Biol* 36:129–149, 1968b.

Leeds SE, Uhley HN, Sampson JJ, Friedman M: A new method for measurement of lymph flow from the right duct in the dog. *Am J Surg* 98:211–216, 1959.

Majno G, Leventhal M: Pathogenesis of histamine type vascular leakage. *Lancet* 2:99, 1967.

Majno G, Shea SM, Leventhal M: Endothelial contraction induced by histamine type mediators. An electron microscopic study. *J Cell Biol* 42:647, 1969.

Mawhinney HJD, Roddie IC: Spontaneous activity in isolated bovine mesenteric lymphatics. *J Physiol (Lond)* 229:339–348, 1973.

Mayerson HS: The physiologic importance of lymph. In Hamilton WF, Dow P (eds): *Handbook of Physiology*. Sect 2: *Circulation II*. Bethesda, MD, American Physiological Society, 1963, vol II, pp 1035–1073.

Mayerson HS, Patterson RM, McKee A, LeBrie SJ, Mayerson P: Permeability of lymphatic vessels. *Am J Physiol* 203:98–106, 1962.

McHale NG, Roddie IC: The effect of transmural pressure on pumping activity in isolated bovine lymphatic vessels. *J Physiol (Lond)* 261:255–269, 1976.

McMaster PD: Changes in the cutaneous lymphatics of human beings and in the lymph flow under normal and pathological conditions. *J Exp Med* 65:347–372, 1937.

Nicoll PA, Hogan RD: Pressures associated with lymphatic capillary contraction. *Microvasc Res* 15:257–258, 1978.

Ohhashi T, Azuma T, Sakaguchi M: Active and passive mechanical characteristics of bovine mesenteric lymphatics. *Am J Physiol* 239:H88–H95, 1980a.

Ohhashi T, McHale NG, Roddie IC, Thornbury KD: Electrical field stimulation as a method of stimulating nerve or smooth muscle in isolated bovine mesenteric lymphatics. *Pflügers Arch* 388:221–226, 1980b.

Olszewski WL, Engeset A: Intrinsic contractility of prenodal lymph vessels and lymph flow in human leg. *Am J Physiol* 239:H775–H783, 1980.

Pappenheimer JR, Soto-Rivera A: Effective osmotic pressure of the plasma proteins and other qualities associated with the capillary circulation in the hindlimb of cats and dogs. *Am J Physiol* 152:471–491, 1948.

Parker JC, Falgout HJ, Parker RE, Granger DN, Taylor AE: The effect of fluid volume loading on exclusion on interstitial albumin and lymph flow in the dog lung. *Circ Res* 45:440–450, 1979.

Parsons RJ, McMaster PD: The effect of the pulse upon the formation and flow of lymph. *J Exp Med* 68:353–376, 1938.

Patterson RM, Ballard CL, Wasserman K, Mayerson HS: Lymphatic permeability of albumin. *Am J Physiol* 194:120–124, 1958.

Prather JW, Bowes DN, Warrell DA, Zweifach BW: Comparison of capsule and wick techniques for measurement of interstitial fluid pressure. *J Appl Physiol* 31:942–945, 1971.

Renkin EM: Lymph as a measure of the composition of interstitial fluid. In Fishman AP, Renkin EM (eds): *Pulmonary Edema*. Bethesda, MD, American Physiological Society, 1979.

Richardson PDI, Granger DN: Capillary filtration coefficient as a measure of perfused capillary density. In Granger DN, Bulkley GB (eds): *Measurement of Blood Flow*. Baltimore, Williams & Wilkins, 1981.

Russell JA, Zimmerman K, Middendorf WF: Evidence for $\alpha$-adrenergic innervation of the isolated canine thoracic duct. *J Appl Physiol* 49:1010–1015, 1980.

Rusznyák I, Földi M, Szabó G: *Lymphatics and Lymph Circulation*. Oxford, Pergamon, 1960.

Scholander PF, Hargens AR, Miller SL: Negative pressure in the interstitial fluid of animals. *Science* 161:321–328, 1968.

Smith RO: Lymphatic contractility: a possible intrinsic mechanism of lymphatic vessels for the transport of lymph. *J Exp Med* 90:497–509, 1949.

Starling EH: The influence of mechanical factors on lymph production. *J Physiol (Lond)* 16:224–267, 1894.

Starling EH: On the absorption of fluids from the connective tissue spaces. *J Physiol (Lond)* 19:312–326, 1896.

Taylor AE: Capillary fluid filtration. Starling forces and lymph flow. *Circ Res* 49:557–575, 1981.

Taylor AE, Gibson WH, Granger HJ, Guyton AC: The interaction between intracapillary and tissue forces in the overall regulation of interstitial fluid volume. *Lymphology* 6:192–208, 1973.

Uhley HN, Leeds SE, Sampson JJ, Friedman M: Role of pulmonary lymphatics in chronic pulmonary edema. *Circ Res* 11:966–970, 1962.

Webb RC, Starzl TE: The effect of blood vessel pulsations on lymph pressure in large lymphatics. *Bull Johns Hopkins Hosp* 93:401–407, 1953.

White JC, Field ME, Drinker CK: On the protein content and normal flow of lymph from the foot of the dog. *Am J Physiol* 103:34–44, 1933.

Wiederhielm CA: The interstitial space. In Fung YC, Perrone N, Anliker M (eds): *Biomechanics: Its Foundations and Objectives*. Englewood Cliffs, NJ, Prentice-Hall, 1972, pp 273–286.

Wiederhielm CA, Weston BV: Microvascular, lymphatic, and tissue pressures in the unanesthetized mammal. *Am J Physiol* 225:992–996, 1973.

Yoffey JM, Courtice FC: *Lymphatics, Lymph and the Lymphomyeloid Complex*. London, Academic Press, 1970.

# 6

# *Abnormal Peripheral Lymphatics*

## THOMAS F. O'DONNELL, JR., M.D.

Most investigators have accepted the basic classification of lymphedema into primary and secondary forms as described by Allen et al. (1946). Secondary lymphedema is usually acquired while primary lymphedema is related to an in utero developmental defect. Kinmonth et al. (1957) further subdivide the primary lymphedemas by age of onset: congenital, present at birth; praecox, present before age 35; and tarda, occurring after age 35. The utility of this latter classification relates to the clinical diagnosis, management, and prognosis of primary lymphedema. This subdivision also recognizes that developmental defects in the lymphatic system are present at birth but may express themselves later in life (praecox or tarda).

After the development of clinical lymphography, Kinmonth (1969) proposed another method of classifying the primary lymphedemas—by lymphographic pattern. Not only did this method permit further subdivision along anatomic lines, but also it provided an approach for investigating the etiology of primary lymphedema.

On the basis of lymphography, the lymphedemas are divided into: *aplasia*, no demonstrable lymphatic vessels; *hypoplasia*, a decreased number of lymphatic vessels; and *hyperplasia*, an increased number of lymphatic vessels. The advantages of lymphography are that it: determines definitively whether the process is indeed lymphatic in origin; has important prognostic value (for example, hyperplasia may be associated with lesser degrees of lymphedema and may be more frequently bilateral than hypoplasia); and assesses the feasibility of surgical therapy (that is, whether a lymphovenous shunt is possible).

## ETIOLOGY

### Primary Lymphedema

Like other vascular dysplasias, primary lymphedema is probably due to a developmental defect in the lymphatic system. Lymphatic abnormalities are often associated with arterial and venous dysplasia in the same limb (O'Donnell, 1977), as well as other congenital anomalies. Lymphographic examinations of a few congenital cases of lymphedema have demonstrated aplasia or severe hypoplasia. Why some forms of lymphedema are delayed in their clinical expression is less clear. Certainly, other factors must influence the appearance of the functional abnormality—edema formation. Bilateral lymphography of a patient with only unilateral lymphedema frequently demonstrates hypoplastic lymphatics in the clinically normal leg. The predilection for the left lower extremity, female preponderance, and peak incidence at puberty suggest that hormonal changes may be associated with the appearance of clinical lymphedema. In contrast, the development of lymphedema after minor surgery or trauma implicates possible damage to functioning collateral pathways.

Two groups have favored an acquired cause of primary lymphedema. Olszewski and his colleagues (1972a, b) suggested that inflammatory changes within the lymphatic vessels or lymph nodes may result in primary lymphedema. Biopsy specimens from 30 patients with primary lymphedema demonstrated that all layers of the wall were normally developed but that the lumen was obstructed by a thickened intima. In addition, 50% of their patients had a hypoplastic lymphographic pattern and exhibited lymph stasis changes similar to those observed in lymphedema secondary to postinflammatory states. Basing their interpretation on these histological and radiological findings, Olszewski and his colleagues argued that inflammation, most likely related to recurrent infection, caused hypoplasia by progressive obliteration of the lymphatic vessels. By contrast, histological findings in the hyperplastic form were characterized by a hypertrophied muscular layer with an unobstructed vessel lumen. Increased contractility was observed on cinelymphography. These investigators offered a different explanation for the hyperplastic type of primary lymphedema, that it was a consequence of obstruction.

In their sequential histological studies of patients with primary lymphedema, Fyfe and others (1982) demonstrated that fibrosis of the lymph node might be a significant factor in primary lymphedema. They felt that fibrosis of the lymph node obstructed lymph flow and therefore caused secondary lymph stasis. Based on this hypothesis, they infused steroids via an intralymphatic route to 20 patients with primary lymphedema. Subsequently the limb girth of the 20 patients decreased, and the subcutaneous tissue became more supple. While their finding suggests that lymph node fibrosis, an acquired lesion, plays a role in primary lymphedema, the basic defect, a lack of development of lymphatic vessels and nodes, occurs in utero.

An alternate theory has been forwarded by Calnan (1968). He challenged the belief that in utero alterations in the lymphatics were the basic cause of primary lymphedema. Since lymphedema has its highest incidence of onset during puberty with many cases presenting later, an acquired cause seemed more likely. The preponderance of females affected and the predilection for involvement of the left leg suggested that an anatomic defect was responsible. Subsequent experiments conducted by Calnan and Kountz (1965) and by Burn (1968) demonstrated that structural and functional lymphatic abnormalities resulting in lymphedema could develop after venous obstruction. Perhaps the left iliac vein was compressed by the right iliac artery and the resultant obstruction led to increased venous pressure and subsequent lymphatic abnormalities. This theory gained support from observations of increased femoral vein pressure in several patients with primary lymphedema (Rigas et al., 1971).

Unfortunately, the venous obstruction theory could not be substantiated by other investigators.

Negus et al. (1969) disproved two links in the chain of events. In a series of 12 patients with primary lymphedema, they found normal femoral vein pressures. Both on acrylic injection casts of the left iliac vein and on femoral venograms, these investigators noted indentation of the vein but no true obstruction. Moreover, the fundamental weakness of the venous obstruction theory is that it is difficult to rationalize hypoplasia, the most common (90%) pattern of lymphography, as a result of lymphatic obstruction. In view of the evidence to date, primary lymphedema, particularly of the hypoplastic type, appears to be due to a developmental defect. Factors that can be construed as secondary may modify its expression.

## Secondary Lymphedema

Although the causes of secondary lymphedema are varied (Table 6.1), interruption of lymphatic continuity by obstruction or by extirpation is the usual cause. This may occur either at the nodal or truncal level. For example, removal of the major lymphatic trunks and regional nodes of the arm may be followed by significant limb swelling in 10–30% of cases. Other factors, such as secondary infection or radiation, modify the incidence of lymphedema. In an experimental preparation of secondary lymphedema (Olszewski, 1973), removal of skin, subcutaneous tissue, and lymphatics was followed by transient edema within the first month in all animals (acute surgical lymphedema). This edema resolved by 6 weeks, but 35% of the animals had significant lymphedema at 2 years and 55% at 5 years. Serial lymphograms revealed progressive dilatation of lymph vessels and numerical hyperplasia. Lymph protein content was tripled. After surgery for cancer, especially radical mastectomy, several factors other than removal of lymph nodes and vessels have been suggested as responsible for secondary lymphedema. Trauma to the axillary vein with subsequent perivenous fibrosis and obstruction, postoperative infection

TABLE 6.1.
CAUSES OF SECONDARY LYMPHEDEMA

| Cause | Pathophysiology | Lymphographic Pattern |
|---|---|---|
| Malignant disease | Obstruction of node by tumor | Obstruction with collateral circulation |
| Radiation | Obstruction of lymphatic trunks by extrinsic fibrosis at lymph node level | Obstruction |
| Surgery or trauma | Obstruction at lymphatic vessel level | Obstruction with collateral circulation |
| Filariasis | Obstruction at lymph node level | Obstruction—Widened varicose lymphatics with reflux |
| Pyogenic infection | Obliteration of lymphatic trunks | Hypoplasia |

leading to destruction of lymphatic collaterals, and radiotherapy with resultant fibrosis of collaterals have all been incriminated in the development of secondary lymphedema.

Many authors have focused on the role of venous obstruction in relation to secondary lymphedema. In their study of 19 women with postmastectomy edema, Hughes and Patel (1966) found that all had partial or complete obstruction of the axillary vein as well as valvular damage and that 50% showed concomitant damage of their cephalic veins. Larson and Crampton (1973) emphasized that a venogram should be performed in 90% adduction because 34% of normal limbs will show a positional obstruction of the axillary vein. Their series revealed obstruction or nonvisualization of the axillary vein in 8 of 14 patients evaluated for secondary lymphedema. Arnulf (1973) found similar venographic changes in 8 of 13 patients evaluated after radical mastectomy. In contrast to these abnormalities in venous anatomy, we were able to demonstrate significant venous hemodynamic changes in only 2 of 14 patients evaluated for problematic secondary lymphedema (>2 cm) (Raines et al., 1977). Maximum venous outflow examinations, which assess noninvasively venous outflow from the limb and therefore upstream obstruction, were normal in the other 12 patients.

It is evident that venous obstruction is not the sole cause of secondary lymphedema. Collateral lymphatic vessels must develop to bridge the defect caused by surgery. By lymphography performed in postmastectomy patients, Kreel and George (1966) have shown that this collateral lymphatic flow may re-establish itself across the mastectomy site by 1–2 months and even drain to the opposite axilla. Kinmonth and Taylor (1954) had previously emphasized the importance of collateral lymphatic pathways to the supraclavicular nodes, parasternal nodes, and across the operative site. Failure of these collateral pathways to develop, early destruction by infection, or late obliteration by radiotherapy or lymphangitis may be responsible for the development of secondary lymphedema. In our experience hemodynamically significant venous obstruction can aggravate edema caused by lymphatic abnormalities, while venous insufficiency alone can cause edema, much as it does in the lower extremity.

Filarial infection, an uncommon cause of secondary lymphedema in the United States, is related to obstruction of the node or lymphatic vessel by the adult worm. That this infection is directly lymphatic and not blood-borne has been suggested by Gooneratne (1969). He linked the site of inoculation by the mosquito to the regional area eventually involved by lymphedema.

Although the infections or inflammation are less a cause than a consequence of lymphedema, in patients with chronic dermatitis or chronic venous insufficiency recurrent infection may lead eventually to secondary lymphedema. In several patients with the post-thrombotic syndrome, we have observed obliteration of the superficial lymphatics. Vitek and Kaspar (1973) revealed obliteration of the deep lymphatic in 3 of 16 patients undergoing lymphograms of the deep lymphatic system for post-thrombotic syndrome.

## CLINICAL CONSIDERATIONS

Since many of the symptoms and physical findings are similar in primary and secondary lymphedema, they are discussed together here.

### Symptoms

In either the initial presentation or less advanced cases of lymphedema, the patient usually observes the cosmetic defect produced by limb swelling (Table 6.2). The edema generally involves the ankle or hand first, is worse at the end of the day, and resolves somewhat with elevation of the limb at night. As the degree of edema increases and involves more of the limb, it may not diminish with simple elevation. This lack of fluctuation with elevation or with simple compressive measures correlates well with the development of subcutaneous fibrosis.

As the degree of lymphedema increases further, the patient may experience a sensation of heaviness in the limb. The additional weight of fluid-filled tissue may actually encourage the patient to drag his or her foot or to avoid use of the upper limb in the performance of daily tasks. Mild aching discomfort or fatigue is common. By contrast, intense or severe pain is unusual in lymphedema and signifies a rapid increase in the degree of edema or massive swelling. Differentiation of the discomfort caused by accumulation of edema fluid from that caused by nerve injury is particularly important in the patient with secondary lymphedema. Ganel and associates

TABLE 6.2.
CLINICAL DIAGNOSIS OF LYMPHEDEMA

| Symptoms | Physical Findings | Helpful Concomitant Physical Findings | Methods of Evaluation |
|---|---|---|---|
| Limb swelling | Limb edema | Distichiasis | Lymphography |
| Heaviness | Dorsal buffalo hump | Pedal angiomata | Measurement of limb |
| Recurrent | Elephantine | Hyperplastic form | circumference |
| lymphangitis | distribution | Amelogenesis imperfecta | Volume displacement |
| Skin changes | Pinkish-red skin color | Congenital cardiac deformities | Xeroradiography |
| Fungal infections | Lichenification | Gonadal dysgenesis | $^{131}$I-albumin disappearance |
| | Peau d'orange | Pes cavus | curves |
| | Subcutaneous tissue | Changes in long bones | Computed tomography |
| | lacks resilence | | |

(1979) showed that following radical or modified mastectomy 28% of patients had carpal tunnel syndrome and another 28% suffered from brachial plexus entrapment on the side of surgery. By contrast, only 8% had carpal tunnel and 5% brachial plexus symptoms on the nonoperated side. Over 10% of the patients had both types of entrapment on the operated side. Of the 90 women evaluated, nearly 45 (50%) had lymphedema of some degree. In contrast to the sharp, burning neuritic pain with a dermatomic distribution caused by nerve involvement, the patient with pain secondary to lymphedema often describes her discomfort as bursting: "My leg feels like it is going to blow up." The pain is heavy or dull in quality and is not localized. Lymphangitis, a frequent complication of lymphedema, also may produce a painful limb, but it is described as "prickly" and the pain is localized to the skin.

With further progression of the disease process, the patient may observe changes either in the skin, such as thickening and lichenification, or in the subcutaneous tissue, ligneous fibrosis. These changes are aggravated by fungal, bacterial or viral infections common to lymphedema. The development of these infections may be favored by pruritis-induced excoriation of the skin. The patient's scratching may lead to linear shallow areas or skin breakdown, but it is unusual for the patient with lymphedema to present with a frank ulcer.

## Physical Findings

The dimension and shape of the lymphedematous limb are characteristic (Fig. 6.1) and should provide the major clue to diagnosis. The dorsum of the forefoot demonstrates a pathognomonic increase in tissue with loss of normal contour. This distribution of edema is called a

*buffalo hump* because the anterior margin of the ankle joint may be spared out of proportion to the degree of edema. There is usually a crease across the ankle joint and less edema distally at the metatarsal-phalangeal joint line. Both areas of sparing create a humping up of tissue over the dorsum when viewed from the side (Fig. 6.2). Due to the presence of edema fluid in the digits, particularly in the toes, the skin cannot be tented up over the dorsum of the toes in the patient with lymphedema. This physical finding is a pathognomonic physical sign of lymphedema, a positive Stemmer's sign. The lower limb may be shaped like a tree trunk in a roughly cylindrical shape (Figs. 6.1 and 6.3). This contrasts with the distribution of edema in congestive heart failure or in venous insufficiency, where the edema is most severe in the dependent or ankle area. To take issue with an old clinical axiom, lymphedema, especially in the early stages, will pit. It is only when the degree of subcutaneous fibrosis becomes markedly increased that diminished tissue compliance prevents pitting (Young et al., 1976).

The type of skin changes observed in a lymphedematous limb may be helpful in the differential diagnosis as well as in grading the severity of the process. In mild lymphedema the skin is near normal in texture, although the color may be salmon-pink due to cutaneous vasodilatation and increased cutaneous blood flow. Digital pressure will show pitting and yield a doughy sensation. A peau d'orange effect may be observed (Fig. 6.4). Moderate lymphedema is associated with skin thickening, definite peau d'orange, and episodic bouts of cutaneous erythema (Figs. 6.2 and 6.3). The latter is due to lymphangitis attacks. Mild lichenification may be present, and fungal infection may be observed in the interdigital clefts. More resiliency in the subcutaneous

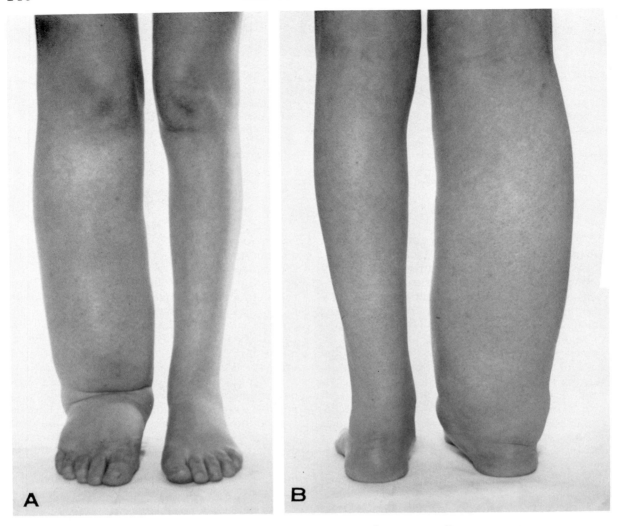

FIGURE 6.1. VIEWS OF LOWER EXTREMITY AND LYMPHEDEMA PRAECOX

tissue indicates fibrosis. In severe lymphedema, hyperkeratosis, lichenification, and fissures are observed in the skin. The subcutaneous tissue is firm.

Distichiasis (duplication of the eyelashes) and blotchy angiomata frequently accompany the hyperplastic form of lymphedema (Shammas et al., 1979). *Amelogenesis imperfecta* may also be present. A variety of cardiac lesions, including pulmonic stenosis, atrial septal defect, and patent ductus arteriosus, have been associated with lymphedema. Careful auscultation of the heart should be performed to rule out previously unrecognized cardiac lesions in patients with primary lymphedema. In Kinmonth's series (1972), 7% had gonadal dysgenesis in association with hypoplastic lymphatics. Four patients had the

chromosomal pattern of Turner's syndrome, the characteristic webbed neck, and the increased carrying angle of the arms. In addition, pes cavus and abnormalities of the long bones of the lower leg have been described in association with primary lymphedema (Jackson and Kinmonth 1970).

In 1892 Milroy described a type of hereditary lymphedema characterized by what he termed its "congenital origin." Unfortunately, in practice Milroy's disease has become a synonym for any form of primary lymphedema. The term should be reserved for those rare cases of primary lymphedema (2% of 100 cases studied by Kinmonth, 1972), which are congenital, familial, and usually involve the lower limb. Kinmonth has reviewed the sex incidence of patients and their

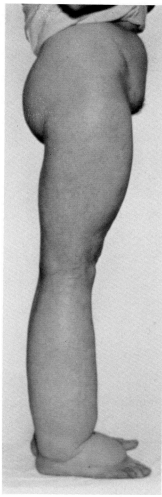

FIGURE 6.2. LATERAL VIEW OF PATIENT WITH MODERATE
LYMPHEDEMA PRAECOX

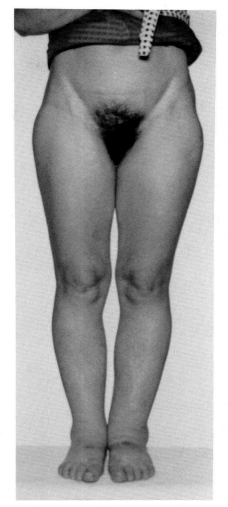

FIGURE 6.3. MILD LYMPHEDEMA

affected relatives and described a ratio of 48 males to 49 females. The genetics of Milroy's disease has not been fully elucidated, but an autosomal dominant mode of transmission is favored. Esterly (1965) ruled out a different mode of inheritance. In Kinmonth's series (1972) lymphography revealed aplasia in the majority of cases. Two cases showed severe hypoplasia, however. The degree of lymphedema is progressive and usually extends to involve the entire limb.

## METHODS OF EVALUATION

The purposes of any investigation in a patient with suspected lymphedema are 3-fold: establish the diagnosis; assess lymphatic function; document the degree of lymphedema and its change with therapy. Lymphography is perhaps the most widely accepted definitive form of evaluation.

Some information can be obtained from the preparatory phase of the procedure. Immediately after injection of patent blue dye into the dermis, a blue wheal is formed in the normal limb without any spidery streaming from the central hub. By contrast, in lymphedema, filamentous strands of dye-stained dermal lymphatics (dermal backflow) are observed. Dermal backflow may be more widespread in the obstructive or hyperplastic forms of lymphedema.

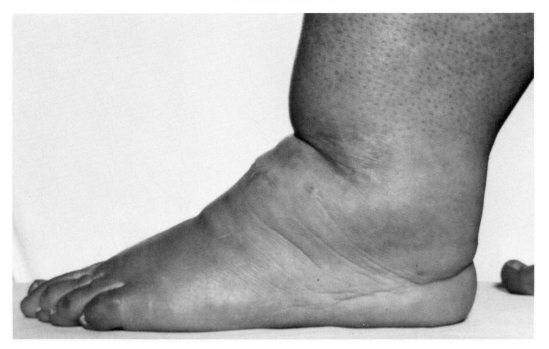

FIGURE 6.4. LATERAL VIEW OF FOOT AND SEVERE LYMPHEDEMA

## Lymphographic Patterns

### Primary Lymphedema

Patients may exhibit aplasia, hypoplasia, or hyperplasia. Eustace and Kinmonth (1976) carried out a detailed analysis of 68 normal lymphangiograms. In this study they described: mean number of lymphatic vessels; mean lymphatic vessel width; number of lymph nodes; and mean inguinal lymph node area. Their data provide a unique reference point for objectively reviewing any lymphangiogram (Table 6.3, Fig. 6.5).

Employing this method O'Donnell et al. (1976a, b) reviewed 20 lymphangiograms in patients with lymphedema associated with mixed vascular deformities. In this series seven patients showed hypoplasia with 2.1 ± 0.8 SE vessels at the upper thigh/inguinal area with a width of 0.63 ± 0.24 mm ± SE. By contrast, the seven limbs with hyperplasia showed a mean of 18.5 ± 3.5 vessels with a width of 1.73 ± 0.53 mm at the upper thigh/inguinal level. Hypo- or hyperplasia can thus be described on the basis of number of lymphatic vessels or trunks, their width, or both. This is less a problem than it appears. In general, lymphedema has been classified by the number of lymphatic vessels. Hypoplasia is defined as a decreased number of lymphatic trunks at a specific reference point (leg, thigh, inguinal, lumbar level). In addition, vessel width is usually decreased or at the upper limits of normal (Fig. 6.6). Occasionally, as in proximal hypoplasia with distal hyperplasia, the width of the numerically hypoplastic trunk may be wider than usual (Figs. 6.7 and 6.8).

By contrast, hyperplasia is defined by an increased number of trunks and may take one of two forms. In unilateral megalymphatics, the more common form, the vessels are increased both in number and in width (Fig. 6.9) and are valveless. They resemble varicose veins. Megalymphatics may be associated with arterial and venous dysplasia, usually an arteriovenous fistula, capillary angiomata, chylous reflux, early presentation of edema, and an equal sex distribution without a family history of edema.

The second form of hyperplasia, which is frequently bilateral, has a striking increase in the *number* of lymphatic trunks (Fig. 6.10). Their width may be normal or only slightly increased. Besides mild bilateral edema, this group has several other unifying clinical findings. They demonstrate blotchy angiomata along the sides of the feet, distichiasis, and other congenital deformities; a family history of edema is common. Shammas and colleagues (1979) described

Table 6.3.
Results of Lymphography in Primary Lymphedema

| Series | No. of Cases | Hypoplasia/Aplasia | Hyperplasia |
|---|---|---|---|
| Buonocore and Young (1965) | 20 | 20 | |
| Thompson (1970) | 50 | 47 | 3 |
| | | (17 prox.*) | |
| Kinmonth (1972) | 100 | 92 | 8 |
| Olszewski et al. (1972b) | 120 | 111 | 9 |
| | | (24 prox.*) | |
| Saijo et al. (1975) | 12 | 7 | 5 |
| Kinmonth (1982) | 562 | 506 | 56 |
| Total | 864 | 783 (91%) | 81 (9%) |

* Proximal hypoplasia with an obstruction.

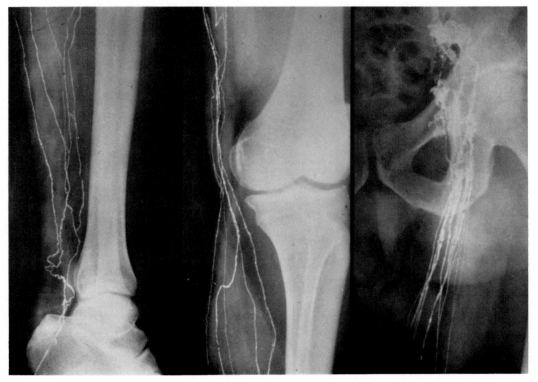

Figure 6.5. Normal Lymphangiogram of the Lower Extremity with Views of Calf and Thigh

two families with this form of lymphedema and distichiasis and related this familial incidence to a pleiotropic gene with a high penetrance and variable expressivity.

Table 6.3 compares the lymphographic findings in various well-known series. Hypoplasia is the commonest abnormality (91%) demonstrated by lymphography. The incidence of aplasia, which Eustace and Kinmonth (1976) view as a severe variant of hypoplasia, usually directly reflects the persistence and patience of the lymphographer.

## Secondary Lymphedema

The pathogenesis of acquired lymphedema and concomitant changes in the lymphograms are discussed in the section on obstruction (Table 6.1). The pattern that develops in patients with clinical lymphedema after cancer surgery is characterized by a progressive increase in the width and number of lymphatic trunks. Kreel and George (1966) demonstrated this pattern of hyperplasia with marked dermal backflow in eight patients following radical mastectomy. Hughes

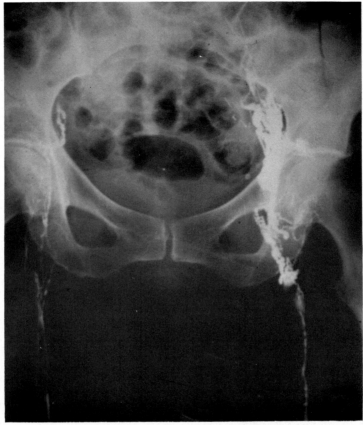

FIGURE 6.6. LYMPHANGIOGRAM ILLUSTRATING HYPOPLASTIC PATTERN OF LOWER EXTREMITY DUE TO PRIMARY
LYMPHEDEMA

and Patel (1966) showed similar lymphographic changes.

Edema of the lower extremity may occur frequently after arterial reconstruction, particularly after femoral-popliteal or tibial bypass. Postoperatively, tissue is reperfused at a higher pressure than preoperatively so that subsequent transcapillary leakage of fluid may occur. The sudden postoperative increase in arterial perfusion pressure has been theorized as an explanation for edema accumulation after vascular reconstruction, but Schmidt and associates (1978) showed partial to total disruption of the lymphatic vessels in 27 of 37 patients after femoral popliteal bypass. Lymphangiograms performed on these patients between the third and ninth postoperative days revealed intact lymph vessels at the knee and the groin. Mild lymphedema (1–2 cm) occurred when at least three lymph vessels were preserved, while moderate to severe lymphedema was noted when all lymph vessels had been divided. Repeat revascularization procedures were associated with the greatest degree of lymphe-

dema. These authors found no correlation with the preoperative condition of the limb, the presence of venous disease, or the degree of postoperative ischemia.

In filariasis, widened varicose lymphatics with numerical hyperplasia and incompetent valves are visible on the lymphangiograms. By contrast, lymphedema due to recurrent lymphangitis or cellulitis results in fibrosis and narrowing of the lymphatic vessels (hypoplasia), while the regional nodes are usually hyperplastic. Lymphography demonstrates small caliber, wispy lymphatic vessels.

## Deep Lymphatics

Since most investigations have focused on the superficial or subcutaneous lymphatics, there is little information on the deep system in lymphedema. Kinmonth (1972) felt that the deep lymphatics were deficient in primary lymphedema, much like the superficial system, and was unable to identify any trunks after injection of patent

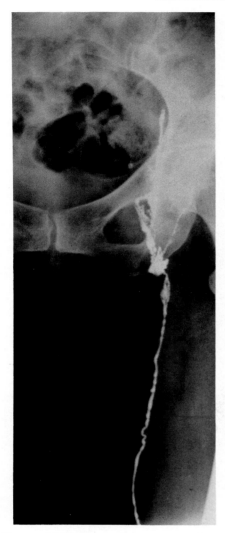

FIGURE 6.7. ANOTHER FORM OF HYPOPLASIA

is crude and subject to many variables, a standardized lymphangiographic technique does afford the opportunity to quantitate lymphatic function. Lipiodol injected into the pedal lymphatics at a rate of 1 ml over 7 min will reach the inguinal nodes by 5 min and the sacroiliac joint by 35 min in a normal lymphatic system. Lymphatic stasis due to decreased vessel caliber (hypoplasia) or increased capacitance (numerical hyperplasia) may slow the transit time. An altered transit time may be the only evidence of lymphatic malfunction in some patients with mild edema and normal lymphatic anatomy by lymphography (Kinmonth, 1972).

One of the main functions of the lymphatic tree is to clear protein from the extravascular extracellular fluid space and return it to the intravascular space. The rate at which labeled albumin is cleared from this site should assess lymphatic function. Indeed, [131]I-albumin disappearance curves are prolonged in the lymphedematous limb. This delayed clearance may be related to trapping of albumin within the interstitial space and subsequent pooling or to reversal of the ratio of normal subcutaneous tissue pressure to muscle compartment pressure. In lymphedema, interstitial fluid protein concentration is elevated and subcutaneous pressure is higher than muscle compartment pressure. Despite this attractive physiological rationale, however, measurements of disappearance curves have little value in the initial assessment of lymphedema (Emmett et al., 1967). This technique has found its greatest use in determining the effects of various surgical procedures for lymphedema (Thompson, 1970).

## Degree of Lymphedema

The two standard methods for assessing the degree of lymphedema are measurement of limb circumference at specific anatomic sites and measurement of limb volume by water displacement. The *amount* of absolute increase in lymphedematous tissue is represented by the abnormal minus the normal dimension, while the *degree* of lymphedema (relative amount of lymphedematous tissue) is related to the [(abnormal-normal)/normal] (Richmand et al., in press). Since there are no tables of normal values applicable to a wide range of limb dimensions, most clinicians use the contralateral limb as the control or normal value. These techniques are hampered by variation of technique, observer error from measurement to measurement, difference in normal limb size (especially in upper limbs), and lack of reproducibility.

Perhaps the most convenient method for cir-

blue. Vitek and Kaspar (1973) carried out lymphography of the deep system in 12 patients with lymphedema. Two of eight patients with primary lymphedema exhibited obliteration of their deep lymphatics with anastomoses to a defective superficial system. One of the four patients with secondary lymphedema showed a similar pattern. The remaining nine patients had normal deep lymphatic systems.

## Lymphatic Function

For clinical purposes transit time and radioactive albumin disappearance curves are the only two techniques that have had widespread use in the functional evaluation of lymphedema. Although measurement of the time taken by a column of contrast media to reach a specific spot

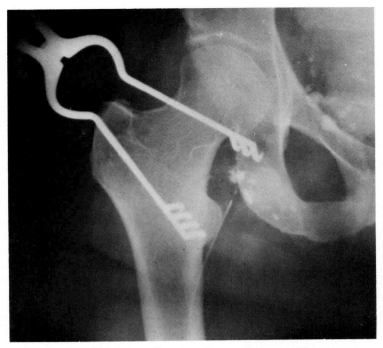

FIGURE 6.8. NODOGRAM SHOWING SEVERE BILATERAL HYPOPLASIA

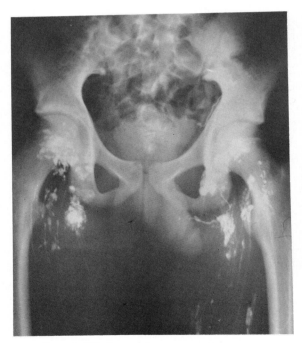

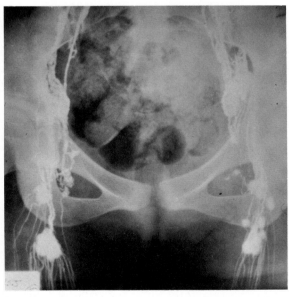

FIGURE 6.10. LYMPHANGIOGRAM FROM PATIENT WITH
NUMERICAL HYPERPLASIA

FIGURE 6.9. LOWER LYMPHANGIOGRAM AND
LYMPHEDEMA OF THE RIGHT EXTREMITY WITH
HYPERPLASIA

cumferential measurements of girth are the pre-made measurement devices used for fitting elastic compression stockings, which consist of a series of paper tapes. Indeed, in our experience

this method of measuring limb girth avoids the variation in technique, observer error, and lack of reproducibility inherent in other methods. For those physicians who see patients with lymphedema frequently, limb volume measurement by water displacement provides objective estimates of total limb edema. The limb is immersed in a large cylinder fitted with a tap so the excess volume of water that escapes through the tap can be volumetrically measured in another container. The volume displacement method does not identify the particular segment of the limb that has increased or decreased in dimension.

Soft tissue x-ray or xeroradiography provides an objective means for measuring skin and subcutaneous thickness independently. In a series of 11 patients with secondary lymphedema, O'-Donnell et al. (1976a, b) demonstrated a 4-fold increase in skin thickness and a 2-fold increase in subcutaneous tissue. Another important factor assessed by this method is the degree of subcutaneous fibrosis. The amount of subcutaneous scarring or fibrosis is related to tissue compliance and therefore provides a prediction of the limb's responsiveness to compression. Because of radiation exposure inherent in this technique, we have limited its use to a yearly exposure. Tissue tonometry measurement, which employs devices similar to those used in assessing glaucoma, is an alternative to xeroradiography for determining the degree of subcutaneous tissue fibrosis. This method is particularly important in assessing the effects of pharmacological treatment of subcutaneous fibrosis.

## Computed Tomography

Computed tomography (CT) scanning is an important new adjunct to the evaluation and management of lymphedema. In my practice the number of lymphangiograms performed has been decreased by substituting CT for lymphographic assessment of lymph node size and number. CT allows noninvasive, objective classification of primary lymphedema patients into aplastic, hypoplastic, or hyperplastic types depending on the number of lymph nodes. In patients with secondary lymphedema, CT is a powerful diagnostic tool for determining whether recurrent neoplasm or other inflammatory processes have caused the lymphedema. Finally, CT scanning is useful in assessing the cause of proximal extremity enlargement. We now employ CT as our standard method for assessing patients with lymphedema.

## NONSURGICAL TREATMENT

In our experience over 90% of patients can be managed without surgery. The goals of nonoperative therapy are: reduction of limb size, preservation and improvement in skin quality, softening of subcutaneous tissue, and prevention of lymphangitis (Table 6.4).

### Reduction in Limb Size

The degree of lymphedema is reduced by improving the function of existing lymphatics and utilizing alternative pathways for fluid transport. Simple elevation of the leg at night by placing blocks under the foot of the bed or suspending

the arm in a sling is associated with moderate success, particularly in soft lymphedemas. The use of a pillow to elevate the leg is usually ineffective because the limb slips off the pillow in the middle of the night. Compression therapy with either elastic stockings or pneumatic devices is fundamental to reducing limb girth. Conventional forms of compression by elastic hose maintain the limb at its initial girth when measured for the hose. Therefore, the patient should be measured in the morning, preferably at home before much edema has accumulated. I generally employ 40–50 mm Hg gradient stockings (Sigvaris) but may use 30–40 mm Hg compres-

TABLE 6.4.
TREATMENT OF LYMPHEDEMA

| Nonoperative | Operative | |
|---|---|---|
| Reduction of Limb Size | Physiological | Excisional |
| Elevation | Buried dermal flap | Skin and subcutaneous tissue excision |
| Elastic compression | Lymphovenous shunt | with split thickness skin graft coverage |
| Massage | Full thickness skin bridge | Staged excision of subcutaneous tissue |
| External pneumatic compression | Omental transposition | with vascularized local flaps |
| | Subcutaneous tunnels | |
| Improvement in skin quality | Lysis of fibrotic venous | |
| | obstruction | |
| Skin lotion | | |
| Benzopyrones | | |
| Treatment of fungal and bacterial | | |
| infections | | |

sion stockings initially when the patient feels that the firmer stocking is too tight. The length of the stocking is matched to the distribution of edema. In patients with ankle, forefoot, and calf edema, below-the-knee stockings are much more comfortable because they do not bind at the popliteal fossa. In patients with concomitant thigh edema, however, panty hose or thigh-high stockings are preferable.

By applying two elastic hose, we have used relatively high pressures in selected patients. Initially, eight of our patients with lymphedema (seven primary and one secondary) were fitted to two full length 30–40 mm Hg elastic compression stockings (Sigvaris). The compression was gradually increased at 2-month intervals: 30–40 mm Hg inner, 40–50 mm Hg outer at 4 months; 40–50 mm Hg inner and 50–60 mm Hg outer at 6 months. Hemodynamic studies with digital plethysmography showed no deleterious effects on arterial flow when the two stockings were applied. Sequential girth measurements were obtained at 10 constant points on the limbs repeatedly during the 10-month trial. As shown in Table 6.5 all limbs had decreased girths. In addition, patients observed that their limbs developed a so-called normal contour. No patient discontinued treatment because of discomfort during the 1-year follow-up. The acceptance of double compression treatment may be attributed to the gradual increase in circumferential pressure, which must be paced differently for each patient. During the initial course of double compression therapy, it was not unusual to see increases in thigh girth, which then decreased progressively after 4 months. In those young patients who can tolerate the pressure and the difficulty in putting these stockings on, double compression therapy is a helpful adjunct.

In over 100 patients with lymphedema, followed for 5 years, we observed that conscientious use of elastic stockings will maintain the limb in a reduced state. These findings are similar to those of Zeissler et al. (1972), who followed 183 patients (67%) but unfortunately made no objective measurements.

While single layer elastic stockings may maintain limb size, only the application of high pressure compression will reduce limb size. Van der Mollen and Toth (1974) used a soft rubber tube that was wound around the leg starting from the toes and progressing proximally. This form of high pressure external compression, which they termed *extubation*, develops a pressure of approximately 200–300 mm Hg and can only be carried out when the patient is under anesthesia. With this technique a visible rim of lymphatic fluid within the subcutaneous tissue advances up the leg proximal to the compressing tube. The authors noted "good results."

## External Pneumatic Compression

We initially employed external pneumatic compression with a low pressure. The unicell boot or sleeve was inflated to 60 mm Hg for 12.5 sec of compression alternating with 35 sec of rest. This cycle was different from that of Allenby et al. (1973), who utilized 40 mm Hg pressure at 1 cycle/min. Our pressure waveform was characterized by a fast upstroke and an even sharper down stroke. In a prospective study 17 patients with lymphedema were treated with intermittent external pneumatic compression (Raines et al., 1977). Among the nine patients with lymphedema of the upper extremity, the hands were reduced by nearly 50% following compression, but forearms and upper arms resisted therapy and showed less than a 20% reduction. Those patients with lower extremity lymphedema showed the same pattern, an adequate response at the foot but poor at the calf and thigh. In this study we also correlated the degree of subcutaneous fibrosis, as measured by xerography, with the response to compression. Patients with fibrous subcutaneous tissue responded less well to compression therapy than those with soft subcutaneous tissue. In addition, concomitant venous obstruction lowered the efficacy of compression therapy for lymphedema.

Because the maximum effect of external pneumatic compression was observed at the more

TABLE 6.5.
EFFECT OF DOUBLE COMPRESSION ELASTIC STOCKING IN LOWER EXTREMITY LYMPHEDEMA*

|  | Metatarsal† | Malleolar† | Calf–Low† | Thigh |
|---|---|---|---|---|
| Precompression girth | 25.1 ± 0.7 | 27 ± 1.6 | 35.3 ± 2.1 | 55.5 ± 1.1 |
| Postcompression girth | 21.2 ± 1.2 | 22.4 ± 1.3 | 31 ± 1.8 | 53 ± 2.2 |

\* Girth measurements (mean centimeters ± SE).

† Significant difference to at least $p < .05$ by paired $t$ test.

distal portion of the extremity and because approximately 30–40% of limbs are refractory to this form of therapy due to subcutaneous fibrosis, we sought a more effective method. The development of a high pressure compression device by Zelikovski et al. (1980) appeared to answer those problems. The device is multisegmental so that pressure is distributed in a distal to proximal milking fashion rather than in both centripedal and centrifugal directions as with the unicompartmental device. In addition, higher pressures range up to 110 mm Hg for the upper extremity and 150 mm Hg for the lower extremity, approximately twice the value achieved with the unicompartmental device. A controlled prospective study in our National Institutes of Health Clinical Study Unit examined the efficacy of this device (Richmand et al., in press). Twenty-five patients, seven with upper extremity and 18 with lower extremity lymphedema, underwent 24 hours of treatment. All extremities showed a marked decrease in circumferential measurements. The lower extremity leg volume was reduced by 45%, while the midcalf circumference was reduced by approximately 47%. Table 6.6 shows the results of compression therapy in absolute terms. In addition to the more dramatic decrease in limb girth, sequential compression therapy reduces the limb more rapidly than the unicompartment type. Our present protocol involves application of the compression device so that a significant reduction in limb volume and girth is attained. Elastic compression stockings are then fitted for the individual at the new reduced girth. Approximately 50–70% of our patients have maintained this reduced limb size with faithful wearing of elastic stockings.

TABLE 6.6.
RESULTS OF SEQUENTIAL HIGH PRESSURE PNEUMATIC COMPRESSION FOR LYMPHEDEMA

| Absolute Reduction in Lymphedematous Tissue* | | | |
|---|---|---|---|
| | Wrist | Midforearm | Midupper Arm |
| Arm ($n = 7$) | $0.9 \pm 0.2$ | $1.9 \pm 0.3$ | $1.4 \pm 0.3$ |
| | Ankle | Midcalf | Midthigh |
| Leg ($n = 8$) | $8.4 \pm 1.5$ | $8.1 \pm 1.4$ | $1.5 \pm 0.3$ |

| Percentage (relative) Reduction in Lymphedematous Tissue* | | | |
|---|---|---|---|
| | Wrist | Midforearm | Midupper Arm |
| Arm ($n = 7$) | $45 \pm 14\%$ | $28 \pm 7\%$ | $25 \pm 13\%$ |
| | Ankle | Midcalf | Midthigh |
| Leg ($n = 18$) | $37 \pm 6\%$ | $47 \pm 5\%$ | $36 \pm 7\%$ |

* Mean centimeters ± SE.

## Preservation and Improvement of Skin Quality

The second goal of the nonsurgical treatment of lymphedema is to preserve and improve skin quality. The patient should avoid minor trauma to the skin and should use a water-based lotion twice daily. We prefer Poly-Sorb Hydrate rather than lanolin because the former is certainly less greasy and can be worn with elastic compression stockings. The scaling eczematous skin changes observed in lymphedema can be prevented by consistent use of these skin emollients.

## Softening of Subcutaneous Tissue

Benzopyrones have been shown to soften the subcutaneous tissue of experimentally induced lymphedema (Casley-Smith et al., 1978). Subcutaneous fibrosis appears related to plasma proteins that are deposited in the subcutaneous tissue and cause chronic inflammation. The use of warfarin (Coumadin), a benzopyrone that theoretically enhances the lysis of protein by macrophages, greatly reduces this fibrosis. We have not utilized this pharmacological approach, although it is quite popular in Europe.

## Prevention of Lymphangitis

Approximately 15–20% of patients with lymphedema will present with recurrent lymphangitis as their main symptom. Bacteriological studies of samples obtained by saline aspiration of the cellulitic margin have shown that $\beta$-hemolytic streptococci are the most common bacteria. These patients can become gravely ill because the normal protective immunological barriers to invasive infections are lacking. Indeed, several of our patients have presented in shock. We treat patients with penicillin or oxacillin. Cultures are obtained by saline aspiration so that the antibiotic can be altered pending sensitivity and culture of the organism. In the lower extremity the usual route of entry is through a fungal infection between the toes. Alternatively there may be no obvious sign of entry and the bacteria may have invaded around the hair follicles. An effective course of intravenous antibiotics generally takes 5–7 days, and we maintain the patient on oral therapy for an additional 3 weeks. If a patient has more than two episodes a year, he is placed on prophylactic erythromycin or penicillin. We have found that this greatly reduces the number of infectious episodes. Concomitant with antibiotic therapy, an antifungal powder should be used to prevent fungal infection. If there is active infection, oral griseofulvin should be administered because the powder is preventive only.

## SURGICAL TREATMENT

We have restricted surgery to a small percentage of the patients whom we see for lymphedema. Like evaluating any surgical procedure, the costs of surgery must be offset by the benefits of the procedure. Unfortunately, the most widely performed procedures for lymphedema consist of removing the lymphedematous tissue, and only a small proportion of these patients enjoy long term benefits from this reduction surgery. Indeed, Chilvers and Kinmonth (1975) showed that only 30% of patients had good results, and these benefits were restricted to those patients with the most massive edema. Moreover, the majority of patients regressed to their preoperative girth measurements within 2–4 yr after original surgery. Finally, the surgical morbidity such as major skin necrosis that occurs in nearly a quarter of patients may require both prolonged hospitalization and time lost from work.

Traditionally, the indications for surgery have been: *cosmetic*, to improve the shape and size of the limb, as well as the patient's psychological well-being; *functional*, to reduce limb weight and to improve skin texture; *preventive*, either to minimize the likelihood of angiosarcoma, a lethal complication of lymphedema, or to decrease the number of lymphangitic attacks. We certainly ascribe to the second indication to improve limb function and utilize surgery in patients with massive lymphedema that is unresponsive to compression therapy or in patients with gross skin changes. Surgery should be avoided in patients with: minimal edema (where the difference between the normal and abnormal limb is less than 3 cm); gross obesity; active progression of the disease (the lymphedema has not reached a steady state by girth measurements); and failure to establish a firm diagnosis of lymphedema as the cause of the limb swelling.

Kinmonth (1972) has divided the many forms of surgical treatment into two broad categories: physiological and excisional procedures (Table 6.4).

### Physiological Procedures

The basic purpose of physiological procedures for lymphedema is to promote drainage from the abnormal superficial subcutaneous lymphatics to the normal lymphatics. The latter normal lymphatics may be either deep lymphatics in the limb or lymphatics more proximal to the abnormal lymphatics. Although Kondoleon (1912) believed that excising a wedge of fascia permitted development of superficial to deep lymphatic anastomoses, the reduction in limb size was related more to removing a generous portion of subcutaneous tissue than to functional lymphatic anastomoses. Sistrunk (1918) modified this procedure by excising greater amounts of subcutaneous tissue, which may explain his slightly better results.

Several surgeons have revived Handley's original operation (1908). Subcutaneous tunnels were created by inserting a large silk thread from the lymphedematous hand to the normal shoulder area so that a conduit was fashioned to bypass fluid through the abnormal subcutaneous lymphatics to normal tissue. O'Reilly (1972) used nylon setons in two women with postmastectomy edema with encouraging results but no change in the rate of albumin removal from the lymphedematous tissue. Silver and Puckett (1980) described their subcutaneous tunnel as being quite effective in primary lymphedema, but the lack of objective measurements impaired assessment of this procedure.

### Lymphovenous Shunts

Perhaps the most attractive physiological operation was the lymphovenous shunt first reported clinically by Nielubowicz and Olszewski (1968). An explosion of interest in this procedure followed their report of four patients with secondary lymphedema who had reduced limb size following a lymphovenous shunt. On postmortem examination in one patient who had died from her primary disease, they showed patency in the medullary sinuses, and lymphography showed a functioning lymphovenous anastomosis in the other three patients. Anastomosis of the lymphatic system to the venous system may be carried out in two basic ways: bread-loafing the node and anastomosing the node onto the vein through a venotomy or directly implanting the lymphatic vessels by either microlymphaticovenous anastomoses or by specially constructed tubes (Degni, 1981).

In spite of the excitement and claim for clinical

improvement with lymphaticovenous anasto-moses, objective evidence of successful results is lacking. In 1969, Politowski et al. reported 16 patients who underwent the original procedure of Nielubowicz and Olszewski. These patients had primary lymphedema and were observed for 6–18 months after lymphaticovenous anastomosis. "Good results" were achieved in only eight patients, "fair" in six, and "unsatisfactory" in two. The lack of excellent results was disappointing.

Russian surgeons have been quite enthusiastic about the lymphaticovenous shunt. Milanov et al. (1982) reported on their experiences with 50 patients who underwent lymphovenous anastomoses for treatment of postmastectomy lymphedema. "Good results" were noted in 15 patients and "satisfactory" in another 28. Gong-Kang and associates (1981) showed objective improvement in 13 patients with secondary lymphedema of the upper and lower extremities treated by microlymphaticovenous anastomoses. These limbs demonstrated an average reduction in girth of 6.2 cm. Their results paralleled those of the Australian plastic surgeon O'Brien, who combined microlymphatic surgery with segmental reduction of the limb (O'Brien et al., 1977). O'Brien and Das (1979) showed that three or more lymphaticovenous anastomoses were needed to reduce limb size and also emphasized that technical experience was an important factor in microvascular surgery to achieve good results. They advised caution in evaluating the results of lymphovenous shunts because long term follow-up has not been achieved.

Balanced against these enthusiastic reports are the experimental findings of Puckett et al. (1980). They constructed direct lymphaticovenous anastomoses in a canine model with chronic obstructive lymphedema. Although the early patency of 100% was associated with a significant reduction in lymphedema, by 1 month all lymphovenous anastomoses had occluded. These poor results have been duplicated in other microvascular centers in the United States. In addition, Clodius et al. (1981) have called attention to the problems associated with microlymphatic surgery for lymphedema. They caution that the surgeon should not look at the lymphatic system as a connection of drainage tubes because fibrotic changes in subcutaneous tissue are an important clinical manifestation of lymphedema. Without treatment of both the increased tissue bulk and scarring of fatty tissue, little improvement should be seen. Finally, construction of lymphaticovenous anastomoses presumes that a normal functioning system of lymphatics exists below a block, but such is not the predominant pattern in primary lymphedema. Certainly, lymphaticovenous anastomoses appear to be most ideally suited for obstructive forms of secondary lymphedema.

## Omental Transposition

In an attempt to provide a pathway for normal lymphatics, Goldsmith (1974) employed omental transposition to bridge the area of lymphatic insufficiency, but the long term results were disappointing. In 22 patients followed for 1–7 yr, only 38% showed good results (by very liberal criteria), while 23% had fair results. He wisely suggested that this procedure be used only by a few surgeons experienced with this technique because of a late mortality in a young male. This patient died secondary to a hernia which incarcerated at the site of the omentum's entry into the lower limb.

Various surgeons have revised the original Gillies procedure, which employed a full thickness graft of tissue to bypass lymphatic obstruction. Again, this procedure depends on a local block in the lymphatics and relatively normal lymphatics below the block (Hirshowitz and Goldan, 1971). After extensive experimental work, Kinmonth et al. (1978) used ileum that had been stripped of its mucosa to bridge the area of lymphatic blockage. The submucosal small bowel lymphatics anastomosed with lymphatics in the limb below the block. Kinmonth showed objective improvements in a 22-yr-old patient with lymphedema praecox who underwent this procedure. In addition, we are presently following one of his other patients who has shown very definite improvements in limb size since this operation.

## Buried Dermal Flap

The Thompson procedure or a variation thereof is presently the most widely used surgical procedure for lymphedema (Thompson, 1962). The operation combines excision of subcutaneous tissue with a buried posterior flap that is fixed to the deep fascia. Thompson felt that the buried flap brought the subcutaneous and dermal lymphatics into contact with the deep lymphatics and muscle tissues so that spontaneous lymphatic or lymphovenous anastomoses could develop.

Functional assessment of this procedure with radioactive albumin disappearance curves has led to conflicting results. Thompson (1970) and Harvey (1969) have demonstrated increased disappearance of albumin, which indicated improved function. Sawney (1974) found a reduction in limb circumference and increased albumin clearance only in the immediate postoperative period, but these findings were not present several months later.

Kinmonth (1972) was unable to find any lymphaticolymphatic or lymphovenous anastomoses or lymphangiograms performed after the Thompson procedure. He felt that any improvement beyond what could be expected from simple removal of subcutaneous tissue was related to the compressive massaging effect of the buried flap. He based this conclusion on cinelymphographic studies that showed traction and massaging of the abnormal lymphatics by the calf muscles. The buried dermal flap may also lead to normalization of the reversed subcutaneous to muscle compartment pressure ratio. Table 6.7 summarizes the results of several series for the Thompson procedure.

## Excisional Procedures

Charles (1912), working in an area endemic for tropical elephantiasis, developed an operation that consisted of removing both skin and subcutaneous tissue. Split thickness grafts were applied to cover the exposed deep fascia. At present, the Charles procedure is restricted to those patients with severe skin changes that may prevent the use of vascularized skin flaps or subcutaneous lipectomies (Table 6.8). The thigh area must be tapered to avoid a so-called pantaloon or baseball pants appearance. Late results may be complicated by the development of hyperkeratosis, recurrent sepsis, and condylomata. Dellon and Hoopes (1977) reported the long term results in 10 patients following the Charles procedure. Four of the extremities were examined as late as 20 yr or more following surgery. All patients demonstrated excellent functional results and none demonstrated recurrence of

TABLE 6.7.
PHYSIOLOGICAL OPERATIONS FOR LYMPHEDEMA

| Series | No. of Patients | Type | Results*—No. of Patients | | | Criteria | Length of Follow-up (Yr) |
|---|---|---|---|---|---|---|---|
| | | | Good | Satisfactory (Fair) | Poor | | |
| Buried Dermal Flap | | | | | | | |
| Thompson (1970) | 50 | 1° | 29 | 17 | 4 | Circumference, clearance studies | 1–10 |
| Thompson (1969) | 23 | 2° | 14 | 8 | 1 | Circumference, clearance studies | 1–9 |
| Sawney (1974) | 5 | 1° | No change | 5 | 0 | Circumference, clearance studies | 1 |
| Bunchman and Lewis (1974) | 10 | 1° | 2 | 4 | 4 | Circumference, volume displacement | 1 |
| Kinmonth et al (1975) | 108 | 1° | 29 | 61 | 18 | Circumference, patient's and surgeon's evaluation | 1 |
| Totals | 196 | | 74 (38%) | 95 (48%) | 27 (14%) | | |
| Lymphovenous Anastomosis | | | | | | | |
| Politowski et al. (1969) | 16 | 1° | 8 | 6 | 2 | | |
| Milanov et al. (1982) | 50 | 2° | 15 | 28 | 7 | | |
| Krylov et al. (1979) | 73 | 2° | 25 | 46 | 2 | | |
| Totals | 139 | | 48 (35%) | 80 (58%) | 11 (8%) | | |
| Omental Transposition | | | | | | | |
| Goldsmith (1974) | 22 | Mixed | 10 (46%) | 4 (18%) | 8 (36%) | Size, function, frequency of cellulitis attacks | 1–7 |

* Author's interpretation of varied criteria for each series.

TABLE 6.8
EXCISIONAL OPERATIONS FOR LYMPHEDEMA

| Series | Type of Procedure | No. of Patients | Type | | Results | | Criteria | Length of Follow-up (Yr) |
|---|---|---|---|---|---|---|---|---|
| | | | 1° | 2° | Good | Satisfactory (Fair) | | |
| Fonkalsrud (1979) | Subcutaneous lymphangiectomy | 6 | 6 | 0 | 6 | 0 | Cosmetic, functional | At least 1 |
| Bunchman and Lewis (1974) | Charles (complete excision of subcutaneous tissue and skin) | 14 | 14 | 0 | 14 | (but undesirable pantaloon effect) | | 5 |
| Dellon and Hoopes (1977) | Charles | 12 | 12 | 0 | 12 | 0 | Circumference | 10½ |
| Miller (1975) | Staged subcutaneous excision | 14 | 6 | 8 | 0 | 14 | Circumference | ½–6 (6 for 4) |
| Miller (1977) | Staged subcutaneous excision | 21 | 0 | 0 | 0 | 21 | Circumference | 0 |
| Bunchman and Lewis (1974) | Staged subcutaneous excision | 5 | 5 | 0 | 5 | 0 | | 1½ |
| Feins et al. (1977) | Staged excisions (pediatric age group) | 39 | 39 | 0 | 0 | 39 | Patient interview | 0 |

lymphedema. Miller (1980) found less satisfactory results with the Charles procedure and warned against its widespread use. Of his five patients with lower extremity lymphedema treated by the Charles procedure, three patients eventually underwent amputation because of severe skin changes or chronic cellulitis. He felt that the split thickness graft caused a deformity worse than the original lymphedema.

Many plastic surgeons now employ a variant of the excisional operation first described by Homans of Boston (1936). Subcutaneous tissue excised in stages and well vascularized flaps are developed. Table 6.8 summarizes the results of various recent series that used some form of subcutaneous lipectomy. In many instances, the lack of uniform objective measurements or criteria for assessing the degree of lymphedema and its changes after surgery limits meaningful interpretation of these data. With this procedure large volumes of subcutaneous tissue can be excised, and the incidences of both flap necrosis and sinus formation are lower than with the buried dermal flap.

Miller (1980) has reported his results over 9 yr with 25 patients who underwent staged subcutaneous excision beneath vascularized flaps.

He felt this procedure was associated with a consistent reduction in size and improvement in function. Fonkalsrud (1979) has employed subcutaneous lymphangiectomy in 10 of 28 patients with moderate to severe lymphedema. Because of hypertrophic scarring, he recommends that the procedure be deferred until after the age of 2. He noted good to excellent results in these patients. In a similar pediatric series, Feins et al. (1977) reported on 39 children who underwent staged excisional surgery. They found negligible morbidity and a dramatic reduction in the number of cellulitic and lymphangitic attacks. Again, they restricted the operation to those patients with moderate to severe lymphedema.

Whereas improvement of lymphatic function or removal of tissue bulk is the main target of surgical intervention in primary lymphedema, relief of venous obstruction has been the focus of several procedures for secondary lymphedema. Hughes and Patel (1966) lysed the fibrotic encasement around the axillary vein with "good" results in 15 of 19 patients with postmastectomy lymphedema. Larsen and Crampton (1973) described good results in four of eight patients who underwent a similar procedure.

## GENITAL LYMPHEDEMA

Genital lymphedema is the third most common form of lymphedema, and its classification follows that used for the extremities. Genital lymphedema may be the sole clinical manifestation of lymphedema or associated with: involvement of adjacent tissue, vesicle formation (Fig. 6.11), skin changes, or signs of sepsis (abscess, cellulitis, and inguinal adenopathy). Proximal

hypoplasia with arborization of the more distal subdermal lymphatics is demonstrated on lymphography, which differs from the pattern observed in secondary genital lymphedema. The acquired form is frequently due to filariasis, which lymphography shows as dilated incompetent lymphatics with reflux.

Indications for surgery in genital lymphedema are similar to those for lymphedema of the extremities: gross swelling of the scrotum or penis and recurrent fistula or sepsis. Alternatively, reduction of the mons veneris may be required in women. At St. Thomas Hospital the procedures have ranged from excision of tissue (such as simple circumcision or partial excision of penile and scrotal tissue) to more extensive operations such as scrotal reduction. When the penile skin is severely lichenified, replacement with a split thickness skin graft is favored. Good functional results have been obtained. In a series of 28 patients with genital lymphedema due to filariasis, 18 underwent partial or subtotal scrotectomy, while seven had total scrotectomies with repair by skin graft or by inguinal replacement (Khamma, 1970). Nineteen required some form

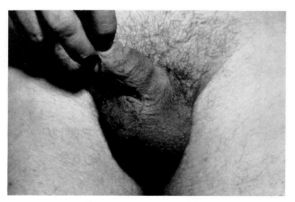

FIGURE 6.11. VIEW OF SCROTAL AREA IN PATIENT WITH CHYLOUS VESICLES

of penoplasty. Other than considerable lymphatic drainage in the early postoperative period, no complications were noted and the later results were quite good.

# CHYLOUS SYNDROMES

The anatomic locations of chylous disorders range from the peritoneal and thoracic cavities, where chyle forms fluid collections, to the neck, urinary tract, and genitalia, where chyle may drain as a fistula. Chylous syndromes, like lymphedema, may be either primary (idiopathic) or secondary. As discussed in the preceding section, obstruction of the main lymphatic vessels by malignancy, infection, or trauma is the chief cause of the chylous syndromes.

## Lower Extremities

The triad of lymphedema (commonly unilateral), cutaneous vesicles, and angiomata is characteristic of chylous syndromes involving the lower extremities. Lymphography demonstrates markedly dilated and capacious lymphatics—megalymphatics (Fig. 6.12). Servelle originally attributed the hyperplastic lymphatics to obstruction of the thoracic duct. In a few patients with megalymphatics, Kinmonth (1972) visualized an abnormally functioning thoracic duct on cinelymphangiography, but obstruction of the thoracic duct was not a consistent finding on all megalymphatics studies. Because of this inconsistency and the frequent finding of unilateral involvement, many have found it difficult to rationalize the mechanism on the basis of thoracic duct obstruction alone. As suggested by Kinmonth et al. (1964), the association of chylous diseases with other congenital anomalies such as angiomata makes in utero developmental error the most likely cause. Ligation of the incompetent lymphatic trunks at the pelvic or inguinal level may prevent reflux and result in both subjective and objective improvement (Fig. 6.12).

## Chylous Ascites

Primary chylous ascites may be fistulous or exudative. A rent in a large and dilated lymphatic vessel leads to formation of a fistula that may be visualized on lymphography. In addition to the fistulous communication with the peritoneal cavity, large capacious megalymphatics are demonstrated by lymphography. Weichert and Jamieson (1970) have described two cases of chylous acites that showed dilated lumbar lymphatics and lymphographic findings suggesting thoracic duct obstruction.

In contrast, exudative chylous ascites is associated with a hypoplastic pattern on lymphography. No discrete site of lymphatic leakage is defined. Before undertaking treatment of chylous ascites, lymphography should be carried out to demonstrate any fistula, which may be corrected by closure of the defect in the lymphatic vessel, its level also being localized by lymphography. The exudative form may require a lymphovenous shunt or a mechanical peritoneal-atrial shunt. In general, chylous ascites secondary to a fistula responds better to therapy than the exudative form does.

Acquired chylous ascites was four times more common than the primary type in the extensive review of 126 cases of chylous ascites by Vasko and Tapper (1967). Twenty-eight cases were due to an inflammatory process, 24 to neoplasm (lymphoma 6, pancreatic carcinoma 4), and 9 to trauma. The authors emphasize the mortality rate among untreated patients: 43% for adults and 29% for children. By contrast, 16 of 28 treated patients recovered.

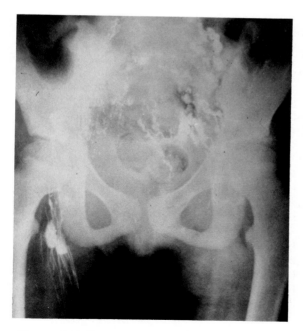

FIGURE 6.12. LYMPHANGIOGRAM SHOWING CHYLOUS REFLUX

## Chylothorax

The causes are similar to chylous ascites: idiopathic, neoplasm, and trauma. Every 24 hr the thoracic duct carries approximately 2400 ml of lymph, rich in protein and fat. Continued loss of this fluid results in electrolyte and nutritional depletion. Lymphography not only assists in localizing the site of the fistulous formation but also defines the anatomy of this highly variable structure.

Treatment of chylothorax is difficult (Selle et al., 1973). The *congenital* or idiopathic form appears to respond well to a more conservative regimen of multiple thoracenteses, advocated originally by Randolph and Gross (1957). When associated with *malignant* disease, chylothorax usually indicates widespread disease, and a conservative approach is warranted. Those cases following trauma, which may require treatment as varied as cardiac surgery, subclavian catheterization, scalene node biopsy, radical neck surgery, and gunshot repair, require the most judgment. An initial nonoperative course is recommended so that surgery is reserved for: large chylous loss (1500 ml/24 hr); no decrease in chyle drainage after 10–14 days; electrolyte or nutritional complications. This latter problem is substantial and was the primary cause of death of a patient in one series (Kinmonth et al., 1964). This patient apparently improved after lymphovenous shunt, but he died from the effects of preoperative depletion by the chylothorax.

## Chyluria

Chyluria is an abnormal condition in which intestinal chyle appears in the urine because of a fistulous communication between the intestinal lymphatics and the urinary tract. Tropical chyluria is a widespread disease of the tropical and subtropical areas of Asia, Africa, Australia, and America, especially along the seacoast and neighboring islands. It is most commonly associated with the filaria parasite, but other parasites have been found in patients with chyluria. Wücherer (1868) discovered the pathogen, and Lewis (1873) in Calcutta found the microfilaria in the blood and urine of a chyluric patient. Manson (1883) pointed to the mosquito as the intermediate host transmitting the larvae to humans. The transmitted larvae migrate into the large lymphatic vessels and nodes and mature. The filarial parasite causes a lymphangitis with lymphocytic and eosinophilic infiltration and fibroblastic proliferation (Cohen et al., 1961). Pos-

sibly the most serious damage occurs from the debris of dead parasites. O'Connor (1932) described a foreign body granulomatous reaction to the dead parasite with obstruction of the lymphatic vessel.

The nontropical form of chyluria is unusual and is frequently associated with conditions that obstruct the thoracic duct. Etiologies associated with this form include malignancy, especially those involving the retroperitoneum, and chronic inflammatory disease such as tuberculosis.

Various theories have been advanced to explain the transit of chyle into the urine. Ackerman (1863) attributed it to obstruction of the lymphatics between the intestines and the thoracic duct, but 42 chyluric patients with completely normal thoracic ducts have been described elsewhere (Koehler et al., 1968; Rajaram, 1970). Nine others had mild abnormalities. In addition, experiments by Drinker and Yoffey (1941) and Blalock et al. (1937) make it apparent that simple obstruction of the lymphatics is difficult to obtain. In only 3 of Blalock's 52 animals could the lymphatics be completely obstructed. Drinker and Yoffey did produce lymphedema by repeated injections of sclerosing material into the lymphatics and repeated ligations of lymphatic vessels.

The most likely explanation for reflux of the chyle into the retroperitoneal lymphatics is obstructive fibrosis in the retroperitoneal lymph nodes with incompetence of the valves and lymphatic dilatation from increased pressure or endolymphatic inflammation.

The final escape of chyle and contrast material from the renal and tubular lymphatics into the collecting system has never been produced experimentally. Presumably, the tubular lymphatics rupture with extravasation of contrast material from the lymphatic vessels into the interstitial space and then into the collecting tubules. Lee (1944) showed that fluid escapes through an intact lymphatic wall when the intralymphatic pressure is sufficiently elevated. The method of escape from the interstitial space into the collecting tubules is far from clear, however.

Clinically, the onset of chyluria is sudden and may be associated with trauma or straining. Many patients experience back pain and weakness. Renal colic may occur, and there may be associated hematuria. The character of the urine is typical. Without associated hematuria, the urine is milky in color and clears dramatically by shaking the urine with ether or chloroform. Another simple test is the Sudan III fat stain. The duration of chyluria is rarely more than 2 weeks and in the majority of cases 1 week or less. There is loss of plasma protein and an increased susceptibility to infection. There is no correlation between an abnormal blood urea nitrogen or serum creatinine and chyluria. The disease is accompanied frequently by impaired renal function with decreasing glomerular filtration, especially when there is associated infection and pyuria.

Intravenous urography is rarely abnormal. Hilar lymphatics may be seen on retrograde urography, but they are also seen occasionally in normal patients. The lymphographic findings are related to the degree of involvement. The pelvic and retroperitoneal vessels increase in size and number and may become tortuous. When there is elephantiasis, dilated tortuous vessels may be found in the leg, groin, and genitalia. Contrast material transit in the lymphatic vessels and various collateral lymphatics is prolonged. Contrast material may reflux into the renal and tubular lymphatics with demonstration of lymphaticourinary fistulae (Kittredge et al., 1963; Choi and Weidemer, 1964; Koehler et al., 1968; Rajaram, 1970) (Fig. 6.13). Treatment is either by direct ligation of abnormal communicating lymphatics (Llyod-Davies et al., 1967) or by injection of sclerosing solutions into the renal pelvis. The former is the favored approach.

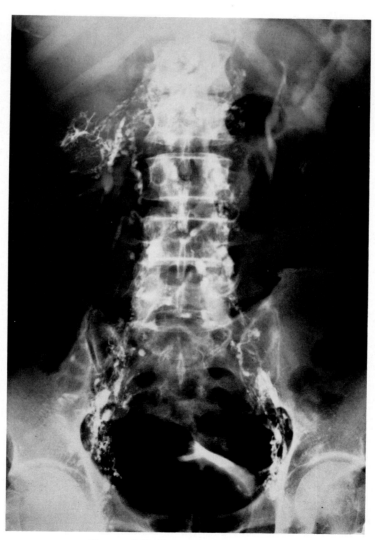

FIGURE 6.13. PARASITIC CHYLURIA

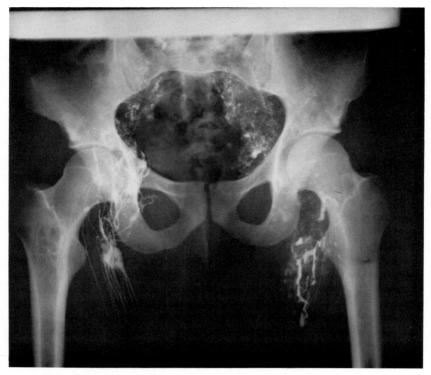

FIGURE 6.14. LYMPHANGIOGRAM FROM 21-YR-OLD WHITE MALE WITH LYMPHANGIOMA OF THE RETROPERITONEAL SPACE

## NEOPLASMS OF THE LYMPHATIC VESSELS

The most common tumors arising from the lymphatic vessels are benign and are of three types (Kinmonth, 1982): lymphangioma simplex, cavernous lymphangioma, and cystic hygroma. Whether these abnormalities deserve the designation *neoplasm* is debated. They probably originate from sequestrated or poorly developed analages rather than from actively proliferating neoplasms. By contrast, cavernous lymphangiomas may communicate with the main lymphatic trunks. For example, we noted communication with the inguinal and pelvic lymph vessels in one 21-yr-old male with a cavernous lymphangioma (Fig. 6.14).

The treatment of cystic hygromas and large cavernous lymphangiomas is usually excision, but care must be taken to avoid injury to adjacent vital structures. Because of this threat, radiation and injection of sclerosing solutions have been advocated by some surgeons. Incomplete excision of the lesion is a common problem and may result in recurrence of the lymphangioma.

The appearance of reddish-brown nodules and plaques in a limb with chronic lymphedema may represent sarcomatous change. Angiosarcoma has been called Kaposi's sarcoma, but the latter is a distinct entity. Kaposi's sarcoma may arise in a nonedematous limb, is slow growing, and on histological examination consists of spindle cells (Kinmonth, 1972). By contrast, angiosarcoma appears to be rapidly growing, especially when first clinically detected, and metastasizes widely. It originates from endothelial cells. Despite radiation and surgical treatment, the outlook at present is bleak for most patients with such tumors.

# Obstruction and Collateral Flow

**MELVIN E. CLOUSE, M.D.**

Obstruction of the lymphatics may not lead to edema if competent collateral pathways are available. Reichert (1926) completely transected the lymphatics and demonstrated a decrease in edema after the fourth preoperative day. This decrease correlated with regeneration and bridging of the superficial lymphatics at the incision site. Edema had cleared completely on the fifth postoperative day (after bridging the deep lymphatics at the incision). Blalock et al. (1937) found patent collateral lymphatic pathways in the immediate vicinity of the obstruction after multiple attempts to completely ligate the thoracic duct, the right lymphatic duct, and the cisterna chyli.

In conventional foot lymphangiography, the contrast material is injected into the lymphatics draining into the superficial inguinal nodes. When those nodes are obstructed, the deep inguinal nodes fill. Occasionally, the deep nodes fill in normal subjects as well, however, so their filling alone cannot be considered abnormal. When the obstruction is more complete, collateral lymphatic channels in the thigh, perineum, external genitalia, and anterior abdominal wall may fill (Fig. 6.15). If the obstruction is higher in the iliac area, backflow may occur into the presacral, hypogastric, and lumbar areas (Fig. 6.16).

Obstruction and increased intralymphatic pressure result in the dilatation, stasis, and valvular insufficiency visible on the lymphangiogram (Yune and Klatte, 1969; Escobar-Prieto et al., 1971). Flow in the lymph vessel sometimes reverses in search of an alternate pathway (Figs. 6.15 and 6.17), and occasionally the vessels rupture with extravasation of lymph and contrast material into the interstitial spaces of the leg (Fig. 6.18) or the pleural and peritoneal cavities. Cunningham (1969) demonstrated extensive collateral lymphatic pathways and peritoneal extravasation of contrast material in a patient with malignant disease of the pelvis. Peritoneal extravasation has also been noted by Camiel et al. (1964), Cook et al. (1966), Craven et al. (1967),

Fuchs and Zuppinger (1965), and Takahashi et al. (1968).

Dilatation and local extravasation may occur in normal lymphatic vessels after too rapid an injection during lymphangiography. Small droplets appear as beads along the lymphatic vessel. This should not be interpreted as obstruction in an otherwise normal lymphangiogram.

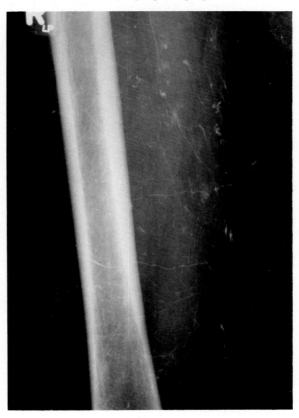

FIGURE 6.15. OBSTRUCTION: INGUINAL LYMPHATICS
A 74-yr-old man presented with right leg and scrotal edema. Urography showed a rigid area on the inferior and right lateral wall of the bladder that was a transitional cell carcinoma. Lymphangiography showed complete obstruction of the inguinal lymphatics with retrograde filling of superficial channels in the thigh and scrotum. The inguinal and iliac nodes showed central filling defects of metastatic tumor.

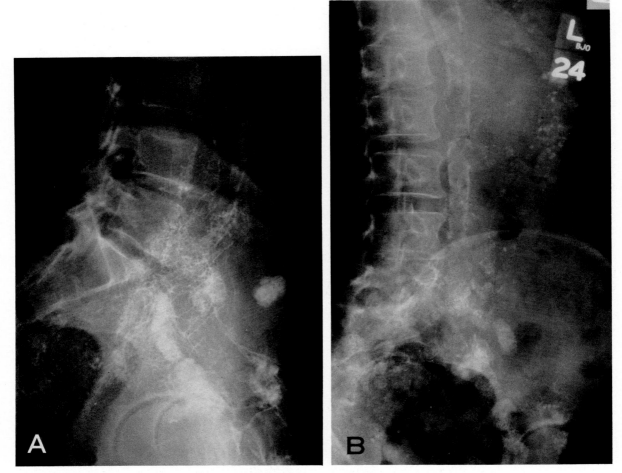

FIGURE 6.16. OBSTRUCTION: PERIAORTIC LYMPHATICS

A 58-yr-old woman noted swelling of her feet and ankles for 1 month. She had been treated 2 yr previously for stage 2A Hodgkin's (lymphocyte depletion). *A*: Lymphangiogram showed almost complete obstruction above L5. Note calcium in the aorta. There is marked reflux of contrast material into the presacral and hypogastric lymphatics. *B*: Film at 24 hr shows contrast material in mesenteric lymph nodes.

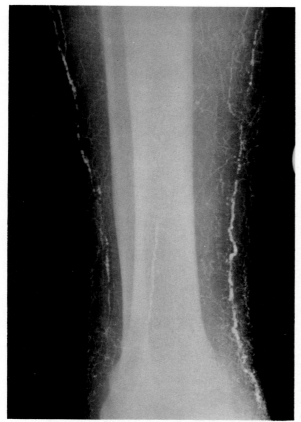

FIGURE 6.17. OBSTRUCTION: DERMAL LYMPHATIC FILLING
Obstruction of inguinal lymphatics with marked reflux of contrast material into dermal lymphatics in lower leg.

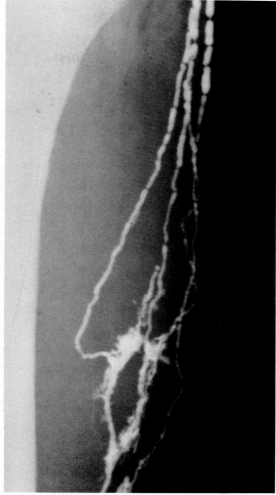

FIGURE 6.18. OBSTRUCTION WITH LYMPHATIC RUPTURE
A 55-yr-old man presented with metastatic sarcoma obstructing the inguinal lymphatics. The lymphangiogram shows dilatation of the lymphatic vessels and rupture with extravasation of contrast material.

Backflow and drainage via the collateral circulation are the final alternatives of the lymphatic system to bypass an obstruction. The pattern of collateral flow is unpredictable and not specific for any particular disease. There may be changes in the lymph nodes, however, which suggest a benign or malignant disease as the cause. Wallace (1968) and Wallace and Jing (1972) have shown that metastatic spread of carcinoma is not haphazard but rather an orderly response depending upon the development of collateral lymphatic flow.

## LYMPHATICOVENOUS COMMUNICATION

When the lymphatic system is overwhelmed and edema develops, there may be an attempt to decompress by lymphaticolymphatic and lymphaticovenous shunts. These routes are most often functional in chronic obstructive states such as neoplastic invasion of lymph nodes with complete obstruction, surgical resection, or certain benign conditions such as retroperitoneal fibrosis (Figs. 6.19 and 6.20). Most authors conclude that the lymphaticovenous communications are enlarged pathways normally present, which function only under stress from increased

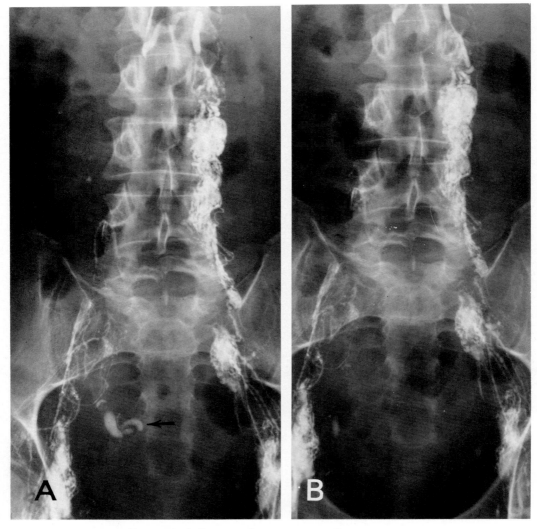

FIGURE 6.19. SYSTEMIC LYMPHOVENOUS COMMUNICATION

A 60-yr-old man had 6 months of progressive right leg edema and testicular pain after an acute episode of right flank and back pain. *A*: Lymphangiogram. There is complete obstruction of right iliac lymphatics. A lymphovenous communication fills a pelvic vein (*arrow*). The examination was terminated. *B*: A film 15 min later shows a second lymphovenous communication with venous filling. The venous collection of contrast material seen in *A* has passed centrally. Retroperitoneal fibrosis was found at operation.

volume or pressure within the lymphatic system (Yoffey and Courtice, 1956; Rusznyak et al., 1960).

Communications between lymphatics and veins have been discussed periodically in the literature, but until the advent of clinical lymphography the concept was controversial. In 1834 Wutzer demonstrated communication between the thoracic duct and the azygous vein in a women whose thoracic duct was obstructed. Silvester (1911–1912) described openings of the

lymphatic from the mesentery and lower limbs into the inferior vena cava near the renal vein in monkeys. Also in 1911, Baum declared the existence of lymphaticovenous communications in the sacral, jugular, and cephalic veins of canine and bovine animals. Pressman et al. (1962) and Mayerson (1962) demonstrated communication between the lymphatic and venous systems within lymph nodes. Their findings provide one explanation for the observation that considerably more lymph is produced in the body than

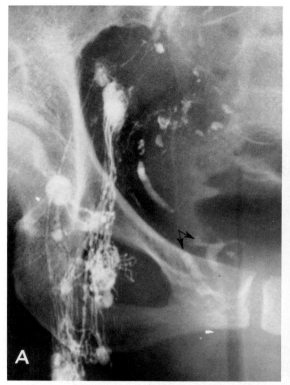
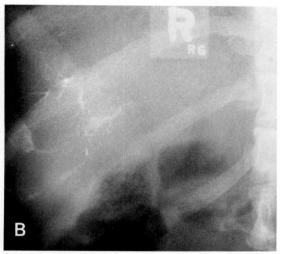

FIGURE 6.20. PORTAL LYMPHOVENOUS COMMUNICATION

A 60-yr-old woman with postradiation therapy for carcinoma of the cervix with recurrent disease. *A*: Lymphangiogram. Film after 5 ml of Ethiodol shows lymphovenous communication with the hemorrhoidal veins (*arrows*). The injection was terminated. *B*: Abdominal film 30 min later shows Ethiodol in right hepatic branch of the portal vein.

can be explained by measurement of total lymphatic flow from the thoracic and mediastinal trunks (Bollman et al., 1948; Kubik, 1952).

A number of authors have noted a marked decrease in circulating lymphocytes after ligation of the thoracic duct with return to normal levels within 4–6 days after establishment of collateral flow (Biedl and Decastello, 1901; Lee, 1922; Drinker and Yoffey, 1941). Threefoot et al. (1963), using plastic corrosion models of the lymphatic system, demonstrated lymphaticovenous and lymphaticolymphatic communications after prolonged ligation of the cisterna chyli. The venous channels involved were vena cava, renal, adrenal, iliac, and hemiazygous veins. Shanbrom and Zheutlin (1959) demonstrated accessory lymphatics draining directly into the jugular vein without traversing the lymph nodes. Bron et al. (1963) and Wallace et al. (1964) demonstrated these communications fluoroscopically while performing lymphography on clinical subjects.

Wolfel (1965) demonstrated a direct communication between the para-aortic lymphatics and the inferior vena cava after complete obstruction of the retroperitoneal nodes by metastatic seminoma. Roentgenographically these communications are most frequently seen in the iliac and para-aortic areas. They may also occur peripherally when there is complete obstruction of the inguinal or axillary nodes (Fig. 6.21).

When performing lymphography, especially when obstruction is suspected, it is imperative to film frequently and possibly fluoroscope to demonstrate lymphaticovenous communications and thus prevent extensive oil embolization. The flow in the vein is considerably more rapid than in the lymphatic vessel, and the contrast material appears as tiny droplets in the dependent portion of the vein. In a dependent vein or in the presence of venous stagnation, the contrast material may outline the entire vein (Fig. 6.20).

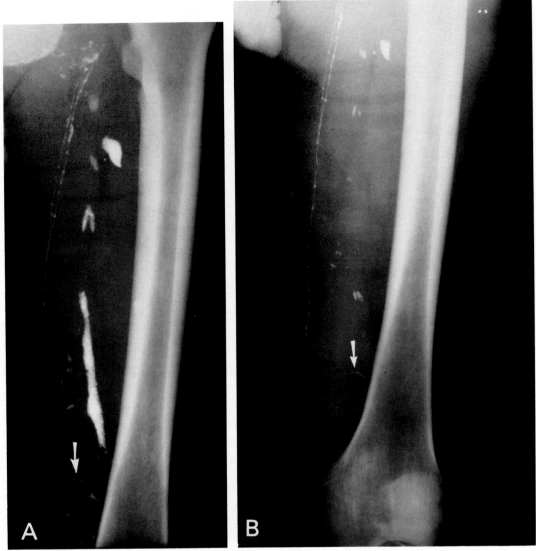

FIGURE 6.21. PERIPHERAL LYMPHOVENOUS COMMUNICATION

This 56-yr-old man had Kaposi's sarcoma and leg edema for 3 months. *A:* Lymphangiogram, left leg. fluoroscopy was delayed on the left because of difficulty in cannulating right pedal lymphatics. Fluoroscopy after 4 ml of Ethiodol revealed complete obstruction of the inguinal lymphatics with a large amount of contrast material in the femoral vein. Contrast material could be seen passing from the lymphatic vessel transversely across the leg (*arrow*) to the femoral vein. *B:* Injection was discontinued. Contrast material remained in the communication (*arrow*). The contrast material in the vein passed centrally. Oil pneumonitis cleared in 1 week.

## PERINEURAL AND PERIVASCULAR SPACES

Considerable controversy exists concerning the presence and functional significance of the perivascular and perineural spaces. These potential spaces are soft tissue planes which surround the nerves and blood vessels and which have no endothelial lining. Included are the Virchow-

Robbins space surrounding the cerebral blood vessels, perineural and perivascular spaces around nerves and blood vessels, and the intra-adventitial space surrounding branches of the pulmonary arterioles.

Larson et al. (1966) were unable to demonstrate any communication between the peri-neural space and the lymphatic system after injecting sky blue dye, vinyl acetate, and India ink into the soft tissue and nerves. There was no communication with the perineurium when contrast material was injected into the lymphatics. When contrast material was injected into the perineurium, it passed both proximally and distally in the nerve sheath without communication with the lymphatic vessels.

According to Sidney Wallace (1968) the concept of paralymphatics was proposed by Ottoviani. Wallace demonstrated contrast material in the perivascular space during lymphography. These spaces are more frequently seen in patients with edema (Fig. 6.22), although they have been demonstrated in patients without lymphatic obstruction. The pattern of opacification follows the contour of the particular vessel and occasionally the nerve.

The perivascular space usually fills in an orthograde manner. The perivenous space is occasionally filled after the intradermal injection with patent blue violet dye during pedal lymphography, usually when there is a decrease in number of lymphatics. This may necessitate another incision to find a suitable lymphatic for cannulation.

Perivascular contrast material is rarely seen even in patients with lymphedema, and one must agree with Larson that tumor and lymph progress along tissue planes of least resistance. The lymphatic vessels lie in close proximity to the neurovascular bundle, and it is understandable that tumor enters the perineural and venous space by direct extension.

Wallace believes, however, that lymphographic findings support the concept of a functionally significant paralymphatic system even though contrast material may remain in these locations for 5 months (Kusick, 1971). These spaces may not be artifactual as suggested by Larson et al. (1966); however, the long term absence of perineurial contrast material in the findings of Larson et al. indicates that the perivenous and perineural spaces have limited functional significance for transport of lymph and tumor cells.

The intra-adventitial spaces in the lung are those potential spaces surrounding the pulmonary arterioles. As with the perivascular and perineural spaces, there is no endothelial lining. They were first described by Ivanov (1936) and demonstrated by Földi et al. (1954) in patients with pulmonary edema. These spaces contain the

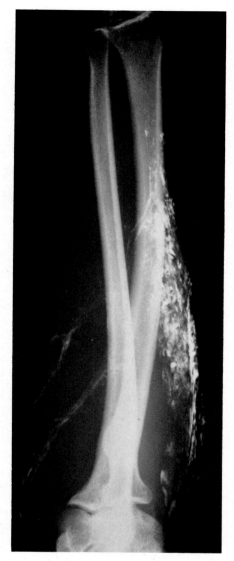

FIGURE 6.22. PERIVENOUS LYMPHATICS
A 32-yr-old woman developed edema of the arm after surgical removal of a subcutaneous nodule on the forearm. The lymphangiogram shows extensive perivenous contrast material with extravasation into the soft tissue. (Courtesy of W. G. Eklund, M.D., Portland, Oregon).

same edema fluid as the pulmonary lymphatics and alveoli. Ivanov's original concept was that this space served as a communication between lymphoid slits (the connective tissue) and endothelium-lined lymphatic capillaries (Kondoleon, 1912). Investigators to date have failed to demonstrate a connection between the lymph vessels and the intra-adventitial space.

## LYMPHOCELE AND LYMPH FISTULAE

Injury to lymphatic vessels, such as surgery or blunt trauma, leads to passage of lymph into soft tissues of body cavities. The lymph may be confined and form a lymphocele or may exit through an operative wound. The lymphocele may be small, such as those resulting from inguinal node biopsy (Fig. 6.23). After renal transplantation, lymphoceles may be very large, compressing the renal vein and requiring drainage (Madura et al., 1970; Koehler and Kyaw, 1972; Moreau et al., 1973; Sampson et al., 1973; Rashid et al., 1974). Untreated, they may lead to renal failure, venous thrombosis, and pulmonary embolism (Lorimer et al., 1975).

Lymph fistulae may be insignificant with minor drainage from the incision site after scalene node biopsy. Severe lymph fistulae with a large amount of lymphatic drainage may follow thoracic duct injury due to radical chest surgery. Storen et al. (1974) have demonstrated lymph extravasation and fistulae in the lower leg after arterial reconstructive surgery (Fig. 6.24). Lymph fistulae may occur spontaneously when tumor completely replaces the lymph nodes and obstructs the lymph channels (Fig. 6.25).

Lymphatic damage is encountered frequently in the pelvic area after radical surgery for carcinoma of the cervix. The surgeon is faced with the dilemma when performing a radical node dissection. If all of the lymphatics are removed and ligated, there may be obstruction and postoperative edema in the lower leg. If dissection is not extensive, nodes may be left behind. Transection of lymphatic channels that are not ligated may result in considerable lymph escape into the peritoneal cavity. In these cases the degree of edema depends upon the number of lymphatic vessels ligated and the adequacy of the collateral circulation to bypass the interrupted channels.

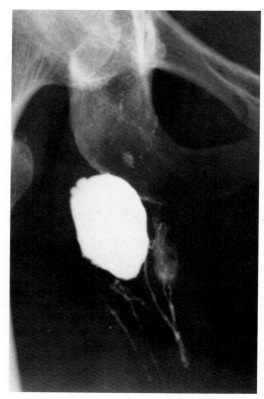

FIGURE 6.23. LYMPHOCELE

This 63-yr-old woman had a right inguinal node removed that proved to be Hodgkin's disease. Eight months later she noted swelling in the same area. The lymphogram revealed a lymphocele that was subsequently excised.

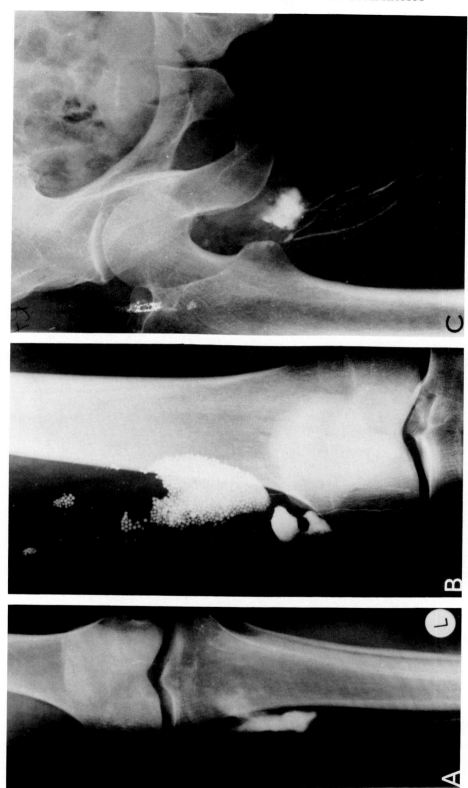

FIGURE 6.24. LYMPH FISTULA AFTER ARTERIAL SURGERY

Lymphangiogram 2 weeks after arterial reconstruction of the lower limb shows interruption of lymphatic vessels and formation of lymphoceles at dissection sites. (Courtesy of Drs. E. J. Storen, H. O. Myhre, and G. Stiris, Oslo, Norway.)

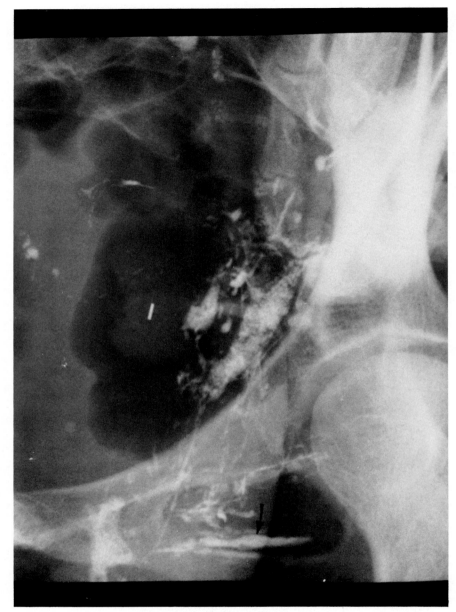

FIGURE 6.25. LYMPH FISTULAE

A 55-yr-old woman following postirradiation and surgery for carcinoma of the cervix with recurrent disease. Lymphangio-gram demonstrated obstruction high in the external iliac nodes. There is extravasation of contrast material above the ischial tuberosity (*arrow*).

## PRIMARY INTESTINAL LYMPHANGIECTASIA

Intestinal lymphangiectasia is characterized by marked tortuosity and irregular dilatation of the mesenteric and mucosal lymphatics. Clinically, an extreme loss of protein in the gastrointestinal tract results in hypoalbuminemia, hypogammaglobulinemia, edema, and pleural effu-sion. There appears to be a poor correlation between the extent of edema and severity of hypoalbuminemia. Lymphocytopenia is an almost universal accompaniment of the syndrome. Mucosal jejunal biopsy shows dilated lymphatics in the mucosa.

The cause of hypoproteinemia in patients with intestinal lymphangiectasia appears to be rupture of dilated lymphatic vessels with loss of lymph into the bowel lumen or exudation through the lymphatic capillaries. Discharge of lymph into the intestinal lumen has been demonstrated by intestinal intubation (Stoelinga et al., 1963) and extravasation of contrast material into the intestinal lumen by pedal lymphography (Mistilis et al., 1965).

Intestinal lymphangiectasia may be part of a systemic lymphatic dysplasia (Stoelinga et al., 1963; Bookstein et al., 1965). Pomerantz and Waldmann (1963) demonstrated systemic lymphatic abnormalities in four patients with intestinal lymphangiectasia by lymphography. Studies of the arteries and veins in primary intestinal lymphangiectasia have not been reported.

Shimkin et al. (1970) analyzed nine pedal lymphangiograms of patients with intestinal lymphangiectasia. The findings included hypoplasia of lower extremity lymphatics, dermal backflow in the skin, possible thoracic duct obstruction with a tortuous and dilated thoracic duct, and a

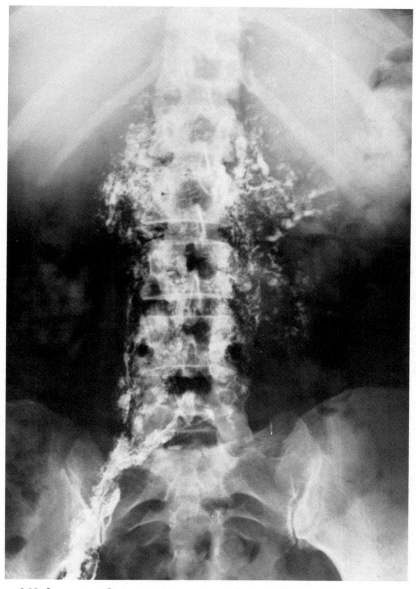

FIGURE 6.26. INTESTINAL LYMPHANGIECTASIA WITH PROTEIN-LOSING GASTROENTEROPATHY
Lymphangiogram shows marked reflux into numerous dilated mesenteric lymphatic vessels. (Courtesy of Joseph J. Bookstein, M.D., Ann Arbor, Michigan.)

stippled appearance of the contrast material in the lymph nodes. Others have reported dilated and varicose lymphatics (Pomerantz and Waldmann, 1963; Bookstein et al., 1965) (Fig. 6.26).

Although the exact pathogenesis is obscure, lymphangiectasia is probably due to a congenital malformation with symptoms developing in childhood and a family history of hypoproteinemia with effusion. The associated protein-losing gastroenteropathy may also be seen in a number of acquired lesions, including constrictive pericarditis, congestive heart failure, retroperitoneal fibrosis, and pancreatitis (Waldmann, 1966).

In constrictive pericarditis venous hypertension obstructs the flow of lymph into the venous angle, increasing intralymphatic pressure and decreasing lymphatic flow. Takashima and Takekoshi (1968) have reported hypoproteinemia

and intestinal lymphangiectasia as presenting symptoms in a patient with constrictive pericarditis.

The mechanism of protein-losing enteropathy associated with congestive heart failure is not clear. Davidson and others (1961) have suggested that it is caused by functional obstruction of the lymphatics by increased venous pressure (i.e., similar to constrictive pericarditis) (Peterson and Hastrup, 1963; Peterson and Ottosen, 1964). There is an increase in lymph production in congestive heart failure as well as a later increase in venous pressure; thus a combination of both factors may cause lymphatic hypertension.

In retroperitoneal fibrosis and pancreatitis there is obstruction of the lymphatic channels with dilatation and loss of lymph into the intestinal tract.

# REFERENCES

Ackerman T: Ein Fall Galacturia (urina chylosa). *Deutsch Klin* 15:221, 1863.

Allen EV, Barker NW, Hines EA: *Peripheral Vascular Diseases.* Philadelphia, WB Saunders, 1946.

Allenby F, Calnan JS, Pflug JJ: The use of pneumatic compression in the swollen leg. *J Physiol (Lond)* 231:65, 1973.

Arnulf G: Lymphedema of the upper limb after Halstead's operations of radical mastectomy, lymphography and phlebography. Therapeutic consequences. *Vasc Surg* 7:36, 1973.

Baum H: Können lymphagefässe direkt in Venen einmünden? *Anat Anz* 39:593, 1911.

Biedl A, Decastello A: Über Änderungen des Blutbildes Nach Unterbrechung des Lymph Zuflusses. *Pflugers Arch Ges Physiol* 86:259, 1901.

Blalock A, Robinson CS, Cunningham RS, Gray ME: Experimental studies on lymphatic blockage. *Arch Surg* 34:1049, 1937.

Bollman JL, Cain JC, Grindlay JH: Technique for collection of lymph from the liver, small intestine and thoracic duct of the rat. *J Lab Clin Med* 33:1349, 1948.

Bookstein JJ, French AB, Pollard MH: Protein-losing gastroenteropathy: concepts derived from lymphangiography. *Am J Dig Dis* 10:573, 1965.

Bron KM, Baum S, Abrams HL: Oil embolism in lymphangiography. Incidence, manifestation and mechanism. *Radiology* 80:194, 1963.

Bunchman MM, Lewis SR: The treatment of lymphedema. *Plast Reconstr Surg* 54:64, 1974.

Buonocore E, Young JR: Lymphangiographic evaluation of lymphedema and lymphatic flow. *AJR* 95:751, 1965.

Burn JI: Obstructive lymphopathy. *Ann R Coll Surg Engl* 42:93, 1968.

Calnan J: Lymphoedema: the case for doubt. *Br J Plast Surg* 21:32, 1968.

Calnan J, Kountz SI: Effect of venous obstruction on lymphatics. *Br J Surg* 52:800, 1965.

Camiel MR, Benninghoff DL, Herman PG: Chylous ascites with lymphographic demonstration of lymph leakage into the peritoneal cavity. *Gastroenterology* 47:188, 1964.

Casley-Smith JR, Földi-Börcsök E, Földi M: A fine structural study of the removal of the effectiveness of benzo-pyrone

treatment of lymphoedema by the destruction of the macrophages by silica. *Br J Exp Pathol* 59:116, 1978.

Charles H: In Latham A (ed): *A System of Treatment.* London, Churchill, 1912, vol 3.

Chilvers AS, Kinmonth JB: Operation for lymphedema of the lower limbs. A study of the results in 108 operations using vascularized dermal flaps. *J Cardiovasc Surg* 16:115, 1975.

Choi JK, Weidemer HS: Chyluria: lymphographic study and review of the literature. *J Urol* 92:723, 1964.

Clodius L, Piller NB, Casley-Smith JR: The problems of lymphatic microsurgery for lymphedema. *Lymphology* 14:69, 1981.

Cohen LB, Nelson G, Wood AM, Manson-Bahr PE, Bowen R: Lymphangiography in filaria lymphedema and elephantiasis. *Am J Trop Med Hyg* 10:843, 1961.

Cook PL, Jelliffe AM, Kendall B, McLoughlin MJ: The role of lymphography in diagnosis and management of malignant reticulosis. *Br J Radiol* 39:561, 1966.

Craven CE, Goldman AS, Larson DL, Patterson M, Hendrick C: Congenital chylous ascites. Lymphographic demonstration of obstruction of cisterna chylus reflux into peritoneal space and small intestine. *J Pediatr* 70:340, 1967.

Cunningham JB: The demonstration of an unusual combination of collateral channels during lymphography—a case report. *J Can Assoc Radiol* 20:189, 1969.

Davidson JD, Waldmann TS, Goodman DS, Gordon RR: Protein-losing gastroenteropathy in congestive heart failure. *Lancet* 1:899, 1961.

Degni M: New microsurgical techniques of lymphatico-venous anastomosis for the treatment of lymphedema. *Lymphology* 14:61, 1981.

Dellon AL, Hoopes JE: Charles procedure for primary lymphedema. Long-term clinical results. *Plast Reconstr Surg* 60:589, 1977.

Drinker CK, Yoffey JM: *Lymphatics, Lymph, and Lymphoid Tissue.* Cambridge, Harvard University Press, 1941.

Emmett AJ, Barron JN, Veall N: The use of I-131 albumin tissue clearance measurements and other physiological tests for the clinical assessment of patients with lymphoedema. *Br J Plast Surg* 20:1, 1967.

Escobar-Prieto A, Gonzalez G, Templeton AW, Cooper BR,

Palacios E: Lymphatic channel obstruction. *AJR* 113:366, 1971.

Esterly JR: Congenital hereditary lymphedema. *J Med Genet* 2:93, 1965.

Eustace PW, Kinmonth JB: The normal lymphatic vessels of the inguinal and iliac areas with special emphasis on the efferent inguinal vessels. *Lymphology* 1976.

Feins NR, Rubin R, Crais T, O'Connor JF: Surgical management of 39 children with lymphedema. *J Pediatr Surg* 12:471, 1977.

Field ME, Drinker CK: Permeability of capillaries of dog to protein. *Am J Physiol* 97:40, 1931.

Field ME, Drinker CK: Conditions governing the removal of protein deposited in the subcutaneous tissue of the dog. *Am J Physiol* 98:66, 1931.

Földi M, Kepes J, Papp M, Rusznyak I, Szabo G: Significance of pulmonary lymph circulation in the fluid circulation of the lung. A contribution of the data concerning the pathogenesis of pulmonary oedema. *MTA Biol Orvtud Oszt Kozi Hung* 5:221, 1954.

Fonkalsrud EW: Surgical management of congenital lymphedema in infants and children. *Arch Surg* 114:1133, 1979.

Fuchs WA, Zuppinger A: *Lymphographic and Tumor-Diagnostic.* Berlin, Springer-Verlag, 1965.

Fyfe NC, Rutt DC, Edwards JM, Kinmonth JB: Intralymphatic steroid therapy for lymphedema: preliminary studies. *Lymphology* 15:23–28, 1982.

Ganel A, Engel J, Sela M, Brooks M: Nerve entrapment associated with post-mastectomy lymphedema. *Cancer* 44:2254, 1979.

Goldsmith HS: Long term evaluation of omental transposition for chronic lymphedema. *Ann Surg* 180:847, 1974.

Gong-Kang H, Ru-Qui H, Zong-Zhao L, Yao-Liang S, Tie-De L, Gong-Ping P: Microlymphaticovenous anastomosis for treating lymphedema of the extremities and external genitalia. *J Microsurg* 3:32, 1981.

Gooneratne BWM: Lymphography of filarial infections. Lecture, St. Thomas Hospital, 1969.

Handley WS: Lymphangioplasty. *Lancet* 1:783, 1908.

Harvey RF: The use of I-131 labelled human serum albumin in the assessment of improved lymph flow following buried dermis flap operations in cases of post-mastectomy lymphedema of the arm. *Br J Radiol* 42:260, 1969.

Hirshowitz B, Goldan S: A bi-hinged chest-arm flap for lymphedema of the upper limb. *Plast Reconstr Surg* 48:52, 1971.

Homans J: Treatment of elephantiasis of legs. *N Engl J Med* 215:1099, 1936.

Hughes JH, Patel AR: Swelling of the arm following radical mastectomy. *Br J Surg* 53:4, 1966.

Ivanov GF: Pulmonaire de la circulation lymphatique. *Bull Histol Appliquee Physiol Pathol* 13:401, 1936.

Jackson BT, Kinmonth JB: Pes cavus and lymphoedema. *J Bone Joint Surg* 52B:518, 1970.

Khamma NN: Surgical treatment of elephantiasis of male genitalia. *Plast Reconstr Surg* 46:481, 1970.

Kinmonth JB: Primary lymphedemas: classification and other studies based on oleolymphography and clinical features. *J Cardiovasc Surg* (Torino), Special Supplement for XVII Congress of European Society of Cardiovascular Surgeons, 1969.

Kinmonth JB: *The Lymphatics: Diseases, Lymphography and Surgery.* Baltimore, Williams & Wilkins, 1972.

Kinmonth JB: *The Lymphatics: Surgery, Lymphography and Diseases of the Chyle and Lymph Systems.* London, Edward Arnold, 1982.

Kinmonth JB, Taylor GW: The lymphatic circulation in lymphedema. *Ann Surg* 139:129, 1954.

Kinmonth JB, Taylor GW, Tracy GD, March JD: Primary lymphoedema. *Br J Surg* 45:1, 1957.

Kinmonth JB, Taylor GW, Jantet GM: Chylous complications of primary lymphoedema. *J Cardiovasc Surg (Torino)* 5:327, 1964.

Kinmonth JB, Patrick JH, Chilvers AS: Comments on operations for lower limb lymphedema. *Lymphology* 8:56, 1975.

Kinmonth JB, Hurst PA, Edwards JM, Rutt DD: Relief of lymph obstruction by use of a bridge of mesenteric and ileum. *Br J Surg* 965:829, 1978.

Kittredge RD, Hashin S, Roholt HB, Van Itallie TB, Finby M: Demonstration of lymphatic abnormality in a patient with chyluria. *AJR* 90:159, 1963.

Koehler PR, Kyaw MM: Lymphatic complications following renal transplantation. *Radiology* 102:539, 1972.

Koehler PR, Chiang TC, Lin CT, Chen KC, Chen KY: Lymphography in chyluria. *AJR* 102:455, 1968.

Kondoleon E: Die Chirurgische Behandlung der Elephantiastichen Oedeme. *Munch Med Wochenschr* 59:525, 1912.

Kreel L, George P: Post-mastectomy lymphangiography: detection of metastases and edema. *Ann Surg* 163:470, 1966.

Krylov VS, Rabkin IE, Milanov NO, Ermakov NP, Alekseev VI: Rol'limfografii pri opredelenii pokazanii k nalozheniiu priamogo limfovenoznogo anastomoza. *Khirurgiia (Mosk)* 9:3, 1979.

Kubik I: Die Hydrodynamischn und Mechanischen Faktoren in der Lymphzirkulation. *Acta Morphol Acad Sci Hung* 2:95, 1952.

Kusick H: *Technique of Lymphography and Principles of Interpretation.* St Louis, Warren H Green, 1971, p 174.

Larson DL, Rodin AE, Roberts DK, O'Steen WK, Rappaport AS, Lewis SR: Perineural lymphatics: myth or fact. *Am J Surg* 112:488, 1966.

Larson NE, Crampton AR: A surgical procedure for post-mastectomy edema. *Arch Surg* 106:475, 1973.

Lee FC: Establishment of collateral circulation following ligation of the thoracic duct. *Bull Johns Hopkins Hosp* 33:21, 1922.

Lee FC: Permeability of lymph vessels and lymph pressure. *Arch Surg* 48:335, 1944.

Lewis TR: On a hematazon inhabiting blood, its relation to chyluria and other diseases. *Ind Ann Med Sci* 16:504, 1873.

Lloyd-Davies RW, Edwards JM, Kinmonth JB: Chyluria: a report of five cases with particular references to lymphography and direct surgery. *Br J Urol* 39:560, 1967.

Lorimer WS, Glassford DM, Sarles HE, Remmers AR, Fish JC: Lymphocele: a significant complication following renal transplantation. *Lymphology* 8:21, 1975.

Madura JA, Dunbar JD, Cerilli JG: Perirenal lymphocele as a complication of renal homotransplantation. *Surgery* 68:310, 1970.

Manson P: *The Filaria Darginis-hominis.* London, HK Lewis, 1883.

Mayerson P: Permeability characteristics of the lymph node. Senior thesis, presented at the 12th annual Senior Scientific Session of Tulane University School of Medicine, New Orleans, Louisiana, May 9, 1962.

Milanov NO, Abalmasov KG, Lein AP: Correction of lymph flow disturbances following radical mastectomy. *Vestn Khir* 128:63, 1982.

Miller TA: Surgical management of lymphedema of the extremity. *Plast Reconstr Surg* 56:633, 1975.

Miller TA: A surgical approach to lymphedema. *Am J Surg* 134:191, 1977.

Miller TA: Charles procedure for lymphedema: a warning. *Am J Surg* 139:290, 1980.

Milroy WF: An undescribed variety of hereditary oedema, *NY State J Med* 505, 1892.

Mistilis SP, Skyring AP, Stephen DD: Intestinal lymphangectasia: mechanism of enteric loss of plasma-protein and fat. *Lancet* 1:77, 1965.

Moreau JF, Leski M, Beurton D, Cukier J, Michel JR, Kreis J, Lacombe M: Lymphoceles obstructives apres transplantation renale. *Ann Radiol (Paris)* 16:471, 1973.

Negus D, Edwards JM, Kinmonth JB: The iliac veins in relation to lymphedema. *Br J Surg* 56:481, 1969.

Nielubowicz J, Olszewski W: Surgical lymphaticovenous shunts in patients with secondary lymphedema. *Br J Surg* 55:440, 1968.

O'Brien BM, Das SK: Microlymphatic surgery in management of lymphoedema of the upper limb. *Ann Acad Med Singapore* 8:474, 1979.

O'Brien BM, Sykes P, Threlfall GN: Microlymphaticovenous anastomoses for obstructive lymphedema. *Plast Reconstr Surg* 60:197, 1977.

O'Connor FW: The aetiology of the disease syndrome in *Wuchereria bancrofti* infection. *Trans R Soc Trop Med Hyg* 23:13, 1932.

O'Donnell TF: Congenital mixed vascular deformities of the lower limbs: the relevance of lymphatic abnormalities to their diagnosis and treatment. *Ann Surg* 185:162, 1977.

O'Donnell TF, Edwards JM, Kinmonth JB: Lymphography in the mixed vascular deformities of the lower extremities. *J Cardiovasc Surg (Torino)* 17:1976a.

O'Donnell TF, Kalisher L, Raines JK, Darling RC: Assessment of lymphedema by xeroradiography. *Physiologist* 19:3, 1976b.

Olszewski W: On the pathomechanism of development of postsurgical lymphedema. *Lymphology* 6:35, 1973.

Olszewski W, Machowski Z, Sawicki A, Wielubowicz J: Clinical studies in primary lymphedema. *Pol Med J* 11:1560, 1972a.

Olszewski W, Machowski Z, Sokolowski J, Sawicki Z, Zerbino D, Nielubowicz J: Primary lymphedema of lower extremities. I. Lymphangiographic and histologic studies of lymphatic vessels and lymph nodes in primary lymphedema. *Pol Med J* 11:1564, 1972b.

O'Reilly K: Treatment by nylon setons of lymphedema of the arm following radical mastectomy. *Med J Aust* 1:1269, 1972.

Peterson VP, Hastrup J: Protein-losing enteropathy in constrictive pericarditis. *Acta Med Scand* 173:401, 1963.

Peterson VP, Ottosen P: Albumin turnover and thoracic-duct lymph in constrictive pericarditis. *Acta Med Scand* 176:335, 1964.

Piller NB: Lymphedema, macrophages, and benzopyrones. *Lymphology* 13:109, 1980.

Politowski M, Bartkowski S, Dynowski J: Treatment of lymphedema of the limbs of lymphatic-venous fistula. *Surgery* 66:639, 1969.

Pomerantz M, Waldmann TA: Systemic lymphatic abnormalities associated with gastrointestinal protein loss secondary to intestinal lymphangiectasia. *Gastroenterology* 45:703, 1963.

Pressman JJ, Simon MB, Hand K, Miller J: Passage of fluids, cells and bacteria via direct communications between lymph nodes and veins. *Surg Gynecol Obstet* 115:207, 1962.

Puckett CL, Jacobs GR, Hurvitz JS, Silver D: Evaluation of lympho-venous anastomoses in obstructive lymphedema. *Plast Reconstr Surg* 66:116, 1980.

Raines JK, O'Donnell TF, Kalisher L, Darling RC: Selection of patients with lymphedema for compression therapy. *Am J Surg* 133:430, 1977.

Rajaram PC: Lymphatic dynamics in filarial chyluria and prechyluric state—lymphographic analysis of 52 cases. *Lymphology* 3:114, 1970.

Randolph J, Gross R: Congenital chylothorax. *Arch Surg* 74:405, 1957.

Rashid A, Posen G, Couture R, McKay D, Wellington J: Accumulation of lymph around the transplanted kidney (lymphocele) mimicking renal allograft rejection. *J Urol* 111:145, 1974.

Reichert FL: The regeneration of lymphatics. *Arch Surg* 13:871, 1926.

Richmand DM, O'Donnell TF, Zelikovski A: Sequential pneumatic compression for lymphedema: a controlled trial. *Arch Surg*, in press.

Rigas A, Vomoyannis A, Gianoulis K, Antipas S, Tsardakas E: Measurement of the femoral vein pressure in edema of the lower extremities. Report of 50 cases. *J Cardiovasc Surg (Torino)* 12:411, 1971.

Rusznyak I, Foldi M, Szabo G: *Lymphatics and Lymph Circulation.* New York, Pergamon Press, 1960.

Saijo M, Munro IR, Mancer K: Lymphedema: a clinical review and follow-up study. *Plast Reconstr Surg* 56:513, 1975.

Sampson D, Winterberg AR, Murphy GP: Lymphoceles complicating renal allotransplantation. *NY State J Med* 73:2710, 1973.

Sawney CP: Evaluation of Thompson's buried dermal flap operation for lymphedema of the limbs: a clinical and radioisotopic study. *Br J Plast Surg* 27:278, 1974.

Schmidt KR, Welter H, Pfeifer KJ, Becker HM: Lymphangiographische Untersuchungen zum Extremitatenodem nach rekonstruktiven Gefasseingriffen im Femoropoplitealbereich. *ROEFO* 128:194, 1978.

Selle JG, Synder WM, Schreiber JT: Chylothorax: indications for surgery. *Ann Surg* 177:245, 1973.

Shammas HJ, Tabbara KF, Der Kaloustian VM. Distichiasis of the lids and lymphedema of the lower extremities: a report of ten cases. *J Pediatr Ophthalmol Strabismus* 161:129, 1979.

Shanbrom E, Zheutlin N: Radiographic studies of lymphatic system. *AMA Arch Intern Med* 104:589, 1959.

Shimkin PM, Waldmann TA, Krugman RL: Intestinal lymphangiectasia. *AJR* 110:827, 1970.

Silver D, Puckett J: Lymphangiogplasty: a ten year evaluation. *Surgery* 80:748, 1980.

Silvester CF: On the presence of permanent communications between the lymphatics and the venous system at the level of the renal vein in adult South American monkeys. *Am J Anat* 12:447, 1911–1912.

Sistrunk WE: Modifications of the operation for elephantiasis. *JAMA* 71:800, 1918.

Stoelinga GBA, van Munster PJJ, Sloof JP: Chylous effusions into the intestine in a patient with protein-losing gastroenteropathy. *Pediatrtrics* 31:1011, 1963.

Storen EJ, Myhre HO, Stiris G: Lymphangiographic findings in patients with leg edema after arterial reconstruction. *Acta Chir Scand* 140:385, 1974.

Takahashi M, Takeda K, Ishibashi T, Kawanami H: Peritoneal extravasation of oily contrast medium following lymphography. *AJR* 104:652, 1968.

Takashima T, Takekoshi N: Lymphographic evaluation of abnormal lymph flow in protein-losing gastroenteropathy secondary to chronic constricting pericarditis. *Radiology* 90:502, 1968.

Thompson N: Surgical treatment of chronic lymphedema of the lower limb. *Br Med J* 2:1566, 1962.

Thompson N: The surgical treatment of advanced postmastectomy lymphedema of the upper limb. With the later results of treatment by buried dermis flap operation. *Scand J Plast Reconstr Surg* 3:54, 1969.

Thompson N: Buried dermal flap operation for chronic lymphedema of the extremities. Ten year survey of results in 79 cases. *Plast Reconstr Surg* 45:541, 1970.

Threefoot SA, Kent WT, Hatchett BF: Lymphaticovenous

and lymphaticolymphatic communications demonstrated by plastic corrosion models of rats and by post mortem lymphangiography in man. *J Lab Clin Med* 61:9, 1963.

Van der Molen HR, Toth LM: The conservative treatment of lymphedema of the extremities. *Angiology* 25:470, 1974.

Vasko JS, Tapper RI: The surgical significance of chylous ascites. *Arch Surg* 95:355, 1967.

Vitek J, Kaspar Z: The radiology of the deep lymphatic system of the leg. *Br J Radiol* 46:120, 1973.

Waldmann TA: Protein-losing enteropathy. *Prog Gastroenterol* 50:422, 1966.

Wallace S: Dynamics of normal and abnormal lymphatic systems as studied with contrast media. *Cancer Chemother Rep* 52:31, 1968.

Wallace S, Jackson L, Dodd GD, Greening RR: Lymphatic dynamics in certain abnormal states. *AJR* 91:1187, 1964.

Wallace S, Jing B: Testicular malignancies and the lymphatic system. In Johnson D (ed): *Testicular Tumors.* Flushing, NY, Medical Examination Publishing, 1972.

Weichert RF, Jamieson CW: Acute chylous peritonitis. A case report. *Br J Surg* 57:230, 1970.

Wolfel DA: Lymphatico-venous communications. *AJR* 95:766, 1965.

Wücherer O: Filaria. *Gaz Med da Bohia*, 1868.

Wutzer CW: Einmundung des Duct Thoracicus in die Vena Azygos. *Arch Anat Phys* 311, 1834.

Yoffey JM, Courtice FC: *Lymphatics, Lymph and Lymphoid Tissue.* Cambridge, MA, Harvard University Press, 1956.

Young AE, Rutt DC, Kinmonth JB: The objective measurement of skin thickness in lymphedema. *Eur Surg Res* 8:31, 1976.

Yune HY, Klatte EC: Lymphography in lymphatic obstruction. *Radiology* 92:824, 1969.

Zeissler RM, Rose G, Nelson PA: Postmastectomy lymphedema: late results of treatment in 385 patients. *Arch Phys Med Rehabil* 53:159, 1972.

Zelikovski A, Melamed I, Kott I: The Lympha-Press—A new pneumatic device for the treatment of lymphedema: clinical trial and results. *Folia Angio* 28:165, 1980.

# 7

# *Malformations of the Mesenteric Lymphatics*

MARCEAU SERVELLE, M.D.*

Between 1964 and 1982, we studied 310 patients with malformation of the mesenteric lymphatics, 80 of whom were checked at laparotomy after a fat meal. All 80 patients had lymphography and lymphochromeas of the small intestine. The study led us to the following conclusions:

1. Clinical diagnosis of mesenteric lymphatic malformations is quite easy with the hyperlipidemia test.

2. Lymphograms of the mesenteric lymphatics reveal collateral channels for chyle flow not only in the abdomen but also in the thorax.

Table 7.1 enumerates the diseases that occur secondarily to malformations of the mesenteric lymph vessels, and Table 7.2 lists the diseases associated with mesenteric lymph vessel malformations but not caused by this malformation.

## TWO FUNDAMENTAL LESIONS

Lymphograms of the lower limb were performed by pedal or inguinal lymph node injection. Lymphograms of the small intestine were obtained during laparotomy after a fat meal. The cisterna chyli was almost never opacified. The

* Figures 7.1–7.24 are from Servelle M, Nogues C: *The Chyliferous Vessels.* Expansion Scientifique Francaise, 15, rue Saint-Benoit, 75006 Paris, 1981.

A 16-mm, English-speaking movie entitled "Congenital Malformations of the Chyliferous Vessels" and written by M. Servelle can be borrowed free of charge from Service du film de la Recherche Scientifique, 96 Boulevard Raspail, 75272 Paris Cedex 6.

mesenteric nodes were commonly hypoplastic, and many were no larger than a grain of wheat. Occasionally a node would be much larger than normal, sometimes as large as a tangerine.

For our mesenteric lymphograms, we frequently injected a radiopaque medium mixed with Evans blue dye into one of the mesenteric nodes. These injections showed a thickening of the capsule due to additional muscle fibers and to histological alterations of the interior of the node. On two occasions, the radiopaque medium injected into the node remained totally intranodal; it did not enter afferent or efferent lymphatics. In a normal subject, the mesenteric nodes make up the largest group in the organism (130–150 nodes).

To sum it up, malformation of the cisterna chyli and mesenteric lymph node abnormalities were the two basic anatomic lesions involved in

TABLE 7.1.

COMPLICATIONS DUE TO MALFORMATIONS OF THE MESENTERIC LYMPHATICS IN 165 PATIENTS*

| | |
|---|---|
| Protein-losing enteropathy | 14 |
| Chyloperitoneum and chyle cyst of the mesentery | 12 |
| Chyluria | 11 |
| Lymphedema with chyle reflux in the lymphatics of the leg and its complications (chylorrheas, chylarthrosis, intraosseous lymphatics, anovulvar excrescences) | 45 |
| Chylothorax and chyle cysts of the mediastinum | 15 |
| Chylopericardium | 9 |
| Chyle reflux in the pulmonary lymphatics | 12 |
| Simple hypoproteinemia | 2 |
| Isolated food allergies | 17 |

* From Servelle M, Nogues C: *The Chyliferous Vessels.* Expansion Scientifique Francaise, 15, rue Saint-Benoit, 75006 Paris, 1981.

TABLE 7.2.

MALFORMATIONS OF THE MESENTERIC LYMPHATICS ASSOCIATED WITH OTHER DISEASES IN 165 PATIENTS

| | |
|---|---|
| Common lymphedema | 31 |
| Lymphedema of the genitals | 4 |
| Milroy's disease | 8 |
| Klippel-Trenaunay syndrome | 30 |
| Common edema | 4 |
| Vascular complications from use of birth control pills | 10 |

lymph vessel malformations in our patients. These two changes gave rise to alterations of upstream lymphatics in the mesentery and in all walls of the small intestine. Furthermore, since the lymph could not evacuate normally in these patients, various collateral channels in both the abdomen and the thorax were used for evacuation. These nodal modifications in lymph vessel malformations probably are responsible for changes in the white blood cell count usually observed and for the lack of resistance to infection in children handicapped by such abnormalities.

## PATHOPHYSIOLOGY

In the presence of malformation of the mesenteric lymphatic vessels, the developmental pathology is the same as that found in all domains involving lymph vessels: loss of valvular function secondary to dilatation of the lymphatic vessels due to lymph stasis. Our diagram sums up the importance of valvular function in the presence of vessel interruption, such as surgical intervention or a congenital malformation (Fig. 7.1).

### Mesenteric Lymph Vessel Modifications in the Abdominal Cavity

Malformations of the cisterna chyli and of mesenteric nodes hinder evacuation via the mesenteric lymphatics; beneath this barrier, the vessels become thick, sinuous, and taut white varices. On both aspects of the mesentery, their tangles form whitish patches the size of the palm

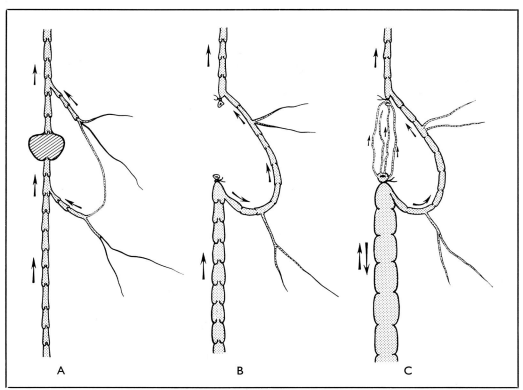

FIGURE 7.1. DEVELOPMENTAL PATHOLOGY

*A*: A normal lymphatic vessel with a node and collateral vessels. The two branches are linked by fine anastomoses. *B*: The node has been resected. The lymphatic trunk below the resection dilates, but its valves remain competent. The collateral below the resection dilates and loses its valvular function. Lymph in the subjacent lymphatic trunk flows against the stream, enters this collateral, then via the anastomoses reaches the overlying branch and returns to the lymphatic trunk above the resection. *C*: If this substitute circulation proves to be insufficient, the subjacent lymphatic trunk dilates further, and its valves no longer come into contact with one another. The lymph may then flow back toward the periphery. Often, in the place of the resected segment, a small substitute circulation develops.

of the hand. Dilatation can be localized to a chyle cyst of the mesentery. These distended mesenteric lymphatics are likely to rupture into the peritoneal cavity and cause chyloperitoneum. If this rupture remains subperitoneal, a chyloma forms, which may either rupture into the peritoneal cavity or be resorbed. On the small intestine, dilated lymphatics form a characteristic meshwork pattern and usually lose their valvular function. The opaque medium spreads every which way, filling all of the meshes in the net as well as the equally dilated lymphatics of the muscular and mucosal layers of the intestine. In normal subjects, contrast medium fills the lymphatic vessels in a single direction. Among patients with lymphatic abnormalities, dilatation of the vessels involves all intestinal layers. In the mucosa, dilatations of the central lymphatics

cause the villi to be club-shaped. Their rupture into the intestinal lumen produces protein-losing enteropathy and a direct communication between the inside of the mesenteric lymphatics and the intestinal cavity, which is always septic. This accounts for the development of mesenteric lymphangitis.

The cistern of Pecquet is the ultimate recipient not only of the mesenteric lymphatics but also of the lymphatics of the stomach and colon. Lymphochromea brings out dilatation of the gastric and colonic lymphatics in patients with malformations. Such increases in caliber can result in chyle reflux into the rectosigmoid lymphatics.

Compensating somewhat for these blocked vessels, collateral neolymphatics develop on the mesocolon and other sections of the colon. These vessels contain chyle, and they drain toward the lymphatics of the abdominal and thoracic walls.

The hepatic and pancreatic lymphatics also drain into the cistern of Pecquet and become dilated in the presence of mesenteric lymphatic malformations. On our intestinal lymphograms, the Lipiodol injected into a mesenteric lymphatic drained not only into the liver lymphatics but also into those of the pancreas (which had increased in caliber and in number) and ended in the diaphragmatic lymphatics.

A blocked cisterna chyli also hinders evacuation of lymphatics of the intrapelvic genital organs and urinary bladder. They dilate, and sometimes chyle reflux appears in the bladder and in the uterus and its adnexa. This disruption of flow is often complicated by vulvar chylorrheas and, in one patient, by a chyle cyst of the ovary.

## Chyle Reflux in Subperitoneal Lumbar Region and Lower Limbs

Besides the mesenteric lymphatics, the following channels also lead to the cisterna chyli: the two lumbar lymphatic trunks that drain lymph from the lower limbs, external genital organs, kidneys, adrenal glands and abdominal wall, and the iliac lymphatics that drain part of the lymphatics of the uterus and its adnexa and those of the bladder.

In malformations of the cistern of Pecquet (Fig. 7.2), the two lumbar trunks, like the mesenteric lymphatics, cannot evacuate normally; they dilate and gradually lose their valvular function. Thus, the mixture of chyle and lymph in the cisterna chyli can flow back against the stream in these lumbar lymphatic trunks. In a first phase, this reflux is stopped by the nodes of Bogros' space in the inguinal region, but this stoppage is only temporary. The various

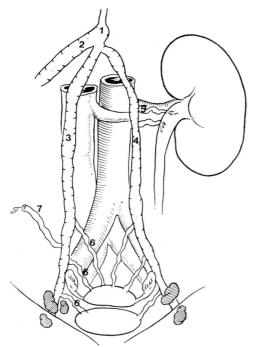

FIGURE 7.2. MECHANISMS OF CHYLE BACKFLOW AS FAR AS THE INGUINAL REGIONS

When there is malformation of the cistern of Pecquet (1), the intestinal lymphatic trunk (2) and the two lumbar trunks (3 and 4) dilate and then lose their valvular function. The mixture of chyle and lymph contained in the cistern of Pecquet first flows back as far as the inguinal regions. Lymphatics of the kidney (5), also hindered in their draining functions, dilate, lose their valvular function, and finally rupture into the renal pelvis (chyluria). In the pelvis, some thick collaterals (6) of the iliac lymphatics flow back into the bladder, the uterus, and its annexes. An external collateral (7) of the iliac lymphatics can open directly to the skin of the abdominal wall.

branches of the lumbar trunks also dilate and lose their valvular function. The highest placed of these collateral channels are the renal lymphatics, into which the chyle refluxes. The lymphatics of the renal pelvis dilate and then rupture into the calyces; this is the most common cause of chyluria. When severing the renal lymphatics, we have noted that lymphatics of the adrenal glands are often dilated and filled with chyle as well.

The two lumbar trunks also drain lymphatics of the abdominal wall. In one patient, chyle reflux into these parietal lymphatics resulted in isolated chylorrheas in the abdominal wall.

The same mechanism (reflux following dilatation and loss of valvular function) also can be observed in collaterals of the iliac lymphatics, particularly those which partly drain the intrapelvic genital organs and bladder. We have seen chyle reflux in some enormous internal iliac and gluteal lymphatics give rise to edema in one buttock and gluteal chylorrhea.

The pressure in the standing patient's thick lumbar and iliac lymphatics filled with chyle forces the barrier formed by the external iliac and inguinal nodes. Step by step, the chyle flows back into the lymphatics of one or, less frequently, both of the lower limbs, resulting in lymphedema with reflux of chyle into the leg lymphatics (Fig. 7.3). Rather rapidly, this reflux of chyle involves the cutaneous lymphatics in the foot and external genitals. Small white vesicles or transcutaneous lymphatic blisters appear on the skin (Fig. 7.4) and then rupture, producing chylorrhea. These vesicular ruptures bring the interior of the lymphatic vessels into contact with a cutaneous surface that is always septic, hence the appearance of lymphangitis or erysipelas. The chyle reflux in the leg lymphatics involves both superficial and deep lymphatics. Dilated lymphatics of the joints may rupture, resulting in chylarthrosis. Chyle reflux may also spread to lymphatics of the muscles and especially to those of the bones: sizable intraosseous geodes appear along the tibiae, femora, pelvic bones, or lumbar vertebrae. We have examined five patients with this phenomenon.

## Chyle Drainage Channels through Thorax to Cervical Region

Between 1943 and 1963, our first lymphograms of the lower limbs showed that in malformations of the cisterna chyli, chyle mixed with lymph from the lower limbs is evacuated in the thoracic area through two newly formed lymphatic channels located on either side of the spine. These

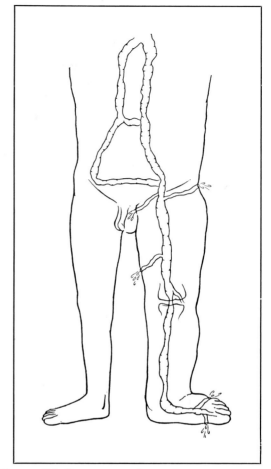

FIGURE 7.3. DIAGRAM OF CHYLE BACKFLOW IN THE LOWER LIMB

We have observed chylorrheas in the genitals, thigh, foot, and knee joint (chylarthrosis).

channels develop at the expense of anastomoses connecting terminations of the intercostal lymphatics (Fig. 7.5). Due to circulatory overload in these newly formed laterovertebral lymphatic channels, the intercostal lymphatics leading to them have more trouble evacuating, and some of them dilate, losing their valvular function. Chyle in these two laterovertebral channels can then move (against the current) into these dilated valveless intercostal lymphatics. In certain cases (Fig. 7.6), this chylous fluid reaches the lateral wall of the thorax and then returns to the base of the neck via laterothoracic, axillary, and subclavian lymphatics. Loss of valvular function involves the entire length of the intercostal lymphatic. Still moving against the stream, the chylous fluid reaches the internal mammary lymphatics and returns to the cervical region via the lymphatic of the first intercostal space (Fig. 7.7).

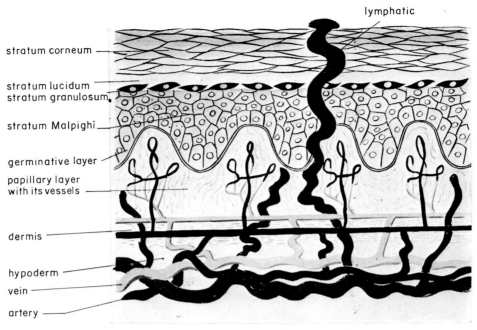

stratum corneum

stratum lucidum
stratum granulosum

stratum Malpighi

germinative layer

papillary layer
with its vessels

dermis

hypoderm

vein

artery

lymphatic

FIGURE 7.4. CHYLE BACKFLOW IN THE CUTANEOUS LYMPHATICS
The cutaneous vesicles observed in lymphedema with chyle backflow are transcutaneous lymphatic hernias.

FIGURE 7.5.   COLLATERAL FLOW SECONDARY TO
MALFORMATION OF CISTERN OF PECQUET
   When there is a malformation of the cistern of
Pecquet, two large laterovertebral lymphatics de-
velop at the expense of anastomoses between ter-
minations of the intercostal lymphatics.

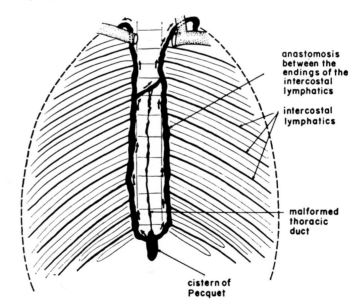

anastomosis
between the
endings of the
intercostal
lymphatics

intercostal
lymphatics

malformed
thoracic
duct

cistern of
Pecquet

   When the cistern of Pecquet does not function
normally (due to malformation, rupture, tumor,
or parasitic invasion) or when the mesenteric
nodes are abnormal, chyle absorbed by the small
intestine must be evacuated through collateral
channels, consisting mainly of diaphragmatic
lymphatics and their drainage channels leading
to the cervical region. Some dilated lymphatics
run directly from the cisterna chyli to the diaphragm. Intestinal lymphograms show that Lipiodol injected into the mesenteric lymphatics
often evacuates first through the hepatic lymphatics, then travels via vessels of the suspensory
ligaments, and finally enters the diaphragmatic
lymphatics. This oily contrast medium, contained in lymphatics of the small intestine, also
traces the course of numerous peripancreatic
lymphatics that drain backward and upward

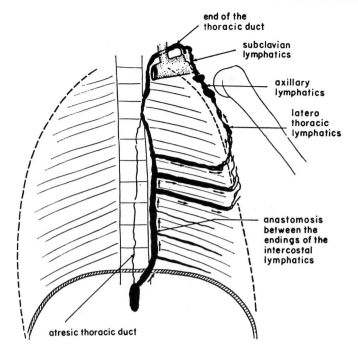

**FIGURE 7.6. LOSS OF FUNCTION IN INTERCOASTAL LYMPHATICS SECONDARY TO MALFORMATION OF CISTERN OF PECQUET**

Development of circulation in these laterovertebral lymphatics hinders evacuation of the intercostal lymphatics. They dilate and lose their valvular function, and the chyle can flow against the stream and enter their lumina. This backflow may only go as far as the lateral wall of the thorax. It is evacuated first via the laterothoracic lymphatics and then via the axillary and subclavian lymphatics toward the base of the neck.

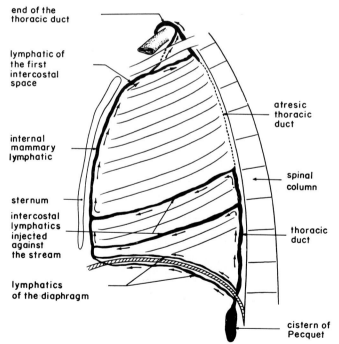

**FIGURE 7.7. CHYLE BACKFLOW IN INTERCOSTAL LYMPHATICS**

In some cases, the backflow takes place over the entire length of the intercostal lymphatics. The chyle is evacuated toward the neck via internal mammary lymphatics.

through lymphatics of the subdiaphragmatic cellular tissue and finally along the course of lymphatics of the diaphragm. In other words, the diaphragm becomes a chyle derivation zone, and its numerous lymphatics dilate considerably. Those vessels that are covered by the pleura become thick, whitish lymphatic varices with very thin walls capable of rupturing into the pleural cavity and causing spontaneous chylothorax. Those vessels that are located on the inferior surface of the diaphragm and are covered by the peritoneum may also rupture, causing chyloperitoneum.

Thoracic radiographs obtained after injection

of Lipiodol into the malformed mesenteric lymphatics show that these dilated diaphragmatic lymphatics evacuate toward the base of the neck by two different channels—in front, via the thick internal mammary lymphatics; and further back, in the mediastinosagittal region, via thick ascending mediastinal lymphatics and lymphatics of the triangular ligaments of the lung. These mediastinal paths ascend via nodes of the bifurcatio tracheae (Fig. 7.8) and then run toward the peritracheal lymphatics. These same nodes of the tracheal bifurcation also receive the pulmo-

nary lymphatics. Due to circulatory overload created by this chyle derivation in the lymphatics of the tracheal bifurcation, these pulmonary lymphatics have difficulty evacuating.

First, lymphatics of the lung dilate (Figs. 7.9–7.11) and then lose their valvular function. Thus, chyle contained in lymphatics of the bifurcation can reflux upstream into the pulmonary lymphatics, both subpleural and peribronchial. The lymphatics located under the pleura can rupture into the pleural cavity, causing spontaneous chylothorax (Fig. 7.12). The peribronchial lymphat-

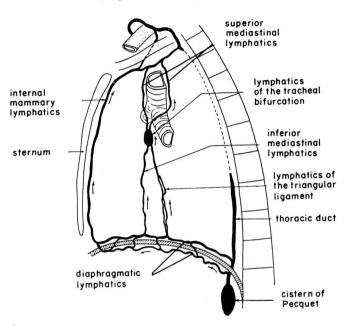

FIGURE 7.8.   DILATED DIAPHRAGMATIC LYMPHATICS

Lymphatics of the diaphragm, abnormally filled with chyle, drain toward the cervical region—in front, via the internal mammary lymphatics; farther back, via the inferior lymphatics of the mediastinum and the triangular lymphatics toward the tracheal bifurcation and then via the peritracheal lymphatics.

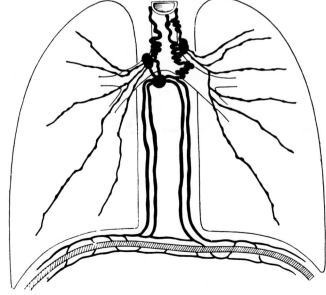

FIGURE 7.9.   RETROGRADE COLLATERAL FLOW TOWARD THE TRACHEAL BIFURCATION

Frontal view of evacuation of diaphragmatic lymphatics toward the tracheal bifurcation and peritracheal lymphatics.

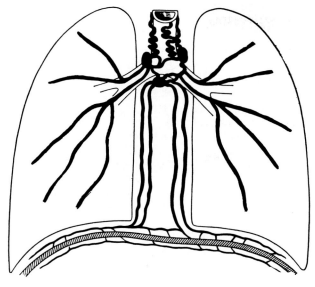

FIGURE 7.10.   DILATATION OF PULMONARY LYMPHATICS
Drainage of chyle toward the tracheal bifurcation hinders evacuation of pulmonary lymphatics, which dilate and then lose their valvular function.

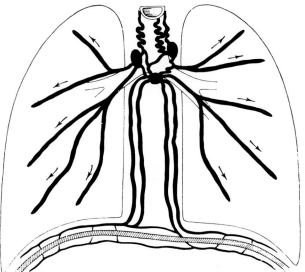

FIGURE 7.11.   RETROGRADE FLOW INTO PULMONARY LYMPHATICS
As a result of the loss of valvular function, chyle can flow back into pulmonary lymphatics.

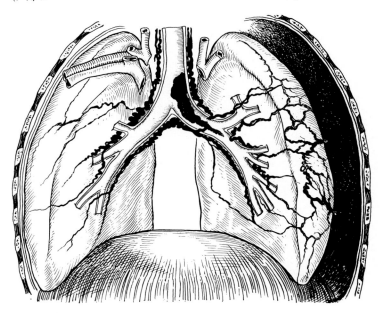

FIGURE 7.12.   SPONTANEOUS CHYLOTHORAX—LYMPHOBRONCHIAL FISTULA
Rupture of pulmonary lymphatics filled with chyle: in the pleura, chylothorax, in the bronchi, pseudovomiting.

187

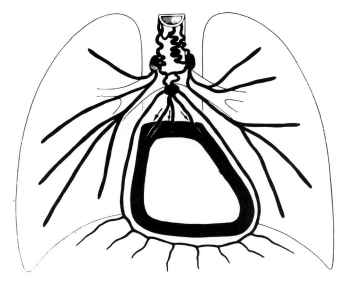

FIGURE 7.13.  CHYLOPERICARDIUM
In the event of derivation of chyle in the tracheal and pulmonary lymphatics, due to the familiar mechanism (stasis→dilatation→loss of valvular function), the chyle flows back into the cardiac lymphatics. Their rupture causes chylopericardium.

ics, also dilated by chyle, first herniate through the bronchial mucosa, sometimes rupturing into the bronchus and causing pseudovomiting. Chyle from the intestine can bring bacterial organisms to the lungs, giving rise to pulmonary lymphangitis. Normally, cardiac lymphatics also drain into lymphatics of the tracheal bifurcation to a considerable extent. In the event of chyle moving via the inferior mediastinal lymphatics toward the tracheal bifurcation (triggered by the same mechanism of dilatation and loss of valvular function), the chyle may reflux into cardiac lymphatics, which may rupture and cause chylopericardium (Fig. 7.13).

## STUDYING MALFORMATIONS OF MESENTERIC LYMPHATICS

Most of our patients were referred to us by pediatricians. Therefore, they had had all of their clinical and biological examinations (in particular, tests with radioiodinated polyvinylpyrrolidone or with labeled macromolecules). In addition, as a means of diagnosis, we used the hyperlipidemia test.

### Hyperlipidemia Test

After taking a blood sample during fasting (t0) for quantity determination of lipids and optical density, the patient absorbs 60 g of butter (40 g for children), and blood samples are taken every hour for 5 hr for the same quantity determinations (t1, t2, t3, t4, t5). From these measurements a total lipids curve and an optical density curve can be constructed.

### Total Lipids Curve

In normal subjects (Fig. 7.14), lipemia in the fasting state (t0) occurs at 6 g. After that, the levels are t1 = 6.4 g, t2 = 7 g, t3 = 7.3 g, t4 = 6.5 g, and t5 = 5.5 g. In cases of mesenteric lymphatic malformations, the total lipids curve permits easy diagnosis in almost every case; it almost always shows a plateau with no postprandial peak. Table 7.3 shows the variations in total lipids in patients with mesenteric lymphatic malformations.

### Optical Density Curve

In normal subjects (Fig. 7.15), the optical density level in the fasting state (t0) is 4.5; after that, the levels are t1 = 7, t2 = 13, t3 = 18, t4 = 14, t5 = 10. Variations in this optical density curve in cases of mesenteric lymphatic malformations are presented in Table 7.4.

To sum it up, the induced hyperlipidemia test provides a very easy diagnosis of malformations of mesenteric lymphatics because 98% of patients will have a total lipids curve with a low plateau, while the optical density curve will be above the reference curve in 70% of patients. The diagnostic value of such biochemical data was unerringly confirmed in the course of our 80 laparotomies performed on patients who had absorbed a fat meal.

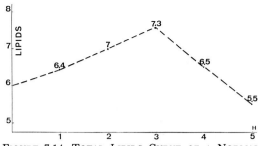

FIGURE 7.14. TOTAL LIPIDS CURVE OF A NORMAL SUBJECT AFTER ABSORPTION OF 60 G OF BUTTER
Blood samples were taken every hour for 5 hr. The summit is 7.3 g/liter at T3.

TABLE 7.3.
VARIATIONS OF TOTAL LIPIDS CURVE IN 165 MALFORMATIONS OF MESENTERIC LYMPHATICS

| | |
|---|---|
| Typical plateau well below reference curve | 70% |
| Plateau level with reference curve's peak | 15% |
| Plateau clearly above highest point of reference curve | 9% |
| Low double plateau | 4% |
| Normal progress curve but well below reference curve | 2% |

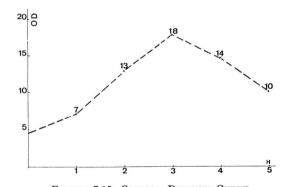

FIGURE 7.15. OPTICAL DENSITY CURVE
Normal optical density curve under the same conditions as for the lipids curve: summit = 18.

## Laparotomy after Fat Meal

Four hours before surgery, the patient absorbs 40 g of melted butter in a glass of lukewarm milk to assure that the abnormal mesenteric lymphatics will be definitely colored white by chyle and will be easy to observe. On the small intestine itself, the meshwork pattern is a pathognomonic sign of mesenteric lymphatic malformations. In the mesentery, lymphatic vessels have a very abnormal appearance; they are dilated, sinuous, and intertwined. The anatomy of mesenteric nodes and the abnormal course of mesenteric lymphatics in front of the mesocolon or

TABLE 7.4.
VARIATIONS OF OPTICAL DENSITY CURVE IN 165 CONGENITAL MALFORMATIONS OF MESENTERIC LYMPHATICS

| | | |
|---|---|---|
| Curve well above reference curve | 44% | |
| Very high curve with two peaks | 20% | 70% |
| Plateau level with reference curve | 6% | |
| Normal curve | 8% | |
| Normal progress curve but well below reference curve | 8% | |
| Plateau well below reference curve | 14% | |

colon and in front of the pancreas, aorta, left renal vein, or hepatic pedicle are easy to observe, although the abnormalities vary greatly from one individual to another. Intestinal lymphography completes the surgical exploration. It, too, reveals polymorphous malformations.

## Intestinal Lymphography and Lymphochromea

Lymphography by the pedal or inguinal approach cannot opacify the mesenteric lymphatics, but it can supply a few elements suggesting malformations—considerable stasis in lumbar lymphatics; no opacification of the cistern of Pecquet; opacification of pancreatic, diaphragmatic, hepatic, or renal lymphatics; only occasional passage of Lipiodol in the intestinal lumen; and, on the thoracic films, opacification of the diaphragmatic, internal mammary, mediastinal, or pulmonary lymphatics.

Intestinal lymphography can be performed only during laparotomy after the patient has absorbed a fat meal. We use 8 ml of Lipiodol and 2 ml of Evans blue dye aspirated in a 10-ml syringe. Most of the time, puncture of a lymphatic on the small intestine is easy: first, a bit of dye is injected to make sure that the needle is in the lymphatic; then the opaque medium is injected. If such an injection is impossible, a node is punctured in the upper part of the mesentery. If the needle tip is in the lymphatic circulation, a small amount of Evans blue dye injected through the needle will diffuse into the afferent or efferent lymphatics. When the diffusion becomes apparent, the piston of the syringe is turned upward in order to propel the oily contrast.

As soon as the injection is completed, small intraperitoneal radiographs are taken using 9 × 12 cm or 6 × 6 cm film sterilized in plastic envelopes. Then 30 × 40 cm cassettes are slipped under the patient's abdomen and thorax. Filming is repeated as required by progression of the contrast medium, which is often slow. As soon as the abdomen is closed, full face and profile radiographs of the abdomen and thorax are taken. These films are repeated every 4–6 hr for the first postoperative day and once daily during the next 6–8 days. When lymphatics of the liver or lung are injected, the radiopaque product may remain in the lymphatics for several days, hence the need for delayed films.

In very thick lumbar or iliac lymphatics, the ultrafluid Lipiodol forms droplets and becomes a poor indicator of vessel caliber. For this reason Lipiodol is supplemented or replaced by the water-soluble opaque medium used for intravenous urography. Sometimes 50–60 ml are needed to fill these large dilated lymphatics, good visualization of which is useful to the surgeon who must resect them.

These intestinal lymphograms have shown a number of abnormalities associated with congenital chylous malformation—absence of opacification or a very marked abnormality of the cisterna chyli; a few malformations of the thoracic duct, particularly a considerable mass of mesenteric lymphatics in front of the lumbar aorta; upstream reflux in the mesentery; persistent opacification of very thick mesenteric lymphatics on the injected intestinal loop; opacification of lymphatics found in postoperative radiographs of many areas: pancreatic, hepatic, diaphragmatic, mediastinal, intercostal, and pulmonary.

## Clamped Biopsy of Small Intestine

Histological examination of samples from total superficial lymphangiectomies in 700 patients treated for elephantiasis of the lower limbs almost never revealed the same sizable dilatations of superficial lymphatics brought out by the lymphograms. This is due to the fact that during the operation lymph escapes from distended lymphatics, which collapse. The histologist only sees some rather inconclusive vascular fissures. Thus, in cases of mesenteric lymphatic malformation, we isolate a short segment of the small intestine between two clamps that shut off all blood and lymph circulation (Fig. 7.16). These clamps are left in place during fixation. Thus, the examining histologist is able to observe intestinal lymphatics in their normal diameter, something which no other sampling method permits. Thus, my colleague, Dr. Noguĕs, has been able to show dilatation of the lymphatics not only in the mucosa but also in the submucosa and in the muscular and cellular layers of the small intestine. This dilatation of mesenteric lymphatics may be more marked in either one or another layer of the intestinal wall, depending upon the patient. Such histological modifications are usually more marked in the upper third of the small intestine, from the duodenojejunal angle upward. We strive to study the segment that appears to be the most seriously altered.

## FREQUENCY OF MESENTERIC LYMPHATIC MALFORMATIONS

Mesenteric lymphatic malformations are very common. Between 1966 and January 1980, we made 165 observations. During the 2 yr that followed, we studied 145 new cases. We were able to do so thanks to the hyperlipidemia test, not only in the disorders illustrated in Table 7.1 but also in cases of malformation of the deep veins (Klippel-Trenaunay syndrome), in various forms of elephantiasis, in vascular accidents due to the contraceptive pill, and in food allergies. Such malformations of the mesenteric lymphatics may be observed from childhood or discovered only in adulthood after a long latency period. Although such a condition is not hereditary, on several occasions we encountered two or three cases in the same family.

## CLINICAL ASPECTS OF MESENTERIC LYMPHATIC MALFORMATIONS

### Protein-losing Enteropathy

This condition has particular importance to pediatricians. In 1964, a girl of 18 was referred to us for considerable loss of chyle in the duodenal region. Four years earlier, this girl had been observed by pediatricians and described as having enteropathy with loss of proteins and steatorrhea subsequent to Gordon's test and the iodine-131 triolein test. At age 18, chyloperitoneum appeared, and duodenal intubation yielded a sizable quantity of chyle. Pedal lymphography

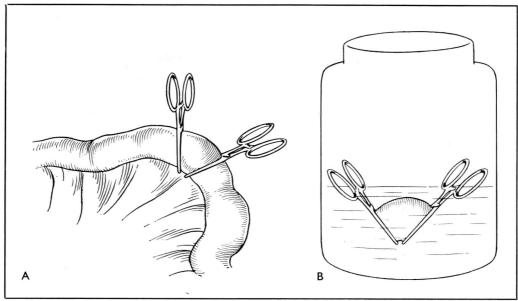

FIGURE 7.16. DIAGRAM OF A CLAMPED BIOPSY

*A*: Positioning of the clamps on the small intestine. *B*: The section is performed on the outer side of the clamps. The excised part of the small intestine with the two clamps in place is then immersed in fixative after injection with a fine needle of a small amount of fixative fluid into the short intestinal lumen.

did not opacify the cistern of Pecquet (Fig. 7.17) or the loop of the small intestine (Fig. 7.18). At subsequent right thoracolaparotomy, we resected all chyle-filled lymphatics leading to the duodenum and pancreas, front and back. Immediately the proteins, which had been low for 4 yr, returned to normal. Six weeks later chylothorax developed due to rupture of a thick chyle-filled diaphragmatic lymphatic, which we sutured by thoracotomy. Surgical occlusion of the chyloduodenal fistula had overloaded the lymphatic circulation of the diaphragm. Today, 17 yr after our operations, this patient is feeling very well, and her proteins are near normal. The total lipids curve (Fig. 7.19) is quite typical of blocked mesenteric lymphatics. What was involved was an ultra-acute form of protein-losing enteropathy occurring on top of a chronic form. This observation led us to become interested in malformations of the mesenteric lymphatics.

In 1974, Professor Rossier, a pediatrician, sent us a child aged 10 yr suffering from lymphedema with chyle reflux in the lymphatics of the legs and genitals as well as Klippel-Trenaunay syndrome. The pedal lymphogram revealed thick iliac and lumbar lymphatics, no opacification of the cisterna chyli, and opacification of the lymphatics of the pancreas, left kidney, and left diaphragmatic cupola, then of the lungs. The total lipids curve reached a plateau that was level with the peak of the reference curve. Because of the chyle backflow in the leg lymphatics, we performed a subperitoneal resection of the highly dilated and chyle-filled lateroaortic lymphatics. After this resection, we opened the peritoneum and observed the typical meshwork pattern of mesenteric lymphatics on the small intestine, a greater than normal number of mesenteric nodes, and numerous chylous varices on the mesentery. The intestinal lymphogram showed drainage of the mesenteric lymphatics through the liver (Fig. 7.20).

After viewing the lymphograms, we asked the boy's mother whether he had ever had diarrhea. She revealed that between the ages of 18 and 24 months, he had suffered from exudative enteropathy. After resection of the laterocaval lymphatics, we operated on his lymphedema of the genitals using our total superficial lymphangiectomy technique. For the 2 yr that followed, the boy was in good health. Then, marked anemia developed along with hypoproteinemia and blood in the stools. For 1 yr, every 4 months, we subjected him to albumin perfusions and transfusions, but his condition remained serious. Blood was still found in the stools. We then located the most pathological segment during laparotomy after a fat meal with an intestinal lymphogram and lymphochromea. We resected the 50 cm that featured highly altered lymphat-

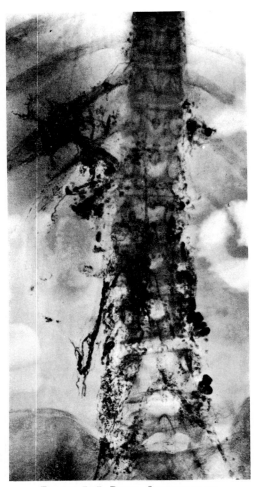

FIGURE 7.17. PEDAL LYMPHOGRAM

The cistern of Pecquet and the thoracic duct are not opacified. There is considerable stasis in the lumbar lymphatics. A large patch of lymphatic varices is in front of the right tenth and eleventh ribs.

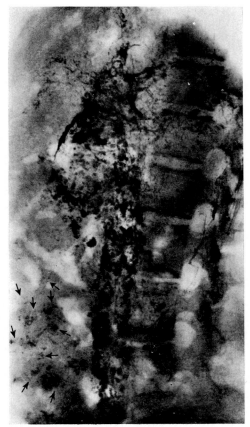

FIGURE 7.18. LYMPHOGRAM: LATERAL VIEW 8 HR AFTER INJECTION

The radiopaque medium has moved into the small intestine (*arrows*). Sizable aortocaval lymphatics are visible anterior to the first and second lumbar vertebrae, anterior to and above the aortocaval lymphatics, which in Figure 7.17 overlie the tenth and eleventh right ribs.

ics. For the past 2 yr, this boy has felt very well. The red blood cell count and blood proteins have been normal, and there is no longer any blood in the stools.

We have since operated on 14 other patients with protein-losing enteropathies; each operation included intestinal lymphography and clamped biopsy. These explorations have revealed that protein-losing enteropathy is not an isolated disease affecting only the intestinal mucosa but rather a complication of mesenteric lymphatic malformations. Malformations of the cistern of Pecquet and of the mesenteric nodes block the circulation of chyle. The central lymphatics of the intestinal villosities become distended. Their rupture into the intestinal lumen causes considerable loss of chyle, producing exudative enteropathy.

## Chyloperitoneum

Since 1965, we have operated on 17 patients for spontaneous chyloperitoneum. We have found that there can be no chyloperitoneum without congenital malformation of the mesenteric lymphatics. The extravasation of chyle in the peritoneal cavity may appear as an isolated incident, or it may be preceded by other clinical manifestations. Associated abnormalities are most often further consequences of mesenteric lymphatic malformations—exudative enteropathy, chylothorax, chyle reflux in the leg lymphatics, or chyluria. The chyle-dilated mesenteric lymphatics may rupture directly into the peritoneal cavity. Sometimes this rupture takes

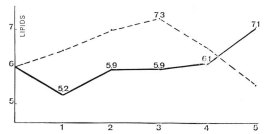

FIGURE 7.19. TOTAL LIPIDS CURVE

The total lipids curve is plateau-shaped in the vicinity of 6 g until the fourth hour and then rises to 7.1 g at the fifth hour. This is a typical contour for a mesenteric lymphatic malformation. The *dotted line* is the curve of a normal subject.

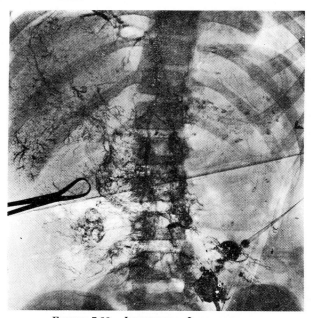

FIGURE 7.20. INTESTINAL LYMPHOGRAM

Drainage of the chyliferous vessels through the liver toward the diaphragmatic muscle is shown. A thick mesenteric lymphatic is visible overlying the right half of the first two vertebrae. The cistern of Pecquet is not visible. The thoracic duct is normal.

place in two steps. First, a subperitoneal chyloma forms, and secondarily, this chyloma opens into the peritoneum. Diagnosis is usually easy. We observe peritoneal extravasation, a puncture yields chyle, and the hyperlipidemia test results feature a plateau-like total lipids curve.

One of our patients, first seen at age 5 months, had been given a diagnosis of essential hypoproteinemia. We examined this same patient 16 yr later for edema of the lower limbs with a 1-cm increase in the length of the right lower limb. The venogram revealed a malformation of the popliteal vein, on which we operated. Six months later, the peripheral edema had decreased, but the abdomen was still swollen. Ascites was of medium amplitude. The puncture yielded chyle. Blood proteins were 49 g/liter. Lymphography (via inguinal injection) revealed dilatation of the iliolumbar lymphatics but no opacification of the cisterna chyli. There was reflux of the opaque medium into the leg lymphatics. During laparotomy, we discovered chyloperitoneum of medium amplitude, but the upper portion of the small intestine was white, as though it had been dipped in wet plaster. There was no mesenteric lymphatic in front of the left renal vein and no mesenteric node; there were only two large ileocolic nodes. Despite this highly unusual appearance of the small intestine, 8 yr after our intervention, this patient is well; she has married and borne a child. This was the only one of our patients found to suffer from both chyloperitoneum and chylothorax at the same time.

Chyloperitoneum may also appear in adults, sometimes as late as 55 yr. One woman presented at 38 and then at 42 yr with chylothoraxes that corrected with surgery. One year later, chyloperitoneum appeared. In each instance, the hyperlipidemia test was positive. Mesenteric lymphatic malformations may have remained latent until chyle appeared in the peritoneal cavity. When chyloperitoneum has existed for some time, the omentum majus has often lost its fat tissue and is frequently fenestrated or, in fact, reduced to a solely vascular structure.

Chyloperitoneum may be complicated by intestinal obstruction; the small intestine becomes engulfed in coagulated chyle and must be resected. One of our patients developed two intestinal obstructions during the evolution of chyloperitoneum, which finally occurred at age 40 yr (hypoproteinemia count, 44 g). At the time of the first attack, the coagulated chyle enclosed only the last 30 cm of the small intestine. Eighteen months later, intervention for a second intestinal obstruction revealed that the entire intermediate portion of the small intestine was enveloped in a white membrane formed by coagulated chyle and requiring resection. In this case, histological examination of the clamped biopsy showed partial thickening of the edematous submucosa. This submucosa and the muscularis mucosa contained a lymphangiectatic network. Fatty acid crystals were also observed in the lamina propria and muscularis mucosa.

Treatment of chyloperitoneum first consists of simple aspiration through a very fine drain inserted in a small trocar. Sometimes the chyloperitoneum can disappear after several days of aspiration. Otherwise, laparotomy must be performed on the patient after a fat meal. If the hypoproteinemia is very marked, albumin infusions will be required. As soon as the abdomen is opened, chyle in the peritoneum is aspirated, lesions are noted and assessed, and the small intestine and mesentery are examined for rupture of a dilated mesenteric lymphatic. This rupture is not always easy to detect. If such is the case, a peritoneal lavage with lukewarm serum will help identify the place through which the chyle is escaping. After careful suture of the escape hole, the drainage tubes are left in place in the parietocolic grooves and in Douglas' cul-de-sac.

## Lymphedema with Chyle Reflux in Leg Lymphatics

We operated on 49 patients suffering from lymphedema with reflux of chyle into the lymphatics of the leg. Diagnosis is usually easy because the patient complains of lacteous discharges, and small white vesicles appear on the skin of the affected limb.

In nearly all such cases, lymphography by direct puncture of a lymphatic or cutaneous vesicle is very easy and may be repeated at will. The lymphograms bring out lymphatics of considerable diameter (3–10 mm) in the lower limb and in the iliac and lumbar regions, which accounts for the chyle reflux and loss of valvular function. There is invariably a malformation of the cistern of Pecquet and of the mesenteric lymphatics. In all patients coming to surgery over the past 18 yr the hyperlipidemia test yielded the characteristic plateau-like curves. In treating these patients with lymphedema and chyle reflux, total superficial lymphangiectomy must be completed by subperitoneal resection (right, then left) of the lateroaortic, then of the laterocaval lymphatics, after the patient has had a fat meal. These lumbar lymphatics are highly dilated and colored white by chyle. Since 1964, after completing these subperitoneal resections, incision and examination of the peritoneum have invariably revealed mesenteric lymphatic malformations with the familiar meshwork pattern on the small intestine. Lymphography of the mesenteric lymphatics has always confirmed this diagnosis. So we can indeed assert that behind every lymphedema with chyle reflux in the leg lymphatics there are mesenteric lymphatic malformations.

In the first phase, the chyle reflux in the lumbar and iliac lymphatics goes no further than the nodes of Bogros' space and the inguinal nodes. The renal lymphatics that empty into the lumbar trunks have trouble evacuating. They dilate and lose their valvular function, allowing the chyle to flow back into the lymphatics of the kidneys and pelvis renalis. Finally, the latter vessels rupture in the calyces, causing chyluria, which in some of our patients preceded the appearance of lymphedema with chyle reflux. Likewise, in the pelvis, the iliac lymphatics receive chyle from the collaterals draining lymph from the bladder and intrapelvic genital organs. By the same mechanism (dilatation and loss of valvular function), the chyle refluxes into the lymphatics of the bladder, uterus, and adnexa. Chyle backflow in the uterine region gradually triggers vaginal and vulvar lymphorrheas, which may appear before the lymphedema with chyle reflux. Our present experience, based on nine observations, suggests that vaginal or vulvar chylorrhea does not occur without malformation of the mesenteric lymphatics.

Reflux of chyle stops at the inguinal fold only temporarily. Lymphatics of the lower limbs drain with increasing difficulty, dilate, and lose their valvular function. The chyle then flows all the way back to lymphatics of the foot and may also dilate lymphatics of the skin. One of these dilated vessels may herniate on the surface and cause a whitish cutaneous vesicle to appear. This vesicle may rupture, causing chylorrheas and bringing the interior of the lymphatic into contact with the cutaneous surface, which is always septic. The result is lymphangitis, which can sometimes be very serious. Several of our patients developed septicemia after such vesicular ruptures, and one died when the infection was neglected for a month. Families of these patients must always be warned of the gravity of lymphangitic infections and realize the necessity of using an antiseptic on the patient's skin in case of chylorrhea. If the patient runs a fever, an efficient and prolonged antibiotic treatment must be applied.

Sometimes chylorrheas do not appear until late in the disease process. In 1952, a youth of 20 yr consulted us for lymphedema of the lower limb. Examination revealed definite fluctuation in the popliteal fossa. Puncture with a large needle yielded 2.5 liters of chylous fluid, which we replaced with 50 ml of a water-soluble opaque medium. The lymphogram showed enormous popliteal and crural lymphatics (as thick as a finger) and retrograde opacification of lymphatics of the leg. This patient underwent surgery for lymphedema of the lower limb and genitals after several lymphangitic infections and two episodes of septicemia.

Our first diagnosis of lymphedema with chyle reflux was made in 1945 on a 33-yr-old patient presenting with lymphedema but no cutaneous vesicles and no chylorrhea. During denudation of the external saphenous vein behind the peroneal malleolus with a view to performing a venography, we discovered, in contact with this vein, a large lymphatic filled with chyle. After injection of opaque dye into this thick lymphatic, the radiographs revealed superficial and deep lymphatics the size of a saphena magna with retrograde filling of the lymphatics of the foot.

Generally, patients consult us for edema of the lower limbs or genitals accompanied by white cutaneous vesicles and, often, chylorrhea. Dilatation of the lymphatics with reflux of chyle is not confined to superficial lymphatics, however; the deep lymphatics (muscle, joint, bone) may be involved. One of our surgical patients had had three extravasations of chyle in the knee joint. Evacuation of the chyle by puncture followed by elastic bandage compression cured these chylarthroses.

A boy of 7 yr had surgery in 1948 for Klippel-Trenaunay syndrome. At 17 yr sizable edema of the buttock developed with abundant gluteal chylorrhea that continued for 28 yr. In 1976, a hyperlipidemia test confirmed the diagnosis of malformation of the mesenteric lymphatics. In 1977, laparotomy following a fat meal provided further confirmation and enabled us to discover enormous white lymphatic varices (6 mm in diameter) in front of the inferior vena cava and iliac vessels. Resection of these markedly dilated lymphatics stopped the gluteal chylorrheas, which have not recurred for 5 yr (Figs. 7.21 and 7.22).

In patients with lymphedema and reflux of chyle, three special complications must be borne in mind—vulvar and vaginal chylorrheas, genitoanal verrucose formations, and intraosseous lymphatics.

### Vulvar and Vaginal Chylorrheas

In one of our observations, vulvar chylorrhea appeared only at the time of menstruation and disappeared with menopause. Most of the time, they have appeared in girls aged 8 to 12 yr and have raised serious therapeutic problems. In 1974, a girl of 12 was referred to us for vulvar chylorrheas accompanied only by edema of the labia majora. The vulvar lymphogram showed evacuation toward the pelvis via a central lymphatic and bilaterally via the inguinal, then the iliac lymphatics. After subperitoneal resection of the periaortic and pericaval lymphatics, chylorrheas became rarer and less abundant. The patient underwent laparotomy after a fat meal. We resected the lymphatics in front of the sacral concavity. Mesenteric lymphatic malformation was pronounced with reflux of chyle in the sigmoid and around the uterus and tubes. One year later, chyloperitoneum with hypoproteinemia at 55 g and a red blood cell count of 2,900,000 made a second laparotomy imperative for suture of a ruptured mesenteric lymphatic and resection of a chyle cyst of the ovary. After a few months, a third sizable chyloperitoneum appeared, accompanied by deterioration of the general condition and proteins at 42 g. Six months later, thrombosis of the sylvian artery had brought on left hemiplegia. Finally, 2 yr after the vulvar chylorrheas had first appeared, chylothorax by reflux of chyle in the lungs caused death.

In light of our lymphographic and surgical experience, these vulvovaginal chylorrheas can be divided into two groups. In the first group, the lymphedema involves only the labia majora, reflux of chyle comes from the inguinal regions, and resection of both labia majora yields good results. In the second group, losses of chyle occur not only in the labia majora but also inside the vagina, and reflux of chyle has invaded the lymphatics of the uterus and adnexa with secondary propagation to the vaginal lymphatics. In this second group it is necessary to resect the lateroaortic, laterocaval, and iliac lymphatics. It is very difficult to eliminate completely the reflux of chyle in all the vaginal lymphatics.

### Genitoanal Verrucose Formations

Reflux of chyle into lymphatics of the external genitals and anal region sometimes causes verrucose formations. Often they are voluminous and very annoying. They must be resected, although they may recur. The presence of these verrucose formations should suggest mesenteric lymphatic malformations, which can be confirmed by the hyperlipidemia test.

### Intraosseous Lymphatics

Since 1944, we have operated on 570 patients with lymphedema of the limbs but without chyle reflux. In none of these patients did we note intraosseous lymphatics. Conversely, in our 49 cases of lymphedema with chyle reflux into lymphatics of the lower limbs, we observed five instances of intraosseous lymphatics containing chyle like the superficial and deep lymphatics. At the same time, these five patients presented

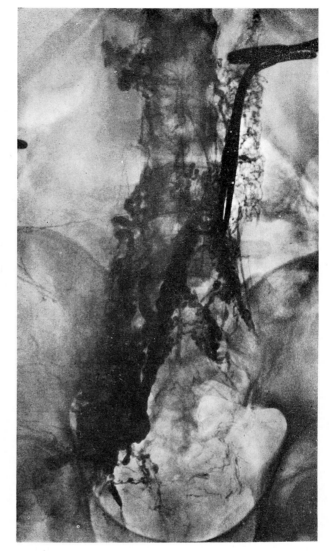

FIGURE 7.21. ABDOMINAL LYMPHOGRAM
Enormous right lumbar and iliac lymphatic varices are shown. A clamp obliterates the point of injection. In front of the right head of the femur, note the opacification of some very large gluteal lymphatics.

with Klippel-Trenaunay syndrome (malformation of the deep veins with lengthening of the limb). Two of them died, one from infectious complications and the other from coagulation disorders. A third patient, aged 12 yr, is in critical condition with considerable chyle reflux in the pelvis, lower limb, and vulva complicated by coagulation disorders for which there is no remedy. Therefore, observation in a child of intraosseous lymphatics, chyle reflux, and Klippel-Trenaunay syndrome necessarily prompts us to exercise great reserve in the prognosis.

## Chyluria

When chyle flows back into the two lumbar lymphatic trunks, the first collaterals it meets

are the lymphatics of the kidneys and pelvis renalis. Therefore, these lymphatics cannot evacuate normally; they dilate and then lose their valvular function. The chyle contained in the lumbar lymphatic trunks, running upstream, enters these distended renal and renopelvic lymphatics, causing them to rupture into the pyelic cavity, causing chyluria.

We have operated on 12 patients with chyluria. In half of these cases, we were dealing with isolated incidents occurring with no other prodrome. Chyluria may last for several months, then disappear, only to recur a few months or years later. Our most recent surgical patient had first presented with chyluria at age 20 yr. The symptoms disappeared a few months later but

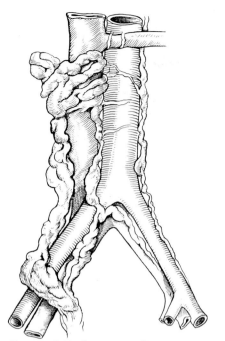

FIGURE 7.22. OPERATIVE DRAWING
Very thick lymphatic varices surround the inferior vena cava and right iliac vessels.

reappeared for a month at age 21 yr and again at 30 yr. When it appeared for the fourth time, it lasted for 9 months until we operated. The patient's medical history revealed nothing more than intolerance to fatty foods and, especially in more recent years, rather frequent spells of diarrhea.

In the other half of our observations, the chyluria appeared in either child or adult, but in the medical histories we found phenomena that pointed to malformation of the mesenteric lymphatics—exudative enteropathy, chyloperitoneum, chylothorax, or reflux of chyle in the lymphatics of the leg. In some cases, the chyluria had a filarial origin with parasites destroying the appendant valvules of the lumbar lymphatic trunks, causing reflux and chyluria.

The diagnosis of chyluria is usually easy. The urine is lacteous and contains lipids and proteins. The patient has no functional disorders. Sometimes blood is mixed with chyle. In certain cases, rapid examination of the urine suggests albuminuria. As soon as the lipids are detected, a hyperlipidemia test is ordered; the plateau-like curve will identify mesenteric lymphatic malformation. Cystoscopy with urine separation reveals the side on which the chyluria has occurred. After taking a sample of urine from each kidney, the ureteral probe is advanced further on the side of lacteous urine until it enters the renal pelvis.

After external compression of this lumbar ureter with a balloon applied in front of the external iliac fossa, some opaque media is injected into this renal pelvis. The radiographs will show the thick lymphatics of the kidney.

Pedal lymphography shows considerable dilatation, first of the iliac, then of the lumbar lymphatics, and, almost invariably, opacification of the lymphatics of both kidneys, which are always dilated. Sometimes the opaque medium penetrates into the renal pelvis on the side affected by chyluria. The cistern of Pecquet is never opacified, but lymphatics of the pancreas, liver, diaphragm, and mediastinum stand out distinctly.

In 1951, we operated on an 8-yr-old boy for Klippel-Trenaunay syndrome (malformation of the popliteal vein). One year later, chylothorax appeared on the left side. At thoracotomy, we sutured a rupture in a thick diaphragmatic lymphatic containing chyle. At age 13, his urine was lacteous and pink for 5 months. Examination of the urine indicated albuminuria and hematuria. At 14 and 15 yr, the urine became lacteous again; the diagnosis at that time was chyluria. A surgeon stripped and severed an inferior polar artery that had been compressing the renal lymphatics. The hematochyluria remained copious, however. At age 18 yr pedal lymphography showed thick iliac, then lumbar lymphatic varices, opacification of the lymphatics of the left kidney, and passage of the opaque medium into the left renal pelvis. The cistern of Pecquet was not injected, but the mesh-like network of diaphragmatic lymphatics was clearly outlined along with the three intercostal lymphatics and those of the right lung. The following year we resected the lymphatics of the right kidney, but the same operation proved difficult on the left side and was not completed because of the surgery performed 4 yr earlier.

At age 21 yr, lymphedema occurred with reflux of chyle into the lymphatics of the leg and genitals, requiring surgery. At 23 yr, chyluria recurred. Unable to isolate the kidney, we had to perform a nephrectomy. Finally, at 31 yr, protein-losing enteropathy appeared with diarrhea and fever. The total lipids curve was a plateau. The laparotomy after a fat meal revealed the typical mesh-like aspect of malformation of the mesenteric lymphatics on the small intestine. There was considerable stasis of lymph in the rectosigmoid without reflux of chyle. The proteins were at 50 g, and there were numerous attacks of mesenteric lymphangitis, obliging us to maintain the patient on oral antibiotic therapy.

In this patient, chyluria appeared after chylothorax and was followed first by lymphedema with reflux of chyle and then by protein-losing enteropathy. We have had eight patients in whom chyluria was an isolated phenomenon. In all of these patients, the hyperlipidemia test featured a plateau-like total lipids curve. At surgery we noted considerable dilatation of the lumbar lymphatics and mesenteric lymphatic malformations. We have concluded that chyluria only occurs in the presence of mesenteric lymphatic malformations.

### Treatment of Chyluria

Absorption of 40 g of butter 4 hr prior to surgery with a subperitoneal approach provides a distinct view of some thick white lymphatic varices along the aorta or inferior vena cava. The renal lymphatics also feature a milky coloration. At first, the kidney is left in place. Loops of catgut are drawn around the renal artery and then around the renal vein and the renal pelvis. All of the lymphatics located in front of the pedicle, definitely colored white, are resected between the ligatures. At this point, the kidney is tilted forward in order to ligate and resect the posterior lymphatics of the renal pedicle. Then the kidney is set upright again, and a single catgut loop is threaded under the three parts of the pedicle. After this, the kidney is rotated forward again. Finally the two ends of the loop are pulled back to make sure that all of the renal lymphatics have indeed been severed. At this time the lateroaortic or laterocaval lymphatics are resected between L1 and L5. Even when chyluria is unilateral, lymphography shows that the lymphatics of both kidneys are still dilated: this is why we perform the operation on both sides, but with 2–3 months between operations. At the end of the operation, after opening the peritoneum, we invariably have observed malformations of the mesenteric lymphatics.

These resections of the lymphatics of both kidneys have always brought about complete and final disappearance of chyluria with no subsequent disorders. Accordingly, after kidney transplantation, there are no complications secondary to resection of the renal lymphatics, whereas in small intestine transplants, severing of the mesenteric lymphatics explains systematic failures.

## Chylothorax and Chylous Cyst of Mediastinum

### Clinical Course

We have examined and operated on 15 patients for spontaneous chylothorax. On four occasions, chylothorax was an isolated phenomenon. Clinical examination revealed pleural extravasation, and puncture yielded chyle. On 11 occasions, the patient's family history included disorders that strongly suggested malformations of the mesenteric lymphatics. Chylothorax may be associated with chylopericardium or chyloperitoneum, or it may occur in a patient suffering from lymphedema with chyle reflux or from chyluria. As soon as the pleural puncture has yielded a chylous fluid with high concentrations of proteins and total lipids, a hyperlipidemia test must be requested. In all of our cases of spontaneous chylothorax, the total lipids curve was a plateau. The lymphatics of the diaphragm are highly dilated and filled with chyle when there is malformation of the cistern of Pecquet. In half of our observations, we discovered and sutured ruptures in one of these diaphragmatic lymphatic varices in the pleural cavity during thoracotomy, but these distended diaphragmatic lymphatics evacuate toward the cervical region via the internal mammary and mediastinal lymphatics. The latter evacuate toward the tracheal bifurcation, thereby hampering evacuation of the lung lymphatics, which dilate and lose their valvular function. The chyle flows back into these lung lymphatics. Those located beneath the pleura may rupture, producing chylothorax.

In 1954, we operated on a girl of 18 yr for lymphedema of the lower limb and of the labia majora with chyle reflux. Fourteen years later, her lower limb and vulva were normal, but she consulted us again, complaining of fatigue. Examination revealed a dullness of the left hemithorax, and the pleural puncture yielded chyle. During a left thoracotomy following a fat meal, we discovered and sutured a ruptured lymphatic outside the left subclavian artery. Thirteen years after the chylothorax, the patient is well.

At the age of 15 months, one little boy suffering from chylopericardium recovered spontaneously. When the same patient was 20 yr old, a routine medical examination uncovered a pleural extravasation, although no functional sign existed. A month later, on two occasions, puriform expectorations occurred with a temperature of 40°C. Puncture of this pleural extravasation yielded chyle-like fluid. A few days after that, lymphography of the lower limbs showed dilatation of the iliac and lumbar lymphatics with no opacification of the cisterna chyli. There was a thick lymphatic (diameter 5 mm) along the left edge of the first four thoracic vertebrae and some dilated lymphatics in the two pulmonary fields. During laparotomy following a fat meal a few days later and after aspiration of 2 liters of chylous fluid, we sutured a ruptured lymphatic on the surface of the lung from which chyle was flowing. The preoperative lung lymphogram had revealed very marked dilatation of the lymphatics of both lungs (Fig. 7.23). Thirteen years after this operation, this man is working normally, although when he gets up in the morning, numerous coughing fits bring up chylous sputum.

In 1949, we operated on a 21-yr-old youth for lymphedema with chyle reflux in the right lower limb. Eight years later, chylothorax appeared on the left side. During thoracotomy, we sutured a mediastinal lymphatic rupture above the arch of the aorta. Finally, for 1 month before coming to see us again, he had run a temperature of 40°C. The hemoculture revealed staphylococcic septicemia, and the patient died before antibiotic treatment could get under way. The postmortem examination showed an enormous chyle cyst of the mediastinum (Fig. 7.24).

## Treatment

Chylothorax that is not too voluminous may resorb spontaneously on occasion. Usually the pleural puncture yields a chylous fluid, analysis of which shows that it contains total lipids and proteins. The hyperlipidemia test, with its plateau-like total lipids curve, confirms malformation of the mesenteric lymphatics. Instead of repeating the pleural punctures, we introduce a

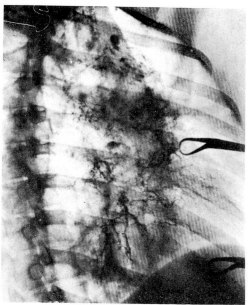

FIGURE 7.23. INTRAOPERATIVE PULMONARY LYMPHOGRAM

The patient is in the right lateral decubitus position. The lymphatic vessels are very large.

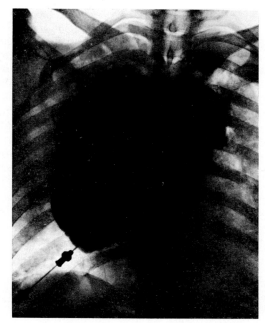

FIGURE 7.24. A LARGE CHYLOUS MEDIASTINAL CYST

very small drain into the pleura through a trocar and begin continuous aspiration. The amount of fluid aspirated is noted daily. In favorable cases, this daily amount decreases rapidly. If so, the drain is left in situ for 2–3 days after the discharge stops, then it is removed. If the amount aspirated daily remains high, an operation is necessary.

There are things one must not do. One must not operate before correcting the hypoproteinemia with albumin perfusions, and during the operation one must not try to ligate the thoracic duct, which plays no part in the pathogenesis of spontaneous chylothorax. Above all, one must not resect the mediastinal lymphangiectasias, for they are useful collateral channels; their resection aggravates the patient's condition. We have seen an exudative enteropathy, a chylothorax on the opposite side, and a chyloperitoneum as a result of such resections. Finally, pleurectomy must be ruled out: there is a risk of injury to the thick, chyle-filled intercostal lymphatics located under the pleura.

On the other hand, there are certain things which must be done. During thoracotomy following a fat meal, the chylous fluid is aspirated and replaced by lukewarm physiological saline. During aspiration, the diaphragmatic cupola must be examined meticulously. In more than half of the patients, chyle can be seen to well up on the diaphragm or in the costodiaphragmatic sinus. This lymphatic rupture must be sutured. If nothing can be seen on the diaphragm, one must meticulously inspect the mediastinal pleura along its entire height, then the intercostal spaces and the hilus of the lung, after which any lymphatic breach must be sutured. If this examination yields nothing, one must examine the surface of each lobe of the lungs, as well as the scissurae, in search of a ruptured subpleural lymphatic. To do so, it is helpful to inject Evans blue dye into the diaphragm and lung. The thorax is closed up, but the little aspiration drains remain. Of our 15 cases of chylothorax, the rupture was on the diaphragm in eight cases, on the lung in five cases, and on the mediastinal pleura in two cases.

## Chylopericardium

In part, lymphatics of the heart evacuate toward the tracheal bifurcation. Therefore, when the lymphatics of the diaphragm evacuate toward the tracheal bifurcation, the same reflux may occur in both the heart and the lung lymphatics. Our intestinal lymphograms in patients with mesenteric lymphatic malformation have shown that often the chyle is evacuated first toward the lymphatics of the liver and then toward those of the diaphragm. Since part of these hepatic lymphatics evacuate into the lymphatics surrounding the suprahepatic veins and inferior vena cava, however, all of these chyle-filled perivenous lymphatics converge to form a veritable ring of thick, chyle-filled lymphatics around the intrapericardiac segment of the inferior vena cava. Often, one of these large lymphatics ruptures into the pericardiac cavity, producing chylopericardium. Fluoroscopy shows a large heart, the surface of which betrays no heartbeat, and echography indicates the existence of fluid in the pericardial cavity. Puncture of the pericardium yields chyle, either pure or mixed with blood. In our 10 operations for chylopericardium the pedal lymphograms showed dilatation of the iliolumbar lymphatics, no opacification of the cisterna chyli, and filling of the lymphatics of the pancreas or liver and of the diaphragm. Each time the hyperlipidemia test was applied, it indicated malformation of the mesenteric lymphatics, and this was confirmed three times by laparotomies.

Thoracotomy is performed 4 hr after the patient has had a fat meal. The pericardium is opened. The chyliform fluid is aspirated, and, after a washing with physiological saline, the point through which the chyle is escaping is located and closed. The pericardial opening must not be too wide, in order not to injure the chyle-filled lymphatics (thymic, mediastinal, or phrenic). We operated on three patients for chylothorax after previous operations for chylopericardium.

## Chyle Reflux in Pulmonary Lymphatics

Among our first 165 observations of mesenteric lymphatic malformation, 12 patients showed chyle reflux in the lymphatics of the lungs and six of them died (four children and two adults). Therefore, this very serious complication of mesenteric lymphatic malformation must be explored further.

Two girls, aged 3 and 17, initially suffered from episodes of acute pulmonary edema, which were treated with intravenous injections of furosemide (Lasix). Both patients produced foamy lacteous expectorations. Analysis revealed that they contained considerable quantities of lipids and proteins. When we attempted thoracotomy on the younger girl, a veritable bronchial flooding by chyle occurred as soon as anesthesia began. The anesthetist was forced to carry out numerous tracheal aspirations. In the older patient, radiology revealed a mediastinal lymphangioma; on two occasions, a surgeon resected mediastinal collateral channels but did not locate the causative mesenteric lymphatic malformation. During the second postoperative phase, chylothorax appeared, and the patient was referred to us. Her total lipids curve showed a plateau. By pleural aspiration using a microcatheter, we drained 220 liters of chyle in 5 months with no pleural cause appearing.

On other occasions, we are faced with cases of protein-losing enteropathy, vaginal lymphorrhea, or lymphedema with chyle reflux in the lymphatics of the legs; in such cases, what first occurs is an unexplainable permanent and progressive dyspnea followed by slight cyanosis. After this chronic respiratory deficiency has evolved over a few years, chylothorax appears, and finally, the patient dies with cyanosis and copious chyliform expectorations. One of these patients, a little girl, suffered for years from unilateral pleural extravasations of a lemon yellowish color. A few weeks before death, this effusion became both bilateral and chylous. At autopsy the lungs were very dense and could not collapse. When this hepatized pulmonary parenchyma was sectioned, chyle flowed out.

There is a great physiopathological analogy between this reflux of chyle in the pulmonary lymphatics and the pleuropulmonary complications that occur in heart patients. Between 1957 and 1973, in the course of mitral valve commissurotomies, we performed 250 lung lymphograms. Study showed that when mitral valve stenosis is very marked, hypertension develops in the arteries of the lung; the lung lymphatics are found to be highly dilated. Those located beneath the pleura let the lymph filter into the pleural cavity—hence the appearance of pleural extravasation in heart patients. The dilated, lymph-filled lung lymphatics located around the bronchi let the lymph flow into the bronchial cavities. This lymph is then partly emulsified by air from respiration, producing the foam characterizing acute edema of the lung. Finally, in mitral valve stenosis with lung infections, the intraoperative lung lymphograms show sclerosed lymphatics; thus, such lung infections in heart patients are actually lymphangitis caused by stasis in dilated, clear lymph-filled pulmonary lymphatics.

Reflux of chyle in the lung lymphatics can occur only in highly dilated lymphatics. Those located under the pleura rupture into the pleural cavity and produce chylothorax. The dilated, chyle-filled peribronchial lymphatics rupture in the bronchial cavities, giving rise, via these lymphobronchial fistulae, to pseudovomiting with chylous sputum containing lipids. A youth of 20 yr, who had surgery for chylothorax and two episodes of pseudovomiting, presented such a reflux of chyle into the pulmonary lymphatics. Thirteen years after our thoracotomy, he still has chronic lymphobronchial fistulae with abundant expectorations upon awakening in the morning.

When these bronchial lymphatics rupture in a fasting patient, expectorations are not very lacteous or not lacteous at all. Clinically, it looks like acute pulmonary edema, but chemical analysis of the sputum shows a large quantity of lipids. Finally, chyle from the intestine may bring microbes with it—hence the appearance of pulmonary lymphangitis.

The very serious evolution of this chyle reflux in the lung lymphatics prompted us to ask Norman Shumway to attempt a lung transplant on the 17-yr-old patient from whom we had aspirated 220 liters of chyle in 5 months, but the patient died before the operation could be performed. At the present time, the Stanford surgeon prefers cardiopulmonary transplant to a simple lung transplant; we concur.

Finally, in certain very rare cases, this chyle reflux in the lung lymphatics is not voluminous. It is limited and gives rise to pneumonopathy with cholesterol crystals.

## Malformation of Mesenteric Lymphatics Associated with Lymphedema without Chyle Reflux

Systematic application of the hyperlipidemia test has enabled us to discover, in 50% of lymphedemas affecting both lower limbs, an association with malformation of the mesenteric lymphatics. The percentage is lower for cases of unilateral elephantiasis. Conversely, it is higher (75%) for lymphedemas of the genitals and Milroy's disease. The fact that mesenteric lymphatic malformation is associated with lymphedema is an important fact to know. It enables us to anticipate the appearance of protein-losing enteropathy, chylothorax, or chyloperitoneum, none of which is ever encountered in lymphedema without mesenteric lymphatic malformation.

## Hypoproteinemia as an Isolated Manifestation of Mesenteric Lymphatic Malformation

In our first 165 cases of mesenteric lymphatic malformation, we observed only two cases of isolated hypoproteinemia. A woman of 39, suffering from thrombosis in varices of the lower limbs, told us that for 5 yr she had had isolated hypoproteinemia. The hyperlipidemia test, yielding a plateau-like total lipids curve, bore out the diagnosis of mesenteric lymphatic malformation, which was further confirmed during laparotomy following a fat meal. One of the sons of this patient also had evidence of hypoproteinemia secondary to mesenteric lymphatic malformation; the clinical manifestations were an intolerance to fat foods and asthenia.

A 42-yr-old nurse was referred to us for lymphedema in one limb; her history included numerous episodes of lymphangitis and two episodes of septicemia. The preoperative checkup revealed hypoproteinemia, and the hyperlipidemia test confirmed malformation of the mesenteric lymphatics.

## Food Allergies and Latent Forms of Mesenteric Lymphatic Malformation

Among our first 165 cases of mesenteric lymphatic malformation, 15 patients presented with a food allergy, and 45 had totally latent forms. In 1967, Waldmann described allergic gastroenteropathy as a cause of excessive loss of proteins at the gastrointestinal level. Our 18 patients were allergic since birth to milk, cream, fats, and cheese. Often, absorption of fats triggered abdominal pains. In all cases, the hyperlipidemia test confirmed the diagnosis of mesenteric lymphatic malformations.

Here again, systematic application of the hyperlipidemia test enabled us to detect the latent forms of mesenteric lymphatic malformations in cases of Klippel-Trenaunay syndrome, in other arterial or venous diseases, and in women who were taking the contraceptive pill. In all of these latent forms, it is possible to anticipate the appearance of a chylothorax, chyloperitoneum, or protein-losing enteropathy.

## CONCLUSION

Lymphography of the mesenteric lymphatics enabled us to opacify abdominal lymphatics of the small intestine secondary to malformations of the cisterna chyli and mesenteric nodes. The thoracic radiographs show the importance of diaphragmatic lymphatics and the channels of evacuation toward the cervical region. Radiography of the small intestine has shown us that protein-losing enteropathy, chyloperitoneum, chyluria, lymphedema with chyle reflux in the leg lymphatics, chylothorax, chylopericardium, and reflux of chyle in pulmonary lymphatics are not independent diseases but merely consequences of mesenteric lymphatic malformation. This new concept calls for modification of the treatment of each of these diseases. These mesenteric lymphatic malformations are very common, but postinfection sclerosis and tumoral invasion of the mesenteric nodes may give rise to the same clinical signs.

Our complete resections of the lymphatics of the kidney have always done away with chyluria without subsequent renal disorders, and this potential is reaffirmed by the many successful kidney transplant operations. On the other hand, the physiological importance of mesenteric lymphatics, as well as the many diseases secondary to their malformation, accounts for the constant failures of small intestine transplants, both experimental and clinical.

# 8

# *Interpretation*

SIDNEY WALLACE, M.D., BAO-SHAN JING, M.D., MELVIN E. CLOUSE, M.D., AND DEWEY A. HARRISON, M.D.

## LYMPHOGRAPHY

Interpretation of the spectrum of lymphographic findings in clinical oncology has two major expectations: to determine if nodes are abnormal and, if so, the extent of dissemination of the disease or its stage.

Technically adequate bilateral pedal lymphangiography consists of opacification of lymphatics and nodes of the inguinal, pelvic, and lumbar regions to the thoracic duct. This can be accomplished in adults by the use of 7 ml of contrast medium injected into a lymphatic in each lower extremity. When this is inadequate to opacify the lymphatic channels to the thoracic duct, a complete series of roentgenograms is done and then repeated after 15–30 min of ambulation. The contrast medium will move from the lower extremities to fill lumbar lymphatics and the thoracic duct.

In analyzing lymphographic characteristics, the most difficult decision of the lymphographer is determining the presence or absence of malignancy in nodes. This can be perplexing when evaluating lymph node changes for lymphoma or solid tumors. The lymphographer must keep in mind the nonspecific response of lymph nodes to a variety of stimuli (Viamonte et al., 1963; Wallace and Greening, 1963; Butler, 1968; Castellino et al., 1974; Parker et al., 1974) and consider the lymphatic system as a functional unit.

Interpretation of the lymphangiogram depends upon the careful scrutiny of both the lymphatic and nodal phases. The lymphatic phase is especially important when evaluating metastases from solid tumors. Under normal circumstances skeletal lymphatics from the lower extremities run a course paralleling the arteries and veins to empty eventually into the left jugulosubclavian venous angle. A primary function of the lymphatic system is transporting fluid; continuity of the vessels through the nodes must be seen in the vascular (lymphatic) phase. With aging, distortion of the lymphatic channels is secondary to dilatation and tortuosity of the adjacent blood vascular tree. The normal emptying time varies but is usually less than 4 hr after the end of the injection, depending upon the patient's activity.

Stasis of contrast material in lymphatics may be associated with obstruction. Frequently, however, the specific etiologic agent is not apparent. Most often stasis is not a clinically significant finding but a technical artifact.

Extravasation of contrast material is usually due to increased intralymphatic pressure either as the result of obstruction or overzealous pressure of injection. If the obstructive process is not obvious, extravasation is also most frequently a technical artifact.

The nodal phase presents a fairly even distribution of contrast material within the nodes in a reticular or granular pattern (Fig. 8.1). The margin of the node is well defined with the hilar area usually demarcated by a smooth indentation. *Lymphatic channels seen on the lymphatic phase must traverse this defect in order to consider the filling defect the hilum of the node.* The node is usually an elongated oval or kidney shape. Alterations in size, number, contour, and architecture occur in disease states. An increase in size and number is frequently interpreted as abnormal, as is the presence of a more rounded contour, but these are nonspecific. Architectural changes are most important.

The afferent, endothelium-lined lymphatics enter the node at the periphery and are continuous with the partially endothelium-lined sinusoids of the node. The efferent channels, completely lined by endothelium, emerge from the hilum of the node. In order to delineate individually the opacified lymphatics and nodes, it is essential to view each by multiple projections to obtain a three-dimensional evaluation. Magnification techniques and tomography are employed to enhance presentation of this information.

Normally, the larger the nodes are, the fewer

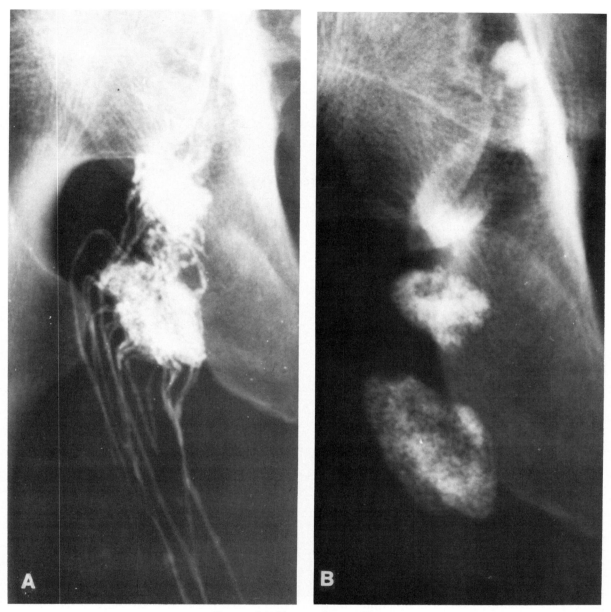

FIGURE 8.1. NORMAL LYMPH NODES

*A:* Lymphatic phase. The afferent lymphatics enter at the marginal sinus. The efferent lymphatics exit at the hilus: *B:* Nodal phase. The defect in the node at the hilus must be confirmed by comparison with the lymphatic phase. The internal architectural pattern is granular and fairly homogeneous.

the number of nodes; and conversely, the greater the number of nodes, the smaller in size the nodes are. The inguinal nodes are generally larger than the iliac nodes, which are in turn larger than the para-aortic nodes. The channel phase is especially important when evaluating metastatic disease because secondary signs of metastatic disease to nodes may be produced by obstruction in a completely replaced node or

obstruction of several afferent and even efferent channels.

Analyzing the nodal phase is important both for solid tumor and lymphomas. The grades of foaminess as outlined by Takahashi and Abrams (1967) are grade 0 for a completely normal node, grade 1 for up to one-third of the node replaced by disease, grade 2 for disease replacing up to two-thirds of the node, and grade 3 for disease replacing greater than two-thirds of the node. Displacement of the nodes from the vertebral body is important. The study is considered abnormal if the nodes are displaced more than 3 cm anterior to the vertebral body in the lateral position or in the frontal position greater than 2 cm lateral to the vertebral body. The accuracy, observing these criteria, should range from 85 to 96% for the lymphomas (Hessel et al., 1977; Castellino, 1982).

When discussing accuracies relating to lymphoma, one should be certain of the criteria used for determining accuracy. If accuracy only relates to positive or negative studies involving para-aortic nodes, the accuracy figures for lymphangiography should be quite high (near 98%). If the accuracy for lymphography is predicated on evaluation of all of the abdominal nodes (i.e., celiac, mesenteric, portal and splenic hilar nodes), the accuracy of lymphography will be much lower.

*Each lymphangiogram must be considered either positive or negative for nodal metastases because equivocal interpretations have little value in management of a patient.* If there is any doubt, the examination should be considered negative and the patient examined with follow-up films and, when necessary, a second lymphangiogram. On the other hand, a definite diagnosis of metastatic disease must have a high degree of accuracy since its influence on patient management is great.

False-positive interpretation of lymph node metastases has provoked considerable adverse criticism of lymphangiography. A proper evaluation must have a three-dimensional display since a false impression of a nodal defect may be due to superimposition of nodes. As previously stated, each node may exhibit a hilar defect which can be properly identified by reviewing the lymphatic phase. Of particular interest is an understanding of the problems that arise in evaluation of the inguinal nodes. These nodes must be carefully scrutinized when they function as the primary site of drainage from neoplasms involving the lower extremities, perineum, and, at times, pelvic viscera. False-positive findings have been reported in the inguinal area because of fatty replacement of nodal parenchyma (Fig. 8.2). False-positive findings also occur in the iliac nodes but are extremely rare (Fig. 8.3). Fibrosis is relatively rare and may occur as the result of repeated insults from minor infection or injuries to the lower extremities. In general these defects will be traversed by lymphatic channels, which may be identified in the lymphatic phase (Fig. 8.2). Because of the difficulty of interpreting the inguinal nodes, the para-aortic nodes assume a

position of unquestioned importance and value to the lymphographer; these nodes are more constant, and the changes are less variable with infrequent filling defects from fat or fibrosis (Viamonte et al., 1963; Abrams et al., 1968; Fuchs, 1971; Kuisk, 1971; Castellino, 1974; Jackson and Kinmonth, 1974).

A false-positive interpretation may also be the result of inflammation. Acute inflammation is usually depicted by enlargement of the node with maintenance of the architecture. The acute reaction to oil-based contrast material may produce temporary generalized enlargement of the lymph nodes. The nodes will spontaneously decrease to normal size within a few months (Steckel and Cameron, 1966). Local defects, such as small abscesses, may also simulate carcinoma.

False-negative interpretation has invoked criticism of lymphography and may occur when microscopic metastases are present but not visible lymphographically. Small nodes, when completely replaced by tumor, may obstruct channels in lower order nodes without evidence of collateral flow (Fig. 8.4). In addition, nodes may contain tumors that are not in drainage areas normally filled by pedal lymphography. This can occur with carcinoma of the testicle that drains to lateral lumbar nodes. In malignant lymphoma, disease may be present in lumbar, celiac, or splenic nodes that do not fill with contrast material (Fig. 8.5).

Another problem for the lymphographer is differentiating malignant lymphoma, leukemia, and solid tumor metastases from reactive hyperplasia and other benign diseases affecting the lymph nodes (Viamonte et al., 1963; Akisada et al., 1969; Raasch et al., 1969; Kuisk, 1971; Renner et al., 1971; Wolfel and Smalley, 1971; Rauste, 1972; Bergstrom and Nevin, 1973; Parker et al., 1974; Walter et al., 1975). Parker et al. (1974) indicate that malignant lymphoma can be differentiated from reactive hyperplasia. They believe that in reactive hyperplasia the nodes in every region are involved to the same degree, whereas lymphomatous nodes usually exhibit gradations of involvement (even though the nodes in all areas may be diseased). The mechanism for the dissemination of reactive hyperplasia in patients with lymphoma may be different from that seen with solid tumors because generalized reactive changes are consistent with generalized inflammatory processes. Reactive hyperplasia associated with solid tumors is more local than in Hodgkin's disease. It begins and is more pronounced in the primary echelon drainage nodes. The nodes downstream from the tumor show reactive changes, while those upstream

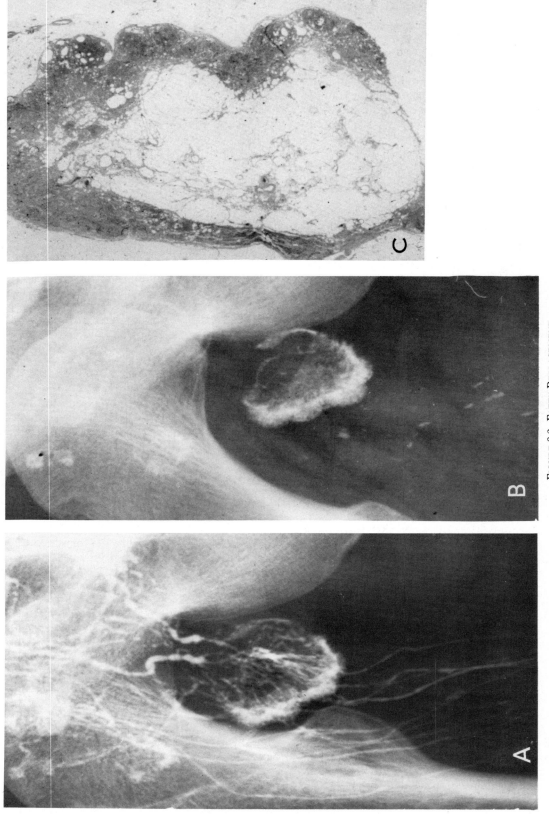

FIGURE 8.2. FATTY REPLACEMENT

*A:* Lymphatic phase. The efferent lymphatics traverse the defect in the node. *B:* Nodal phase. The defect in the node must be further evaluated by comparison with the lymphatic phase. *C:* Specimen. There is deposition of fat in the hilus. The fat is traversed by the lymphatics.

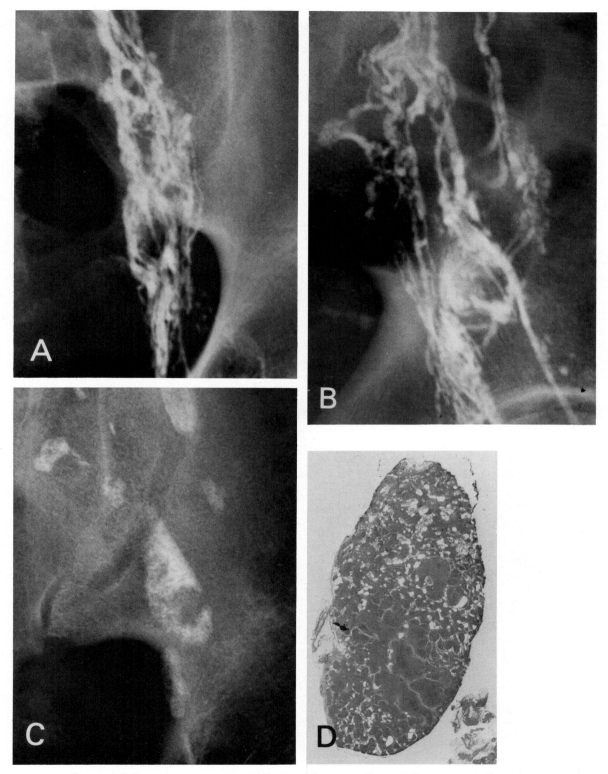

FIGURE 8.3. LYMPHANGIOGRAM ON 55-YR-OLD MALE WITH STAGE B CARCINOMA OF PROSTATE

*A:* Lymphangiogram, frontal view; nodes superimposed over unobstructed lymphatics. *B:* Left posterior oblique view. *C:* Lymph node shows filling defects. Original magnification ×2. *D:* Microscopy. The filling defect was produced by reactive follicular hyperplasia. There is absence of contrast media in the sinusoids. Original magnification ×4.

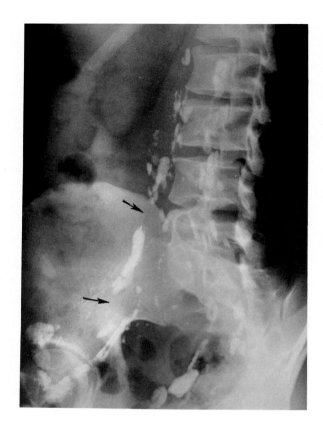

FIGURE 8.4. 23-YR-OLD MALE WITH EMBRYONAL CELL
CARCINOMA OF RIGHT TESTIS

Two nodes in the right common iliac region (*arrows*) were
completely replaced with tumor. The lymphatics did not show
evidence of obstruction. Abnormal nodes could not be identified.

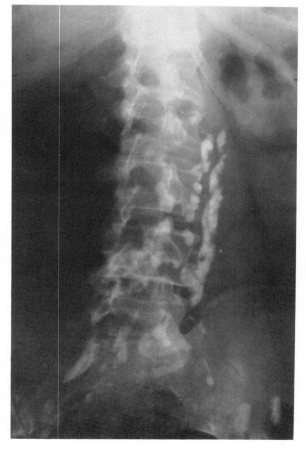

FIGURE 8.5. 55-YR-OLD MALE WITH HODGKIN'S DISEASE
IN SUPRACLAVICULAR NODE

Lymphogram A and B negative. At laparotomy staging
small positive celiac and splenic nodes were found.

have normal architecture. As an example, carcinoma of the bladder may produce reactive hyperplasia in iliac and para-aortic nodes while the inguinal nodes remain normal. The same is true for carcinoma of the testicle (Fig. 8.6). The primary testicular drainage nodes in the aortic area are large and foamy (pseudolymphoma appearance) with reactive changes from seminoma metastases. The nodes of the left iliac and inguinal areas have minimal reactive changes from the orchiectomy. The reactive response in the inguinal and iliac areas after operation is almost always present.

Lymphoid hyperplasia associated with many infections or collagen diseases presents a picture similar to that seen with leukemia. Granulomatous diseases would naturally cause confusion as they do microscopically (i.e., sarcoidosis, tuberculosis, etc.). Hodgkin's disease, especially of the nodular sclerosing variety, and histiocytic lym-

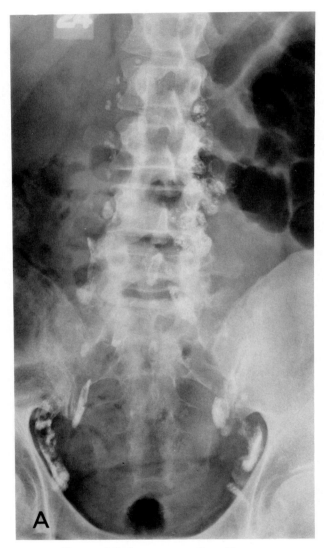

FIGURE 8.6. SEMINOMA OF LEFT TESTICLE

*A:* The nodes in the left para-aortic area are foamy and indistinguishable from lymphoma secondary to reactive changes to seminoma metastases. The nodes in the left external iliac area show acute reactive changes from the orchiectomy. The iliac nodes on the right are normal. Microscopy: *B:* (original magnification ×400) shows areas of pure seminoma cells with little or no reaction, progressing to a histiocytic response (*C*, original magnification ×400). With eventual destruction of the seminoma cells (*D*), there are complete caseation necrosis (*E*, original magnification ×40) and giant cell formation (*F*, original magnification ×400). The giant cells do not represent tumor giant cells.

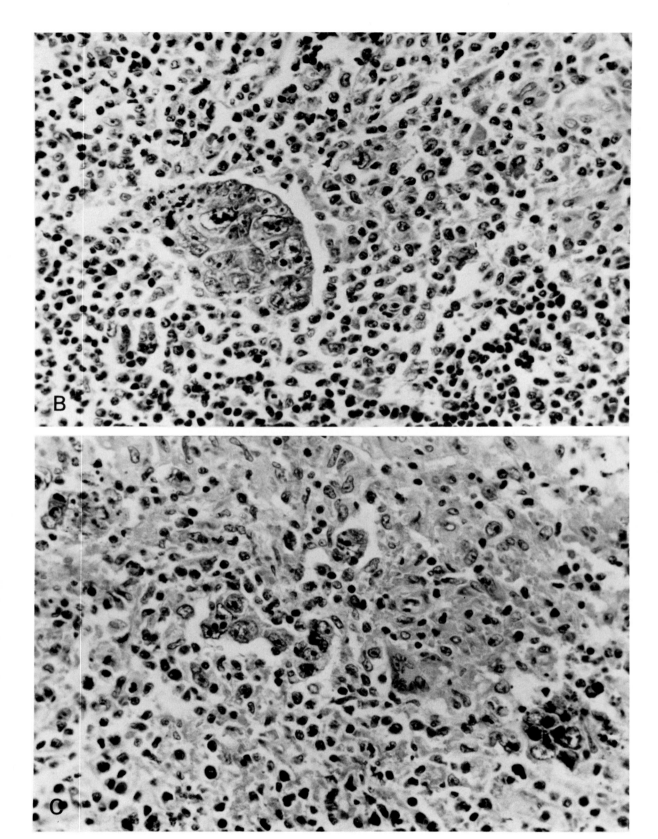

FIGURE 8.6*B* and *C*.

210

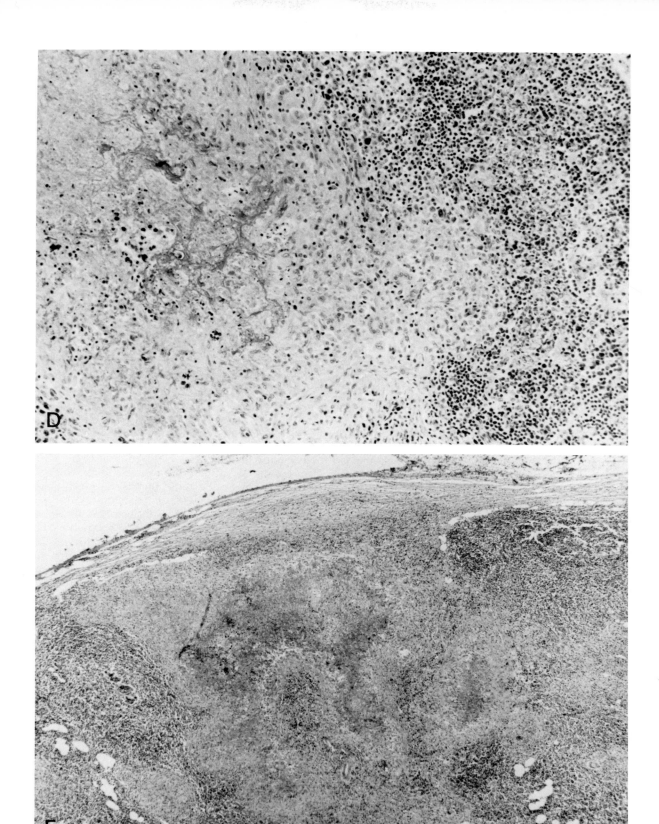

FIGURE 8.6*D* and *E*.

phoma (reticulum cell sarcoma or large cell lymphoma) may result in similar abnormal architectural patterns.

Tuberculosis with cavitation and destruction of a portion of the node (Fig. 8.7) and Hodgkin's disease or histiocytic lymphoma with partial replacement of the lymph nodes at times are difficult to differentiate from carcinoma. Despite these problems, considerable valuable information is offered by lymphangiography in assisting in the formulation of the differential diagnosis and the localization of grossly abnormal lymph nodes. In the presence of a known malignancy, lymphangiography has considerable value in determining the extent of involvement.

## COMPUTED TOMOGRAPHY (CT)

Normal unopacified nodes can be seen on CT, especially in the retroperitoneal and retrocrural areas and occasionally in the pelvis. They appear as soft tissue densities ranging in size from 3–10 mm along the course of the vessels. The internal architecture of the node cannot be evaluated with current CT imaging, and it is doubtful that it ever will be. The para-aortic and caval nodes surround the aorta and inferior vena cava. The external iliac nodes and channels follow the course of the external and common iliac arteries and lie deep in the pelvis adjacent to the obturatorius internus muscle. The obturator node, a member of the medial chain of the external iliac group, is located just above the inguinal ligament and medial to the obturatorius internus muscle. External iliac nodes on CT are frequently confused with internal iliac nodes because of their deep position in the pelvis. The celiac and mesenteric nodes, as well as the splenic hilar and portal nodes, cannot be separated from the adjacent vessels unless they are enlarged in size.

How is large and how large is abnormal? The size of a node is a poor criterion for nodal involvement. Biopsy is frequently necessary. Nodes below 1.5 cm in diameter were once considered normal, and those larger (1–2 cm) were abnormal. Now nodes 1–2 cm are considered suspicious, and those greater than 2 cm are considered definitely abnormal. Enlargement greater than 3 cm is rare but can still be due to reactive hyperplasia (Fig. 8.8). The fewer the nodes in a chain, the larger will be each node. Conversely, the greater the number, the smaller will be each individual node. This concept must be remembered when interpreting abnormality. A cluster of 1-cm nodes (i.e., total mass greater than 2 cm) is probably diseased, whereas an isolated 1–2 cm node should be considered suspicious. Also, inguinal nodes are usually larger than the iliac nodes, and the iliac nodes, in turn, are larger than the para-aortic nodes. The high para-aortic and retrocrural nodes are normally small aggregates of lymphatic tissue 1–3 mm in diameter. Lymph nodes in the retrocrural space are, therefore, considered abnormal if they exceed 6 mm in size (Callen et al., 1977).

Although size of nodes does not confound the interpretation of lymphographs, submacroscopic metastases cannot be appreciated. In addition, nodes may be completely replaced by tumor, and the diagnosis by lymphography must, therefore, be made by the secondary signs of metastatic disease, such as obstructed channels (Fig. 8.9). Figures 8.10–8.12 demonstrate the advantages and disadvantages of both lymphography and CT. In Figure 8.10 nodes in the pelvic area are 0.8 × 1.5 cm or less in size on the lymphograph, hence would be normal by CT; yet a node in the left iliac area is almost completely replaced by tumor and demonstrated by lymphography. Even by redoing CT after lymphangiography, the specific abnormal node could not be definitely demonstrated on 1-cm sections throughout the pelvis. Conversely, CT has a definite advantage as demonstrated by Figure 8.11, which shows extensive disease in the parametrial area from a carcinoma of the cervix. With lymphography, although the abnormality is present, a greater portion of the mass lies outside the confines of the contrast-filled nodes. Hence, CT is a better examination in this patient. Therefore, lymphography and CT should be considered complementary rather than competitive.

In the lymphomas, one can see a large number of nodes all below 1 cm in diameter that are abnormal. Figure 8.12 shows a collection of nodes in the para-aortic area, all much smaller than 1 cm in size, so that if only each individual node is considered, the study would be normal. If the total mass of nodes is considered, however, the study would be interpreted as abnormal.

Massive enlargement in the retroaortic and caval areas may completely obliterate the aorta and cava as well as the mesenteric vessels. Although massive adenopathy around the pancreas and mesentery may mimic tumors of the pancreas, nodal enlargement can be differentiated from primary tumors (Costello et al., 1984). Pitfalls in CT interpretation include confusing an

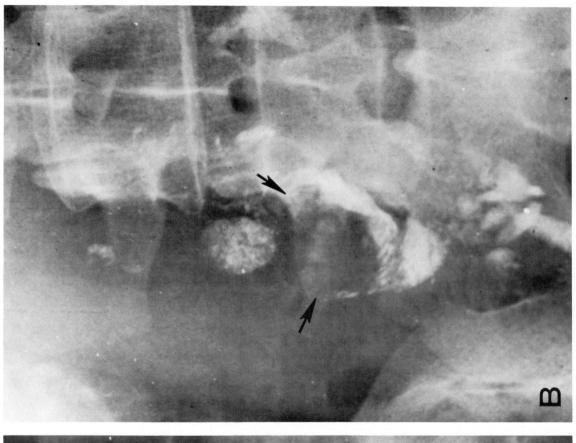

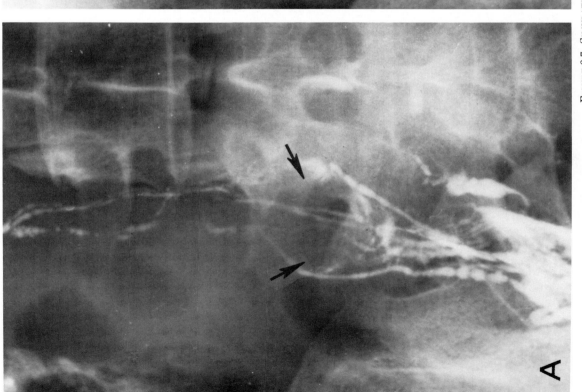

FIGURE 8.7. SIMULATING CARCINOMA PATTERN

*A* and *B*: Tuberculosis. Caseation necrosis produces destruction of a portion of the node (*arrows*). The lymphatics do not traverse the area of caseation. *C* and *D*: Hodgkin's disease, mixed cellularity. The area of involvement was not traversed by lymphatics (*arrows*). Six months later the more classical pattern was obvious in this and the surrounding nodes. *E*: Histiocytic lymphoma (*arrow*) may mimic carcinoma.

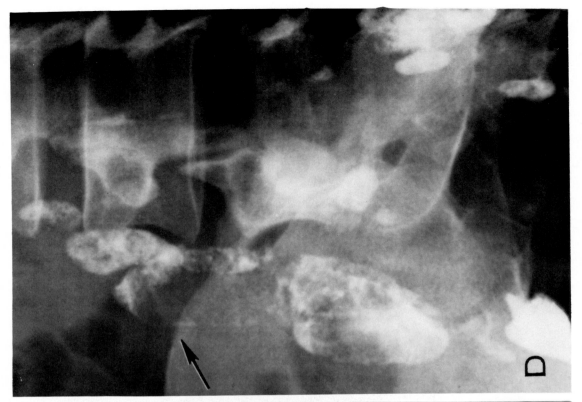

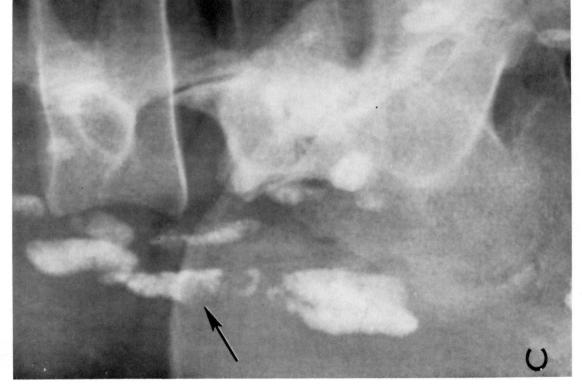

FIGURE 8.7C and D.

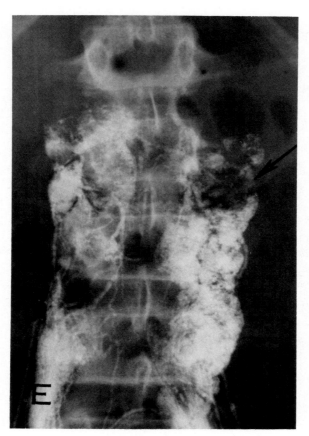

FIGURE 8.7*E*.

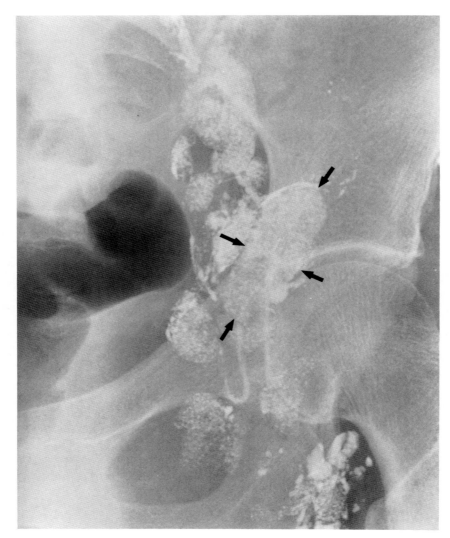

FIGURE 8.8. REACTIVE HYPERPLASIA
A regional lymph node (*arrows*) measured 3.2 × 2 cm in diameter (a 20% magnification is assumed for inguinal nodes) in this 60-yr-old female with cancer of the bladder.

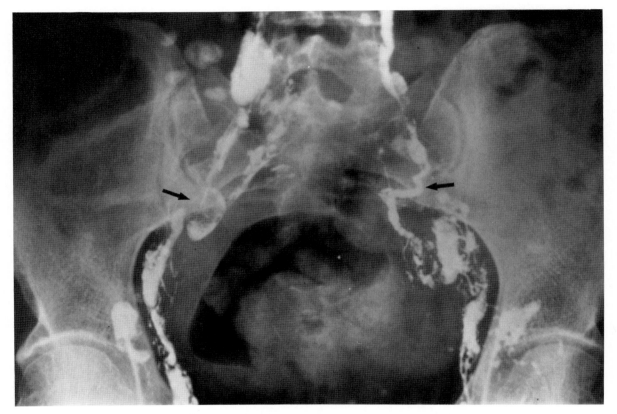

FIGURE 8.9. STAGE 3A CARCINOMA OF THE CERVIX IN A 52-YR-OLD WOMAN

A node in the right iliac chain (*arrow*) is almost completely replaced by tumor, and the channels around it are barely patent. In the left iliac chain the nodes are completely replaced, and only one channel through the area (*arrow*) is patent.

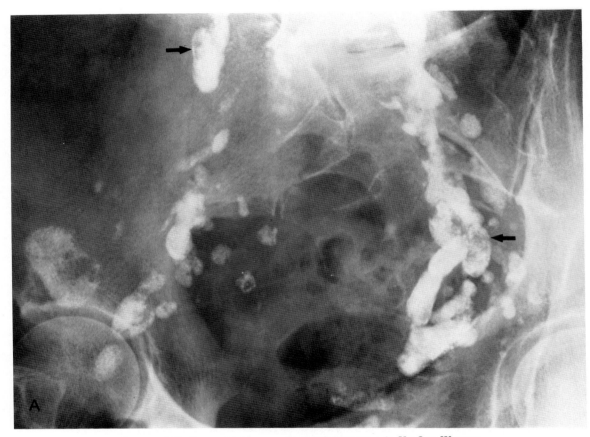

FIGURE 8.10. STAGE 2A CANCER OF THE CERVIX IN A 61-YR-OLD WOMAN

The CT scan performed before lymphangiography was reported as normal. *A:* Lymphogram shows filling defects in the iliac nodes (*arrows*). All nodes are 0.8 × 1.5 cm or less in size. *B:* Repeat CT scan at 1-cm intervals through pelvis shows a questionable node (*arrow*). In this instance, lymphography was the definitive examination. *C:* Analysis of the needle aspirate revealed its positive cytology.

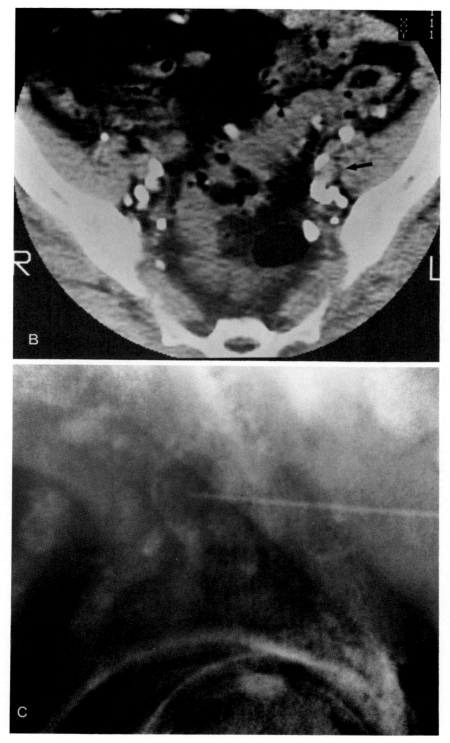

FIGURE 8.10*B* and *C*.

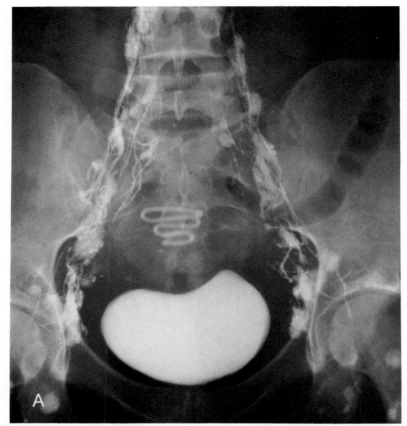

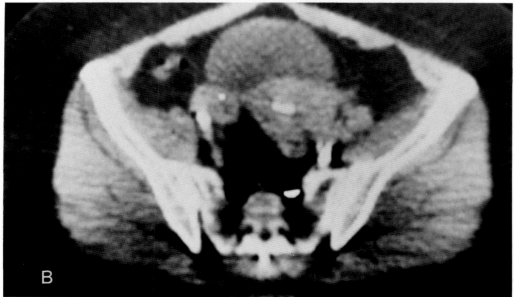

FIGURE 8.11. STAGE 3B CANCER OF THE CERVIX IN A 36-YR-OLD WOMAN

*A:* Lymphangiography shows a decrease in the number of channels in the left external iliac area due to obstruction by tumor. Abnormal nodes are not visible. *B:* CT scan shows large parametrial mass and several nodes completely replaced by tumor. These were not filled or shown by lymphangiography.

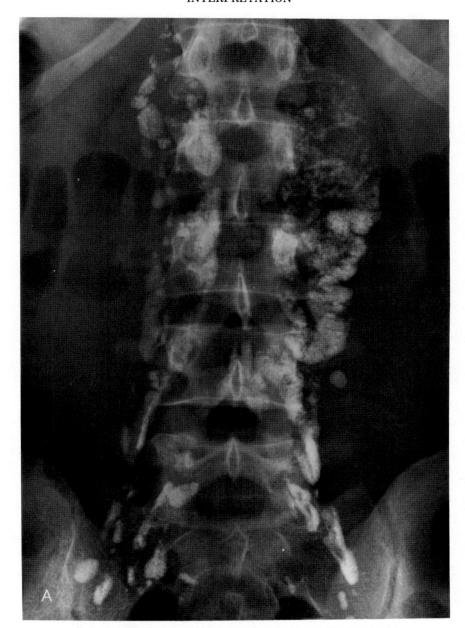

FIGURE 8.12   FEVER OF UNKNOWN ORIGIN IN A 25-YR-OLD MALE

*A:* Lymphangiogram shows large number of abnormal nodes in the para-aortic area. *B:* CT scan of the abdomen after lymphangiography demonstrates contrast medium in normal-sized nodes (all less than 1 cm). Multiple nodes less than 1 cm in diameter are not filled with contrast (*arrows*). Note that each node is less than 1 cm in size, yet the total nodal mass is greater than 1 cm.

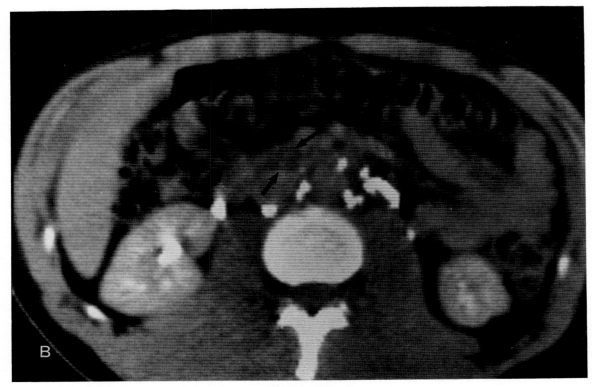

FIGURE 8.12B.

isolated, non-contrast-filled loop of small bowel or blood vessel with disease. In addition, retroperitoneal fibrosis, postradiation therapy changes, or a leaking aortic aneurysm may obliterate retroperitoneal structures. Other sources of confusion include a large crus of the diaphragm (which can be delineated by examining contiguous slices), a large left gonadal vein, and a double inferior vena cava.

# REFERENCES

Abrams HL, Takahashi M, Adams DF: Usefulness and accuracy of lymphangiography in lymphoma. *Cancer Chemother Rep* 52:157, 1968.

Akisada M, Tasaka A, Mikami R: Lymphography in sarcoidosis: comparison with roentgen findings in the chest. *Radiology* 93:1273, 1969.

Bergstrom JF, Nevin JJ: Luetic lymphadenitis: lymphographic manifestations simulating lymphoma. Report of a case. *Radiology* 106:287, 1973.

Butler JH: Nonneoplastic lesions of lymph nodes of man to be differentiated from lymphoma. *Natl Cancer Inst Monogr* 32:233, 1968.

Callen PW, Korobkin M, Isherwood I: Computed tomographic evaluation of the retrocrural prevertebral space. *AJR* 129:907, 1977.

Castellino RA: Lymphographic-histologic correlation in patients with Hodgkin's disease and non-Hodgkin's lymphoma undergoing staging laparotomy. *Lymphology* 7:153, 1974.

Castellino RA: Imaging techniques for staging abdominal Hodgkin's disease. *Cancer Treat Rep* 66:797-700, 1982.

Castellino RA, Billingham M, Dorfman RF: Lymphographic accuracy in Hodgkin's disease and malignant lymphoma

with a note on the "reactive" lymph node as a cause of most false positive lymphograms. *Invest Radiol* 9:155, 1974.

Costello P, Duszlak EJ, Kane RA, Lee RGL, Clouse ME: Peripancreatic lymph node enlargement in Hodgkin's disease, non-Hodgkin's lymphoma, and pancreatic carcinoma. *J Comput Tomogr* 8:1-11, 1984.

Fuchs WA: Neoplasms of epithelial origin. In Abrams HL (ed): *Angiography*, ed 2. Boston, Little, Brown & Co, 1971.

Hessel SJ, Adams DF, Abrams HL: Lymphography in lymphoma. In Clouse ME (ed): *Clinical Lymphography*. Baltimore, Williams & Wilkins, 1977, p 160.

Jackson BT, Kinmonth JB: The normal lymphographic appearances of the lumbar lymphatics. *Clin Radiol* 25:175, 1974.

Kuisk H: *Technique of Lymphography and Principles of Interpretation.* St Louis, Green, 1971, pp 275-278.

Parker BR, Blank N, Castellino RA: Lymphographic appearances of benign conditions simulating lymphoma. *Radiology* 111:267, 1974.

Raasch FO, Cahill KM, Hanna LK: Histologic and lymphangiographic studies in patient with clinical lepromatous leprosy. *Int J Lepr* 37:382, 1969.

Rauste J: Lymphographic findings in granulomatous inflammations and connective tissue diseases. Differential diagnosis between those diseases and lymphomas. *Acta Radiol Suppl* 317:1, 1972.

Renner RR, Nelson DA, Lozner EL: Roentgenologic manifestations of primary macroglobulinemia (Waldenstrom). *AJR* 113:499, 1971.

Steckel RJ, Cameron TP: Changes in lymph node size induced by lymphangiography. *Radiology* 87:753, 1966.

Takahashi M, Abrams HL: The accuracy of lymphangiographic diagnosis in malignant lymphoma. *Radiology* 89:448–460, 1967.

Viamonte M, Altman D, Parks R, Blum E, Bevilacqua M, Recher L: Radiographic-pathologic correlation in the interpretation of lymphangioadenograms. *Radiology* 80:903, 1963.

Wallace S, Greening R: Further observations in lymphangiography. *Radiol Clin North Am* 1:157, 1963.

Walter JF, Soderman TM, Cooperstock MS, Bookstein JJ, Whitehouse WM: Lymphangiographic findings in histoplasmosis. *Radiology* 114:65, 1975.

Wolfel DA, Smalley RH: "Lipoplastic" lymphadenopathy. *AJR* 112:610, 1971.

# 9

# *Benign Lymph Node Disease*

MELVIN E. CLOUSE, M.D.

In the past, lymphography was seldom performed to demonstrate inflammatory disease in the lymph nodes. The most important reason for recognizing inflammatory disease was to distinguish it from lymphoma and metastatic carcinoma. More recently, the usefulness of lymphography in demonstrating sarcoid (Blaudow and Scharkoff, 1972) and tuberculosis (Suramo, 1974) has been reported, but specific indications for lymphography in inflammatory disease have still not been clearly defined.

Ruttner (1967) classified inflammatory diseases according to their morphological appearance: follicular hyperplasia, reactive hyperplasia (hyperplasia of the histiocytes, reticular fibers, and lymphocytic cells), granulomatous inflammation, and abscess-forming or necrotizing inflammation. This is probably the best approach to a classification, but cellular reactions are not always specific even though they may be characteristic of certain inflammatory agents.

The lymphographic patterns of inflammatory reactions are even less specific because the lymph node (composed of lymphoid tissue, reticulum-supporting network, and endothelium-lined sinusoids) has a limited response to some inflammatory agents. The contrast material enters the afferent channels and is distributed throughout the sinusoids. If the inflammatory reaction is purely follicular, the node may appear more granular with a normal marginal sinus. If the response is hyperplastic, the sinusoids may become occluded and produce central filling defects. In both responses the node becomes more foamy and bubbly in appearance and is more difficult to differentiate from lymphoma. The granulomatous and abscess-forming inflammatory reactions interrupt the marginal sinus more frequently and produce filling defects similar to metastatic carcinoma.

## ACUTE INFLAMMATION

Lymph nodes involved by acute inflammation are usually enlarged as a result of hyperplasia of lymph follicles and new follicle formation. The channels leading to and from the node as well as the sinusoids may be enlarged (Fig. 9.1). These changes are reflected in the lymphographic pattern. As the follicles enlarge, they compress the contrast-filled sinusoids. The normal ground-glass appearance gives way to discrete filling defects throughout the nodes, changing it to a more glandular or foamy pattern.

Tjernberg (1956) demonstrated the ability of lymphography to differentiate acute inflammation and metastatic carcinoma. When the sinusoids are dilated, more contrast material can be stored in the node, giving it a more dense, homogeneous appearance. The contrast in the sinusoids may form droplets because it is not compressed by lymphoid follicles. This type of inflammation usually develops in the inguinal and axillary nodes because of infection in the extremities, but it may reflect systemic infection.

Viamonte et al. (1963) showed generalized enlargement of iliac and para-aortic nodes from infectious mononucleosis and enlarged nodes with preservation of nodal architecture in psoriatic arthropathy. Measles, poliomyelitis, rheumatoid arthritis, and ankylosing spondylitis are also known to produce this response.

Wiljasalo et al. (1966) found normal lymph vessels and enlarged, coarsely granular lymph nodes with intact marginal sinuses in the early stages of rheumatoid arthritis and ankylosing spondylitis. The abnormal nodes were located in the iliac and para-aortic areas. The nodes gradually return to normal as inflammation subsides or after several years. Fornier et al. (1969) found inflammatory changes in the lymph nodes to be proportional to the severity of spondyloarthritis. These nodal abnormalities preceded the bony changes.

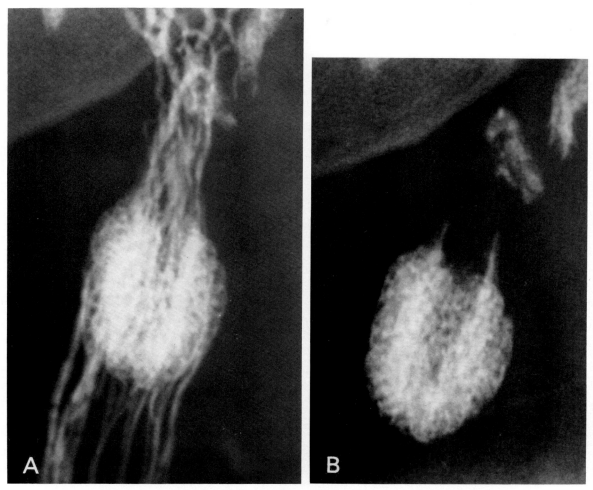

FIGURE 9.1. NONSPECIFIC INFLAMMATORY CHANGES IN LEFT INGUINAL NODES
  *A:* The afferent and efferent channels are enlarged. *B:* The follicles are enlarged. Droplets of contrast material are in enlarged sinusoids. *C:* Large right inguinal node in another patient with chronic dermatitis. There are marginal filling defects, enlarged follicles, and large droplets of contrast material in large sinusoids. *D:* Another patient with generalized exfoliative dermatitis. The inguinal node is most involved because it is the first drainage node. The follicles are enlarged, and a large number of sinusoids are obliterated. The external iliac nodes are involved to a lesser degree.

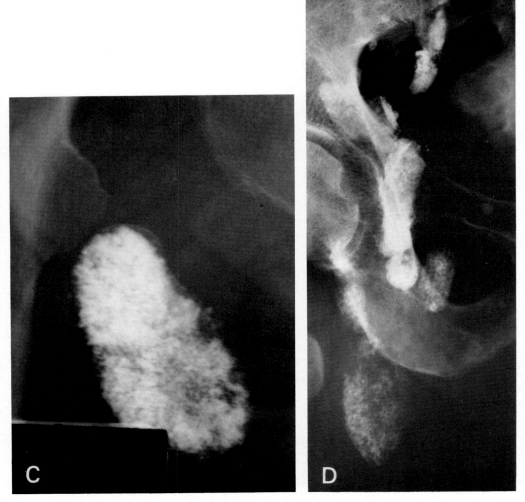

FIGURE 9.1C and D.

## REACTIVE HYPERPLASIA

Reactive hyperplasia is characterized histologically by proliferation of histiocytes, reticulum fibers, and lymphocytes. Hyalinization has also been seen (Castellino et al., 1974). It is regarded as inflammation induced by tumor cells and may imply a defense mechanism within the nodes (Fuchs, 1969). The lymphographic appearance of the lymph node does not differ significantly from nonspecific follicular hyperplastic inflammation. However, the site is important. Reactive hyperplasia is usually observed in areas other than

inguinal drainage nodes unless the inguinal nodes are the primary drainage nodes. The regional lymph nodes are commonly involved in reactive hyperplasia (deRoo, 1973). This can be seen in Figure 9.2, from a patient with carcinoma of the bladder. The iliac nodes showed reactive changes as did all of the downstream drainage nodes, including the common iliac and para-aortic nodes. The changes were more marked in the lower external iliac area. The same criteria hold for other solid tumors, such as the semi-

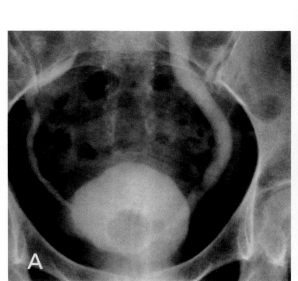

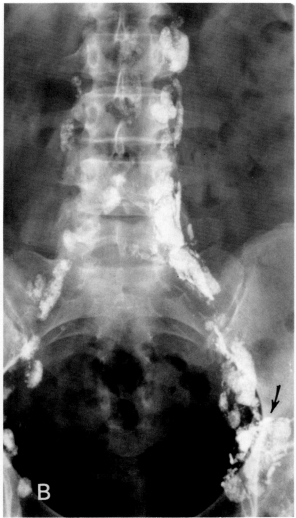

FIGURE 9.2. REACTIVE HYPERPLASIA IN REGIONAL NODES DRAINING BLADDER CARCINOMA
Subject is a 60-yr-old female with carcinoma invading the base of the bladder. *A:* Intravenous pyelogram. Coned view bladder shows dilated, partially obstructed left ureter with carcinoma involving the entire base of the bladder. *B:* Lymphangiogram. The left iliac and para-aortic nodes are enlarged with a foamy appearance. Biopsy (*arrow*) of common iliac node showed reactive hyperplasia. *C:* Left external iliac nodes. Original magnification ×2. *D:* Microscopy. Hematoxylin-eosin stain shows enlarged follicles and proliferation of histiocytic and endothelial lining cells. Original magnification ×40.

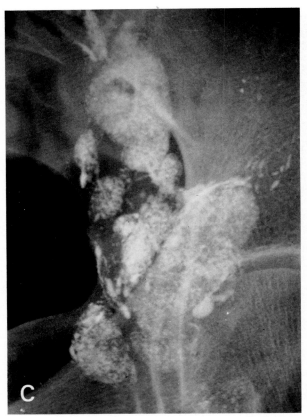 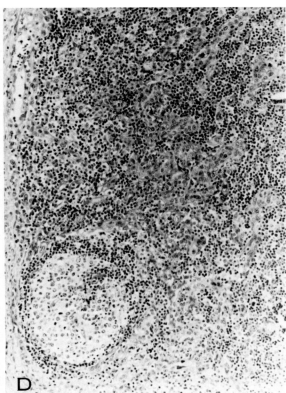

FIGURE 9.2C and D.

noma in Figure 8.6. The primary drainage nodes of the testis showed reactive changes to the tumor that produced a histiocytic response progressing to complete caseation necrosis obliterating the sinusoids and producing the pseudolymphoma appearance. The lymphographic pattern was produced entirely by the inflammatory response and not by tumor cells. It is also interesting that the external iliac nodes show less striking inflammatory changes not related to tumor cells but to the operation.

Lymphographically it is generally possible to distinguish reactive and follicular hyperplastic inflammatory reactions from metastatic carcinoma in lymph nodes, but inflammatory reactions are difficult to differentiate from lymphomas. Ruttner (1967) has suggested that the lymphographic appearance of follicular hyperplasia simulates follicular lymphoblastoma, and Butler (1969) has stated that reactive hyperplasia can

simulate all patterns of lymphoma. Parker et al. (1974) believe that reactive hyperplasia can be differentiated from lymphoma if all of the nodes are involved to the same degree and show a diffuse granular pattern (Fig. 9.3). In lymphoma all of the nodes are seldom involved to the same degree, and the appearance is more bubbly. Although all of the nodes in Figure 9.3 are involved more or less to the same degree, it is very difficult to be absolutely certain that the pattern is not that of follicular lymphoma or Hodgkin's disease other than nodular sclerosis cell type. The reason for the generalized inflammatory changes one sees in lymphoma is not understood. In a systemic inflammatory reaction one sees a generalized inflammatory response in the lymph nodes, whereas in a local inflammatory process one sees inflammatory changes only in the nodes draining the area.

## HYPERPLASIA OF MEDIASTINAL LYMPH NODES

Enlarged mediastinal nodes containing hyperplastic germinal centers and focal areas of hyalinization in addition to scattered plasma cells

have been seen in asymptomatic patients. Lymphographically the node appearance is coarsely granular with intact marginal sinuses. Such find-

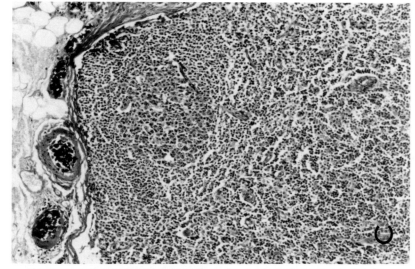

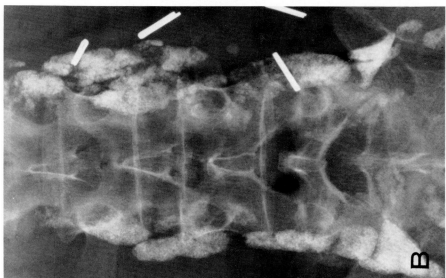

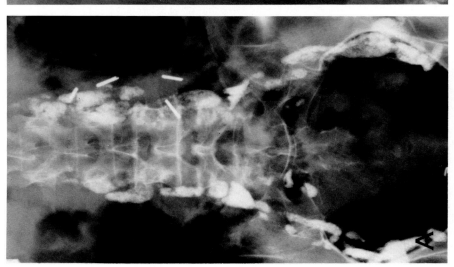

FIGURE 9.3. REACTIVE HYPERPLASIA IN 42-YR-OLD FEMALE WITH LOCALIZED LYMPHOSARCOMA OF STOMACH

A: Lymphogram shows enlarged foamy nodes in the iliac and para-aortic area. All nodes are involved to the same degree. Biopsy taken in area of clips. B: Para-aortic nodes. Original magnification ×2. C: Microscopy. Reactive hyperplasia. Original magnification ×100.

ings may represent a nonspecific inflammatory process (Castleman, 1954; Castleman and Iverson, 1956) or a developmental or growth disturb-ance of lymphoid tissue (Lattes and Pachter, 1962). These changes may also be seen in lymphoma (Nishimine et al., 1974).

## RETROPERITONEAL FIBROSIS

Retroperitoneal fibrosis, first described by Ormond in 1948, is a relatively uncommon clinical entity. The etiology of the disease is unknown but is considered to be related to hypersensitivity or an autoimmune reaction. The disease most frequently occurs in the retroperitoneum. It has also been reported in the mediastinum obstructing the superior vena cava (Kunkel et al., 1954; Barrett, 1958; Hache et al., 1962) as well as involving the inferior vena cava, bile ducts, and duodenum (Schneider, 1964), aorta (Furlong and Connerty, 1958), and mesenteric vessels (Baum, 1972). The colon and bile ducts have also been affected, and an associated vasculitis has been reported (Arger et al., 1973).

The clinical symptoms are nonspecific, and irreversible renal damage may result before a diagnosis is made. Abdominal pain, anorexia, renal dysfunction, hypertension, anemia, and dysproteinemia are suggestive symptoms.

The process may be localized (involving a segment of one ureter) or extensive (involving the entire retroperitoneum from the renal pedicles to the sacrum and encasing all of the retroperitoneal structures). Conventional roentgenograms may reveal loss of the normal contour of the psoas shadows (Holmes and Robbins, 1955).

Urography may reveal delayed excretion of contrast material, dilatation of the collecting system, and a smooth tapered obstruction of one or both ureters. The ureters may taper gradually at the point of obstruction and deviate medially. Medial displacement of the ureters has been considered a significant finding in the diagnosis of idiopathic retroperitoneal fibrosis. Arger et al. (1973) have recently shown that the ureters are encased in the fibrotic process, but there is no medial displacement. The position of the ureters in patients with idiopathic retroperitoneal fibrosis is not statistically different from the position of the ureters in normal patients. The fibrotic process may also obstruct the lymphatics.

The pertinent lymphographic findings in retroperitoneal fibrosis are secondary to obstruction with collateral filling and reflux into lymphatic channels not visualized in normal patients (Fig. 9.4). There is a marked delay in passage of contrast material through the iliac and para-aortic channels. There are frequent, irregular nodal filling defects in delayed films. Lymphatic

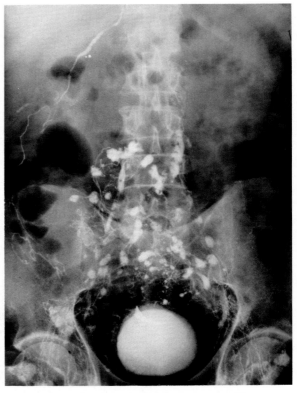

FIGURE 9.4. IDIOPATHIC RETROPERITONEAL FIBROSIS
Lymphangiogram shows no filling of lymphatics above L4 with marked reflux and filling of presacral, bladder wall lymphatic, superficial epigastric (arrow), and a large lymphatic in retroperitoneal area on the right eventually emptying into the thoracic duct.

obstruction predisposes to lymphaticovenous communications, and it is imperative to fluoroscope and film routinely, especially in the pelvis, during the procedure (Fig. 9.5). Patients presenting these lymphographic findings have been reported (Clouse et al., 1964; Suby et al., 1965; Bookstein et al., 1966; Hahn, 1966; Lemmon and Kiser, 1966; Gregl et al., 1967). The lymphatics above L4 are usually not visualized.

Aortography and cavography also have diagnostic importance in retroperitoneal fibrosis. The fibrotic process compresses and obstructs the major vessels, resulting in complete obstruction of the inferior vena cava. Collateral circulation develops in the venous system similar to

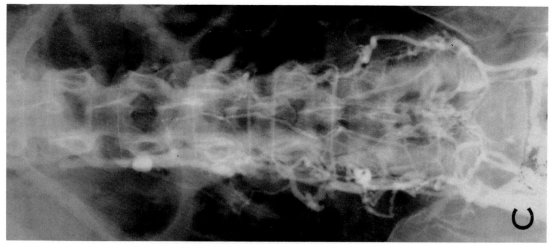

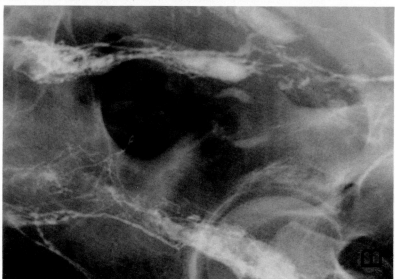

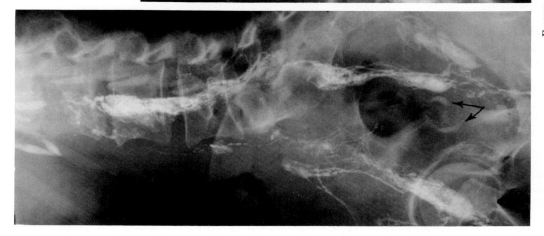

FIGURE 9.5. ANOTHER PATIENT WITH IDIOPATHIC RETROPERITONEAL FIBROSIS

A: The right common iliac lymphatics are obstructed. Contrast material outlines a pelvic vein (arrows). B: Coned view of lymphaticovenous communication. C: Bilateral femoral venogram shows obstruction of the inferior vena cava with extensive filling of lumbar veins. D: Retrograde urogram shows obstruction and encasement of the ureter at the exact site of obstruction of the right common iliac lymphatics (arrow). E: Lymphogram 24 hr after injection shows no nodal filling on the right above L4.

the lymphatic collateral circulation. It is most frequently seen in the second to fourth lumbar area (Fig. 9.5C).

Microscopic examination reveals fibrous tissue and granulomatous fibroelastic areas, containing histiocytes, lymphocytes, and plasma cells. There may be secondary fatty degeneration with areas of necrosis.

## RETROPERITONEAL PANNICULITIS

Retroperitoneal panniculitis is presumed to be related to mesenteric panniculitis and may represent an early stage of retroperitoneal fibrosis (Rogers et al., 1961; Harbrecht, 1967). It is characterized by fat necrosis (Clemett and Tracht, 1969) and inflammation of adipose tissue containing lymphocytes, plasma cells, and fibro-cytes. The lymphographic findings include central and peripheral filling defects in the nodes similar to the inflammatory changes of retroperitoneal fibrosis, granulomatous processes, and metastatic disease (Giustra et al., 1973). The lymphatic channels are not disturbed (Fig. 9.6).

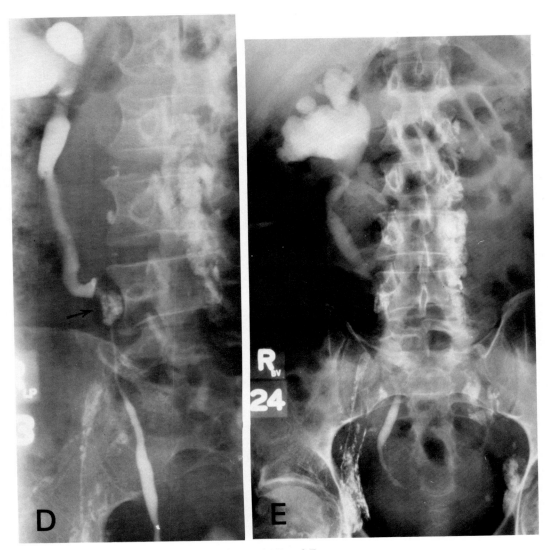

FIGURE 9.5D and E.

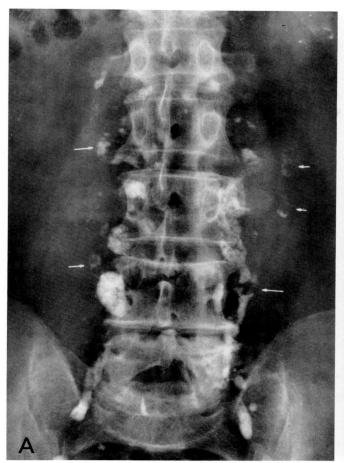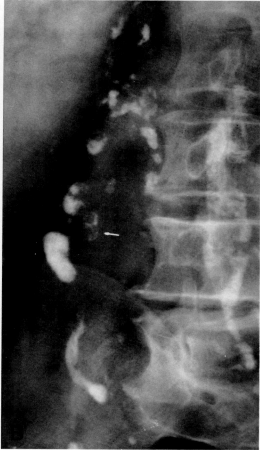

FIGURE 9.6. RETROPERITONEAL PANNICULITIS

Common iliac and para-aortic lymph nodes after 24 hr are abnormal with areas of peripheral and central "replacement" (*arrows*). The filling defects resulted from an inflammatory process with loss of normal architecture. *A:* Frontal view. *B:* Right posterior oblique view. (Courtesy of Peter E. Giustra, M.D., Rockland, ME.)

## FIBROLIPOMATOSIS

Infiltration of the lymph node by fat and fibrous tissue is a degenerative change related to the process of aging and is seen in patients of middle and older age groups. The center of the lymph node is replaced by fat and fibrous tissue, leaving an incomplete rim of lymphatic tissue at the periphery (Fuchs et al., 1960; Fischer et al., 1962; Ditchek et al., 1973). The appearance on the lymphogram is that of a large central filling defect with contrast material in the peripheral lymphatic tissue (Fig. 9.7).

The findings must be differentiated from metastatic carcinoma. Fibrolipomatosis is most commonly seen in the inguinal and axillary nodes because they are the first order drainage nodes of the extremities. It may also be seen in the common iliac nodes following pelvic inflammatory disease.

## LIPOPLASTIC LYMPHADENOPATHY

This process is associated with aging, is more common in women, and is characterized by mature adipose cells in the hilum of the lymph node. Morehead and McClure (1953) and Morehead (1965) have described the excessive accumulation of fat within axillary nodes. The nodes are usually normal in size, but they may become large enough to bother the patient. Wolfel and

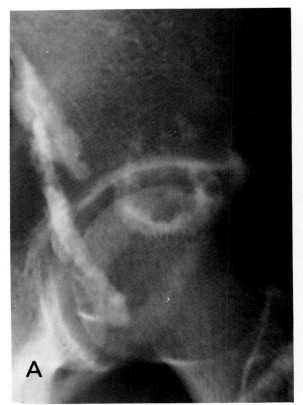

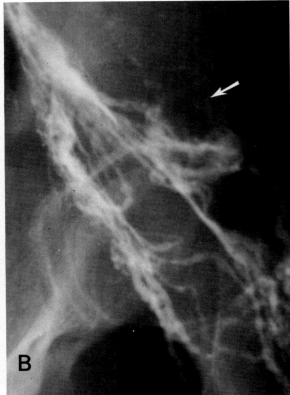

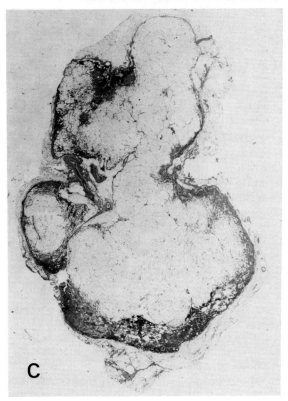

FIGURE 9.7.   FIBROLIPOMATOUS LYMPH NODE CHANGES IN
34-YR-OLD MALE WITH HODGKIN'S DISEASE IN
SUBMANDIBULAR LYMPH NODE

*A:* Coned view of lymphogram. Early channel filling shows
paucity of efferent vessels in external iliac node. *B:* Nodal phase
shows large filling defect (*arrow*). *C:* Microscopy, whole node
mount, shows fatty replacement. Original magnification ×4.

Smalley (1971) and Platzbekder et al. (1973) have reported marked enlargement due to lipo-plastic changes in the external iliac and para-aortic nodes. The etiology is obscure.

## GRANULOMATOUS EPITHELIOID INFLAMMATION

Granulomatous reactions are produced by a large variety of organisms, including:

1. Sarcoidosis
2. Bacterial infections: tuberculosis, leprosy, tularemia, *Treponema pallidum*, brucellosis
3. Fungi: histoplasmosis, coccidioidomycosis
4. Protozoan: toxoplasmosis, leishmaniasis
5. Parasites: filariasis
6. Regional enteritis

### Sarcoidosis

Sarcoidosis is a systemic disease of unknown etiology. The patients have an altered immuno-logical response with hypergammaglobulinemia (Goldstein et al., 1971) and nonspecific hyper-complementemia (H50, C4, C2) (Sheffer et al., 1971). Viamonte et al. (1963) described the lym-phographic changes in sarcoid and reported six cases (Fig. 9.8). Albrecht et al. (1967) reported abnormal pelvic and retroperitoneal nodes in 55% of 20 patients in whom there was no other clinical evidence of node enlargement. Bacsa and Mandi (1966) in lymphography of 12 patients and Rauste (1974) in 136 patients observed a correlation of hilar node enlargement with ab-normal pelvic and retroperitoneal nodes.

Blaudow and Scharkoff (1972) in 96 cases of sarcoid also found concomitant retroperitoneal involvement in 33% of patients with stage 1

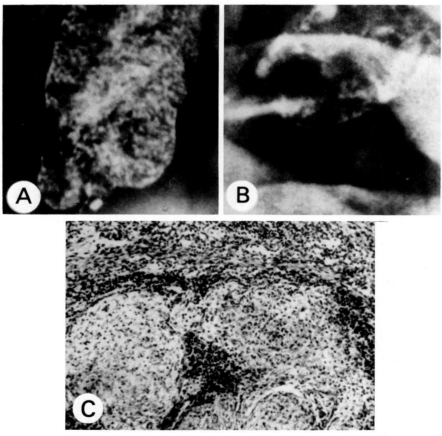

FIGURE 9.8. SARCOIDOSIS

*A:* Right inguinal node changes indistinguishable from lymphoma. *B:* Left supraclavicular node. *C:* Magnification shows discrete noncaseating granulomas. Original magnification ×100. (Courtesy of Manuel Viamonte, Jr., M.D., Miami, FL.)

disease. In stage 2, 45% had retroperitoneal node involvement when the disease was present less than 1 yr and 75% when the disease had been present for more than 1 yr. In contrast, Akisada et al. (1969) and Zalar (1973) found no consistent relationship between abnormal paratracheal and mediastinal nodes and severity of lung changes with abnormal retroperitoneal nodes.

LaMarque et al. (1971a, b) described the lymphographic changes in sarcoid as occurring in three stages. The first stage of adenitis produces a granular appearance to the nodes with droplets of contrast material in slightly dilated sinusoids. An intermediate stage produces a foamy appearance. In the late stage the node undergoes fibrosis with obstruction of sinusoids and lymph channels between the nodes, resulting in nodes which may be only partially filled.

Blaudow and Scharkoff (1972) consider the occurrence of a granular pattern with sharply defined filling defects to favor spontaneous remissions. They recommend lymphography only in therapy-resistant and reactivated cases as well as the suspicion of intra-abdominal sarcoidosis. The lymphographic pattern is not specific for sarcoid in any stage of the disease. It mimics acute and reactive hyperplastic inflammatory reactions or lymphomas. In contrast, Strickstrock and Weissleder (1968) do not recommend routine lymphography in patients with histologically verified pulmonary sarcoidosis because demonstration of retroperitoneal nodes has no therapeutic importance. The response to therapy in this disease is best followed by chest roentgenograms.

## Tuberculosis

Infections with the tubercle bacillus produce central and marginal filling defects of varying sizes on the lymphograms. The nodes may be normal to enlarged. The bacilli enter via the afferent channels, lodge in the marginal sinus or sinusoids, and produce a caseous area of necrosis with obstruction of the sinusoids. The node appearance more closely resembles metastatic carcinoma, but it may also be indistinguishable from lymphoma (Schaffer et al., 1963; Viamonte et al., 1963; Ruttiman, 1964; Babeau and Fourier, 1965; Betoulieres et al., 1968).

Albrecht et al. (1967) studied 15 patients with tuberculosis and only cervical adenopathy; six were found to have abnormal retroperitoneal nodes. They suggest that tuberculosis infection should not be considered a regional disease. In support of this concept Gregl and Kienle (1969) reported a case of carcinoma of the breast with ipsilateral old tuberculous node involvement that was indistinguishable from metastatic carcinoma.

In 100 patients with tuberculosis Suramo (1974) found diseased lumbar nodes in 71 and iliac nodes in 11. In 61 patients the nodes were normal in size. Abnormal iliac and lumbar nodes were present in 41 of 52 patients with cervical or axillary lymph node tuberculosis and in 17 of 18 patients with urogenital tuberculosis. The diagnosis of tuberculosis was considered reasonably certain when the nodes were enlarged, when they showed marginal filling defects produced by caseation necrosis, and when the central architecture of the node was destroyed. When the central architecture of the node is disrupted, the appearance more closely resembles lymphoma. The diagnosis of tuberculosis is less certain when the sinusoids are mildly dilated and not disrupted. The caseating areas produce filling defects slightly larger than normal follicles. These changes result in a lymph node that is more granular or foamy without marginal filling defects (Fig. 9.9).

## Other Granulomatous Diseases

The lymphographic pattern in brucellosis, syphilis, and histoplasmosis also simulates lymphoma. LaMarque et al. (1971a, b) described the lymphographic changes in 11 patients with brucellosis. The study showed generalized lymph node involvement associated with nonspecific adenitis and lymph node fibrosis. During the acute stage of brucellosis, the lymph nodes are moderately enlarged in a coarse granular lymphographic pattern. In the chronic stage the nodes increase in size; as irregular filling defects increase, the pattern becomes more foamy.

In syphilis, capsular fibrosis, vascular endothelial proliferation, granuloma, and follicular hyperplasia with sheets of plasma cells produce a generalized pattern throughout the nodes that is indistinguishable from lymphoma (Kerk and Schilling, 1969; Bergstrom and Navin, 1973). Histoplasmosis also produces changes in the lymph node indistinguishable from the malignant lymphoma. Viamonte et al. (1963) observed a nonspecific inflammatory reaction with preservation of the internal architecture of the lymph nodes. Bottcher (1974) reported toxoplasmosis lymphadenitis superimposed on Hodgkin's disease. The nodes were slightly enlarged with small follicular filling defects characteristic of inflammatory disease.

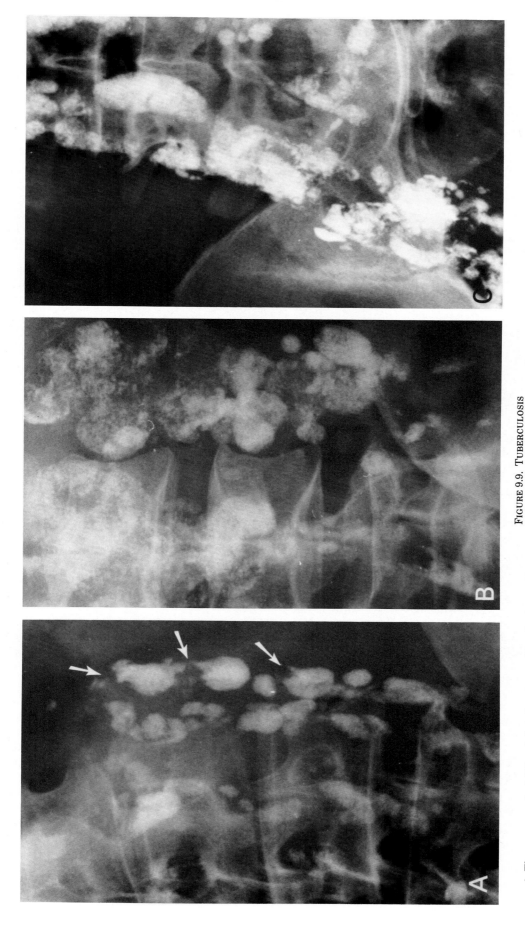

FIGURE 9.9. TUBERCULOSIS

*A:* There are marginal filling defects in para-aortic nodes (*arrows*). *B:* The para-aortic nodes are more foamy with destruction of central nodal architecture. *C:* Common iliac nodes show uneven granular nodes, coarser than normal with large globules of contrast material in large sinusoids. (Courtesy of Ilkka Suramo, M.D., Oulu, Finland.)

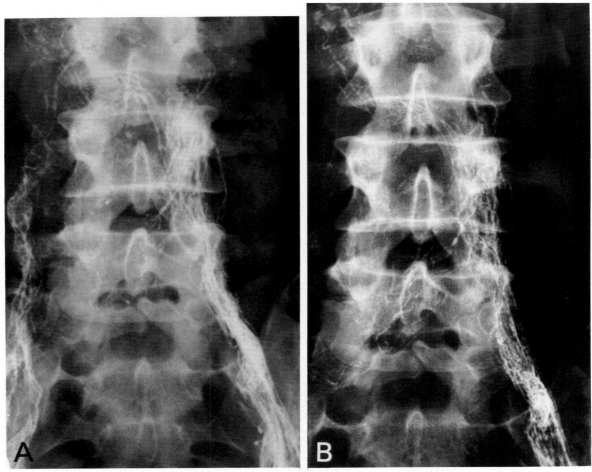

FIGURE 9.10. RADIATION CHANGES IN LYMPHATICS
*A:* Normal para-aortic lymphatics. *B:* Lymphatics 3 yr after 3500 roentgens.

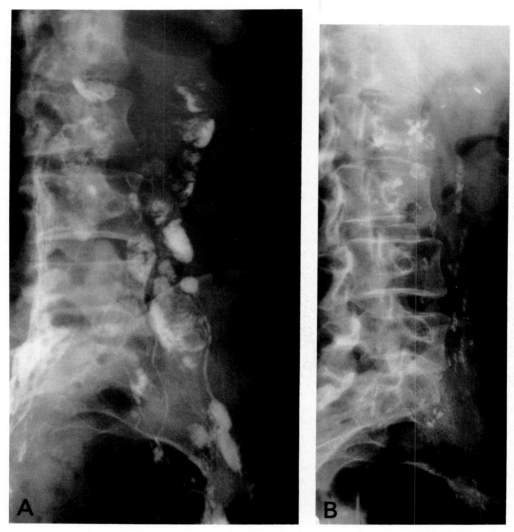

FIGURE 9.11. RADIATION CHANGES IN LYMPH NODES IN 26-YR-OLD FEMALE WITH STAGE 4E HODGKIN'S DISEASE
*A:* Lymphogram (1969) showing extensive involvement of the para-aortic nodes. *B:* Lymphogram 6 yr later (1975) showing small atrophic lymph nodes without recurrent Hodgkin's disease.

## RADIATION CHANGES

The sensitivity of lymphocytes to irradiation was described by Heineke (1905). Excellent papers have described the rapid death of lymphocytes in lymphoid tissue and decrease in circulating lymphocytes after irradition. Trowell (1952), using the light microscope, described the changes of chromatin clumping followed by nuclear vacuolization, pyknosis, and fragmentation. Cytoplasmic disintegration follows nuclear disruption (Trowell, 1952; Schrek, 1961). Histiocytes containing cellular debris can be seen 3 hr after 300 roentgens, are more numerous after 8 hr, and disappear after 24–48 hr (DeBruyn, 1948).

Smith et al. (1967), using the electron microscope, demonstrated prominent histiocytic pseudopodia near damaged lymphocytes within 30 min after 500 roentgens of whole body irradiation. Damaged lymphocytes showed aggregation of chromatin near the nuclear membrane, electron-dense mitochondria, and widening of the perinuclear space with separation of the nucleus and cytoplasm. Three hours later the chromatin had condensed near the nuclear membrane, and the center of the nucleus became electron-lucent. Nuclear disintegration was complete within 6 hr, and remnants of nuclei and other cytoplasmic organelles were noted within histiocytes. Similar findings have been reported by Holsten (1970).

Irradiation of the lymph nodes causes destruction of lymphocytes even in low doses of 50–800 roentgens (Cottier, 1966). Engeset (1964) irradiated the lymph nodes of rats with a single dose of 3000 roentgens. Lymphocyte destruction was complete within 24 hr, and after 9 months the node was replaced by fibrous tissue with no follicles or sinuses. The ability of the lymph node to regenerate appears to be variable, however. Hall and Morris (1964) have reported re-establishment of node lymphocyte population by circulating lymphocytes.

There has been considerable controversy as to the ability of irradiated nodes to filter particulate matter and tumor cells. Virchow (1863) suggested that lymph nodes are effective barriers to particulate matter. Many investigators confirmed his observation (Drinker et al., 1934; Engeset, 1962; Ludwig and Titus, 1967), while others (Yoffey and Sullivan, 1939; Dettman et al.,

1966; Herman et al., 1968) have seen no effective barrier by the nodes. The same type of experiments using live tumor cells have resulted in additional conflicting data (Engeset, 1964; Fisher and Fisher, 1967). Ujiki et al. (1970), using V2 rabbit carcinoma, found that the irradiated lymph node acted as an effective barrier for 2–3 weeks. Three weeks after tumor infusion, distant tumor growth was increased in rabbits receiving 1000–3000 roentgens, but after 6 weeks both groups had a similar incidence of distant tumor growth. They concluded that the earlier presence of distant metastases in the irradiated rabbit was the result of a decrease in barrier function allowing immediate passage of tumor cells during the process of infusion and that irradiated nodes are unable to retain growing cancer cells for the same length of time as the normal nodes.

The effect of irradiation on lymphatic vessels has been studied extensively. Van Den Brenk (1957), using the Sandison-Clark type of ear chamber on rabbits, observed lymphatic vessel regeneration with doses of 1000 roentgens but not doses of 2000 roentgens. Preformed lymphatics survived after doses of 4000 roentgens, and irradiation failed to produce swelling of the lymphatic endothelium and obstruction. Lenzi and Bassani (1963), studying pelvic organs after irradiation, found tortuous vessels but no obstruction after doses of 15,000 roentgens. Obstruction was only found in areas receiving 25,000–30,000 roentgens with tissue necrosis.

Other authors reviewing clinical material (Wiljasalo and Perttala, 1966; Ariel et al., 1967) also report no obstruction in normal lymphatics after therapeutic doses of radiation. Reduction in size of lymph nodes secondary to fibrosis and fine delicate lymphatic vessels are seen on second-look lymphography (Fig. 9.10). The lymph nodes do not retain large amounts of contrast material (Fig. 9.11). Irradiation of lymph nodes and vessels infiltrated by tumors may produce obstruction by tumor and tissue necrosis, fibrosis, or recurrent tumor. In these patients constant monitoring is necessary in order to observe collateral lymphatic circulation and to discontinue the procedure when lymphovenous communications are present.

## REFERENCES

Akisada M, Tasaka A, Mikami R: Lymphography in sarcoidosis: comparison with roentgen findings in the chest. *Radiology* 93:1273, 1969.

Albrecht A, Taenzer V, Nickling H: Lymphographische befunde sei Sarkoidose und Lymphkrotentuberkulose. *Fortschr Roentgenstr* 106:178, 1967.

Arger PH, Stolz JL, Miller WR: Retroperitoneal fibrosis. An analysis of the clinical spectrum and roentgenographic signs. *AJR* 119:812, 1973.

Ariel IM, Resnick MI, Oropeza R: The effect of irradiation (external and internal) on lymphatic dynamics. *Radiology* 99:404, 1967.

Babeau P, Fourier A: Rapport clinique de la lymphographie lipiodolee dans certaines formes de lymphadenite tuberculereuse. *J Belge Radiol* 48:332, 1965.

Bacsa S, Mandi L: Abdominal lymphography in thoracic sarcoidosis. *Scand J Respir Dis* 47:244, 1966.

Barrett NP: Idiopathic mediastinal fibrosis. *Br J Surg* 46:207, 1958.

Baum S: Case records, Massachusetts General Hospital. *N Engl J Med* 287:33, 1972.

Bergstrom JF, Navin JJ: Luetic lymphadenitis: lymphographic manifestations simulating lymphoma. *Radiology* 106:287, 1973.

Betoulieres P, LaMarque JL, Ginestie JF, Caubes C: Etude des aspects lymphographiques de la tuberculose ganglionnaire. *J Radiol Electrol Med Nucl* 49:1, 1968.

Blaudow K, Scharkoff T: Lymphographie des retroperitonealen Lymphsystems bei Sarkoidose. *Z Erkr Atmungsorgane* 136:311, 1972.

Bookstein JJ, Schroeder KF, Batsakis JG: Lymphangiography in the diagnosis of retroperitoneal fibrosis: case report. *J Urol* 95:99, 1966.

Bottcher J: Lymphographie bei dem Zusammentreffen von Lymphknoten-Toxoplasmose und Stationarer Lymphogranulomatose. *Roentgenblaetter* 27:257, 1974.

Butler JJ: Non-neoplastic lesions of lymph nodes in man to be differentiated from lymphomas. *Natl Cancer Inst Monogr* 32:233, 1969.

Castellino RA, Billingham M, Dorfman RF: Lymphographic accuracy in Hodgkin's disease and malignant lymphoma with a note on the "reactive" lymph node as a cause of most false-positive lymphograms. *Invest Radiol* 9:155, 1974.

Castleman B: Case records of the Massachusetts General Hospital: hyperplasia of mediastinal lymph nodes. *N Engl J Med* 250:26, 1954.

Castleman B, Iverson L: Localized mediastinal lymph node hyperplasia resembling thymoma. *Cancer* 9:822, 1956.

Clemett AR, Tracht DG: The roentgen diagnosis of retractile mesenteritis. *AJR* 107:787, 1969.

Clouse ME, Fraley EE, Lituim SB: Lymphographic criteria for diagnosis of retroperitoneal fibrosis. *Radiology* 83:1, 1964.

Cottier H: Histopathologie der Wirkung ionisierender Strahlen auf hohere Organismen (Tier und Mensch). In: *Encyclopedia of Medical Radiology II/2*. New York, Springer-Verlag, 1966, p 100.

DeBruyn PPH: Lymph node and intestinal lymphatic tissue. In Bloom W (ed): *Histopathology of Irradiation from External and Internal Sources*. New York, McGraw-Hill, 1948, pp 348–445.

deRoo T: *Atlas of Lymphography*. Sandoz, 1973, p 34.

Dettman PM, King ER, Zinberg YH: Evaluation of lymph node function following irradiation or surgery. *AJR* 96:711, 1966.

Ditchek T, Blahut J, Kittelson AC: Lymphadenography in normal subjects. *Radiology* 80:175, 1973.

Drinker CK, Field ME, Ward HK: The filtering capacity of lymph nodes. *J Exp Med* 59:393, 1934.

Engeset A: Barrier function of lymph glands. *Lancet* 1:324, 1962.

Engeset A: Irradiation of lymph nodes and vessels. *Acta Radiol Suppl* 229, 1964.

Fischer HW, Lawrence MS, Thornbury JR: Lymphography

of the normal adult male. *Radiology* 78:399, 1962.

Fisher B, Fisher E: Barrier function of lymph node to tumor cells and erythrocytes. II. Effect of x-ray, inflammation, sensitization and tumor growth. *Cancer* 20:1914, 1967.

Fornier AM, Denizet D, Delagrange A: La lymphographie dans la spondylarthrite ankylosante. *J Radiol Electrol Med Nucl* 50:773, 1969.

Fuchs WA: In Rentchnick P (ed): *Lymphography in Cancer*. New York, Springer-Verlag, 1969, p 94.

Fuchs WA, Ruttiman A, DelBuono MS: Zur Lymphographie bei Chronischen sekundaren Lymphodemen. *Fortschr Geb Roentgenstr Nuklearmed* 92:608, 1960.

Furlong JH Jr, Connerty HV: Compression of the aorta and ureters by a retroperitoneal inflammatory mass; case report. *Del Med J* 30:63, 1958.

Giustra PE, Killoran PJ, Opper L, Root JA: Abnormal excretory urogram and lymphangiogram in retroperitoneal panniculitis. *Radiology* 106:545, 1973.

Goldstein RA, Israel HL, Rawnsley HM: Effect of race and stage of disease on the serum immunoglobulins in sarcoidosis. In Levinsky L, Macholda F (eds): *5th International Conference on Sarcoidosis, Prague Karolinum June 16–21, 1969*. Prague, Universita Karlova Praha, 1971, p 178.

Gregl A, Kienle J: Axillary lymph node tuberculosis presenting lymphographic signs of metastasis from ipsilateral breast cancer. *Radiology* 93:1107, 1969.

Gregl A, Truss F, Grabner F, Kienle UJ: Lymphographie und Cavographie bei der idiopathischen retroperitonealen Fibrose. *Fortschr Roentgenstr* 107:329, 1967.

Hache L, Woolner LB, Bernatz PB: Idiopathic fibrous mediastinitis. *J Dis Chest* 41:9, 1962.

Hahn BD: The use of lymphangiography for the diagnosis of idiopathic retroperitoneal fibrosis. *Am J Obstet Gynecol* 14:539, 1966.

Hall JG, Morris B: Effect of x-radiation of the popliteal lymph node on its output of lymphocytes in immunological responsiveness. *Lancet* 1:1077, 1964.

Harbrecht PJ: Variants of retroperitoneal fibrosis. *Ann Surg* 165:388, 1967.

Heineke H: Experimentelle Untersuchungen uber die Einwirkung der Roentgenstrahlen auf inner Organe. *Mitt Grenzgeb Med Chir* 14:21, 1905.

Herman PG, Benninghoff DL, Mellins HZ: Radiation effect on the barrier function of the lymph node. *Radiology* 91:698, 1968.

Holmes GW, Robbins LL: *Roentgen Interpretation*, ed 8. Philadelphia, Lea & Febiger, 1955, p 372.

Holsten DR: Die Strahleneinwirkung auf den lymphnoten, eine elektronenmikroskopische Untersuchung. *Strahlentherapie (Munchen)* 139:41, 1970.

Kerk L, Schilling T: Lymphographische Befunde bei Uenerischen Erkrankungen. *Fortschr Geb Roentgenstr Nuklearmed* 111:22, 1969.

Kunkel WM, Clagett OT, MacDonald JR: Mediastinal granulomas. *J Thorac Cardiovasc Surg* 27:565, 1954.

LaMarque JL, Ginestie JF, Senac JP, Harson B: Etude lymphographique de la brucellose. *Ann Radiol (Paris)* 14:79, 1971a.

LaMarque JL, Ginestie JF, Senac JP, Mathieu F: Apport de la lymphographie dans la maladie de Besnier-Boech-Schaumann. *Ann Radiol (Paris)* 14:437, 1971b.

Lattes R, Pachter MR: Benign lymphoid masses of probable hamartomatous nature. *Cancer* 15:197, 1962.

Lemmon WT, Kiser WS: Idiopathic retroperitoneal fibrosis. Diagnostic enigma: report of a case simulating diabetes insipidus and a review of the literature. *J Urol* 96:658, 1966.

Lenzi M, Bassani G: The effect of radiation on the lymph

and on lymph vessels. *Radiology* 80:814, 1963.

Ludwig J, Titus JL: Experimental tumor cell emboli in lymph nodes. *Arch Pathol* 84:304, 1967.

Morehead R: *Human Pathology.* New York, McGraw-Hill, 1965, p 1307.

Morehead R, McClure S: Lipoplastic lymphadenopathy (abstr.). *Am J Pathol* 26:615, 1953.

Nishimine M, Sako M, Kubota A, Okada S: Lymphography in mediastinal lymph node hyperplasia: report of two cases. *Lymphology* 7:22, 1974.

Ormond JK: Bilateral ureteral obstruction due to involvement and compression by inflammatory retroperitoneal process. *J Urol* 59:1072, 1948.

Parker BR, Blank N, Castellino RA: Lymphographic appearance of benign conditions simulating lymphoma. *Radiology* 111:267, 1974.

Platzbekder H, Kohler K, Hanefeld M, Kunze D: Zur sogenannten, Lipomatose der Lymphknoten im Lymphogramm. *Radiol Diagn (Berl)* 6:677, 1973.

Rauste J: Lymphography in granulomatous inflammations. *Scand J Respir Dis (Suppl)* 89:186, 1974.

Rogers CE, Demetrakopoulos NJ, Hyamns V: Isolated lipodystrophy affecting the mesentery, the retroperitoneal area and the small intestines. *Ann Surg* 153:277, 1961.

Ruttiman A: Die Lymphographie. In: *Ergebnisse der medizinischen Strahlenforschung,* Neue Folge, Band I, Hrsg. Schinz-Glauner-Ruttimann. Stuttgart, G Thieme, 1964.

Ruttner JR: Pathological anatomy of "benign" lymph node disease. In: *Progress in Lymphology.* Stuttgart, G Thieme, 1967, p 98.

Schaffer B, Koehler RP, Daniel CR, Wohl GT, Rivera E, Meyers WA, Skelley JF: A critical evaluation of lymphography. *Radiology* 80:917, 1963.

Schneider CF: Idiopathic retroperitoneal fibrosis producing vena caval, biliary, ureteral and duodenal obstruction. *Ann Surg* 159:316, 1964.

Schrek R: Qualitative and quantitative reactions of lymphocytes to x-rays. *Ann NY Acad Sci* 95:839, 1961.

Sheffer AL, Ruddy S, Israel HL: Serum complement levels in sarcoidosis. In Levinsky L, Macholda F (eds): *5th International Conference on Sarcoidosis, Prague Karolinum, June 16–21, 1969.* Prague, Universita Karlova Praha, 1971, ch 5, p 195.

Smith EB, White DC, Hartsock RJ, Dixon AC: Acute ultrastructural effects of 500 roentgens on the lymph node of mouse. *Am J Pathol* 50:159, 1967.

Strickstrock KH, Weissleder H: Lymphographische Diagnose und Differentialdiagnose bei der Sarkoidose. *Fortschr Roentgenstr* 108:576, 1968.

Suby HJ, Kerr WS, Grahm JR, Fraley EG: Retroperitoneal fibrosis: a missing link in the chain. *J Urol* 93:144, 1965.

Suramo L: Lymphography in tuberculosis. *Acta Radiol Suppl* 339:1, 1974.

Tjernberg B: Lymphography as an aid to examination of lymph nodes. *Acta Soc Med Upsalien* 61:207, 1956.

Trowell OA: The sensitivity of lymphocytes to ionising radiation. *J Pathol Bacteriol* 64:687, 1952.

Ujiki GT, O'Brien PH, Moss WT, Putong P, Towne W: The lymph node barriers to viable tumor cells before and after irradiation. *J Surg Oncol* 2:193, 1970.

Van Den Brenk HAS: The effect of ionizing radiations on the regeneration and behavior of mammalian lymphatics. *Radiology* 78:837, 1957.

Viamonte M, Altman D, Parks R, Blum E, Bevilacqua M, Recher L: Radiographic-pathologic correlation in the interpretation of lymphangioadenograms. *Radiology* 80:903–1963.

Virchow R: *Cellular Pathology.* London, John Churchill, 1863.

Wiljasalo M, Perttala Y: Lymphographic changes caused by radiotherapy. *Ann Med Intern Fenn* 55:57, 1966.

Wiljasalo M, Julkunen H, Saluen I: Lymphography in rheumatic diseases. *Ann Med Intern Fenn* 55:125, 1966.

Wolfel DA, Smalley RH: Lipoplastic lymphadenopathy. *AJR* 112:610, 1971.

Yoffey JM, Sullivan ER: The lymphatic pathways from the nose and pharynx. *J Exp Med* 69:133, 1939.

Zalar J: Limfografija u Dijagnostici Retroperitonealne Sarkoidoze. *Plucne Bolesti Tuberk* 25:183, 1973.

# 10

# *Lymphoma—The Functional Approach to the Pathology of Malignant Lymphoma*

ROBERT J. LUKES, M.D.*

In the two decades since the Rye Conference on Hodgkin's disease, there has been remarkable progress in understanding the pathology of the disease and the effectiveness of therapy; however, in the non-Hodgkin's lymphomas little progress occurred until the past decade.

Through the decades the non-Hodgkin's lymphomas have been involved in disputes over terminology and classification, apparently as a result of a lack of fundamental understanding of lymphopoiesis and the associated imprecision in cytological characterization and identification. The traditional terms lymphosarcoma and reticulum cell sarcoma have been applied in an extraordinarily variable fashion. Each term included a number of cytological types and presently has achieved a meaningless status in communication (Gall, 1958; Lukes, 1968). In addition, follicular lymphoma was regarded as a lymphoma of the follicular structure in the traditional cytological classification but apparently accounted for only 50% of the nodular proliferations (Jones et al., 1973). The approach of Rappaport et al., proposed in 1956 long before the modern developments in immunology, provided important emphasis on cytological features and the significance of nodularity. Its clinical and prognostic value only recently became appreciated. Unfortunately, the classification of Rappaport does not appear conceptually relevant since it lacks a relationship to our modern understanding of lymphocytes and immunology.

Lukes and Collins (1973) and Collins and Lukes (1971) initially outlined the basis for a new functional approach for the malignant lymphomas, relating these neoplasms to the recent remarkable developments in immunology, the T

and B cell systems, and alterations in lymphocyte transformation. A functional approach was outlined subsequently for redefinition of the lymphomas applying a variety of immunological and cytochemical techniques to characterize these processes according to the T and B cell systems (Lukes and Collins, 1974a). In these initial publications it was proposed that (a) malignant lymphomas principally involve the T and B lymphocytic systems; (b) lymphomas of "true" histiocytes are rare, and reticulum cell sarcoma and histiocytic lymphoma of the past, with rare exceptions, are lymphomas of transformed lymphocytes of either the T or B cell systems; and (c) lymphomas commonly develop as a block or a "switch on" (derepression) in lymphocyte transformation. A functional classification initially was presented at the Congress of Radiologists meeting in 1972 in Freiburg, West Germany, and subsequently defined in detail (Lukes and Collins, 1974a, b). On the basis of this conceptual approach, the lymphomas are regarded as aggregates of immune-deficient cells that migrate, target, and function to varying degrees similar to their normal counterparts. It was suggested also that the study of lymphomas from an immunological approach might lead to a better understanding of the basic mechanism of these disorders and eventually permit design of a more ideal biological approach for therapy.

Following the presentation of our new functional approach and classification at a series of international meetings in 1973 (Lukes and Collins, 1974b, 1975), a number of other classifications were proposed (Bennett et al., 1974; Dorfman, 1974; Gerard-Marchant et al., 1974; Lennert et al., 1975), but all of the authors were reluctant to relate the lymphomas to the T and B cell systems. With the exception of the Kiel classification (Gerard-Marchant et al., 1974), these new classifications are modifications of the

* The reporting of this investigation has been supported in part by National Institute of Health training grants PO1 CA-19449-01 and CA-09025-01A1. There was partial support by the Beaumont Foundation.

Rappaport approach. The results of a number of studies using immunological surface markers on non-Hodgkin's disease and related leukemias support the T and B cell nature of lymphomas (Aisenberg and Long, 1975; Braylan et al., 1975; Brouet et al., 1975; Gajl-Peczalska et al., 1975; Green et al., 1975; Leech et al., 1975; Berard et al., 1976; Davey et al., 1976). Our studies, using an ever expanding array of techniques in our multiparameter approach, have demonstrated that lymphomas with few exceptions mark as T and B cells and rarely as histiocytes (Lukes and Collins, 1977; Lukes et al., 1978a, b, 1982, 1983). The lymphomas of large cells for the most part mark as transformed lymphocytes. The addition of monoclonal antibodies to the armamentarium of the multiparameter approach has increased greatly our capability of characterizing lymphoma and leukemia cells. They give every indication that the expanding number and value of new monoclonal antibodies will extend the precision of defining the level of lymphocyte developmental blocks and the function of both normal cells and their lymphomatous counterparts.

In this presentation, I review briefly: the immunological and morphological basis of our proposal; the functional classification and cytological types of both Hodgkin's and non-Hodgkin's lymphomas; the functional approach and the results of our multiparameter studies; clinical-pathological correlations; and the Working Formulation for Pathology (Rosenberg et al., 1982).

## IMMUNOLOGICAL AND MORPHOLOGICAL BASIS

Malignant lymphomas now appear established as neoplasms of the immune system. From our studies lymphoma cells can be related to their normal counterparts according to their morphological features, distributional characteristics, and immunological surface markers (Lukes and Collins, 1977; Lukes et al., 1978a, b, 1982, 1983). There has been dramatic progress in immunology in the past 15 yr—particularly the establishment of the T and B lymphocytic systems in man with their distinctive functions and the remarkable phenomenon of lymphocyte transformation—which is fundamental for our understanding of malignant lymphomas. The terminology and classifications of the past, including that of Rappaport et al. (1956), lack any relationship to modern immunology since they were all proposed long before these phenomena were demonstrated.

### Lymphocytic Systems

The recent progress in immunology has been a subject of numerous reviews, and its relationship to malignant lymphomas has clearly been emphasized by Hansen and Good (1974). The T and B lymphocytic systems, originally discovered through ablation experiments in animals, were confirmed in man through studies of immune deficiency states. A third lymphocytic system, the precursor cell for T and B lymphocytes, possibly the marrow stem cell, also appears to exist. We have proposed the term, *U cell* (undefined or unmarked), since it lacks both T and B cell markers. The U cell includes, therefore, the theoretical null cell and those cells presently without specific demonstrable surface markers or definable characteristics or functions. In all three systems the remarkable lymphocyte transformation phenomenon apparently occurs, and each has small, intermediate, and transformed cells. Recognition of these three systems with their individual variants accounts for the remarkable diversity of the morphological and functional expressions of both normal lymphocytes and their lymphomatous counterparts.

The proposed development of the T and B cell systems is well documented in experimental animals. The T cell acquires its membrane characteristics when the precursor cell or U cell migrates to the thymus during a limited period in immunological development and comes in contact with thymic epithelium, at which time the cell membrane is modified in an unknown fashion. In a similar manner in the avian species, the precursor cell, after migrating to the bursa of Fabricius, acquires its B cell characteristics. The precise location of the bursal equivalent in man has never been identified in spite of extensive search, although it apparently exists in some form, possibly in Peyer's patches. The precursor cell seems to possess the membrane characteristics of both T and B cells that apparently are uncovered selectively in the thymus and the bursa of Fabricius. Using monoclonal antibodies, the evolving changes in the display of surface and cytoplasmic antigens are currently being elucidated, but it will be some time before the sequence of events in both T and B cell lines will be established.

The T cell or thymic-dependent system is involved in cellular immunity and is measured clinically by delayed hypersensitivity responsiveness and in vitro lymphocyte transformation response to certain mitogens. T cell function is associated with the formation of a variety of soluble substances known as lymphokines, and the functional cells producing the substances are designated as suppressor and helper T cells. The diversity and complexity of the functioning T cells only now are becoming appreciated, although their morphological expressions are unknown. Undoubtedly malignant lymphomas of T cells at times may possess some of these functions, as has been suggested by Broder et al.'s (1976) proposal of the helper T cell nature of the cells in Sézary's syndrome. The B cell system, also known as the bursal equivalent system, is involved in immunoglobulin and antibody production.

The topographical distribution of the T and B lymphocytic system is now well established and is important morphologically in the understanding of normal immune reactions in various tissues and the morphological interpretation of malignant lymphomas. From the ablation experiments in animals and parallel findings in congenital immune defects in man, the B cell system has been related to follicular centers and the distribution of plasma cells, while the T cell system is distributed in the paracortical areas of lymph nodes, perivascular regions of the spleen, and in small foci in the gastrointestinal tract. B cells are found in primary and secondary follicles wherever they exist and in the Malpighian bodies of the spleen, the lamina propria of the gastrointestinal tract, and interspersed in the bone marrow. The lymphocytic systems are not static. The T lymphocytes circulate four to six times a day and account for approximately 70% of normal peripheral blood lymphocytes. It is estimated that 20–25% of peripheral blood lymphocytes are B cells, although recent studies suggest that the proportion of B cells may be considerably lower. Thus, there is an extremely complex daily circulating traffic of lymphocytes through blood and tissue with a highly selective "homing" phenomenon of the T and B cell systems to preferential anatomic sites throughout the body. From our morphological studies the lymphomas essentially are distributed in a highly predictable fashion parallel to the migration and distributional characteristics of their normal counterparts.

## Lymphocyte Transformation

This remarkable phenomenon has been studied extensively in vitro, but its morphological expressions and implications, both in normal immunological reactions and the malignant lymphomas, were unappreciated by pathologists until our published proposals (Lukes and Collins, 1974a, b). Lymphocytes under the influence of certain plant mitogens, such as phytohemagglutinin, pokeweed, concanavalin A, and antigens to which an individual has been immunized, change from a small lymphocyte to a large hyperbasophilic blast cell or transformed lymphocyte. The exact mechanism of initiating transformation is not established (O'Brien et al., 1977). Phytohemagglutinin and concanavalin A are thought to be highly selective transformers of T cells, while pokeweed is believed to transform both T and B cells. The only selective mitogen for human B cells appears to be *Nocardia apaca*, although the EB virus is a B cell transformer in human lymphoblastoid cell lines. From our morphological studies, both the small lymphocyte and the fully transformed cell are regarded as expressions of lymphocytes. The small lymphocyte represents the dormant form, and the transformed lymphocyte represents the metabolically active dividing state. Lymphocytes in vivo seem to modulate between the dormant and the dividing forms. The morphological expression encountered is contingent upon the immunological requirements. If our proposal is correct, the concept of morphological differentiation in lymphocytes is inappropriate with the exception of the change to functional expressions, such as the plasma cell in the B cell system. In this situation the use of a term for differentiation does not appear as meaningful as the use of a functional designation.

The transformed lymphocyte is four to six times the size of a small lymphocyte and has primitive, finely distributed chromatin, one or more prominent nucleoli, and abundant deeply basophilic cytoplasm in Romanowski's stained preparations. The cytoplasm is intensively pyroninophilic. The in vitro transformed lymphocytes grow in cohesive clusters. In sections of concentrated specimens these cells present wide variations in cell size and resemble a primitive appearing neoplastic process with numerous mitotic figures. Upon comparison study we were impressed by the remarkable resemblance of in vitro transformed lymphocytes and the large cells in both normal reactive lymphoid tissue and malignant lymphomas with the exception of obvious macrophages. Large transformed lymphocytes (immunoblasts) were identified in small numbers in the interfollicular tissue in benign reactions and in severe degrees in infectious mononucleosis, and in the regional lymph nodes of smallpox vaccination. Binucleated transformed immunoblasts, indistinguishable from diagnostic Reed-Sternberg cells of Hodgkin's disease, were found in every case of infectious mononucleosis on which morphological material was available for study (Lukes et al., 1969; Tindle et al., 1972). There are also transformed lymphocytes in reactive follicular centers, varying in size and number, apparently as a reflection of the state of reactivity. The morphological features of transformed lymphocytes most effectively are demonstrated in methyl green pyronine and Giemsa-stained sections. The follicular center is established as a B cell region, and, therefore, we regard the large transformed lymphocyte of the follicular center as a transformed B cell. Transformed lymphocytes (immunoblasts) of both T and B cell types apparently occur in the interfollicular tissue and are presently difficult to differentiate in histological sections, although it seems likely that the B immunoblast is larger and possesses more densely staining amphophilic cytoplasm which at times may have plasmacytoid features.

## B Cells

In lymph nodes normal B cells principally are found in primary and secondary follicles, in the peripheral blood in small numbers, and in the medulla of lymph nodes in functional expression as plasma cells. Transformed B cells are located in follicular centers, in interfollicular tissue with transformed T cells, and in widespread sites of reaction often with plasma cells. Following the recognition of transformed B cells in follicular centers, we proposed the follicular center cell (FCC) concept (Lukes and Collins, 1973, 1974a, b, 1975). Camera lucida studies of normal follicular centers revealed four cell types (*a*) cleaved FCC, (*b*) noncleaved FCC, (*c*) tingible body macrophages, and (*d*) dendritic reticulum cells. The wide range in size of both the cleaved and noncleaved cell revealed by the camera lucida drawings (Fig. 10.1) of normal FCC was attributed to stages in B cell transformation. Identification of nuclear cleavage planes depends upon the technical quality of the fixation, processing, and histological sections. In the average formalin-fixed, thick lymph node section, the cytological features, particularly nuclear cleavage planes, are not readily discernible. Methyl green pyronine-stained, well fixed tissue most ideally demonstrates the character of the noncleaved (transformed) FCC.

In the FCC concept we proposed the sequence in B cell transformation from the small B lymphocyte of the lymphocytic mantle to the large noncleaved FCC as illustrated in Figure 10.2. In this concept, the small lymphocyte, under the influence of antigen trapped in the follicular center primarily on the surface of dendritic reticulum cells illustrated schematically as a perifollicular center, is induced to undergo transformation as shown by Nossal et al. (1968). In the

## NORMAL FOLLICULAR CENTER CELLS

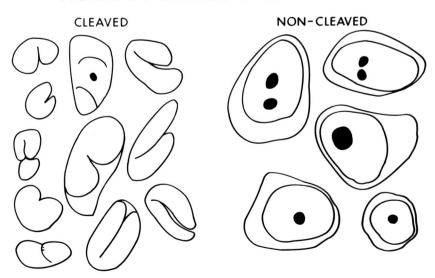

FIGURE 10.1.

SCHEMATIC REPRESENTATION OF DEVELOPMENT OF MALIGNANT LYMPHOMAS
OF FOLLICULAR CENTER CELLS

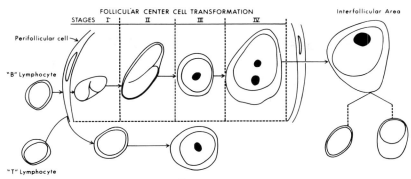

FIGURE 10.2.

first stage the small lymphocyte changes to the small cleaved FCC. By gradual enlargement and acquisition of a small amount of pyroninophilic cytoplasm, it reaches the second stage, the large cleaved FCC.

In the third designated stage, the small noncleaved FCC, the nucleus becomes round, the nuclear chromatin is finely dispersed in association with a small nucleolus, and the cytoplasm is prominently pyroninophilic. In the fourth stage, the large noncleaved FCC is similar, but larger, has more abundant pale acidophilic cytoplasm, and one to three more prominent nucleoli are often situated on the nuclear membrane. The cleaved cells of the follicular center are essentially nondividing cells, while the noncleaved cells are dividing cells. From the studies of Dr. Clive Taylor, of our group, cytoplasmic immunoglobulin initially can be demonstrated in the large cleaved FCC in small amounts and with increasing prominence in the small and large noncleaved FCC stages (Taylor and Mason, 1974; Taylor, 1976). The large noncleaved FCC appears in histological sections to migrate out of the follicular center into the interfollicular tissue where we have designated it an immunoblast of B cell type. This apparent migration is supported by the ultrastructural studies of follicular centers of tonsils by Kojima and Tsunoda (1976), also using the immunoperoxidase technique. The demonstration of cytoplasm immunoglobulin in FCC and some immunoblasts of the interfollicular tissue provides strong supportive evidence of their relationship and B cell nature. The proposed direction of in vivo transformation of B cells in the follicular center is in contradiction to the generally held view. Our proposal is based on our in vitro lymphocyte transformation experience. The in vitro phenomenon occurs from the small lymphocyte to the transformed lym-

phocyte in both T and B cell systems. The proposed sequence in the FCC concept also parallels the evolution observed in FCC lymphomas in which the process is observed initially as the small cleaved FCC type with limited aggressiveness, and later there is change to the highly aggressive noncleaved FCC type. The FCC concept provides the basis for relating the cytological types of FCC neoplasms to their normal counterparts and permits an understanding of the evolution of the process in the B cell system.

## T Cells

The morphological differentiation between T and B cells remains a subject of debate even though functional studies are beginning to provide strong support for the distinctiveness of some cytological types in both systems. The transformed lymphocytes (immunoblasts) of the T and B cell systems are generally similar, but the B immunoblast at times may be larger, have more abundant, denser, amphophilic cytoplasm, and even have plasmacytoid features. The demonstration of cytoplasmic immunoglobulin by the immunoperoxidase technique developed by Taylor and Mason (1974) is a helpful method for distinguishing transformed T and B cell types of the interfollicular tissue because of the cytoplasmic content of immunoglobulin in B cells. Transformation in T cells occurs in a somewhat parallel fashion to B cells but outside of the follicular center in the paracortical region without the formation of cleaved nucleated cells or plasma cells. The intermediate stage of transformation consists of medium-sized cells with round nuclei, finely dispersed chromatin, small nucleoli, and a moderate amount of pyroninophilic cytoplasm. The T cell lymphomas observed thus far possibly may represent extreme expansions of defective counterparts of normal cells that ordinarily occur in small numbers and as yet have not been described. The convoluted T cell we described in children and young adults possibly is a development abnormality of the pre-T cell (Barcos and Lukes, 1975; Stein et al., 1976). The cerebriform cell of Sézary's syndrome has been proposed as lymphoma of helper cells by Broder et al. (1976). Lymphomas of T cells as characterized by monoclonal antibodies are discussed briefly later in this chapter.

## A FUNCTIONAL CLASSIFICATION OF MALIGNANT LYMPHOMAS

The immunological basis of the functional classification of malignant lymphomas outlined briefly in the previous section can be summarized in the following points: (a) malignant lymphomas are neoplasms of the immune system; (b) they involve primarily T and B cell and U cell (undefined) systems and rarely histiocytes and monocytes; (c) malignant lymphomas possibly develop as a block or a "switch on" (derepression) of lymphocyte transformation in the various lymphocytic systems; and (d) the cytological types of lymphoma are counterparts to normal immunological cells and are similar in varying degrees morphologically and functionally. The cytological types of lymphoma are related to positions in B and T cell transformation illustrated in Figure 10.2, with the exception of the true histiocytic lymphoma, the convoluted lymphocyte that possibly represents a pre-T cell (Barcos and Lukes, 1975; Stein et al., 1976) and the cerebriform cell of Sézary's syndrome and mycosis fungoides, the precise nature of which remains uncertain. The involved cell in Hodgkin's disease is unknown.

Our functional classification initially was proposed before the application of multiparameter studies. The results of our studies on over 1300 cases of lymphomas and related leukemias using these techniques have confirmed the immunological approach and the cytological types (Lukes et al., 1983). Only the lymphoma of small T lymphocytes, the lymphoepithelioid T lymphocyte, and immunoblastic sarcoma of T cells have been added to the original cytological types. It is acknowledged that the final acceptance of any classification is dependent upon the soundness of the conceptual basis as well as the clinical relevance and effectiveness of its application. Acceptance may require a number of years of trial by numerous centers.

The classification of malignant lymphoma is listed in Table 10.1 according to the following major groups: (a) U cell (undefined), (b) T cell, (c) B cell, (d) histiocytic, (e) cell type of uncertain origin—Hodgkin's disease; and (f) unclassifiable. The U cell (undefined) type is hypothetical and was developed for the proliferations of cells that lack discriminating primitive morphological features and have undetectable immunological or cytochemical markers according to presently available techniques. It includes the theoretical null cell and the primitive lymphocytes or true stem cells, such as those found in acute lymphocytic leukemia (ALL) in childhood without specific markers. The unclassifiable type is designed for those lymphomatous appearing proliferations on which the histological and cytological findings are indistinct or obscured for technical reasons, and the process cannot be classified precisely.

In both the T and B cell group there is a small lymphocytic type and a large transformed lymphocytic type or immunoblastic sarcoma. The T cell group also includes cytological types with the extraordinary nuclear configuration, the

**TABLE 10.1.**
FUNCTIONAL CLASSIFICATION

*U cell* (undefined)
*T cell*
  Small lymphocyte
  Convoluted lymphocyte
  Cerebriform lymphocyte (mycosis
    fungoides and Sézary's syndrome)
  Lymphoepithelioid T cell
  Immunoblastic sarcoma of T cells
*B cell*
  Small lymphocyte
  Plasmacytoid lymphocyte
  Follicular center cell (FCC)
    Follicular, diffuse, follicular and diffuse, and with or
      without sclerosis
    Small cleaved
    Large cleaved
    Small noncleaved
    Large noncleaved
  Immunoblastic sarcoma B cells
  Hairy cell leukemia
*Histiocytic*
*Cell of uncertain origin*
  Hodgkin's disease
    Lymphocyte predominance
    Mixed cellularity
    Lymphocyte depletion
    Nodular sclerosis
*Unclassifiable*

primitive appearing convoluted T cell and the cerebriform cell of Sézary's syndrome and mycosis fungoides. The B cell group contains the FCC variants which are regarded as plasma cell precursors and the plasmacytoid lymphocytic type which is frequently associated with dysglobulinemias, such as Waldenström's syndrome. The histiocytic type refers to those disorders that lack the immunological surface markers and features of T or B cells and exhibit the cytochemical expression of histiocytes for which we have used the $\alpha$-naphthyl butyrate cytochemical method (Yam et al., 1971b) and the cytoplasmic immunoperoxidase technique for muramidase, $\alpha$-1-antitrypsin, and $\alpha$-1-antichymotrypsin. Hodgkin's disease is subclassified according to the well established and accepted types of the Rye classification (Lukes et al., 1966b), which is a modification of the original Lukes-Butler classification (Lukes et al., 1966a, b). The classification and cytological types have been described in detail in a number of publications (Lukes et al., 1966a; Lukes, 1971). Only the essential features are considered in this chapter.

## T Cell Types

### Small Lymphocyte (T Cell)

The existence of a lymphoma-leukemia of small T cells has been documented by multiparameter studies in a small number of cases, but the distinctiveness of the morphological features has not been established. The cytological features we have observed in a small group of cases appear to represent three subtypes: (*a*) The *nobby* subtype has compact basophilic nuclear chromatin with irregular nodular nuclear borders and scanty pale cytoplasm. (*b*) The *cytoplasmic* subtype resembles the type I Downey cell with compact basophilic nuclear chromatin, abundant pale cytoplasm with scalloped cytoplasmic borders, and azurophilic granules. (*c*) The *prolymphocytic* subtype is a primitive appearing cell with a medium-sized nucleus with fine acidophilic chromatin, a large, well demarcated central nucleolus, and a moderate amount of lightly basophilic cytoplasm.

### Convoluted Lymphocyte

This process is a diffuse proliferation of primitive appearing noncohesive cells occurring in widely infiltrated masses or in partially or totally involved lymph nodes (Fig. 10.3). The lymphoma cells vary in size from that of a small lymphocyte to four to five lymphocyte nuclear diameters.

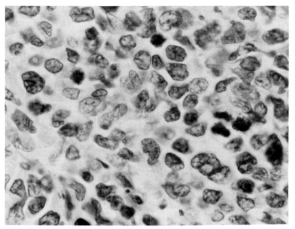

FIGURE 10.3. CONVOLUTED LYMPHOCYTIC TYPE
The nuclei vary widely in size and configuration, have finely dispersed chromatin, numerous fine linear subdivisions, and no apparent nucleoli. The cytoplasm is scant.

The nuclei have distinctive, finely distributed chromatin and inconspicuous or small nucleoli. The nuclei of the smaller cells are round in configuration, while the larger cells commonly have deep subdivisions of varying prominence. At times these subdivisions present an image of a "chicken footprint." Usually the linear subdivisions resemble a convolutional phenomenon in a round nucleus, but the nucleus may be irregular and almost lobated from the deep convolutions. The small and large cells vary in frequency. The frequency of mitoses typically ranges from five to seven per high power field and is proportional to the number of large cells. The cytoplasm is indistinct or scanty and relates to the noncohesive character of the cells. Occasionally, reactive "starry-sky" phagocytes are interspersed, and for this reason the proliferation may be mistaken for a Burkitt lymphoma in overly thick sections.

### Cerebriform Cell of Sézary's Syndrome and Mycosis Fungoides

The lymphoma cells in these closely related conditions are medium size and approximately one to two normal lymphocytes in diameter. They have barely discernible linear subdivisions in cells found in the peripheral blood and tissue, but in the later aggressive stage the cells may be large, the chromatin finely dispersed and the configuration outline remarkably abnormal. There is only a narrow rim of cytoplasm that usually contains numerous periodic acid-Schiff (PAS)-positive globules at times in a "necklace" distribution. Ultrastructural studies dramatically demonstrate the deep cerebriform subdivisions (Rosas-Uribe et al., 1974; Lutzner et al., 1975).

### Lymphoepithelioid T Cell

This cytological type of lymphoma is still debated because of its rarity and the infrequency of immune phenotyping studies. In our experience with 18 cases characterized by multiparameter studies, the cells vary considerably in size and expression, and the disease often evolves to immunoblastic sarcoma. This type of lymphoma is characterized by a special association with epithelioid cells, the significance of which is as yet uncertain. The abnormal lymphocyte is larger than a normal small lymphocyte. The nuclear chromatin is loosely dispersed, and the nucleus is enlarged and often twisted, giving a squiggly appearance. Immunoblasts are associated in varying numbers, but plasma cells are rare. Large lobated cells raise the question of Reed-Sternberg cells and call for differentiation from Hodgkin's disease—lymphocytic and histiocytic types (Lukes, 1971).

### Immunoblastic Sarcoma of T Cells

We are just becoming acquainted with this proliferation (Levine et al., 1981). It exhibits a lymphocytic spectrum ranging from a small irregular peculiar lymphocyte to the fully transformed lymphocyte. The medium and large cells closely resemble in vitro transformed lymphocytes and in histological sections have pale staining to almost water-clear cytoplasm with well defined, cohesive, interlocking cytoplasmic membranes. The nucleus is round to oval with finely distributed chromatin and usually one central prominent nucleolus. The process generally extends throughout the lymph node and is unassociated with follicle or nodule formation. The small peculiar lymphocyte appears to be a definite component of an evolving process.

## B Cell Types

### Small Lymphocyte of B Cells

This is a diffuse proliferation of noncohesive small lymphocytes closely resembling normal lymphocytes. They have uniform round nuclei with compact basophilic chromatin, inapparent nucleoli, and a small rim of pale staining cytoplasm. Plasma cells essentially are absent. Lymphomatous follicles or nodules are absent, but scattered ill-defined pale foci composed of large transformed lymphocytes and accompanied by

mitoses, representing proliferative foci (so-called pseudofollicles), at times are prominent.

### Plasmacytoid Lymphocytic Type

This lymphomatous proliferation is generally similar to the small lymphocyte of B cells with the exception of an abnormal plasma cell component but with a nucleus that resembles a lymphocyte (Fig. 10.4). There is also a component of cells intermediate between the small lymphocyte and the abnormal plasma cell. A large pale acidophilic staining globule which is PAS-positive occasionally overlies the nucleus (Dutcher body) in Waldenström's macroglobulinemia (Dutcher and Fahey, 1959). A similar cellular proliferation is found with other types of dysglobulinemias, but often no dysglobulinemia is detected (Levine et al., 1980).

### FCC Types

The four FCC types may occur with follicular, follicular and diffuse, or diffuse histological patterns, with or without sclerosis. The small cleaved FCC type usually is associated with some degree of follicle (nodular) formation, the large cleaved FCC in approximately one-half of the cases, and the noncleaved FCC occasionally (10%).

**Small Cleaved FCC.** The range in size and configuration of normal cleaved FCCs is illustrated schematically in Figure 10.1. The small cleaved FCC varies in size from a small lymphocyte to that of a reactive histiocyte nucleus (Fig. 10.5). The nuclei are basically of irregular con-

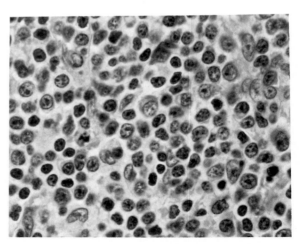

FIGURE 10.4. PLASMACYTOID-LYMPHOCYTIC TYPE
The proliferation appears predominantly lymphocytic, but a proportion of the cells have plasmacytoid cytoplasm in varying amounts.

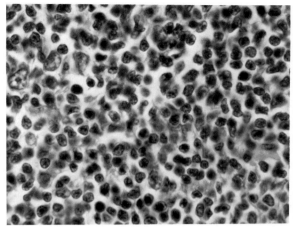

FIGURE 10.5. SMALL CLEAVED FOLLICULAR CENTER CELL
TYPE

These cells are small and have irregular nuclei often with
a single linear subdivision. Mitoses are rare. The cytoplasm
is scanty.

figuration, and a variable portion of the cells
exhibit typical nuclear cleavage planes similar to
normal cells. The degree of irregularity and
cleavage increases in prominence with nuclear
size. The nuclear chromatin is compact and basophilic, and nucleoli are inconspicuous. Mitotic
figures are rare. The cytoplasm is scanty or indistinct. A small proportion of noncleaved
(transformed) FCCs is intermixed, usually in
small numbers, but on occasion reaching 10–
20%. The small cleaved cells usually extend
throughout the lymphomatous follicles into the
interfollicular tissue and commonly infiltrate the
capsule.

**Large Cleaved FCC.** The nucleus of the
large cleaved cell is larger than a reactive histiocyte nucleus and consistently irregular in configuration. Often the nuclear cleavage planes result
in exaggerated nuclear forms. The cytoplasm is
moderate in amount and pyroninophilic, and
frequently this proliferation is associated with a
deposit of pale staining intercellular material and
early sclerosis. Small and large cleaved FCCs
commonly occur together in different parts of a
lymphomatous proliferation when the large
cleaved FCC is prominent, particularly with sclerosis.

**Small Noncleaved (Transformed) FCC.**
This lymphoma is composed of medium-sized
cells with features of small transformed lymphocytes. The nuclei are round and regular in configuration, and the nuclei predominantly do not
exceed the size of the phagocyte nucleus. The
nuclear chromatin is finely dispersed, and there
are several small nucleoli. There is a narrow rim
of pyroninophilic cytoplasm, and the cellular

borders are cohesive in well fixed tissue. Reactive
phagocytes of "starry-sky" type commonly are
regularly interspersed throughout the tumor.
This lymphoma fulfills the criteria of the Burkitt
lymphoma of Africa when the cells are uniform
in size and configuration (Berard et al., 1969).
In the United States the small noncleaved FCC
usually exhibits considerably more variation in
cytological features and is designated commonly
as the non-Burkitt type. In a few reported cases
of the Burkitt lymphoma, a follicular (nodular)
pattern has been observed in a small portion of
the proliferation (Mann et al., 1976). This observation provides support for our proposal that the
Burkitt lymphoma is of FCC type (Lukes and
Collins, 1973, 1974a, b, 1975).

**Large Noncleaved (Transformed) FCC.**
This lymphoma in general possesses similar cytological features to the small noncleaved FCC
type with the exception that the cells are larger
and have more abundant cytoplasm, the nuclei
are larger, and the nucleoli are more prominent.
Often two prominent nucleoli are found situated
on the nuclear membrane in a characteristic
pattern on the short axis of an oval nucleus.
Mitoses are numerous. Both individual cell necrosis and areas of necrosis are common.

*Immunoblastic Sarcoma of B Cells*

This lymphoma of transformed B cells resembles the large noncleaved FCC, but in general it
is a larger cell with more dense amphophilic
cytoplasm and often exhibits plasmacytoid features (Fig. 10.6). It lacks the typical features of

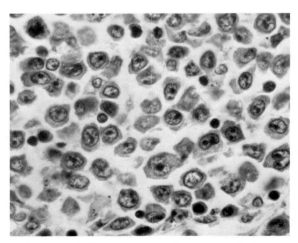

FIGURE 10.6. IMMUNOBLASTIC SARCOMA OF B CELLS

The cells are large and resemble the in vitro transformed
lymphocytes. The nuclei are round to oval and occasionally
irregular in configuration. The chromatin is finely dispersed,
and the nucleoli are prominent. The cytoplasm is abundant
and deeply staining.

the FCC types, specifically the cleaved FCC component and follicular pattern. The process often initially is observed partially involving an abnormal immune process of various types and presents as monomorphous areas (clones) of large abnormal immunoblasts. Later in the process the proliferation may totally involve and replace the lymph node or present as a tumor mass. The immunoblasts of B cell types are differentiated from T immunoblasts on the basis of the density of the amphophilic cytoplasm and their frequent plasmacytoid character. The demonstration of the cytoplasmic immunoglobulin by the immunoperoxidase technique (Taylor and Mason, 1974; Taylor, 1976) offers supportive evidence, particularly if monoclonal in character. Similarly, monoclonal surface immunoglobulin substantiates its B cell nature.

### Histiocytic

A true histiocytic type appears to exist as an interrelated histiocyte-monocyte proliferation. The number of proven cases with functional studies is too small at the present time to establish an accurate description of its morphological expressions. To be acceptable as a true histiocytic type, the lymphoma cells in our view require cytochemical demonstration of their macrophage-monocyte enzyme with the $\alpha$-naphthyl butyrate esterase (Yam et al., 1971a). Ideally, the lack of immunological surface markers for T and B cells also is shown. The small number of proven cases we have had the opportunity to study have been variable in their histological appearance but have had both an identifiable histiocyte component, such as a macrophage, and also a monocyte component. Several of these cases have terminated with a leukemic process resembling a monocytic leukemia.

### Uncertain Cell Type—Hodgkin's Disease

The precise nature of the Reed-Sternberg cell remains controversial, although the histological types of the Rye classification (Lukes et al., 1966b) adapted from the original Lukes and Butler types (Lukes et al., 1966a) have long been accepted. The histological types of both classifications are designed to characterize the host response and are based on our concept that the basic process in Hodgkin's disease is a struggle between host and the factors involved in the induction of Reed-Sternberg cells. The lymphocyte predominant, histological type is regarded as an expression of an extremely effective host response, characterized morphologically by a predominance of lymphocytes and a rarity of diagnostic Reed-Sternberg cells and clinically by disease of limited extent.

The lymphocyte depletion type, by contrast, is associated with an ineffective host response reflected morphologically by decreased numbers of lymphocytes associated with either a distinctive type of diffuse fibrosis or numerous diagnostic Reed-Sternberg cells and clinically by stage III or IV disease. The mixed cellularity type occupies an intermediate position between lymphocyte predominance and lymphocyte depletion and indicates a failing host response expressed clinically by changing disease. Nodular sclerosis is regarded separately as a result of its dominant association with the anterior superior mediastinum and adjacent cervical, hilar, and axillary lymph nodes and is regarded as a regional expression of Hodgkin's disease. It includes cases with both quiescent and aggressive disease. The spread of nodular sclerosis appears to be contiguous and predictable, while in the remaining types it usually skips the mediastinum and is noncontiguous in its spread.

In the following, each histological type of the Rye classification is briefly defined.

**Lymphocyte Predominance.** This type includes both the lymphocytic and histiocytic, nodular and diffuse types of our original classification (Lukes et al., 1966a). The proliferation may be composed dominantly of lymphocytes or histiocytes or in varying proportions, although a predominance of lymphocytes is most commonly encountered. In approximately half of the cases the proliferation is aggregated into large vague nodules and is associated usually with stage I disease. The lymphocytic and histiocytic components are regarded as reactive host responses. The lymphocytes are small and have round to irregular nuclei and scanty cytoplasm. The histiocytes occur singly or in small clusters and at times resemble small sarcoid-like aggregations. Scattered throughout the lymphocytic and histiocytic proliferation is a prominent component of large polyploid appearing cells with pale cytoplasm, folded and overlapping large nuclei, and small or inconspicuous nucleoli. We have designated these cells the L & H variants of the Reed-Sternberg cell, since they have proved extremely reliable in recognizing this histological type (Lukes, 1971). By contrast the diagnostic Reed-Sternberg cell with huge nucleoli typically is extremely rare in this type.

**Mixed Cellularity.** This type, as the name implies, contains a variety of components in variable degrees. Diagnostic Reed-Sternberg cells with large nucleoli are conspicuous; histiocytes, eosinophils, and disorderly fibrosis are also commonly prominent. The mixed type also provides a category for those cases in which the histological findings do not fulfill the criteria for any of the other histological types.

**Lymphocyte Depletion.** This type includes the diffuse fibrosis and reticular types of our original classification (Lukes et al., 1966a). In the former there is typically marked reduction in cellularity associated with a distinctive type of disorderly fibrosis characterized by loose, amorphous, poorly formed connective tissue that extends throughout the majority of the lymph node. Diagnostic Reed-Sternberg cells are often difficult to find. Lymphocytes may be infrequent or limited to a portion of the node. In the reticular variant, diagnostic Reed-Sternberg cells are extremely numerous and, on rare occasions, appear sarcomatous. Features of both the reticular and diffuse fibrosis types at times may be found together.

**Nodular Sclerosis.** This histological type exhibits numerous variations in expression both in the degree of sclerosis and in its cellular composition. The sclerosis varies from a single broad collagen band extending from a thickened lymph node capsule to almost total sclerosis of a mass. The cellularity varies from predominantly lymphocytic to a dominance of lacunar cell variants of the Reed-Sternberg cell. There are two essential criteria for the diagnosis of the nodular sclerosing type: (*a*) thick birefringent collagen bands and (*b*) typical lacunar cells with well demarcated cellular borders, abundant water-clear cytoplasm, and a tendency to multiple lobation with small nucleoli. Often the lacunar cells occur in distinctive cohesive clusters in the center of lymphocytic nodules that are often surrounded by a collagen band. Central necrosis of these lacunar cell clusters associated with mature granulocyte infiltration is common. Using our approach in Hodgkin's disease, Bennett et al. (1981) successfully related eight subtypes of nodular sclerosis to survival. Almost 100% of patients with a predominence of lymphocytes survived 5 yr, while those with few lymphocytes and numerous diagnostic Reed-Sternberg cells fared poorly. The remainder of subtypes arrayed themselves in an orderly intermediate fashion.

## RESULTS OF FUNCTIONAL STUDIES

The functional approach employs a variety of techniques in the study of lymphomas and related leukemias, including special morphology, cytochemistry, electron microscopy, and immunological surface marker techniques to characterize the type of proliferation. Since 1981, monoclonal antibody studies either by flow cytometry or by immunoperoxidase labeling on special frozen tissue sections have greatly augmented our capability. Over the past 2 yr such studies have become the central focus and thrust of our investigation and have essentially replaced the rosette techniques. When possible, other techniques, such as immunoglobulin synthesis and cell kinetics, are used to evaluate their functional capacity. The immunological surface marker techniques have been helpful in the study of immune abnormalities and defects for a number of years, and more recently they have been applied to the study of malignant lymphomas and their leukemic expressions. The results of these studies in general support our initial proposal that these disorders, with the exception of a portion of ALL, mark as T or B cells and rarely as histiocytes. The morphological features of our cytological types of lymphoma are predictive of the T and B cell type in a high proportion of cases (Lukes and Collins, 1977; Lukes et al., 1978a, b, 1982, 1983).

The most commonly employed and effective techniques in the study of malignant lymphomas until monoclonal antibodies became available are listed in Table 10.2. These techniques have been the subject of numerous reviews (Braylan et al., 1975; Green et al., 1975; Kunkel, 1975; Lukes et al., 1978a, b, 1982, 1983) and are only

TABLE 10.2.

TECHNIQUES FOR IDENTIFICATION OF T AND B CELLS AND HISTIOCYTES

|  | T Cells | B Cells | Histiocytes-Monocytes |
|---|---|---|---|
| Sheep red blood cell rosettes |  |  |  |
| E | + | − | − |
| EAC (IgM)* | − | + | + |
| EA (IgG) | − | − | + |
| Surface Ig† | − | + | − |
| Cytoplasmic immunoperoxidase |  |  |  |
| Immunoglobulin | − | + | − |
| Muramidase | − | − | + |
| Antiserum |  |  |  |
| HTLA‡ | + | − | − |
| HBLA‡ | − | + | − |
| α-Naphthyl butyrate | − | − | + |

* The convoluted T cell has been observed with complement receptors.

† T cells have a small amount of surface Ig.

‡ HTLA, human T lymphocyte antibody; HBLA, human B lymphocyte antibody.

briefly summarized here. Fresh biopsies of lymph nodes or masses, or specimens of peripheral blood, are essential for all except the immunoperoxidase technique on paraffin sections. Suspensions of live cells are required for the immunological surface marker techniques and freshly prepared imprints and unfixed frozen tissue for most of the cytochemical techniques. These include a battery of stains that are distinctive for granulocytes, histiocytes, monocytes, and special cells, such as those of hairy cell leukemia and ALL. Ideal fixation for histopathology is achieved with the collection of fresh biopsy material by the preparation of thin (2–3 mm) tissue blocks which permit rapid and thorough penetration by the fixative. We have found a modified Zenker's solution to be the best fixative for hematopoietic tissues.

Sheep erythrocytes attach to lymphocytes in suspension and form rosettes under a variety of controlled conditions and help in the discrimination between T and B cells and histiocytes (Jondal et al., 1972). Spontaneous rosettes of sheep erythrocytes (E) form consistently about T cells. Similar rosette formation of complement-dependent type (EAC) occurs with B cells, histiocytes, and convoluted T cells if the sheep erythrocytes are previously exposed to antibody IgM and complement, whereas rosette formation (EA) occurs with histiocytes and monocytes, if the erythrocytes are pretreated with antibody (IgG) only. Application of the EAC and EA techniques to frozen unfixed tissue sections effectively identifies the B cell nature of reactive follicles and lymphomatous nodules as well as the distributional character of histiocytes and monocytes in lymph nodes and spleen (Jaffe et al., 1974). The detection of surface immunoglobulins is generally regarded as the most effective method of identifying B cells (Kunkel, 1975). Immunoglobulin is identified on live cells using fluorescent-labeled monospecific antibodies for heavy and light immunoglobulin chains. The population of B cells found in the peripheral blood of normal individuals and in reactive lymphoid tissue exhibits a variety of immunoglobulins (polyclonal immunoglobulin) on their surface. Typically the lymphomas and leukemias of B cell type display monoclonal surface immunoglobulins (i.e., a single heavy and a single light chain on their surface). Monoclonicity is interpreted as evidence of a neoplastic clonal proliferation similar to the immunoglobulin production observed typically in myeloma.

Demonstration of immunoglobulin synthesis is acknowledged as the most precise method for characterizing a B cell proliferation. In paraffin sections of fixed tissue, it is possible to demonstrate cytoplasmic immunoglobulin and to characterize the immunoglobulin monospecifically according to heavy and light immunoglobulin chains using the immunoperoxidase technique as described by Taylor and Mason (1974) and Taylor (1976). The basis of the technique is similar to the fluorescent method with horseradish peroxidase substituted for the fluorescent label on the specific antibody. The stained peroxidase serves as the marker for the site of the immunoglobulin. The immunoperoxidase technique may also be used on fixed paraffin sections for the demonstration of cytoplasmic muramidase (lysozyme), an enzyme found normally in histiocytes, monocytes, granulocytes, and a variety of tissues other than T and B cells. The $\alpha$-naphthyl butyrate cytochemical technique detects an enzyme found in histiocytes and monocytes and identifies a somewhat wider range of histiocytes and monocytes than the immunoperoxidase for muramidase, but this cytochemical technique is limited to relatively fresh tissue imprints, peripheral blood, bone marrow smears, and unfixed frozen tissue sections (Yam et al., 1971a). Prior exposure of the specimen to sodium fluoride blocks the staining of monocytes and permits the distinction between histiocytes and monocytes. The tartrate-resistant acid phosphatase technique of Yam et al. (1971b) is a useful method of precisely identifying cases of hairy cell leukemia through its demonstration of a single isoenzyme.

Monoclonal antibodies have been produced against a variety of antigens and cell types. These antibodies provide great specificity for antigens, but some antigens may be shared by several types of cells, and, thus, monoclonal antibodies may not always be as specific for cell types as initially thought. There is currently a rapid expansion in the number of monoclonal antibodies. As a result it seems likely that in time most normal and neoplastic cells and their functional products will be identified and characterized by monoclonal antibodies. Such antibodies may be employed in fluorescent form on cell suspensions using the flow cytometer or in immunoperoxidated labeled form on special frozen tissue sections. Cytofluorometry studies permit the evaluation of large numbers of cells by a variety of antibodies used sequentially, but there is uncertainty of the identity of the positively labeled cells. Using labeled monoclonal antibodies on frozen sections, the positively labeled cells can be evaluated morphologically and also related to the structure of the tissue as studied in parallel by light microscopy techniques.

The results of many studies on malignant lymphomas and leukemias of lymphocytes evaluated by the various surface marker techniques have now appeared in the literature (Brouet et al., 1973; Aisenberg and Long, 1975; Braylan et al., 1975; Gajl-Peczalska et al., 1975; Green et al., 1975; Leech et al., 1975; Berard et al., 1976; Davey et al., 1976). In general, the results of these studies support our original proposal that (a) malignant lymphomas are neoplasms of the immune system, (b) for the most part these proliferations mark as T and B cell types, and (c) lymphomas of histiocytes as macrophages are rare. It is clear from these reports and our experience that the techniques are complex procedures vulnerable to erroneous and at times confusing results. Unquestionably, refinement of these techniques and the development of more perience that the techniques are complex procedures vulnerable to erroneous and at times confusing results. Unquestionably, refinement of these techniques and the development of more precise methods will ultimately add greater preder my colleague, Dr. Robert Collins, and by my group at the University of Southern California School of Medicine using essentially similar techniques—have provided verification of the cytological types of our functional classification and the value of the immunological approach outlined in this presentation (Lukes and Collins, 1977; Lukes et al., 1978a, b, 1982, 1983). The results of these studies are briefly summarized here and related to the other recent reports.

The non-Hodgkin's lymphomas and the closely related leukemias of past classifications appear to be groups of disorders rather than homogeneous entities. ALL of childhood has been demonstrated to be heterogeneous (Kersey et al., 1973; Haegert et al., 1975), 20–25% of cells are of T cell type, a small portion are of B cell type resembling small noncleaved FCC, and the remainder that fail to mark are included in our U cell group. Chronic lymphocytic leukemia (CLL) and its tissue counterpart, the lymphoma of small lymphocytes, also are heterogeneous, although only 1–2% are of T cell type and the remainder mark as B cells.

We regard both T and B cell types of CLL as lymphomas of small lymphocytes that have a propensity for peripheral blood and bone marrow involvement. The cerebriform cell of Sézary's syndrome (Brouet et al., 1973) and mycosis fungoides is accepted as a T cell (Lutzner et al., 1975). Broder et al. (1976) have shown evidence of the possible helper T cell character of Sézary cells, and a monoclonal antibody has been developed that identifies a distinctive antigen on the cerebriform (Sézary) cells which is also pres-

ent on normal helper T cells. Similarly, the T cell nature of the convoluted lymphocyte appears to be confirmed from our studies (Lukes and Collins, 1977; Lukes et al., 1978a, b, 1982, 1983) and from those of Stein et al. (1976), who also demonstrated strong focal acid phosphatase positivity. Similar strong acid phosphatase positivity also was found by Catovsky et al. (1974) in a small group of proven T cell ALL cases. It is acknowledged that the degree of convolutional nuclear change varies widely from case to case in both lymphomatous and leukemic expressions. Recognition of nuclear convolutions also may be difficult in less than optimal histological sections. The combination of variable frequency and technical factors may account for the difference in the findings reported by Nathwani et al. (1976). Nuclear convolutions are more difficult to discern in smear preparations. This proliferation is interrelated with the T cell type of ALL of childhood mentioned above (Kersey et al., 1973). Monoclonal antibody studies have revealed an evolving display of changing antigens as T cells develop from the earliest pre-T cell to the mature thymocyte. More time and more ideal monoclonal antibodies are needed before the precise relationship between specific antigens and distinctive morphological features is elucidated. T cell ALL and convoluted T cell lymphoma are either closely related or identical, but the exact status remains unestablished. The cerebriform T cell usually displays a helper T cell antigen on its surface, while studies on a small number of cases of T immunoblastic sarcoma reveal marking for helper or suppressor T cell antigen. Finding a helper or suppressor membrane antigen on T cells does not necessarily relate to their functional state.

The study of lymphomas previously included in the histiocytic type of Rappaport has presented a problem in investigation, apparently because of the fragile nature of these high turnover rate types of cellular proliferations and the difficulty of cell separation. Nevertheless, in our study these cells have marked almost always as T or B cells when a sufficient number of viable cells was obtained for evaluation (Lukes and Collins, 1977; Lukes et al., 1978a, b, 1982, 1983). Morphologically these cells usually presented the features of transformed lymphocytes either as immunoblastic sarcoma of T or B cell types or as large noncleaved (transformed) FCCs. Only eight cases in our study marked as the histiocytic types, and these were distinguishable morphologically from the lymphomas of transformed lymphocytes. However, as a result of their studies of transplantable lymphomas in nude mice,

Epstein and Kaplan (1974) believe that the large cells essentially are of histiocytic type. However, these lymphomas were not evaluated prior to transplantation by the multiparameter techniques.

Lymphomas with a follicular (nodular) histological pattern have been shown by Jaffe et al. (1974), using the frozen section EAC and EA rosette techniques, to be of B cell type. In our study of FCC lymphomas with follicular or diffuse histological patterns, monoclonal type surface immunoglobulin was demonstrated in the majority of cases (Lukes and Collins, 1977; Lukes et al., 1978a, b, 1982, 1983). The follicular nature of lymphomatous follicles was demonstrated in the comparative ultrastructural studies of normal and lymphomatous follicles by Glick et al. (1975). In the same study the morphological identity of FCC lymphomas, whether nodular or diffuse, was also observed. The ultrastructural similarity of normal follicular centers and nodular lymphomas also was reported by Levine and

Dorfman (1975). These studies confirm the views of Lennert (1973) and the original ultrastructural findings of Kojima et al. (1973) that nodular lymphomas consist of lymphomatous follicles.

The controversial nature of hairy cell leukemia seems to have been clarified by demonstrations of monoclonal surface immunoglobulin in the majority of cases we reported (Lukes and Collins, 1977; Lukes et al., 1978a, b, 1982, 1983) and by the observation of immunoglobulin synthesis following trypsinization by Dr. Collins' group.

In Hodgkin's disease the results of surface marker studies have provided further evidence in support of a possible T cell abnormality. A reduction in the number of T cells has been reported by a number of observers, but evidence has been reported by Fuks et al. (1976) of a serum factor that interferes with E rosette formation. The possibility of interference with T cell function by this serum factor has considerable potential significance.

## CLINICAL AND MORPHOLOGICAL CORRELATIONS

In the past the morphological types of malignant lymphomas and related leukemias included a number of cytological types as a result of the lack of precision in methodology. Homogeneous cell proliferations have now been recognized using the multiparameter approach, and a number of new clinical, morphological, immunological entities have emerged, such as the convoluted T cell type, the FCC types, and the immunoblastic sarcomas of both T and B cell types (Lukes and Collins, 1977). It is possible that there are as many as 9 or 10 entities presently included in malignant lymphomas. Unquestionably, the identification and investigation of homogeneous cell proliferations will permit an improved understanding of their biological character and an appreciation of their clinical expressions and therapeutic responsiveness that previously have been obscured in the heterogeneous groups.

The degree of aggressiveness of the T and B cell types can be related to their morphological features and presumed proliferative rates. The cytological types are arranged according to their aggressiveness in Table 10.3, together with their potential evolutionary changes. In general the small cells of both T and B cells are of limited aggressiveness, while the larger cells, the transformed lymphocytic types, are highly aggressive.

The change in the small cell types from the low aggressive to the highly aggressive expres-

sions occurs in varying frequency with the cytological types. This change, we believe, represents a "switch on" derepression) of the lymphocyte transformation mechanism. In the seven types included in the B cell groups, four are of limited aggressiveness (low turnover rate proliferations): the small B lymphocyte, the plasmacytoid lymphocyte, and the small and large cleaved FCC types. There are three highly aggressive (high turnover rate) proliferations: the small and large noncleaved (transformed) FCC types and immunoblastic sarcoma of B cells. Both the small and large cleaved FCC types commonly evolve into the highly aggressive proliferations of the noncleaved FCC type in the later phases of the disease after variable periods of time up to many years. The plasmacytoid lymphocytic type occasionally terminates as immunoblastic sarcoma of B cells, while the small B lymphocyte, including CLL, rarely evolves to immunoblastic sarcoma of B cells. In the past, the latter has been designated as the Richter syndrome. The degree of aggressiveness of the T cell types has not been established. In the cerebriform lymphocyte of Sézary's syndrome and mycosis fungoides, the limited aggressiveness of the prolonged earlier phases is well known and is associated predominantly with small cells. The later highly aggressive tumor phase is accompanied by either large cerebriform cells or large T cells. The convoluted

TABLE 10.3.
EVOLUTION OF CYTOLOGICAL TYPES OF MALIGNANT LYMPHOMA IN RELATIONSHIP TO AGGRESSIVENESS*

| Low Aggressiveness | High Aggressiveness |
|---|---|
| T cell types | Convoluted lymphocyte |
| Small lymphocyte | IBS (T cell) |
| Cerebriform lymphocyte | |
| Lymphoepithelioid cell | |
| B cell types | |
| Small lymphocyte ——— rare | IBS† (B cell) |
| Plasmacytoid lymphocyte | |
| (Myeloma) | |
| Small cleaved FCC ——— rare | Small noncleaved FCC |
| ——— common | Large noncleaved FCC |
| Large cleaved FCC | |

* The position of histiocytic lymphoma is unknown.
† Most cases of IBS (immunoblastic sarcoma) of B cell type evolve from previous non-neoplastic abnormal immune states.

T cell has a high turnover rate proliferation throughout its course. The full range of T cell expressions and the evolution of T cell immunoblastic sarcoma have yet to be elucidated. Successful therapy of the low aggressive types in our view depends to a large extent on prevention of the evolution to the highly aggressive types or prevention of the "switch on" (derepression) of the transformation mechanism.

Clinically, in our experience the low aggressive T and B cell types both have an insidious onset; are generally widespread when initially evaluated, apparently because of their noncohesive, mobile character; and have prolonged median survivals. The lymphoma of the small B lymphocyte, the prototype of the lymphomas of low aggressiveness, predominantly is expressed as CLL. The plasmacytoid lymphocytic lymphoma at times is associated with IgM gammopathy and Waldenström's syndrome, but occasionally it is associated with IgG gammopathy, commonly without any serum globulin abnormality (Levine et al., 1980). The small cleaved FCC type usually has a follicular pattern and presents with asymptomatic lymphadenopathy. On detailed clinical staging, over 70% of the cases have widespread disease involving bone marrow, spleen, and retroperitoneal nodes. The large cleaved FCC type has a follicular pattern of limited degree in approximately 50% of the cases, is often associated with a sclerosing component, and has a lower frequency of widespread disease. The large cleaved FCC lymphoma with sclerosis most commonly presents in the retroperitoneum, mesentery, and inguinal region and is widespread in less than half of the cases. The sclerosing lym-

phomas were initially described by Bennett and Millett (1969) in the retroperitoneum under the term *nodular sclerosing lymphosarcoma* as a slowly progressive process. The highly aggressive Burkitt's lymphoma of Africa and the American counterparts appear to be included in the small noncleaved FCC type and, on rare occasions, have a follicular pattern (Mann et al., 1976; Levine et al., 1983; Pavlova et al., 1984).

In American children from our experience, the proliferation is more variable but is of the small noncleaved FCC type and usually diffuse. Clinically, over 70% of the cases have an abdominal presentation, often in the terminal ileum or cecum or as a mesenteric or retroperitoneal mass. It is in dramatic contrast to the convoluted T cell type, the most common cytological type in this childhood case series, that presented primarily with either a mediastinal mass, peripheral lymphadenopathy, or a bone lesion. The large noncleaved FCC and the immunoblastic sarcoma of B cells are somewhat similar morphologically but usually present clinically in different situations. The large noncleaved FCC represents the later aggressive phase of the small cleaved FCC type and at times may be the initially observed presentation in lymph nodes, tonsils, or gastrointestinal tract. It may represent the initial site or a primary lymphoma in the tonsil or gastrointestinal tract and offers the opportunity for effective therapy, if observed sufficiently early. We have observed immunoblastic sarcoma of B cells, on the other hand, usually developing in a variety of abnormal immune states, including immunoblastic lymphadenopathy (Lukes and Tindle, 1975; Levine et al., 1981), systemic lupus erythematosus, immunosuppressed states for graft rejection, malabsorption disease, both alpha chain disease and sprue, in the thyroid in Hashimoto's disease, and Sjögren's syndrome (Lukes and Collins, 1974a, b, 1975). Senescence also appears to represent a failing or defective immune state. Immunoblastic sarcoma also is found at times with the plasmacytoid lymphocyte in Waldenström's macroglobulinemia, rarely with the small B lymphocytes associated with CLL, and on a few occasions in younger individuals without an apparent underlying immunological abnormality. Thus far, immunoblastic sarcoma of T cells has been preceded only occasionally by an abnormal immune state in our experience. The distinctiveness of immunoblastic sarcoma as a clinical morphological entity has been supported by Mathe and associates (1975).

Of the T cell types, the cerebriform lymphocytes of Sézary's syndrome and mycosis fungoides are well known clinically and generally accepted as T cell types. On the other hand, there is an insufficient number of cases of lymphoma of small T lymphocytes to define their clinical expressions with certainty, although there are suggestive features of their distinctiveness. The convoluted T cell lymphoma is the prototype of the new emerging entities and was previously included in ALL or one of several types of the lymphomas depending upon the initial clinical manifestations and the available material for diagnosis. The process principally is observed in children and, more commonly, in teenagers. It presents with a prominent mediastinal mass in over half the cases but at times with lymphadenopathy and bone lesions or a diffusely leukemic marrow (Barcos and Lukes, 1975; Stein et al., 1976). The initial presentation often is outside of the marrow, such as a mediastinal mass or lymphadenopathy, and involves the marrow in a leukemic fashion during relapse. In our original study both lymphoid masses and leukemic marrows were observed at times in individual cases and demonstrated the potential for both lymphoma and leukemic expressions (Barcos and Lukes, 1975). For this reason, we regard the convoluted T cell as a lymphoma-leukemic process. In our experience the convoluted T cell process dramatically responds to ALL therapy, but it relapses generally within 6 months. The central nervous system commonly is involved either initially or at relapse. The L-asparagine dependence of T cell ALL reported by Ohnuma et al. (1976) demonstrates the distinctive biological characteristic of this T cell neoplasm that in our view interrelates closely with the convoluted T cell type.

The clinical expressions of the new histiocytic lymphoma defined as a macrophage by enzymatic studies are uncertain since only a small number of cases have been identified.

Comparison of our cytological types of the functional classification with those of the classification of Rappaport in terms of clinical pathological correlations demonstrates that most of the emerging entities were lost in the heterogeneous cytological types of Rappaport. The classification of Rappaport et al. (1956) is based essentially on cell size and the potential of each cytological type to occur in either nodular or diffuse histological forms. The nodular proliferations have been demonstrated to be lymphomatous follicles (Jaffe et al., 1974), FCC types (Glick et al., 1975; Leech et al., 1975; Lukes and Collins, 1977) and heterogeneous cytological types (Lukes and Collins, 1977). The prognostic significance in our view relates to the behavior of the FCC types. For example, the small T and B lymphocytes and the plasmacytoid lymphocytic type were included in the well differentiated lymphocytic type. The histiocytic type of Rappaport included the large cleaved FCC, the large noncleaved FCC type, the immunoblastic sarcomas of both B and T cell types, as well as the new histiocytic lymphoma. The convoluted lymphocytic lymphoma apparently was classified variably as either the undifferentiated type or the poorly differentiated lymphocytic diffuse type. When nodular, the poorly differentiated lymphocytic type appears to be essentially similar to the small cleaved FCC type, as do many of the mixed nodular types. The diffuse poorly differentiated lymphocytic and mixed types, however, are of variable composition.

In Hodgkin's disease the correlation of clinical features and the histological types is generally well known (Lukes et al., 1966a). There are three distinctive entities—lymphocyte predominance, lymphocyte depletion, and nodular sclerosis. Lymphocyte predominance is observed principally in asymptomatic males in clinical stage I with disease presenting most commonly in the upper cervical region. The median survival is prolonged, and there is an excellent chance of cure. Lymphocyte depletion presents a contrasting type, occurring in older males with symptomatic febrile disease, often with pancytopenia and lymphocytopenia, and disease principally in abdominal lymph nodes, spleen, liver, and bone marrow. The median survival is 4 months, and response to therapy generally is poor (Neiman et al., 1973). Nodular sclerosis predominantly occurs in younger individuals, and there is a definite sex association since the majority of women exhibit the nodular sclerosing type. It also has a regional association with the mediastinum, even though it may be observed initially in any stage. Those patients with disease of limited extent have a prolonged median survival and an excellent opportunity for cure.

## WORKING FORMULATION FOR PATHOLOGY OF NON-HODGKIN'S LYMPHOMAS

The proposal of our functional approach evoked a rash of new classifications as indicated earlier and led to considerable confusion in the minds of clinicians regarding the most appropriate classification for clinical usage and therapy protocol studies. An international study supported by the National Cancer Institute on over 1000 cases was proposed to test the effectiveness of the six classifications. The design of the study and the results of the morphological and clinical studies have been reported in considerable detail (Rosenberg et al., 1982). In Table 10.4 the relationship between the working formulation and Lukes-Collins classification is shown. Comparison of the cytological designation in the working formulation and those of the Lukes-Collins classification reveals that many of the cytological terms are essentially identical. Malignant lymphoma, mixed follicular, and mixed diffuse are included in the working formulation and are likely to be troublesome diagnostic areas. The inherent difficulty in defining the morphological criteria and the resultant heterogeneity in the case populations included under these terms will produce confusion. It is unfortunate also that there was reluctance to include T and B cell designations because it was intended as a morphological basis for diagnosis. With the dramatic development in the effectiveness of monoclonal antibodies, particularly in the immunoperoxidase-labeled form on both frozen and paraffin sections, it appears that the working formulation is already outmoded.

## SUMMARY

1. The non-Hodgkin's lymphomas of past decades have been involved in terminological and conceptual disputes with lack of progress. By comparison, advances in pathology and therapy of Hodgkin's disease have been dramatic.

2. Recently we outlined a functional approach for the malignant lymphomas with the goal of relating these disorders to the T and B cell systems and alterations in lymphocyte transformation. Five general groups were proposed: (*a*) U cell (undefined); (*b*) T cell; (*c*) B cell, including the FCC types; (*d*) histiocytic; and (*e*) cell of uncertain origin—Hodgkin's disease.

3. A multiparameter investigative approach—including special morphology, cytochemistry, electron microscopy, immunological surface marker, in vitro, and immunoperoxidase techniques—has been employed in the redefinition of these disorders according to the T and B cell systems. The results of a number of studies including our own reveal that the majority mark as T or B cells with the exception of a portion of ALL and the rare true histiocytic type. Our studies indicate that the majority of lymphomas previously regarded as reticulum cell sarcoma or histiocytic lymphoma involve transformed lymphocytes with the exception of the true histiocytic type. Of major importance is the predictive nature of the morphological types, but it is dependent upon excellent histological material and an experienced observer.

4. The results of the functional studies demonstrate the heterogeneity of the histological types of the past, including the histiocytic type and the diffuse types of Rappaport and ALL of childhood. A number of homogeneous cytological types have been identified and are emerging as clinical, morphological, immunological entities, such as the convoluted T cell lymphoma-leukemia that interrelates with T cell ALL, the plasmacytoid lymphocyte type often associated with dysglobulinemias of various types, the cerebriform type associated with Sézary's syndrome and mycosis fungoides, the FCC types, and immunoblastic sarcoma of B cells that commonly develops in abnormal immune disorders. In Hodgkin's disease the long suspected immunological abnormality has been related to decreased numbers of T cells in the peripheral blood and to a recently identified serum factor that interferes with E rosette formation.

5. The implications of the functional approach, both immediate and future, are important and far reaching. Use of the new approach by pathologists will require a change in the collection and processing of biopsy material to

TABLE 10.4.

A WORKING FORMULATION OF NON-HODGKIN'S LYMPHOMAS FOR CLINICAL USAGE (AND EQUIVALENT OR RELATED TERMS IN THE LUKES-COLLINS CLASSIFICATION)

| Working Formulation | Lukes-Collins Equivalent or Related Terms |
| --- | --- |
| Low grade | Low grade |
| A. Malignant lymphoma | ML* small B or T lymphocyte (CLL) |
|     Small lymphocytic | ML plasmacytoid lymphocytic (B cell) |
|       consistent with CLL | |
|       plasmacytoid | |
| B. Malignant lymphoma, follicular | ML small cleaved FCC, follicular (B cell) |
|     Predominantly small cleaved cell | |
|       diffuse areas | |
|       sclerosis | |
| C. Malignant lymphoma, follicular | ML small cleaved FCC, follicular (B cell) |
|     Mixed, small cleaved and large cell | ML large cleaved FCC, follicular (B cell) |
|       diffuse areas | |
|       sclerosis | |
| Intermediate grade | Intermediate grade |
| D. Malignant lymphoma, follicular | |
|     Predominantly large cell | |
|       diffuse areas | ML large cleaved FCC, follicular (B cell) |
|       sclerosis | ML large noncleaved FCC, follicular (B cell) with or without sclerosis |
| E. Malignant lymphoma, diffuse | |
|     Small cleaved cell | |
|       sclerosis | ML small cleaved FCC, diffuse (B cell) |
| F. Malignant lymphoma, diffuse | |
|     Mixed, small and large cell | ML large cleaved FCC, diffuse (B cell) |
|       sclerosis | ML lymphoepithelioid cell (T cell) |
|       epithelioid cell component | ML immunoblastic sarcoma (T cell) |
| G. Malignant lymphoma, diffuse | |
|     Large cell | ML large noncleaved FCC, diffuse (B cell) |
|       cleaved cell | |
|       noncleaved cell | |
|       sclerosis | |
| High grade | High grade |
| H. Malignant lymphoma | |
|     Large cell, immunoblastic | |
|       plasmacytoid | ML immunoblastic sarcoma (B cell) |
|       clear cell | ML immunoblastic sarcoma (T cell) |
|       polymorphous | |
|       epithelioid cell component | Lymphoepithelioid cell lymphoma with immunoblastic sarcoma T cell type |
| I. Malignant lymphoma | ML convoluted T cell |
|     Lymphoblastic | |
|       convoluted cell | |
|       nonconvoluted cell | |
| J. Malignant lymphoma | |
|     Small noncleaved cell | |
|       Burkitt's | ML small noncleaved FCC, diffuse or follicular |
|       follicular areas | Burkitt or non-Burkitt types |
| Miscellaneous | |
|   Composite | |
|   Mycosis fungoides or Sézary's syndrome | Cerebriform lymphocyte (T cell) |
|   Histiocytic | ML true histiocytic plasmacytoma |
|   Extramedullary plasmacytoma | |
|   Unclassifiable | |
|   Other | |

\* ML, malignant lymphoma; FCC, follicular center cell.

achieve the excellent cytological detail required for evaluation. Acquisition of considerable experience with proven cases of new cytological types will be necessary for effective application. The use of a broad spectrum of immunoperoxidase-labeled monoclonal antibodies and antibodies for immunoglobulin light and heavy chains and histiocyte enzymes has extended the capability of pathologists to characterize the nature and function of cells in the hematopoietic system. Application of a battery of these antibodies in the investigation of ALL has confirmed the heterogeneity of ALL and demonstrated the need for such studies in precisely diagnosing these disorders.

6. Relating the malignant lymphomas to modern immunology and the resultant establishment of homogeneous cytological types will permit reliable investigation of the basic biological mechanism of these disorders and ultimately the design of fundamental biological approaches to their therapy.

# REFERENCES

Aisenberg AC, Long JC: Lymphocyte surface characteristics in malignant lymphoma. *Am J Med* 58:300–306, 1975.

Barcos MP, Lukes RJ: Malignant lymphoma of convoluted lymphocytes: a new entity of possible T-cell type. In: *Conflicts in Childhood Cancer*. New York, Alan R Liss, 1975, pp 147–178.

Bennett MH: Sclerosis in non-Hodgkin's lymphomata. *Br J Cancer* 31 (suppl II):44–52, 1975.

Bennett MH, Millett YL: Nodular sclerotic lymphosarcoma: a possible new clinico-pathological entity. *Clin Radiol* 20:339–343, 1969.

Bennett MH, Farrer-Brown G, Henry K, Jelliffe AM: Classification of non-Hodgkin's lymphomas. *Lancet* 2:405, 1974.

Bennett MH, Tu A, Hudson GV: Analysis of grade 1 Hodgkin's disease (report no. 6). Parts 1 and 2. *Clin Radiol* 32:491–498, 1981.

Bernard C, O'Connor GT, Thomas LB, Torloni J: Histopathologic definition of Burkitt's tumor. *Bull WHO* 40:601–607, 1969.

Bernard CW, Gallo RC, Jaffe E, Green I, Devita VT: Current concepts of leukemia and lymphoma: etiology, pathogenesis and therapy. *Ann Intern Med* 85:351–366, 1976.

Braylan RC, Jaffe ES, Berard CW: Malignant lymphomas: current classification and new observations. In Sommers SC (ed): *Hematologic and Lymphoid Pathology Decennial 1966–1975*. New York, Appleton-Century-Crofts, 1975.

Broder S, Edelson RL, Lutzner MA, Nelson DL, MacDermott RP, Durm ME, Goldman CK, Meade BD, Waldmann TA: The Sézary syndrome—a malignant proliferation of helper T cells. *J Clin Invest* 58:1297–1306, 1976.

Brouet J, Flandrin G, Seligmann M: Thymus-derived nature of the proliferating cells in Sézary's syndrome. *N Engl J Med* 289:341–344, 1973.

Brouet J, LaBaume S, Seligmann M: Evaluation of T and B lymphocyte membrane markers in human non-Hodgkin's malignant lymphomas. *Br J Cancer* 31 (suppl II):121–127, 1975.

Catovsky D, Galetto J, Okos A, Milliani E, Galton DAG: Cytochemical profile of B and T leukaemic lymphocytes with special reference to acute lymphoblastic leukaemia. *J Clin Pathol* 27:767–771, 1974.

Collins RD, Lukes RJ: Studies on possible derivation of some malignant lymphomas from follicular center cells. *Am J Pathol* 62:62a, 1971.

Davey FR, Goldberg J, Stockman J, Gottlieb AJ: Immunologic and cytochemical cell markers in non-Hodgkin's lymphomas. *Lab Invest* 35:430–438, 1976.

Dorfman RF: Classification of non-Hodgkin's lymphomas. Lancet 1:1295, 1974.

Dutcher TF, Fahey JL: The histopathology of the macroglobulinemia of Waldenström. *J Natl Cancer Inst* 22:887–916, 1959.

Epstein AL, Kaplan HS: Biology of the human malignant lymphomas. I. Establishment in continuous cell culture and heterotransplantation of diffuse histiocytic lymphomas. *Cancer* 34:1851–1872, 1974.

Fuks Z, Strober S, Kaplan HS: Interaction between serum factors and T lymphocytes in Hodgkin's disease. Use as a diagnostic test. *N Engl J Med* 295:1273–1278, 1976.

Gajl-Peczalska KJ, Bloomfield CD, Coccia PF, Sosin H, Bruning RD, Kersey JH: B and T cell lymphomas. *Am J Med* 59:674–685, 1975.

Gall EA: The reticulum cell, the cytological identity and interrelation of mesenchymal cells of lymphoid tissue. *Ann NY Acad Sci* 73:120, 1958.

Gerard-Marchant R, Hamlin I, Lennert K, Rilke F, Stansfeld AG, Van Unnik JAM: Classification of non-Hodgkin's lymphomas. *Lancet* 2:406, 1974.

Glick AD, Leech JH, Waldron JA, Flexnder JM, Horn RG, Collins RD: Malignant lymphomas of follicular center cell origin in man. II. Ultrastructural and cytochemical studies. *J Natl Cancer Inst* 54:23–36, 1975.

Green I, Jaffe E, Shevach EM, Edelson RL, Frank MM, Berard CW: Determination of the origin of malignant reticular cells by the use of surface membrane markers. In Rebuck JW, Berard CW (eds): *The Reticuloendothelial System*. Baltimore, Williams & Wilkins, 1975, pp 282–300.

Haegert DG, Stuart J, Smith JL: Acute lymphoblastic leukaemia: a heterogeneous disease. *Br Med J* 1:312–315, 1975.

Hansen JA, Good RA: Malignant disease of the lymphoid system in immunologic perspective. *Hum Pathol* 5:567–599, 1974.

Jaffe ES, Shevach EM, Frank MM, Berard CW, Green I: Nodular lymphoma—evidence for origin from follicular B lymphocytes. *N Engl J Med* 290:813–819, 1974.

Jondal M, Holm G, Wigzell H: Surface markers on human T and B lymphocytes. *J Exp Med* 136:207–215, 1972.

Jones SE, Fuks Z, Bull M, Kadin M, Dorfman RF, Kaplan HS, Rosenberg SA, Kim H: Non-Hodgkin's lymphomas. IV. Clinicopathologic correlation in 405 cases. *Cancer* 32:682–691, 1973.

Kersey JS, Sabad A, Gajl-Peczalska K: Acute lymphoblastic leukemic cells with T (thymus derived) lymphocyte markers. *Science* 182:1355–1356, 1973.

Kojima M, Tsunoda R: Localization of immunoglobulins in germinal centers of human tonsils. In Reichard SM,

Escobar MR, Friedman H (eds): *The Reticuloendothelial System in Health and Disease. Part B: Immunologic and Pathologic Aspects.* New York, Plenum Press, 1976, pp 77–86.

Kojima M, Imai Y, Mori N: A concept of follicular lymphoma. A proposal for the existence of a neoplasm originating from the germinal center. In Akazaki K (ed): *GANN Monograph on Cancer Research 15: Malignant Diseases of the Hematopoietic System.* Baltimore, University Park Press, 1973, p 195.

Kunkel HG: Surface markers of human lymphocytes. *Johns Hopkins Med J* 137:216–223, 1975.

Leech J, Glick A, Horn R, Collins R: Immunologic histochemical and ultrastructural studies of malignant lymphomas presumed to be of follicular center cell origin. *J Natl Cancer Inst* 54:11–21, 1975.

Lennert K: Follicular lymphoma. A tumor of the germinal centers. In Akazaki K (ed): *GANN Monograph on Cancer Research 15: Malignant Diseases of the Hematopoietic System.* Baltimore, University Park Press, 1973, p 217.

Lennert K, Mohri N, Stein H, Kaiserling E: Histopathology of malignant lymphomas. *Br J Haematol* 31:193–203, 1975.

Levine AM, Lichtenstein A, Gresik MV, Taylor CR, Feinstein DI, Lukes RJ: Clinical and immunologic spectrum of plasmacytoid lymphocytic lymphoma without serum monoclonal IgM. *Br J Haematol* 46:2799, 1980.

Levine A, Taylor CR, Schneider D, Koehler S, Forman S, Lichtenstein A, Lukes RJ, Feinstein D: Immunoblastic sarcoma of T-cell versus B-cell origin. I. Clinical features. *Blood* 58:52–61, 1981.

Levine AM, Pavlova Z, Pockros A, Teitelbaum A, Paganini-Hill A, Powars D, Lukes RJ, Feinstein DI: Small noncleaved follicular center cell lymphoma: Burkitt's and non-Burkitt variants in the United States. I. Clinical features. *Cancer* 52:1073–1079, 1983.

Levine GD, Dorfman RF: Nodular lymphoma: an ultrastructural study of its relationship to germinal centers and a correlation of light and electron microscopic findings. *Cancer* 35:148–164, 1975.

Lukes RJ: The pathological picture of the malignant lymphomas. In Zarafonetis CJD (ed): *Proceedings of the International Conference on Leukemia-Lymphoma.* Philadelphia, Lea & Febiger, 1968, pp 333–356.

Lukes RJ: Criteria for involvement of lymph node, bone marrow, spleen and liver in Hodgkin's disease. *Cancer Res* 31:1755–1767, 1971.

Lukes RJ, Collins RD: New observations on follicular lymphoma. In Akazaki K (ed): *GANN Monograph on Cancer Research 15: Malignant Diseases of the Hematopoietic System.* Baltimore, University Park Press, 1973, pp 209–215.

Lukes RJ, Collins RD: A functional approach to the classification of malignant lymphoma. *Recent Results Cancer Res* 46:18–30, 1974a.

Lukes RJ, Collins RD: Immunologic characterization of human malignant lymphomas. *Cancer* 34:1488–1503, 1974b.

Lukes RJ, Collins RD: New approaches to the classification of the lymphomata. *Br J Cancer* 31 (suppl II):1–28, 1975.

Lukes RJ, Collins RD: The Lukes-Collins classification and its significance. Conference on the Non-Hodgkin's Lymphomas, San Francisco, September 30-October 2, 1976. *Cancer Treat Rep* 61:971–979, 1977.

Lukes RJ, Tindle BH: Immunoblastic lymphadenopathy. A hyperimmune entity resembling Hodgkin's disease. *N Engl J Med* 292:1–8, 1975.

Lukes RJ, Butler JJ, Hicks EB: Natural history of Hodgkin's disease as related to its pathologic picture. *Cancer* 19:317–344, 1966a.

Lukes RJ, Craver LL, Hall TC, Rappaport H, Ruben P: Hodgkin's disease, report of Nomenclature Committee. *Cancer Res* 26:1311, 1966b.

Lukes RJ, Tindle BH, Parker JW: Reed-Sternberg-like cells in infectious mononucleosis. *Lancet* 2:1003–1004, 1969.

Lukes RJ, Taylor CR, Parker JW, Lincoln TL, Pattengale PK, Tindle BH: A morphologic and immunologic surface marker study of 299 cases of non-Hodgkin's lymphomas and related leukemias. *Am J Pathol* 90:461–486, 1978a.

Lukes RJ, Parker JW, Taylor CR, Tindle BH, Cramer AD, Lincoln TL: Immunologic approach to non-Hodgkin's lymphomas and related leukemias. Analysis of the results of multiparameter studies of 425 cases. *Semin Hematol* 15:322–351, 1978b.

Lukes RJ, Taylor CR, Parker JW: Immunological surface marker studies in the histopathological diagnosis of non-Hodgkin's lymphomas based on multiparameter studies of 790 cases. In: Rosenberg SA, Kaplan HS (eds): *Advances in Malignant Lymphomas: Etiology, Immunology, Pathology.* Bristol-Myers Cancer Symposia, vol 3. New York, Academic Press, 1982.

Lukes RJ, Taylor CR, Parker JW: Multiparameter studies in malignant lymphoma based on studies in 1186 cases. In: Mirand EA, Hutchinson WB, Mihich E (eds): *13th International Cancer Congress, Part E, Cancer Management.* New York, Alan R Liss, 1983.

Lutzner M, Edelson R, Schein P, Green I, Kirkpatrick C, Ahmed A: Cutaneous T cell lymphoma: the Sézary syndrome, mycosis fungoides and related disorders. *Ann Intern Med* 85:534–552, 1975.

Mann RB, Jaffe ES, Brylan RC, Nanba K, Frank MM, Ziegler JL, Berard CW: Non-endemic Burkitt's lymphoma. A B-cell tumor related to germinal centers. *N Engl J Med* 295:685–691, 1976.

Mathe G, Belpomme D, Dantchev D, Khalil A, Afifi AM, Taleb N, Pouillart P, Schwarzenberg L, Hayat M De Vassal F, Jasmin C, Misset JL, Musset M: Immunoblastic lymphosarcoma, a cytological and clinical entity? *Biomedicine* 22:473–488, 1975.

Nathwani BN, Kim H, Rappaport H: Malignant lymphoma, lymphoblastic. *Cancer* 38:964–983, 1976.

Neiman RS, Rosen PJ, Lukes RJ: Lymphocyte-depletion Hodgkin's disease. *N Engl J Med* 288:751–755, 1973.

Nossal GJV, Abbot A, Mitchell J, Lummus Z: Antigens in immunity. XV. Ultrastructural features of antigen capture in primary and secondary lymphoid follicles. *J Exp Med* 127:277–289, 1968.

O'Brien RO, Parker JW, Dixon JFP: Mechanisms of lymphocyte transformation. In Hahn F (ed): *Progress in Molecular and Subcellular Biology.* New York, Springer-Verlag, vol 6, 1977.

Ohnuma T, Orlowski M, Minowada J, Holland JF: Difference in amino acid metabolism of human T- and B-cells in culture. Presented at the Proceedings of the 16th International Congress of Hematology, Kyoto, Japan, September 5–11, 1976.

Rappaport H, Winter WJ, Hicks EB: Follicular lymphoma; re-evaluation of its position in the scheme of malignant lymphoma, based on survey of 253 cases. *Cancer* 9:792–821, 1956.

Rosas-Uribe A, Variakojis D, Molnar Z, Rappaport H: Mycosis fungoides: an ultrastructural study. *Cancer* 34:634–645, 1974.

Rosenberg S, Berard CW, Brown BW, Burke J, Dorfman RF, Glatstein E, Hoppe RT, Simon R, Henry K, Lennert K, Lukes RJ, O'Connor G, Rappaport H, Hartsock R, Kruger G, Nanba K, Robb-Smith AH, Sacks M, Banfi A, Bloomfield C, Bonadonna G, DeLellis R, DeVita VT, Frizzera G, Hu MS, Kaplan HS, Rilke F, Rosai J, Rudders RA, Warnke RA, Ziegler JL: Non-Hodgkin's lymphoma pathologic classification project. National Cancer Institute sponsored study of classifications of non-Hodgkin's lymphomas. *Cancer* 49:2112–2135, 1982.

Stein H, Peterson N, Gaedicke G, Lennert K, Landberg C: Lymphoblastic lymphoma of convoluted or acid phosphatase type—a tumor of T precursor cells. *Int J Cancer* 17:292–295, 1976.

Taylor CR: An immunohistological study of follicular lymphoma, reticulum cell sarcoma and Hodgkin's disease. *Eur J Cancer* 12:61–75, 1976.

Taylor CR, Mason DY: The immunohistological detection of intracellular immunoglobulin in formalin-paraffin sections from multiple myeloma and related conditions using the immunoperoxidase technique. *Clin Exp Immunol* 18:417–429, 1974.

Taylor CR, Parker JW, Pattengale PK, Lukes RJ: Malignant lymphomas: an exercise in immunopathology. In: Crowther DG (ed): *Advances in Medical Oncology.* Proceedings of the 12th International Cancer Congress, Buenos Aires, 1978. New York, Pergamon Press, 1979, pp 125–140.

Tindle BH, Parker JW, Lukes RJ: "Reed-Sternberg cells" in infectious mononucleosis? *Am J Clin Pathol* 58:607–617, 1972.

Yam LT, Li CY, Crosby WH: Cytochemical identification of monocytes and granulocytes. *Am J Clin Pathol* 55:283–290, 1971a.

Yam LT, Li CY, Lam KW: Tartrate resistant acid phosphatase isoenzyme in the reticulum cells of leukemic reticuloendotheliosis. *N Engl J Med* 284:357–360, 1971b.

# 11

# *Lymphoma of Abdomen and Retroperitoneum*

MELVIN E. CLOUSE, M.D.

## HISTORICAL BACKGROUND

### Hodgkin's Disease

Hodgkin's disease was first described in 1832 by Thomas Hodgkin in his paper "On Some Morbid Appearances of the Absorbent Glands and Spleen." Sir Samuel Wilks rediscovered Hodgkin's article and wrote about the disease in 1865, giving it the name Hodgkin's disease. Sternberg in 1898 and Reed in 1902 are credited with first describing the histopathology of Hodgkin's disease. In addition they reviewed the histology of Hodgkin's original patients of 1832, finding the multinucleated cell now called the *Reed-Sternberg cell.*

Histopathology classification of subtypes of Hodgkin's disease comprises four categories, each with its own cellular personality and clinical course (Lukes, 1963; Lukes and Butler, 1966; Lukes et al., 1966a, b). The *lymphocyte predominant* type, which is generally seen at an early stage in young, asymptomatic males, has the most favorable prognosis. Small lymphocytes constitute the most abundant cell form in the stroma, but overall the histiocytes may predominate. Reed-Sternberg cells may be so sparse as to make diagnosis difficult.

The *nodular sclerosing* type has a female predominance and a peak incidence in adolescence and young adulthood (Lukes, 1963; Lukes and Butler, 1966; Lukes et al., 1966a, b). As the description suggests, nodular areas of lymphatic tissue are encircled by large bands of collagenous tissue. These patients often present with stage II disease involving the mediastinum and supraclavicular areas. The prognosis is excellent in early stages of the disease.

The *mixed cellularity* type has a highly cellular and pleomorphic stroma. These patients often present with systemic symptoms. The prognosis is generally less favorable than it is for nodular sclerosing disease.

The *lymphocyte depletion* type is generally seen in older, more symptomatic patients with stage III or IV disease and poses the most unfavorable prognosis. Histologically, profound depletion of lymphocytes in the stroma may take the form of diffuse fibrosis or reticular changes. Both types of changes may occur in the same patient.

### Non-Hodgkin's Lymphoma

Historically, characterizations of the clinical, laboratory, and histopathological features of non-Hodgkin's lymphoma are also interesting. Brill et al. described follicular lymphoma in 1925, and Symmers independently described the same entity 2 yr later; hence the name Brill-Symmers disease. Reticulum cell sarcoma was described by Oberling in 1928. The entity now called Burkitt's lymphoma was described by Burkitt in 1958.

Follicular lymphoma and reticulum cell sarcoma are now considered forms of non-Hodgkin's lymphoma along with other malignant neoplasms of the immune system. Histopathology classifications for these diverse yet related entities include the Rappaport system, which is based on the degree of differentiation of the tumor and on the presence or absence of nodularity (Rappaport et al., 1956). The more recent Lukes and Collins (1977) classification is based on the cell of origin and characterizes the diseased cells of non-Hodgkin's lymphoma as T cells, B cells, histiocytic cells, and U cells (unclassifiable). This system is presented in detail in Chapter 10.

### Pathogenesis

Originally, Hodgkin's disease was considered a disorder of the entire lymphatic system with a multifocal origin and perhaps further extension by spread of a causative agent with de novo infection of disease in different sites. In 1966

Rosenberg and Kaplan proposed a new concept relating to the development of Hodgkin's disease that has become crucial in staging and treatment choice. Their *contiguity theory* was a great help in sweeping away earlier misconceptions concerning the apparently capricious distribution of lymph node involvement with Hodgkin's disease and made possible the systematic maps of disease sites.

The contiguity theory uses the existence of direct connections between pairs of lymph node chains to explain the spread of Hodgkin's disease. The disease metastasizes by movement of tumor cells from a diseased node to an adjacent node via lymphatic vessels. One possible exception to lymphatic spread of Hodgkin's disease occurs in the lymphocyte depletion type, in which vascular invasion and thus hematogenous spread may occur. The clinical tool for developing the contiguity theory, lymphography, became the gold standard for roentgenographic staging because it was the only nonoperative means for assessing the many lymph nodes below the diaphragm. The nodes above the cisterna chyli remained less accessible with images only from inferior vena cavography until the advent of ultrasound and computed tomography.

## Therapy

Although radiation therapy was given to patients with lymphosarcoma in 1902 by Pusey and Hodgkin's disease was treated with x-rays a few years after their discovery, modern radiotherapy for Hodgkin's disease began with the work of Gilbert (Gilbert and Babaiantz, 1931; Gilbert, 1939) and was refined by Kaplan (1962, 1966a, b) at Stanford. Chemotherapy began with the use of nitrogen mustards in 1946 and now includes a wide variety of agents. The most common drug combination was designated by the National Cancer Institute group as MOPP, which is nitrogen mustard, vincristine (Oncovin), procarbazine, and prednisone (DeVita et al., 1970). Using MOPP and high dose radiation after accurately staging and mapping the disease greatly increased survival with Hodgkin's disease, which was universally fatal before the days of specific therapy.

With use of megavoltage radiation and MOPP chemotherapy, present 5-yr and 10-yr survival rates for patients with Hodgkin's disease are 79% and 66%, respectively (Kaplan, 1980b). Importantly, relapses after the fourth or fifth year after treatment are almost nonexistent; most relapses (85%) occur within 3 yr. Patients are considered cured if they are relapse-free for 5 yr (Kaplan, 1980b). A survival analysis of 1225 patients treated between 1961–1977 related 5-yr and 10-yr survival rates to stage at time of diagnosis: for stage I, 90% and 79% survived for 5 and 10 yr, respectively; for stage II, 87% and 74% survived; for stage III, 74% and 57% survived; and for stage IV, 57% and 40% survived (Kaplan, 1980a).

## STAGING

The concept of staging Hodgkin's disease dates back to 1902 when Dorothy Reed described two stages of Hodgkin's disease. Several staging classifications have been proposed since then; the most recent is the classification adopted in Ann Arbor in 1971. This classification distinguishes between the clinical stage (CS)—based solely on limited biopsy, history, physical examination, laboratory radiographic tests, and radioisotope scans—and the pathological stage (PS)—based on anatomic evidence of the extent of disease from laparotomy, laparoscopy, splenectomy, liver biopsy, bone marrow biopsy, and other tissue biopsies (Carbone et al., 1971) (Table 11.1). Constitutional symptoms do not include malaise, fatigue, or pruritus, which are not specific, and do include those that are specific, such as weight loss, night sweats, and fever. Approximately 40% of new cases of malignant lymphoma are Hodgkin's disease and 60% are non-Hodgkin's lymphoma.

## CLINICAL ASSESSMENT

Staging generally begins with a detailed medical history and specific inquiry into systemic symptoms: weight loss of more than 10% of body weight during the preceding 6 months, fever, and night sweats. The lymph node enlargement that prompts the patient to seek care may be palpated in the cervical, submandibular, supraclavicular, axillary, and inguinal regions.

# IMAGING TECHNIQUES

## Chest X-ray and Conventional Tomography

Staging roentgenographically includes a chest radiograph and may include 55° oblique hilar tomography as well as thoracic computed tomography. The chest film has served well for evaluation of mediastinal nodes. Because few of the findings lead to modification of the treatment plan in Hodgkin's disease, full lung tomography is not routinely performed (Castellino et al., 1976). At our institution computed tomography (CT) is performed to evaluate the mediastinum and lungs when there is an equivocal abnormality on the plain film or patients have bulk mediastinal adenopathy requiring precise definition of disease extent.

TABLE 11.1.
CLINICAL STAGING OF LYMPHOMA*

| Category | Description |
| --- | --- |
| Stage I | Involvement of a single lymph node region (I) or of a single extralymphatic organ or site ($I_E$) |
| Stage II | Involvement of two or more lymph node regions (number to be stated) on the same side of the diaphragm (II) or localized involvement of an extralymphatic organ or site of one or more lymph node regions on the same side of the diaphragm ($II_E$) |
| Stage III | Involvement of lymph node regions on both sides of the diaphragm (III) that may also be accompanied by localized involvement of an extralymphatic organ or site ($III_E$) or by involvement of the spleen ($III_S$) or both ($III_{E+S}$) |
| Stage IV | Diffuse or disseminated involvement of one or more extralymphatic organs or tissues with or without associated lymph node enlargement. The reason for classifying the patients as stage IV is identified further by specifying sites according to the following notations: |
| | Pulmonary - PUL   Bone Marrow - MAR |
| | Osseous - OSS   Pleura - PLE |
| | Hepatic - HEP   Skin - SKI |
| | Brain - BRA   Eye - EYE |
| | Lymph Nodes - LYM   Other - OTH |
| Systemic Symptoms | Stage may be subdivided, A for those without defined general symptoms or B for those with general symptoms: |
| | Unexplained loss of over 10% of body weight in previous 6 months |
| | Unexplained fever (> 38°C) |
| | Night sweats |

* Adapted from Carbone et al. (1971).

## Urography

Intravenous pyelography has a low yield of positive results but is routinely included as a roentgenographic staging procedure to demonstrate the anatomy of the urinary system and identify pathology that might demand immediate therapy.

## Inferior Venacavography

Ultrasonography and CT have replaced inferior venacavography as an imaging method in most centers. In its day, cavography was used to demonstrate enlarged lymph nodes high in the para-aortic chain above the cisterna chyli, where lymphography cannot examine adequately. After its introduction in 1959 by Helander and Lindbom, cavography was used in the 1960s by Schwarz et al. (1965), Davidson and Clarke (1968), and DeRoo and van Voorthuisen (1966). The method was evaluated more recently in papers by Pillari (1977) and Resegotti et al. (1983). Most of these papers emphasize the usefulness of cavography, but Schwarz et al. (1965) demonstrated nodal involvement as evidenced by impression into the cava in only 27% of positive cases.

## Radionuclide Studies

Gallium-67 citrate is distributed throughout the body and may be taken up in unexpected sites. In its day, this radiopharmaceutical detected 43% of unsuspected disease sites (Greenlaw et al., 1974; Johnston et al., 1974, 1977). Gallium has been used to detect new sites for biopsy and to measure response to therapy (Higasi and Nakayama, 1972; Henkin et al., 1974; Andrews and Edwards, 1975).

The initial enthusiasm for 67-gallium citrate imaging has waned considerably, however, and it is now used in only a few medical centers. The isotope is relatively expensive, and the procedure is time consuming, requiring scanning over a 72-hr period. Repeated cathartics are needed to cleanse the colon of residual activity, an uncomfortable practice for patients causing poor acceptance. The variable sensitivity of gallium-67 citrate precludes its use for initial detection of patients or as the single test for staging lymphoma (McCaffrey et al., 1976; Potsaid and McKusick, 1977). A thorough review of [67]Ga-citrate is presented by McKusick in Chapter 3.

## Ultrasonography

The enthusiasm for ultrasonic evaluation of the retroperitoneal area has largely diminished because of the advent of CT and the disadvantages of ultrasonography, which is extremely dependent upon the operator and does not give as good global anatomy as CT. In addition, ultrasound is absorbed by gas and bone, causing a large number of retroperitoneal studies (approximately 30% at our institution) to be unsatisfactory. On the other hand, ultrasound is less costly and requires a shorter examination time than CT. It is an excellent modality for studying the superior mesenteric, celiac, portal, and splenic hilar nodes. On balance, however, we no longer use ultrasound in clinical staging of lymphoma.

# LYMPHOGRAPHY

Lymphography has always been highly accurate because it produces direct images of the lymph nodes. The method is useful in directing the surgeon to abnormal or suspicious nodes in order to maximize the value of nodal biopsies at laparotomy and is therefore useful in stages I and II. Its role in patients with widespread disease has always been less clear and is much more so with the advent of CT and ultrasonography. Delineation of extensive retroperitoneal disease or field size for radiation therapy and evaluating response to therapy can now be done by these less invasive modalities. Because lymphographic findings rarely affect therapy for stage III or IV patients, this examination is not usually performed in these Hodgkin's patients. Lymphography is also rarely performed in patients with non-Hodgkin's lymphoma (who do not routinely undergo open abdominal biopsy regardless of the stage).

## Interpretation

Lymphographic criteria for lymphomatous involvement of nodes are generally described as a foamy, lacy, or reticular appearance, which describes the pattern of contrast material filling of the sinusoids displaced by tumor tissue throughout the node. Takahashi and Abrams (1967) quantified the roentgen findings by separating normal from abnormal lymph nodes and defining a structure for evaluating lymph nodes rather than a gestalt type of evaluation. In their grades of foaminess, zero represents the appearance of normal nodes; grade I represents replacement by tumor of up to 33% of the node; grade II represents tumor replacement of up to 66% of the node; and grade III represents greater than two-thirds replacement of the node (Fig. 11.1).

Their criteria also include evaluation for displacement of the node from the lumbar vertebrae. In the lateral view, nodes displaced by greater than 3 cm from the anterior aspect of the lumbar vertebrae are considered abnormal as are those displaced by greater than 2 cm from the lateral aspect of the vertebral body in the frontal view (Fig. 11.2). The uncoiled aorta may drag the nodes laterally, producing a false abnormality because the nodes are in intimate contact with the aorta. Hence caution is advisable in evaluating the position of the nodes in reference to the lumbar vertebrae.

The vascular phase must be evaluated with the nodal phase, especially in solid tumor metastasis, because diseased nodes may be completely replaced by tumor and have obstructed channels. This abnormality will be missed if only the nodal phase is assessed. The vascular phase is less important when evaluating patients with lymphoma because the disease seldom completely obstructs the lymph channels. Lymphaticovenous communications must be sought for they have been associated with a poor prognosis, presumably because of hematogenous spread of the disease (Roxin and Bujar, 1970).

## Pitfalls

Early microscopic disease cannot be detected with lymphography. In addition, benign changes such as reactive hyperplasia may be difficult to differentiate from malignant disease on the lymphograms. It is for these reasons that the rate of false-positive studies exceeds the rate of false-negative studies in most series. In a group of patients examined at the Brigham and Women's Hospital and New England Deaconess Hospital in Boston, there were 16 false-positive and 3 false-negative interpretations. This yielded a true-positive ratio of 95% and a false-positive ratio of 23% with an overall accuracy of 85% (Hessel et al., 1977).

The relative incidence of false-positive and false-negative diagnoses depends on how strictly one applies criteria for abnormality and how frequently one undercalls or overcalls the disease. Applying their criteria strictly, Takahashi and Abrams (1967) were able to achieve an 81%

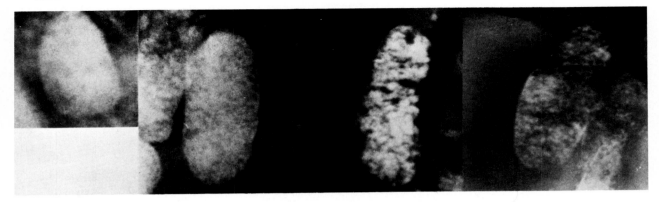

FIGURE 11.1. STANDARD ROENTGENOGRAMS SHOWING FOAMINESS
From left to right: grade 0, grade 1, grade 2, and grade 3.

accuracy in interpreting 206 lymphangiograms for lymphoma. The reported accuracies of lymphography in other series have ranged from 54% (Alcorn et al., 1977) to over 90% (Castellino et al., 1974; Castellino, 1982). Castellino and Marglin (1981) report a sensitivity of 94% and a specificity of 91% with an overall accuracy of 92% in 390 previously untreated patients with Hodgkin's disease. Sensitivity, specificity, and overall accuracy in 209 patients with non-Hodgkin's lymphoma were 88%, 87%, and 88%, respectively. In a more recent study of lymphography at New England Deaconess Hospital and Nassau County Hospital, the sensitivity and specificity were 95% and 89% for 54 patients with Hodgkin's disease and 70% and 100% for 18 patients with non-Hodgkin's lymphoma (Clouse et al., 1985) (Table 11.2).

## COMPUTED TOMOGRAPHY

CT overcomes many of the disadvantages of ultrasound. It gives excellent global anatomy, it is not operator-dependent, and the images are largely not obscured by gas in the bowel or overlying bony structures. The study is also not affected by body habitus or size. Careful interpretation is imperative. When there is not sufficient retroperitoneal fat to contrast with the soft tissue densities of enlarged nodes, ultrasound is superior to CT evaluation. Otherwise, CT is the method of choice for evaluating the retroperitoneal area as well as the superior mesenteric, celiac, portal and splenic hilar nodes.

### Technique

CT staging of patients with biopsy-proven lymphoma is generally performed by scanning the abdomen from the xiphoid to the symphysis pubis at 2-cm intervals with additional scans at intervening 1-cm intervals in any questionable areas. The slice thickness is 1 cm. Oral contrast material is given prior to scanning to opacify the entire bowel and thus to avoid confusing loops of bowel with enlarged nodes. Intravenous contrast material is given when necessary to opacify mesenteric vessels as well as the inferior vena cava.

### Normal

Normal unopacified nodes often can be seen on CT scans, especially in the retroperitoneal and retrocrural areas and occasionally in the pelvis. They appear as soft tissue densities ranging in size from 3–10 mm. The internal architecture of lymph nodes cannot be evaluated with current CT units, and it is doubtful that CT will ever be able to reveal the internal architecture. On the transaxial anatomic sections, nodes completely encircle the aorta as well as the inferior vena cava. In the pelvis, lymphatic channels and vessels lie adjacent to and encompass the iliac vessels. Normal celiac and mesenteric nodes as well as splenic hilar and portal hilar nodes cannot be separated from adjacent vessels. The distribution of retroperitoneal and pelvic nodes is shown in Figures 11.3 and 11.6.

The para-aortic and caval nodes surround the inferior vena cava and aorta. The external iliac nodes follow the course of the external and common iliac arteries and lie deep in the pelvis

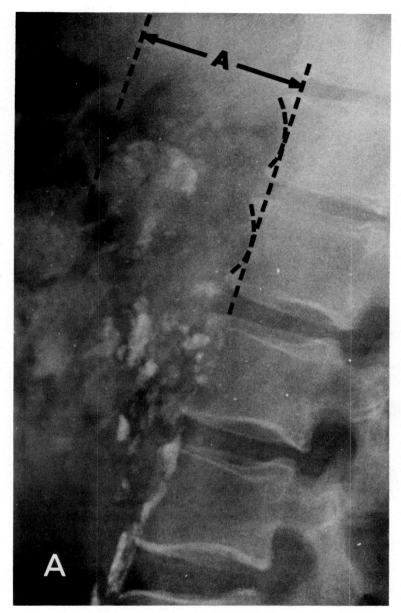

FIGURE 11.2. MEASUREMENT OF LATERAL SPINE TO NODE DISTANCE

*A*: Measurement *A* in this case of Hodgkin's disease is 5.5 cm. The upper limit of normal is 3 cm. If the lateral film had been omitted, correct evaluation of this proven case would have been difficult. *B*: Spine to node distances. The right lateral spine to node distance (measurement *B*) is from the right lateral border of a lumbar vertebral body in its midportion to the most lateral border of the right paracaval node group. In this case, it measures 2.5 cm and is beyond the normal limits of 2 cm. The left lateral spine to node distance (measurement *C*) is the same measurement on the left side. In this case it is within the normal range, measuring 1.8 cm.

adjacent to the obturator internus muscle. The obturator node, a member of the medial chain of the external iliac group of nodes, is located just above the inguinal ligament and medial to the obturator internus muscle (Fig. 11.3). External iliac nodes are frequently confused with internal iliac nodes because of the position deep within the pelvis (Fig. 11.6).

**Abnormal**

Identification of abnormal lymph nodes by CT is based upon recognition of nodal enlargement,

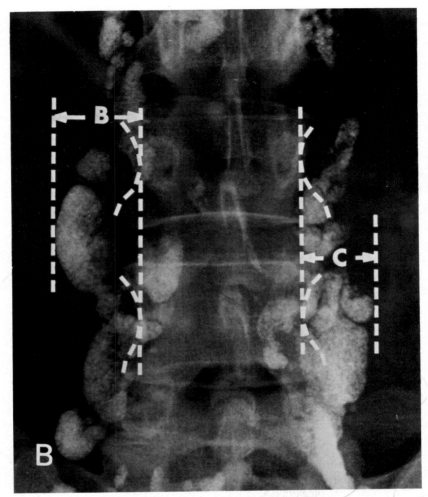

FIGURE 11.2*B.*

TABLE 11.2.
EFFICACY ANALYSES OF LYMPHANGIOGRAPHY, ULTRASONOGRAPHY, AND CT

| Analysis | Lymphangiography | Ultrasonography | CT |
|---|---|---|---|
| Hodgkin's disease | | | |
|   True-positive ratio (sensitivity)* | 95% (18/19) | 30% (3/10) | 36% (5/14) |
|   True-negative ratio: (specificity)† | 89% (31/35) | 100% (17/17) | 91% (21/23) |
|   Overall accuracy‡ | 91% (49/54) | 74% (20/27) | 70% (26/37) |
|   Accuracy of + study§ | 92% (18/22) | 100% (3/3) | 71% (5/7) |
|   Accuracy of − study¶ | 97% (31/32) | 71% (17/24) | 70% (21/30) |
| Non-Hodgkin's lymphoma | | | |
|   True-positive ratio (sensitivity)* | 70% (7/10) | 40% (4/10) | |
|   True-negative ratio (specificity)† | 100% (8/8) | 100% (8/8) | |
|   Overall accuracy‡ | 83% (15/18) | 67% (12/18) | |
|   Accuracy of + study§ | 100% (7/7) | 100% (4/4) | |
|   Accuracy of − study¶ | 73% (8/11) | 57% (8/14) | |

  * Sensitivity: the number of truly positive interpretations divided by the total number of positive cases.

  † Specificity: the number of truly negative interpretations divided by the total number of negative cases.

  ‡ Overall accuracy: the number of imaging studies that were correctly interpreted divided by the total number of studies.

  § Accuracy of positive interpretations: the number of studies correctly interpreted as positive divided by the total number of positive interpretations.

  ¶ Accuracy of negative interpretations: the number of studies correctly interpreted as negative divided by the total number of negative interpretations.

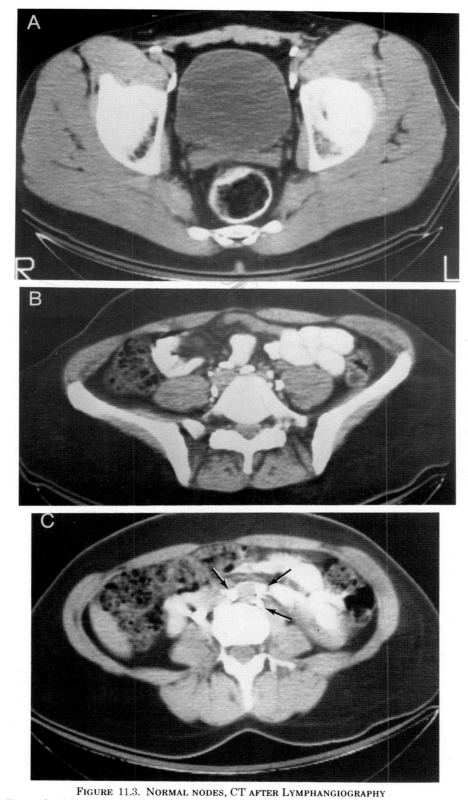

FIGURE 11.3. NORMAL NODES, CT AFTER LYMPHANGIOGRAPHY

*A*: External iliac nodes (obturator) just above inguinal ligament with iliac artery and vein. *B*: Common iliac nodes just below caval and aortic bifurcation. *C*: Para-aortic nodes (*arrows*).

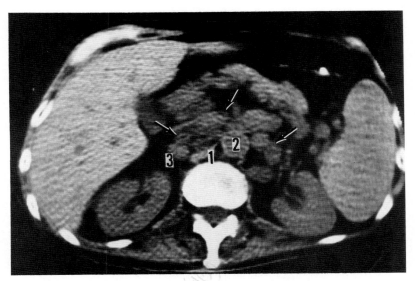

FIGURE 11.4. LYMPHOSARCOMA IN A 63-YR-OLD MALE
Note the peripancreatic adenopathy (*arrows*) with compressed cava (*1*), aorta (*2*), and duodenum (*3*).

which may occur with displacement or obliteration of normal retroperitoneal architecture.
Nodes may vary from a number of isolated enlarged nodes to a large homogeneous mass of
nodes with obliteration of the normal structural
contours and no delineation of individual nodes
(Fig. 11.4). Massive enlargement in the retroaortic and caval areas may completely obliterate the
aorta and cava as well as the mesenteric vessels
(Fig. 11.5*A* and *B*). Mueller et al. (1980) have
described the ultrasonic appearance of the so-
called sandwich sign, an echogenic area of fat
and the superior mesenteric artery sandwiched
between echolucent planes of enlarged nodes.
The sandwich appearance is less distinct on CT.
Generally enlarged masses of nodes have the
density of soft tissues and are located in the
mesentery or mesenteric root (Fig. 11.5*C*).

Lymph nodes below 1.5 cm in diameter were
once considered normal and those above 1.5–2
cm abnormal. Now nodes 1–2 cm are considered
suspicious and those greater than 2 cm definitely
abnormal. Enlargement to greater than 3 cm is
rarely due to reactive hyperplasia. Accommoda-
tions of general guidelines should be made for
node clusters, anatomic area of interest, and age.
As a general rule, the fewer the nodes in a chain,
the larger will be the individual nodes; and conversely, the greater the number of nodes, the
smaller will be each individual node. Thus, a
cluster of nodes 1 cm or greater in size is probably
diseased, whereas an isolated node 1–2 cm in size
should be considered only suspicious (Fig. 11.6).
Also, the inguinal nodes are usually larger than
the iliac nodes, and the iliac nodes are larger

than the para-aortic nodes. The inguinal nodes
may be 1–2 cm in diameter at lymphangiography
due to magnification and filling with contrast
material. The high para-aortic and retrocrural
nodes normally are small aggregates of lymphatic
tissue 1–3 mm in diameter. Lymph nodes in the
retrocrural space are now considered abnormal
if they exceed 6 mm in size (Callen et al., 1977)
(Fig. 11.7).

Like lymphography, CT cannot differentiate
between benign and malignant causes for lymph
node enlargement. Lymph node enlargements
secondary to hyperplasia or granulomatous disease cannot be differentiated from lymphoma.
Other entities such as retroperitoneal fibrosis or
a leaking aortic aneurysm with a large amount
of fibrosis show findings similar to lymphoma.
Other pitfalls for interpreting the CT scan include a large right crus of the diaphragm, which
can be delineated with contiguous slices, an enlarged left gonadal vein, and a double inferior
vena cava coupled with an unopacified loop of
small bowel (Fig. 11.8). All of these presentations
can be evaluated, and pitfalls can be avoided
with forethought of normal anatomy in conjunction with intravenous contrast material.

## Evaluation of Spleen

Splenic involvement by Hodgkin's disease affects stage, prognosis and therapy, and it is the
only identified infradiaphragmatic site of disease
in 8–14% of patients (Desser and Ultmann,
1973). It is perhaps one of the initial abdominal
organs involved with subsequent spread to con-

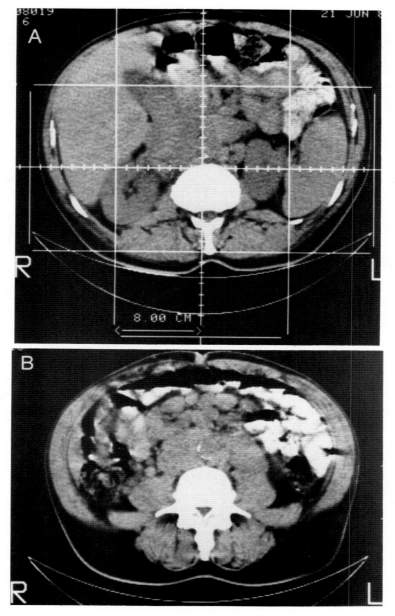

FIGURE 11.5. MASSIVE NODE ENLARGEMENT IN HISTIOCYTIC LYMPHOMA

*A*: Mesenteric nodal enlargement. *B*: Obliteration of aortocaval outlines. *C*: Obliteration of superior mesenteric artery and vein by massive mesenteric adenopathy.

tiguous lymph nodes and the liver. Hepatic involvement without concomitant involvement of the spleen is rare (Rosenberg, 1971; Hessel et al., 1977).

There has never been a good clinical method for evaluating splenic involvement by lymphoma. To date, the data do not indicate that a significant advance has been made even with CT. Blackledge et al. (1980) were able to detect

only 4 of 24 positive spleens in a series of 136 patients with biopsy-proven Hodgkin's disease. Breiman et al. (1978) detected nodular defects greater than 9 mm in diameter in five spleens found to contain lymphomatous nodules histologically but failed to detect nodules less than 9 mm in diameter in five others. Redman et al. (1977) were able to demonstrate splenic parenchymal involvement if the nodules were at least

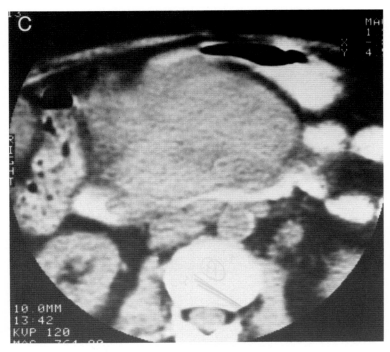

FIGURE 11.5C.

1 cm in diameter. The tumor nodules throughout the spleens in their patients were 1–25 mm in diameter (Fig. 11.9).

### Evaluation of Kidneys and Gastrointestinal Tract

Patients with newly diagnosed Hodgkin's disease seldom have involvement of the kidney or gastrointestinal tract. In contrast, the incidence of kidney and gastrointestinal involvement in newly diagnosed patients with non-Hodgkin's lymphoma has been reported to be 3% and 15%, respectively (Goffinet et al., 1977). In such patients CT scanning of the kidneys may reveal multiple masses of low attenuation value and possibly consequent diffuse enlargement of the entire kidney, reducing function and distorting the collecting system (Fig. 11.10). The kidney may be diffusely infiltrated, and encasement of the renal pelves may obstruct the ureters.

Involvement of the stomach with lymphoma can present as an isolated exophytic mass within the lumen or may cause diffuse thickening throughout the gastric wall (Fig. 11.11). Hodgkin's disease of the small bowel may present with a constricting lesion seen on a small bowel examination. Non-Hodgkin's lymphoma generally produces an aneurysmal appearance with a mass completely encircling the lumen and may show large masses in the mesentery displacing the loops of bowel (Fig. 11.12).

## ACCURACY STUDIES

When evaluating the sensitivity and specificity of diagnostic tests for lymphoma, the applications and usefulness of the test should be evaluated in reference to the disease characteristics one expects to find at initial presentation and should not include a large number of previously treated patients who are clinically known to have stage III or IV disease. In a series of 814 previously untreated patients with Hodgkin's disease, Kaplan (1980a) found that 9.5% were stage I, 47% stage II, 34% stage III, and 9.5% stage IV. In addition, retroperitoneal involvement by Hodgkin's disease tended to occur in a random, nonbulky distribution involving approximately 24% of the patients. Mesenteric nodes were involved in 5%, and the splenic hilum in 28%. In addition, the spleen was diseased in approximately 35% of the patients, the liver in 8%, and the bone marrow in 3%.

The frequency of positive lymphangiograms in

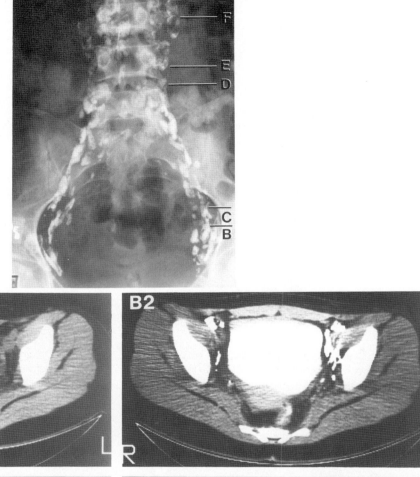

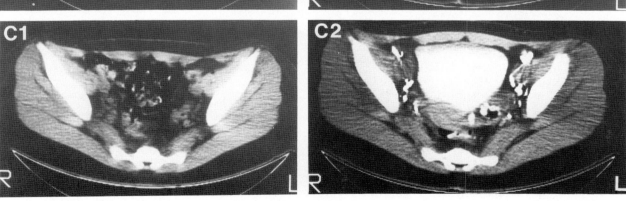

FIGURE 11.6. MIXED CELLULARITY HODGKIN'S DISEASE, CLINICAL STAGE IIA PRIOR TO LYMPHANGIOGRAPHY AND CT
A: Lymphogram reveals abnormal para-aortic nodes. Note the multiple filling defects. The letters on the lymphangiogram indicate the levels of the CT cuts in the rest of this figure. The CT scans were taken before and after lymphangiography for comparison of node size and number. B and C: CT scans show that the external iliac nodes are normal in size but slightly abnormal in texture. These nodes have grade 1 foaminess on the lymphangiogram. D and E: Common iliac nodes at the aorticocaval bifurcation are abnormal in number on these CT scans. The lymphangiogram shows grade 1 foaminess for these nodes. F: Para-aortic nodes at L3 show grade 2-3 foaminess and abnormal number but not abnormal size on the CT scan. G: Para-aortic nodes at the lower border of L2 show grade 1-2 foaminess on the lymphangiogram but are abnormal in number but not size on the CT scans.

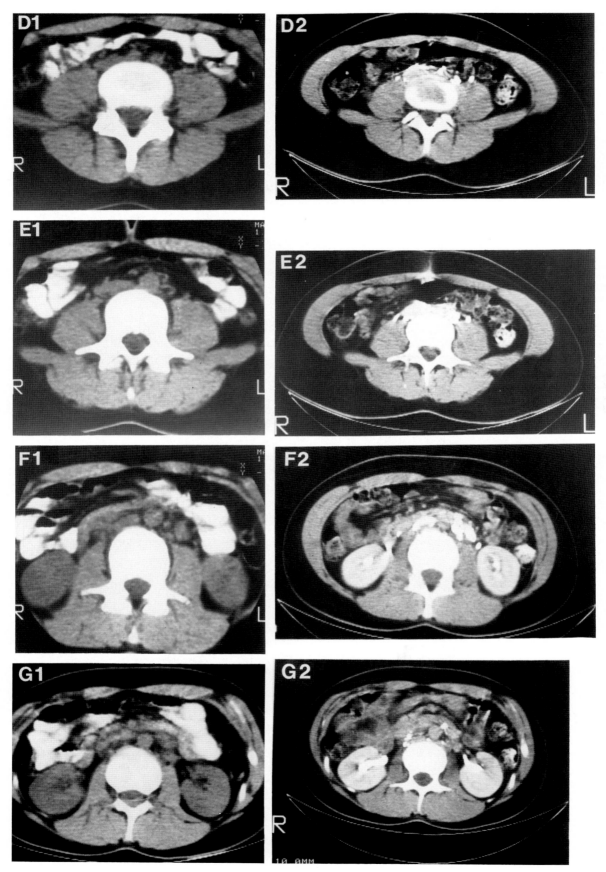

Figure 11.6*D–G*.

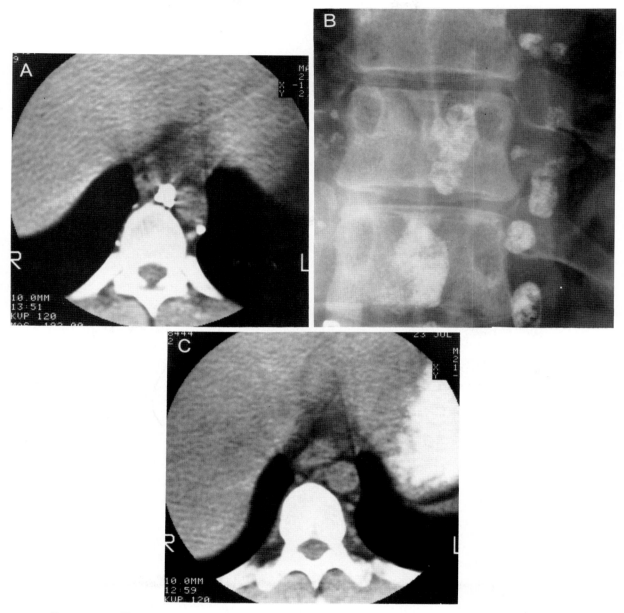

FIGURE 11.7.  NODULAR SCLEROSING HODGKIN'S DISEASE IN LEFT CERVICAL NODES OF A 22-YR-OLD MALE
*A*: CT scan taken before lymphography shows multiple retrocrural nodes 3–7 mm in diameter. *B*: These nodes are shown to be abnormal in architecture by lymphography. *C*: Repeat CT after lymphography shows increase in size of retrocrural node to 2 cm after contrast injection.

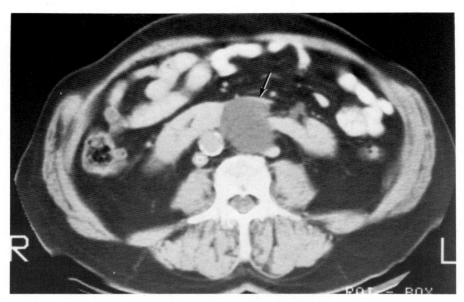

FIGURE 11.8. CT SCAN OF HORSESHOE KIDNEY
Note the cyst over the spine (*arrow*) and the double inferior vena cava filled with contrast material.

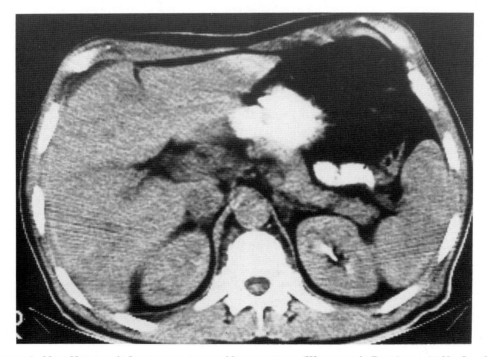

FIGURE 11.9. NON-HODGKIN'S LYMPHOMA OF THE NASOPHARYNX (WALDEYER'S RING) IN A 64-YR-OLD MALE
This abdominal CT scan shows lymphomatous involvement characterized by multiple large low density areas in the liver and spleen.

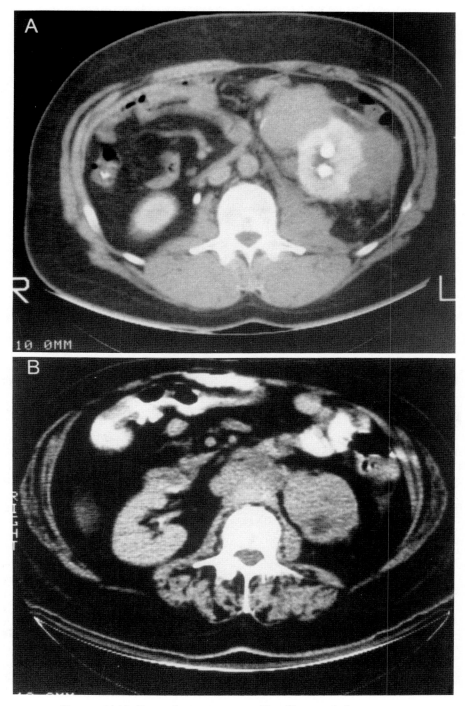

FIGURE 11.10. RENAL INVOLVEMENT IN NON-HODGKIN'S LYMPHOMA

*A*: Complete encasement of the left kidney by tumor. *B*: Low density mass in left kidney. *C*: Multiple low density masses throughout both kidneys.

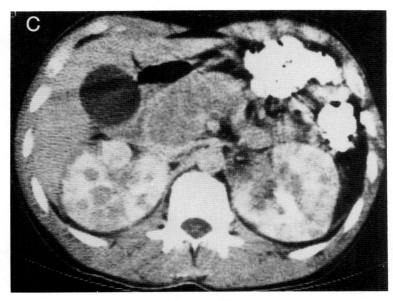

FIGURE 11.10C.

patients initially presenting with Hodgkin's disease also varies with the cell type. Nodular sclerosing, which largely involves the mediastinum, shows a positivity rate of only 26%, whereas lymphocyte-predominant, lymphocyte-depleted, and mixed cellularity show a positivity rate of 58–67% (Hessel et al., 1977). Lymphangiograms in 100 consecutive patients who subsequently had a laparotomy showed nodal involvement in 40% of the patients with left supraclavicular node involvement versus only 8% with right-sided cervical or supraclavicular adenopathy (Kaplan, 1976).

In contrast, non-Hodgkin's lymphoma causes para-aortic, mesenteric, and splenic hilar involvement in 60–70% of the patients with nodular lymphoma (Castellino and Marglin, 1981; Castellino et al., 1980a, b). In diffuse lymphocytic and histiocytic lymphoma, the para-aortic nodes will be involved in 25% of patients and the splenic hilar and mesenteric nodes in 42% and 27%, respectively (Mitchell et al., 1972; Ferguson et al., 1973; Goffinet et al., 1977; Redman et al., 1977; Castellino et al., 1980a, b; Kaplan, 1980a). Also, non-Hodgkin's lymphoma tends to cause large bulky disease diffusely and will often involve all of the retroperitoneal nodes as well as mesenteric nodes.

One would expect that ultrasound as well as CT would be very effective in imaging non-Hodgkin's lymphoma, hence greater sensitivity and specificity than lymphangiography. Conversely, lymphangiography should be more accurate than CT and ultrasound for Hodgkin's disease because the nodes in Hodgkin's disease may be normal to slightly enlarged in size even when the architecture is abnormal and because there is random involvement throughout the retroperitoneum, making detection by CT and ultrasound more difficult.

Any evaluation of accuracy when comparing the various modalities must therefore consider the stages and types of disease included: Are all patients stages I–IV included? Are Hodgkin's disease and non-Hodgkin's disease analyzed together or separately? Accuracy figures for any imaging modality will be higher if clinical stage III and IV patients are included and if the majority of patients have non-Hodgkin's lymphoma rather than Hodgkin's disease. Since 1977 a body of literature has developed comparing CT with lymphography. Unfortunately, in most papers the clinical stage is not specified, and data on Hodgkin's and non-Hodgkin's patients are not presented separately (Table 11.3).

Several interesting papers do specify clinical stage and analyze Hodgkin's disease and non-Hodgkin's lymphoma separately, however (Alcorn et al., 1977; Breiman et al., 1978; Castellino, 1982). Accuracy for lymphography varies in the literature (54–96%), but the range for CT is relatively small (70–83%). Accuracy undoubtedly reflects expertise in performing and interpreting the studies as well as the intrinsic capacity of the test. The reported accuracy of CT for Hodgkin's disease seems surprisingly high, even in

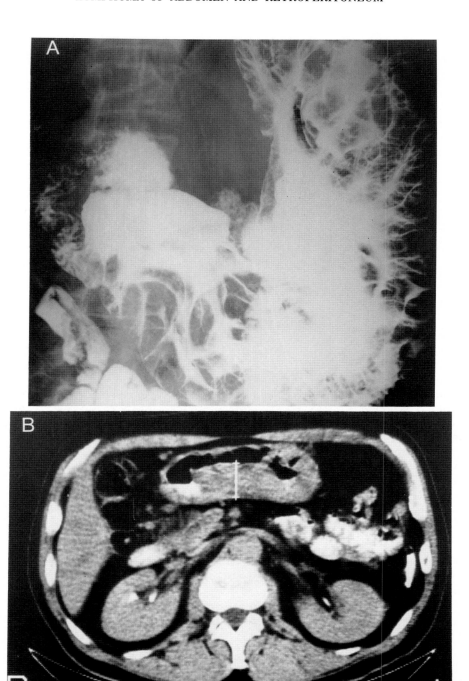

FIGURE 11.11. LYMPHOSARCOMA TREATED 4 YR PREVIOUSLY
This 64-yr-old male presented with gastric recurrence. *A*: Upper gastrointestinal series. *B*: CT scan showing markedly thickened gastric wall.

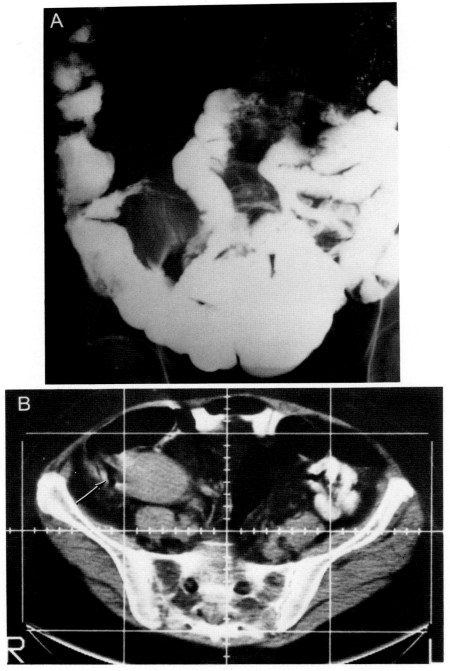

FIGURE 11.12. RIGHT LOWER QUADRANT PAIN AND RECTAL BLEEDING REQUIRING 4 UNITS OF BLOOD IN A 68-YR-OLD FEMALE

*A*: Small bowel shows a mass narrowing and compressing the distal ileum. *B*: CT scan shows mass surrounding and displacing the distal ileum (*arrow*).

TABLE 11.3.
SENSITIVITY, SPECIFICITY, AND ACCURACY OF IMAGING TECHNIQUES IN LYMPHOMA: A REVIEW OF THE LITERATURE*

| Reference | No. Cases Subgroups | Stage | Study | Sensitivity: TP Ratio | | Specificity: TN Ratio | | Accuracy | |
|---|---|---|---|---|---|---|---|---|---|
| Alcorn et al. (1977) | 4 NHL | I-II | CT | 2/4 | 50% | 9/12 | 75% | 11/16 | 69% |
| | 12 HD | Clinical | LAG | 2/3 | 66% | 5/10 | 50% | 7/13 | 54% |
| Best et al. (1978) | 48 HD | Not | CT | 11/11 | 100% | 45/45 | 100% | 56/56 | 100% |
| | 8 NHL | specified | LAG | 9/11 | 82% | 45/45 | 100% | 54/56 | 96% |
| Blackledge et al. (1980) | 76 HD | Not specificied | CT | 10/14 | 71% | 42/62 | 68% | 52/76 | 68% |
| Brascho et al. (1977) | 17 NHL | Not | US | 25/25 | 100% | 24/31 | 77% | 49/56 | 87% |
| | 39 HD | specified | LAG | | | | | 24/33 | 73% |
| Breiman et al. (1978) | 6 NHL | I-II | CT | 6/6 | 100% | 8/10 | 80% | 14/16 | 87% |
| | 12 HD | Clinical | LAG | 6/6 | 100% | 10/10 | 100% | 16/16 | 100% |
| Castellino (1982) | 53 HD | I-II | CT | 10/13 | 77% | 34/40 | 85% | 44/53 | 83% |
| | 52 HD | | LAG | 11/13 | 85% | 39/39 | 100% | 50/52 | 96% |
| Johnston et al. (1977) | 149 HD | Mixed | LAG | 29/64 | 45% | 60/72 | 83% | 89/136 | 65% |
| | sites | | NM | 37/60 | 62% | 57/64 | 89% | 94/124 | 76% |
| Magnusson et al. (1982) | 7 HD | Not | CT | 1/3 | 33% | 6/6 | 100% | 7/9 | 78% |
| | 2 NHL | specified | | | | | | | |
| | 40 HD | Not | LAG | 5/7 | 71% | 24/35 | 68% | 29/42 | 69% |
| | 2 NHL | specified | | | | | | | |
| Redman et al. (1977) | 23 | I-II | CT | 8/9 | 89% | 12/14 | 86% | 20/23 | 87% |
| | | Clinical | LAG | 9/9 | 100% | 13/14 | 93% | 22/23 | 96% |
| Rochester et al. (1977) | 16 | Not | US | 4/6 | 67% | 9/10 | 90% | 13/16 | 81% |
| | 6 | specified | LAG | 0/1 | 0% | 4/5 | 80% | 4/6 | 67% |
| Zelch and Haaga (1979) | 20 | Not | CT | 8/10 | 80% | 9/10 | 90% | 17/20 | 85% |
| | 20 | specified | LAG | 7/10 | 70% | 9/10 | 90% | 16/20 | 80% |
| Totals† | 137 | | CT | 56/70 | 80% | 165/199 | 83% | 221/269 | 82% |
| | 72 | | US | 29/31 | 94% | 33/41 | 80% | 62/72 | 86% |
| | 205 | | LAG | 49/60 | 82% | 149/168 | 89% | 222/261 | 85% |

* NHL, non-Hodgkin's lymphoma; HD, Hodgkin's disease; CT, computed tomography; LAG, lymphangiography; NM, $^{67}$Ga-citrate; US, ultrasonography.

† None of the sensitivity, specificity, or accuracy scores is significantly different ($p < 0.05$; chi square) from the others.

experienced hands, since involvement as seen by lymphography is random and since diseased nodes may be less than 1–2 cm in diameter (Figs. 11.13 and 11.14). With CT sections at 2-cm intervals, small nodes could be missed or even if imaged would be less than the 2 cm size required for abnormality in most areas. The deficits of CT are probably not as critical as the fact that all nodes in a specific area are not opacified with lymphography. The extent of disease is underestimated by lymphography, whereas by CT all nodes in a section are imaged, and if any nodal mass is larger than 2 cm, the study is positive (Figs. 11.6 and 11.13).

Regardless of the reasons, if the accuracy for CT in evaluating Hodgkin's and non-Hodgkin's lymphoma is 83–85% and if the accuracy for lymphography is no greater, one could substitute CT for lymphography in the staging of lymphomas. For those centers where lymphography is performed and interpreted well, however, lymphography has a definite advantage: it is 95–96% accurate.

## IMAGING WORK-UP

The algorithm for work-up of Hodgkin's lymphoma includes physical examination and routine roentgenographic studies followed by bone marrow biopsy. If the bone marrow is positive for Hodgkin's lymphoma, the patient is considered pathological stage IV and a baseline CT is performed prior to therapy. For Hodgkin's patients who are considered to be stage I or II, CT is performed for evaluation of the liver, spleen, and lymph node areas above the cisterna chyli in addition to the para-aortic nodes. Lymphography is performed primarily to assess the ret-

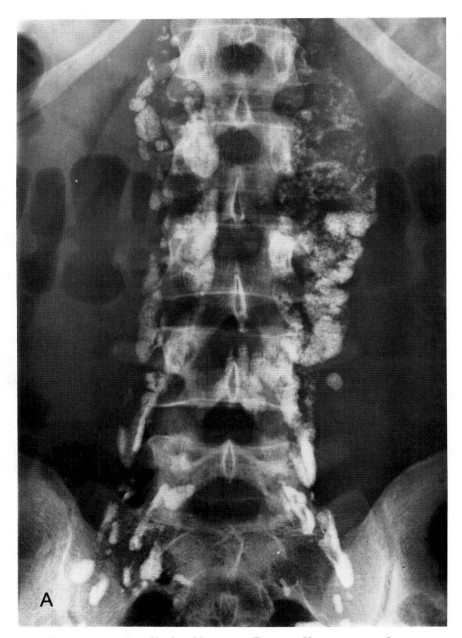

FIGURE 11.13. A 22-YR-OLD MALE WITH FEVER OF UNDETERMINED ORIGIN
*A*: LAG shows abnormal left para-aortic nodes. *B*: CT after LAG shows contrast medium in normal-sized nodes and many nodes without contrast that are smaller than 1 cm. The total nodal mass is greater than 2 cm in diameter, however.

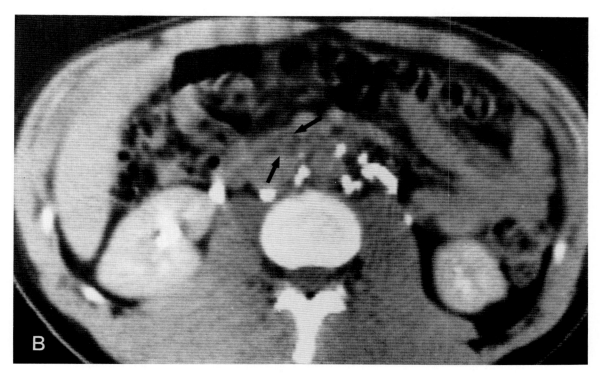

FIGURE 11.13*B*.

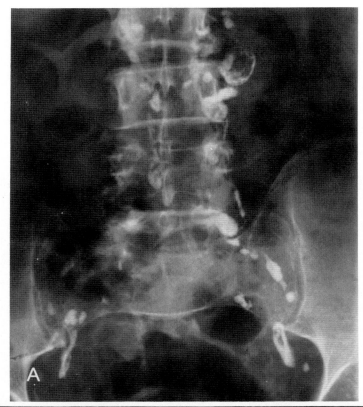

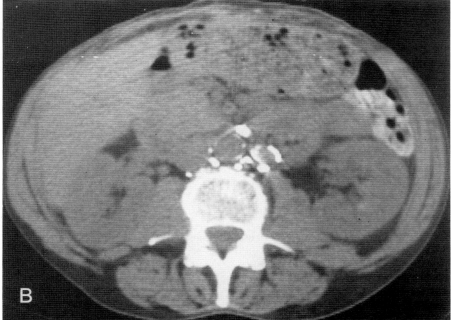

FIGURE 11.14. STAGE IIIB HODGKIN'S DISEASE IN A 62-YR-OLD MAN

The original CT study was interpreted as negative because fat planes were not visible in the retroperitoneum. *A*: LAG shows one abnormal node almost completely replaced by tumor, 1.2 cm in diameter, in left para-aortic area. *B*: CT after LAG shows the same abnormal node.

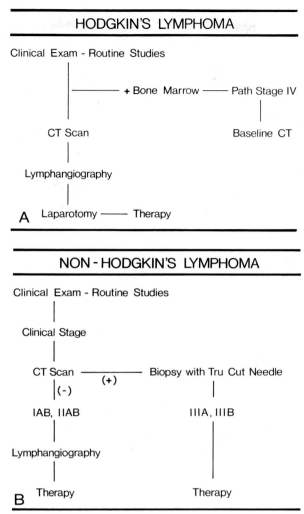

FIGURE 11.15. IMAGING WORK-UP *A*: Hodgkin's disease. *B*: Non-Hodgkin's lymphoma.

roperitoneal nodes as a guide to operative staging and follow-up examination. If CT is positive, lymphography may not be performed, although it is still performed at our institution even when disease is found by CT. After a staging laparotomy with specific sampling of all lymph node areas, including a splenectomy with thorough examination of the spleen at 1-cm intervals, the patient is referred for therapy. Ultrasonography, gallium scanning, and inferior venacavography are not part of our staging algorithm.

The work-up of non-Hodgkin's lymphoma includes clinical examination and routine labora-tory studies as well as CT (Fig. 11.15). Although a case can be made for not performing lymphography in non-Hodgkin's lymphoma because only about 10% of the patients are truly stage I or II at presentation, lymphography should be performed on those patients who have negative CT scans and no other evidence of stage III or IV disease. When the CT scans are positive, a biopsy is made of the retroperitoneal nodes under CT control with a true-cut needle. Inferior venacav-ography, ultrasonography, and gallium scanning are not used in the staging of patients with non-Hodgkin's lymphoma.

## REFERENCES

Alcorn FS, Mategrano VC, Petasnick JP, Clark JW: Contri-butions of computed tomography in the staging and management of malignant lymphoma. *Radiology* 125:717, 1977.

Andrews GA, Edwards CL. Tumor scanning with gallium 67. *JAMA* 233:1100, 1975.

Best JJK, Blackledge G, Forbes WStC, Todd IDH, Eddleston B, Crowther D, Isherwood I: Computed tomography of abdomen in staging and clinical management of lymphoma. *Br Med J* 2:1675, 1978.

Blackledge G, Best JJK, Crowther D, Isherwood I. Computed tomography (CT) in the staging of patients with Hodgkin's disease: a report on 136 patients. *Clin Radiol* 31:143, 1980.

Brascho DJ, Durant JR, Green LE: The accuracy of retroperitoneal ultrasonography in Hodgkin's disease and non-Hodgkin's lymphoma. *Radiology* 125:485, 1977.

Breiman RS, Castellino RA, Harell GS, Marshall WH, Glatstein E, Kaplan HS: CT-pathologic correlations in Hodgkin's disease and non-Hodgkin's lymphoma. *Radiology* 126:159, 1978.

Brill NE, Baehr G, Rosenthal N: Generalized giant lymph follicle hyperplasia of lymph nodes and spleen. A hitherto undescribed type. *JAMA* 84:668, 1925.

Burkitt D: A sarcoma involving the jaws in African children. *Br J Surg* 46:218, 1958.

Callen PW, Korobkin M, Isherwood I: Computed tomographic evaluation of the retrocrural prevertebral space. *AJR* 129:907, 1977.

Carbone PP, Kaplan HS, Musshoff K, Smithers DW, Tubiana M: Report of the committee on Hodgkin's disease staging classification. *Cancer Res* 31:1860, 1971.

Castellino RA: Imaging techniques for staging abdominal Hodgkin's disease. *Cancer Treat Rep* 66:697, 1982.

Castellino RA, Marglin SI: Lymphographic accuracy in 599 consecutive, previously untreated patients with Hodgkin's disease and non-Hodgkin's lymphoma. In Weissleder H, Bartoš V, Clodius L, Málek P (eds): *Progress in Lymphology*, Proceedings of the VII International Congress of Lymphology, Florence, 1979. Prague, Avicenum, Czechoslovak Medical Press, 1981, p 317.

Castellino RA, Billingham M, Dorfman RF: Lymphographic accuracy in Hodgkin's disease and malignant lymphoma with a note on the "reactive" lymph node as a cause of most false-positive lymphograms. *Invest Radiol* 9:155, 1974.

Castellino RA, Filly R, Blank N: Routine full-lung tomography in the initial staging and treatment planning of patients with Hodgkin's disease and non-Hodgkin's lymphoma. *Cancer* 38:1130, 1976.

Castellino RA, Marglin S, Blank N: Lymphoma and leukemia in the retroperitoneum. *Semin Roentgenol* 15:80, 1980a.

Castellino RA, Maylin S, Blank N: Lymphoma and leukemia in the retroperitoneum. In Felson B (ed): *Roentgenology of the Lymphomas and Leukemias*. New York, Grune & Stratton, 1980b, p 80.

Clouse ME, Harrison D, Grassi CJ, Costello PC, Edwards SA, Wheeler HG: Lymphangiography, ultrasonography, and computed tomography in Hodgkin's disease and non-Hodgkin's lymphoma. *J Comput Tomogr* 9:1–8, 1985.

Davidson JW, Clarke EA: Influence of modern radiological technique on clinical staging of malignant lymphomas. *Can Med Assoc J* 99:1196, 1968.

DeRoo T, van Voorthuisen AE: The indications for selective supplementary angiographic examination in lymphography. *Radiology* 97:957, 1966.

Desser RK, Ultmann JE: Staging of Hodgkin's disease and lymphoma. *Med Clin North Am* 57:479, 1973.

DeVita VT Jr, Serpick A, Carbone PP: Combination chemotherapy in the treatment of advanced Hodgkin's disease. *Ann Intern Med* 73:881, 1970.

Edwards CL, Hayes RL: Tumor scanning with 67-gallium citrate. *J Nucl Med* 10:103, 1969.

Ferguson DJ, Allen LW, Griem ML, Morgan EM, Rappaport H, Ultmann JE: Surgical experience with staging laparotomy in 125 patients with lymphoma. *Arch Intern Med* 131:356, 1973.

Gilbert R: Radiotherapy in Hodgkin's disease (malignant granulomatosis): anatomic and clinical foundations; governing principles; results. *AJR* 41:198, 1939.

Gilbert R, Babaiantz L: Notre methode de roentgentherapie de la lymphogranulomatse (Hodgkin): Resultats eloignes. *Acta Radiol* 12:523, 1931.

Goffinet DR, Warnke R, Dunnick NR, Castellino R, Glatstein EJ, Nelson TS, Dorfman RF, Rosenberg SA, Kaplan HS: Clinical and surgical (laparotomy) evaluation of patients with non-Hodgkin's lymphomas. *Cancer Treat Rep* 61:981, 1977.

Greenlaw RH, Weinstein MB, Brill AB, McBain JK, Murphy L, Kniseley RM: $^{67}$Ga-citrate imaging in untreated Hodgkin's disease. Preliminary report of cooperative group. *J Nucl Med* 15:404, 1974.

Helander CG, Lindbom A: Venography of the inferior vena cava. *Acta Radiol* 52:257, 1959.

Henkin RE, Polcyn RE, Quinn JL III: Scanning-treated Hodgkin's disease with $^{67}$Ga-citrate. *Radiology* 110:151, 1974.

Hessel SJ, Adams DF, Abrams HL: Lymphography in lymphoma. In Clouse ME (ed): *Clinical Lymphography*. Baltimore, Williams & Wilkins, 1977.

Higasi T, Nakayama Y: Clinical evaluation of $^{67}$Ga-citrate scanning. *J Nucl Med* 13:196, 1972.

Hodgkin TH: On some morbid appearances of the absorbent glands and spleen. *Med-Chir Trans* 17:68, 1832.

Johnston GS, Benua RS, Teates CD, Edwards CL, Kniseley RM: $^{67}$Ga-citrate imaging in untreated Hodgkin's disease. Preliminary report of Cooperative Group. *J Nucl Med* 15:399, 1974.

Johnston GS, Go MF, Benua RS, Larson SM, Andrews GA, Huber KF: Gallium-67 citrate imaging in Hodgkin's disease: final report of Cooperative Group. *J Nucl Med* 18:692–698, 1977.

Kaplan HS: The radical radiotherapy of regionally localized Hodgkin's disease. *Radiology* 78:553, 1962.

Kaplan HS: Evidence for a tumoricidal dose in the radiotherapy of Hodgkin's disease. *Cancer Res* 26:1221, 1966a.

Kaplan HS: Role of invasive radiotherapy in the management of Hodgkin's disease. *Cancer* 19:356, 1966b.

Kaplan HS: Hodgkin's disease and other human malignant lymphomas: advances and prospects. G.H.A. Clowes Memorial Lecture. *Cancer Res* 36:3863, 1976.

Kaplan HS: *Hodgkin's disease*, ed 2. Cambridge, Harvard University Press, 1980a.

Kaplan HS: Hodgkin's disease: unfolding concepts concerning its nature, management and prognosis. *Cancer* 45:2439, 1980b.

Lukes RJ: Relationship of histological features to clinical stages in Hodgkin's disease. *AJR* 90:944, 1963.

Lukes RJ, Butler JJ: The pathology and nomenclature of Hodgkin's disease. *Cancer Res* 26:1063, 1966.

Lukes RJ, Collins RD: The Lukes-Collins classification and its significance. Conference on the Non-Hodgkin's Lymphomas, San Francisco, Sept 30–Oct 2, 1976. *Cancer Treat Rep* 61:971, 1977.

Lukes RJ, Butler JJ, Hicks EB: Natural history of Hodgkin's disease as related to its pathological picture. *Cancer* 19:317, 1966a.

Lukes RJ, Craver L, Hall TC, Rappaport H, Ruben P: Hodgkin's disease, Report of the Nomenclature Committee. *Cancer Res* 26:1311, 1966b.

Magnusson A, Hagberg H, Hemmingson A, Lindgren PG: Computed tomography, ultrasound and lymphography in the diagnosis of malignant lymphoma. *Acta Radiol [Diagn] (Stockh)* 23:29, 1982.

McCaffrey JA, Rudden RA, Kahn PC, Harvey HA, Delellis RA: Clinical usefulness of $^{67}$gallium scanning in malignant lymphomas. *Am J Med* 60:523, 1976.

Mitchell RI, Peters MV, Brown TC, Rideout D: Laparotomy for Hodgkin's disease: some surgical observations. *Surgery* 71:694, 1972.

Mueller PR, Ferrucci JT, Harbin WP, Kirkpatrick RH, Simeone JF, Wittenberg J: Appearance of lymphomatous involvement of the mesentery by ultrasonography and body computed tomography: the "sandwich sign." *Radiology* 134:467, 1980.

Oberling C: Les reticulosarcomes et les reticuloendotheliosarcomes de la moelle osseuse (sarcomes d'Ewing). *Bull Assoc Fr Etude Cancer* 17:259–296, 1928.

Pillari G: Combined cavography and intravenous pyelography. *NY State J Med* 77:179, 1977.

Potsaid MS, McKusick KA: Radionuclide lymphography. In Clouse ME (ed): *Clinical Lymphography.* Baltimore, Williams & Wilkins, 1977.

Pusey WA: Cases of sarcoma and of Hodgkin's disease treated by exposures to x-rays: a preliminary report. *JAMA* 38:166, 1902.

Rappaport H, Winter WJ, Hicks EB: Follicular lymphoma: re-evaluation of its position in the scheme of malignant lymphoma, based on survey of 253 cases. *Cancer* 9:792, 1956.

Redman HC, Glatstein E, Castellino RA, Federal WA: Computed tomography as an adjunct in the staging of Hodgkin's disease and non-Hodgkin's lymphomas. *Radiology* 124:381, 1977.

Reed DM: On the pathological changes in Hodgkin's disease, with especial reference to its relation to tuberculosis. *Johns Hopkins Hosp Rep* 10:133, 1902.

Resegotti L, Chiarle F, Cogna F, Grosso B, Dolci C, Pistone M: Inferior venacavography for staging of lymphomas. *Acta Haematol* 67:87, 1983.

Rochester D, Bowie JD, Kunzmann A, Lester E: Ultrasound in the staging of lymphoma. *Radiology* 124:381, 1977.

Rosenberg SA: A critique of the value of laparotomy and splenectomy in the evaluation of patients with Hodgkin's disease. *Cancer Res* 31:1737, 1971.

Rosenberg SA, Kaplan HS: Evidence for an orderly progression in the spread of Hodgkin's disease. *Cancer Res* 26:1225, 1966.

Roxin T, Bujar H: Lymphographic visualization of lymphaticovenous communications and their significance in malignant hemolymphopathies. *Lymphography* 3:127, 1970.

Schwarz G, Lee BJ, Nelson JH: Lymphography, cavography and urography in the evaluation of malignant lymphomas. *Acta Radiol [Diagn] (Stockh)* 3:138, 1965.

Sternberg C: Uber Eine Eigenartige unter dem Bilde der Pseudoleukamie verlaufends Tuberculose des lymphatischen Apparates. *Z Heilk* 19:21, 1898.

Symmers D: Follicular lymphadenopathy with splenomegaly. A newly recognized disease of the lymphatic system. *Arch Pathol Lab Med* 3:816, 1927.

Takahashi M, Abrams HL: The accuracy of lymphangiographic diagnosis in malignant lymphoma. *Radiology* 89:448, 1967.

Wilks S: Cases of enlargement of the lymphatic glands and spleen, (or Hodgkin's disease), with remarks. *Guy's Hosp Rep* 11:56, 1865.

Zelch MG, Haaga JR: Clinical comparison of computed tomography and lymphangiography for detection of retroperitoneal lymphadenopathy. *Radiol Clin North Am* 17:157, 1979.

# 12

# *Lymphatic Imaging of Solid Tumors*

BAO-SHAN JING, M.D., AND SIDNEY WALLACE, M.D.

Lymphangiography has had a chaotic course of acceptance. At M. D. Anderson Hospital and Tumor Institute, the peak of 1100 lymphangiograms during 1977 has come to a plateau of 1000 examinations each year since introduction of computed tomography despite an increase in the total number of radiological examinations performed. Approximately one-half of lymphangiographic studies are done on patients with lymphoma, while the others are for patients with solid tumors. A thorough assessment of the extent of neoplastic disease is prerequisite to intelligent management of any patient with cancer.

The most commonly employed techniques for imaging lymph node involvement are lymphangiography (LAG), computed tomography (CT), and ultrasonography (US). Nuclear lymphography and gallium scanning may offer complementary information. Pyelography and venography are employed to define secondary extension of the neoplastic process. Percutaneous lymph node aspiration biopsy can contribute to establishing the histological diagnosis and confirming the imaging findings.

**Lymphangiography.** LAG offers the only direct radiological approach to visualization of the lymph vessels and lymph nodes. The criticisms of lymphangiography are related to both the performance and the interpretation. The technical aspects of this examination can be readily taught to a nurse or a technologist. The medicolegal concerns can be satisfied by the radiologist assuming complete responsibility for the procedure by maintaining close supervision.

Interpretation is by far the most difficult and most critical. With the assistance of clinical information, the radiologist must make a definitive diagnosis (that is, positive or negative for metastatic disease) in order to influence management. An equivocal diagnosis offers little assistance to therapeutic management. The radiologist must not allow the clinician to interpret his degree of indecision. It is essential to be aware of previous therapy, such as surgery, radiation therapy, or chemotherapy, which may influence the size and

integrity of the lymphatics and nodes. Interpretation must be made only if the examination is technically adequate both in the lymphatic and nodal phases. Rigid criteria must be maintained.

To ensure satisfactory results from pedal lymphangiography, an effort should be made in every case to opacify consistently the lymphatics in the pelvic and para-aortic regions up to the cisterna chyli. The LAG opacifies the three major lymphatic channels and lymph nodes in the external and common iliac compartments. The so-called obturator nodes are routinely visible as part of the medial group of the external iliac chain. The hypogastric and presacral lymph nodes are only occasionally opacified. In the lumbar area, three trunks are also demonstrated, one on the lateral aspect of the inferior vena cava (paracaval or right para-aortic), one on the lateral aspect of the aorta (left para-aortic), and one between the aorta and inferior vena cava (interaorticocaval). The lymph nodes anterior and posterior to these major vessels are not as frequently opacified (Fig. 12.1). All other abdominal lymph nodes (such as mesenteric, portahepatic, splenic hilar, renal hilar, and those above the cisterna chyli, including the retrocrural nodes) usually escape detection by LAG.

Pathological changes in the lymphatic system are 3-fold: (*a*) an alteration in lymphatic dynamics; (*b*) a change in the size of the lymph nodes; and (*c*) disruption of the internal architecture of the lymph node. A normal node may vary in size from a few millimeters to as much as 5 cm. There is an inverse ratio between size and number. Therefore, an increase in size is not specific and may be found in normal patients as well as in patients with benign or malignant diseases. Lymph nodes will be increased in size for approximately 2 months after the LAG because the oil-based contrast material produces inflammatory changes, lipogranulomas. Alteration of the internal architecture has paramount importance. LAG is as yet the only radiological method to evaluate the internal architecture of a lymph node. A nodal defect not traversed by the lym-

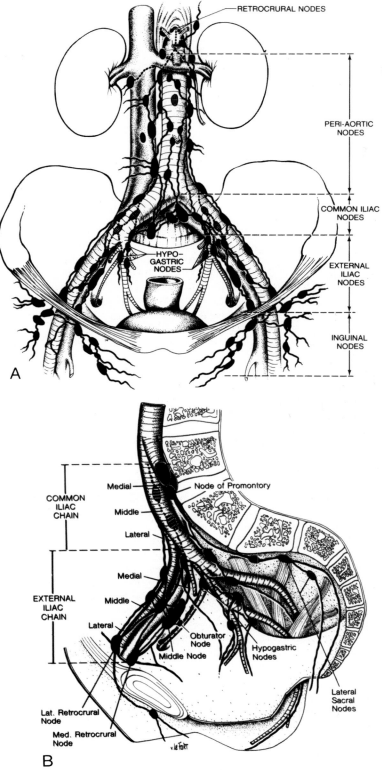

FIGURE 12.1. ANATOMY OF THE PELVIC AND RETROPERITONEAL LYMPHATICS
*A:* Anteroposterior view. *B:* Oblique view. *C:* Various groups of abdominoaortic lymph nodes.

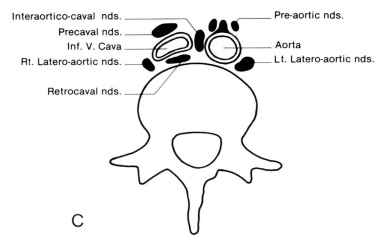

FIGURE 12.1C.

phatics is the most reliable criterion for the diagnosis of metastatic disease in a patient with a known primary neoplasm (Fig. 12.2) although on rare occasions a similar finding may be created by an abscess, caseation necrosis, or fibrosis.

The defects caused by metastases are the result of tumor emboli to the lymph node which subsequently grow to obstruct the marginal sinus and destroy adjacent nodal tissue. Initially these defects are usually in the periphery of the lymph node. The remaining functioning portion of the node is frequently crescent-shaped, and its lymphographic appearance is commonly termed the *rim sign.* A defect as small as 5 mm can be defined as long as it replaces only a portion of a node. If the node is totally replaced by neoplasm, it will not be opacified. Nodal metastases may be suggested by lymphatic vessel abnormalities, notably lymphatic distortion or displacement and lymphatic obstruction with or without collateral channels, including lymphaticovenous anastomosis. A negative LAG does not exclude metastatic disease. False-negative examinations are due to: (*a*) metastasis too small to detect and (*b*) failure to opacify the involved nodes.

The diagnosis of lymph node metastases depends on alteration of nodal architecture with little significance placed on size. This is especially important in diseases frequently accompanied by secondary infection with associated enlarged reactive nodes, as found in carcinoma of the uterine cervix. In a study by Henriksen (1960) on lymph nodes at surgery, 4% of normal-sized nodes contained metastases at histological examination; in a similar study by Plentl and Friedman (1971), 75% of enlarged nodes did not harbor malignancy but resulted from lymphoid hyperplasia. Epithelial neoplasms usually dis-

seminate locally, and the involved nodes need not be enlarged.

LAG identifies lymph node metastases more specifically than other available techniques. It frequently can delineate alteration in internal architecture of the nodes and can detect metastatic deposits in normal-sized or slightly enlarged lymph nodes. The lymphangiographic pattern may suggest the etiology of lymphadenopathy. In advanced lesions with total replacement of the node, the diagnosis of nodal metastases depends on a secondary lymphatic finding which may be best defined by CT or US. The accuracy of LAG in identification of lymph node metastases from carcinomas of various pelvic organs varies from 74–95% and in general relates to limitation of the technique and experience of the interpreters. The results are better in those institutions where LAG is performed routinely and in large volume.

**Computed Tomography.** CT is the computerized reconstruction of an image depicting a radiographic photon-produced slice through the body. This cross-sectional image is composed of many picture elements (pixels). Each pixel represents x-ray absorption measurements of a small area of tissue within the slice and depicts the average attenuation of all of the tissue within the volume elements. Pixel size and slice thickness are important factors in applying CT to the evaluation of tissue absorption numbers.

In a study at M. D. Anderson Hospital, CT images were obtained with a variety of scanners: EMI 5005 18-sec body scanner, GE 8800 10-sec body scanner, Somatom 2 (Siemens) 5–10-sec body scanner, and Somatom DR3 (Siemens) 3–10-sec body scanner. The complete study of the abdomen and pelvis consisted of sections at 1–2-

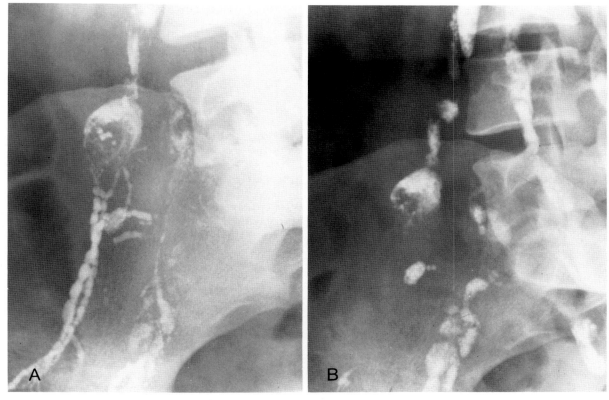

FIGURE 12.2. METASTATIC CARCINOMA FROM THE UTERINE CERVIX
*A:* Lymphatic phase. The lymphatics do not permeate the areas of replacement by metastatic carcinoma. *B:* Nodal phase. The defects in the margin of the nodes are areas of tumor deposition. The remaining functioning portion of the node is opacified, producing a crescent configuration. This represents partial replacement of the nodes by metastatic carcinoma.

cm intervals from the dome of the diaphragm to the symphysis pubis. Additional sections were made when indicated. Oral, rectal, and intravenous contrast media were used, and in women, a vaginal tampon was often used. Identification of lymph nodes by CT depends upon the presence of fat and complete opacification of bowel, blood vessels, and ureters. In the retroperitoneal area, the amount of fat is usually adequate, except perhaps in children and emaciated patients, readily delineating the aorta and inferior vena cava and allowing easy identification of the para-aortic nodes. The pelvic nodes are more difficult to define because of the paucity of fat surrounding the iliac vessels, which are almost inseparable from the nodes.

The external iliac nodes are best demonstrated at the level of the inferior aspect of the sacroiliac joint and about 2 cm superior to the acetabulum. At these levels, it is easy to appreciate the normal separation of external iliac vessels and nodes adjacent to the iliopsoas muscles and anterior to the hypogastric vessels and nodes. The obturator

nodes, the medial chain of the external iliac nodes, are best demonstrated just superior to the acetabulum. The hypogastric or internal iliac nodes are situated around the hypogastric artery and its branches in the dorsal aspect of the pelvis. They are best demonstrated at the level of the inferior aspect of the sacroiliac joint and posterior to the external iliac vessels and nodes.

Lymph nodes in the periaortic region are adjacent to the aorta and the inferior vena cava. Normal-sized para-aortic nodes not opacified by LAG may be seen routinely on CT scans. Usually the aortic contour is well appreciated in its lateral and dorsal aspect on CT, although the vertebral column may partially obscure the dorsal aortic outline. The anterior or ventral aortic margin is variably visualized on CT scan, sometimes being obscured by overlying normal anatomic structures or being insufficiently defined by fatty tissue. The loss of a normal aortic contour, particularly in the lateral and dorsal areas, strongly suggests a pathological process in the para-aortic region, most commonly lymph node enlargement. Primary and metastatic retroperitoneal tumors, vascular disease, and retroperitoneal edema or fibrosis can produce similar alterations. Para-aortic lymph node enlargement can occur without obscuring the aortic contour, however. Some para-aortic nodal groups lie a sufficient distance from the aorta so that even when enlarged, they do not impinge upon the aortic outline.

The margin of the inferior vena cava is not always separable from the surrounding normal structures. Therefore, the lack of a distinct inferior vena caval contour may not be a reliable sign of paracaval disease. The lymph nodes located in the vascular fat angles behind the aorta and inferior vena cava are good indicators of lymph node enlargement. In the early stage of lymph node enlargement, the lymph nodes simply appear as rounded densities somewhat larger than those seen under normal circumstances. With progression of disease, these vascular fat angles are "silhouetted out" so that the margins of the vessels are no longer discernible. Eventually the enlarged lymph nodes can displace the abdominal aorta anteriorly, producing the so-called floating aorta sign. Lymph node enlargement may not involve the para-aortic region but may involve those nodes on the psoas muscles, at the renal pedicle, and in the liver and splenic hila, the superior mesenteric artery, or the celiac axis.

The presentation of enlarged lymph nodes varies from a discrete enlarged node greater than 1.5–2.0 cm in diameter, to a conglomerate of contiguous nodes (Fig. 12.3A), to a large homogeneous mass in which individual nodes are no longer recognizable (Fig. 12.3B). Homogeneous masses that surround the aorta and vena cava may completely obscure the contours of these vessels. Some enlarged nodes may contain zones of decreased attenuation, which may represent tissue degeneration (Fig. 12.3C). This appearance frequently occurs in solid tumors but in only 10% of lymphomas prior to treatment. Following therapy the incidence increases significantly. Because of the lack of fat planes surrounding the iliac vessels, enlargement of pelvic nodes is often difficult to define unless they are opacified by contrast medium. The signs of involvement are enlargement, asymmetry, and obscurity of the contours of neurovascular bundles in the external iliac and hypogastric areas.

Thus far CT offers little specificity. Abnormalities in lymph vessels go undetected. Only gross morphological evaluation of the lymph nodes is possible as defined by size and not internal architecture. In order for retroperitoneal or pelvic metastases to be detected by CT, the diseased nodes must be enlarged. *How big is big? How big is abnormal?* There is a considerable range of normal in the size of lymph nodes, perhaps from 0.5–5.0 cm, and the upper limit of normal is not sharply defined. The cross-sectional diameter will vary depending upon the axis of the lymph node. In the retroperitoneum the long axis of lymph nodes parallels the spine, and the cross-sectional diameter is perhaps the shortest dimension unless there is scoliosis. In the pelvis the long axis of the lymph node is oblique or horizontal in the presence of lordosis; the cross-sectional diameter may be the largest dimension of the lymph node. The cross-sectional diameter of normal para-aortic nodes seldom exceeds 1.5 cm, and most nodes measure less than 1.0 cm. Iliac nodes may be somewhat larger. Consequently, it is difficult, if not impossible, to determine nodal involvement purely on the basis of size.

Nodes involved by disease (infection, inflammation, and neoplasm) are more likely to be enlarged if the arbitrary dimension for enlargement is 1.5 cm. Let us reiterate: Four percent of normal-sized nodes contain metastases (Henriksen, 1960), while 75% of enlarged nodes at surgical exploration do not harbor malignancy but are usually a manifestation of hyperplasia (Plentl and Friedman, 1971). Demonstration of a discrete large node (>1.5 cm), a common finding with pelvic neoplasms, does not absolutely indicate metastasis. Although a characteristic of some granulomatous diseases, such as tuberculosis, clusters of lymph nodes matted together are more likely to be due to metastases in patients with a known primary malignancy. If there are associated findings, including ureteric obstruction or bone destruction, especially in continuity, the diagnosis of metastases is more secure.

Lymph node enlargement outside of that opacified by LAG or that totally replaced by neoplasm can be detected by CT. CT commonly demonstrates the extent of lymph node disease to be significantly greater than what is opacified by LAG. This includes those areas outside the para-aortic region: the renal, splenic, and hepatic hilar nodes, the para-aortic nodes above renal hilar level, and the retrocrural, mediastinal, and supraclavicular nodes.

The information provided by CT is not limited to the lymphatic system; the condition of other pelvic and abdominal structures is also evaluated. Demonstration of primary neoplasm and

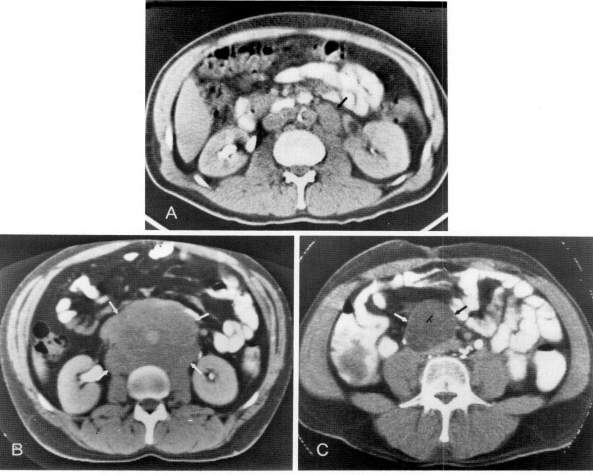

FIGURE 12.3. NODAL METASTASES IN PERIAORTIC AREA

*A:* Discrete enlarged lymph nodes in the left para-aortic area (*arrow*) with mild obstructive uropathy in a patient with carcinoma of the urinary bladder. *B:* Homogeneous conglomerate mantle of enlarged periaortic nodes completely surrounding the aorta and displacing the inferior vena cava anteriorly and laterally (*arrows*) in a patient with seminoma of the testis. There is opacification of the aorta and inferior vena cava. *C:* Enlarged periaortic nodes with zones of necrosis in a patient with carcinoma of the testis.

its local invasion to the pelvic wall and to adjacent organs is a contribution of CT. Secondary involvement of the urinary tract, especially the site and etiology of ureteral obstruction, is best demonstrated by CT. In the screening for liver and adrenal metastases, CT is more accurate and more sensitive than ultrasonography and scintigraphy.

**Ultrasonography.** US utilizes sound waves to demonstrate the image in multidirectional planes. It presents an accurate assessment of the size, shape, location, and internal consistency of the organs or masses and their related abnormalities. The principal advantage of US is the nontraumatic and apparently risk-free nature of this form of energy.

At present, US offers the greatest value in the detection of pelvic gynecological malignancies except in the early stages. Advanced endometrial carcinoma is diagnosed by the presence of uterine enlargement associated with abnormal internal echoes. A multiloculated cystic mass with irregular margins suggests malignant ovarian disease. Any solid mass of the ovary is considered malignant until proven otherwise. The urinary bladder is frequently and easily visible by US, but this is rarely employed clinically for evaluation of bladder carcinoma. Demonstration of a tumor projecting into the lumen adds little to the patient's management. US of the prostate does not as yet yield clinically significant information. Once a suspected pelvic mass is defined by US, the abdomen should be examined for ascites, hydronephrosis, retroperitoneal disease, and liver and adrenal metastases.

Retroperitoneal lymphadenopathy can be detected by US either by demonstration of an enlarged nodal mass or displacement of normal structures (Fig. 12.4). It is, at times, difficult to differentiate fluid-filled bowel loops from nodal masses. Real-time examination revealing peristaltic motion or the change in configuration will be of assistance. US can demonstrate moderate to bulky lymph node enlargement, but it is not sensitive enough to detect abnormal nodes of normal size. Bowel gas frequently interferes with optimal use of this procedure.

US does play a role in following the patient's response to therapy, but it is only valuable if lymphadenopathy is clearly identified.

**Pyelography.** Pyelography is a complementary examination in evaluation of the retroperitoneal area in that it may confirm the existence of totally replaced nodes by displacement or obstruction of the urinary tract. Asymmetry of ureters is a common normal occurrence. Enlarged nodes usually displace the upper ureters laterally and the lower portions of the ureters medially. In conjunction with lymphangiography, obstructed or distorted lymphatics and abnormal nodes can be more definitely implicated if they produce an associated change in the urinary tract. This occurred in a patient with carcinoma of the cervix, clinically stage II, whose lymphangiogram revealed small abnormal iliac nodes in the junctional areas between the common and external iliac lymph nodes. Intravenous pyelography demonstrated obstruction of the

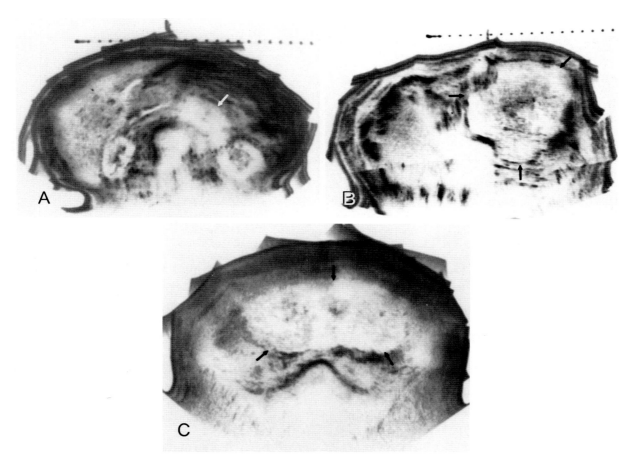

FIGURE 12.4. ULTRASONOGRAM OF RETROPERITONEAL LYMPHADENOPATHY AND MESENTERIC METASTASES
*A:* Transverse ultrasonogram through the upper abdomen. There is slight enlargement of lymph nodes due to metastases in the left para-aortic area (*arrow*). The nodes are larger than normal and are clearly shown without evidence of gas interference. *B:* Transverse ultrasonogram through the midabdomen. A large nodal metastasis is clearly demonstrated in left para-aortic area (*arrows*). *C:* Transverse ultrasonogram of the lower abdomen. A large saucer-shaped mass due to mesenteric metastases is well shown in the middle part of the abdomen (*arrows*).

right ureter with nonvisualization of the right kidney, presumably due to obstruction of the right ureter, supporting the diagnosis of metastases (Fig. 12.5). In patients with carcinoma of the cervix previously treated by radiation therapy, the obstruction of a ureter is most likely due to recurrent neoplasm.

**Venography.** Venography may offer considerable assistance in establishing the etiology of lymphatic obstruction by demonstrating masses distorting or obstructing the adjacent veins. The limitations of venography depend upon the size and position of the involved nodes in relationship to the opacified veins. The studies available include (a) bilateral iliac venography, (b) inferior vena cavography, (c) compression inferior vena cavography for retrograde opacification of the internal iliac and sacral veins, and (d) selective renal, ovarian, or testicular venography. Selective catheterization of either ovarian vein, usually the left, will opacify the ovarian, adnexal, and uterine veins bilaterally. Inferior vena cavography can only evaluate the right side of the retroperitoneal space. In the region of L2 where the lumbar trunks usually drain into the cisterna chyli, vena cavography is of utmost importance. It may also assist in establishing the extent of involvement above the point of lymphatic obstruction as well as in the detection of enlarged nodes not ordinarily opacified by lymphangiography. Distortion and obstruction of veins are nonspecific as to etiology. Invasion of veins is usually neoplastic in origin (Fig. 12.6). Difficulties may be encountered by the presence of thrombophlebitis.

**Percutaneous Transabdominal Lymph Node Aspiration Biopsy.** Selective lymphadenectomy has found increasing application in conjunction with LAG and CT for staging prior to therapy. The percutaneous approach to the retroperitoneal and pelvic lymph nodes with a fine caliber needle represents a simple technique to confirm the presence of neoplasm, thereby obviating the need for exploratory laparotomy in selected cases. In view of the relative position of the para-aortic and pelvic lymph nodes in relation to the great vessels, an anterior transabdominal approach seems most suitable. The site of biopsy in a patient with a metastatic disease is just above the crescentic configuration. Percutaneous transabdominal lymph node aspiration biopsy involves passage of a no. 22–23 gauge needle into the peritoneal cavity through solid and hollow viscera. In our series of more than 400 biopsies, such potential problems as intra-abdominal bleeding, pancreatitis, and bile peritonitis were not encountered. The possibility of disseminating neoplasm by aspiration does not seem to present a significant problem as concluded by laboratory investigation and clinical experience with percutaneous biopsies of lung and kidney neoplasms using even larger caliber needles.

Percutaneous transabdominal lymph node aspiration biopsy has enhanced the value of LAG and CT. Percutaneous biopsy of lymph nodes suspected of metastases represents further application of both LAG and CT. The LAG can better localize the metastatic focus as a defect in an opacified lymph node (Fig. 12.7). Biopsy under CT guidance is of inestimable assistance in totally replaced or nonopacified lymph node, abdominal masses, and liver metastases (Fig. 12.8). This technique yields an accuracy of 75–85% in lymph nodes containing metastatic carcinoma but only 50% with lymphoma. Epithelial metastases, especially those originating in the pelvic viscera, are frequently highly cellular, poorly vascularized, and readily distinguishable from the normal lymphocytes of a lymph node.

## MECHANISM OF LYMPH NODE METASTASIS

In a patient with carcinoma, the nodes involved by metastasis should be along the primary and secondary echelons of the lymphatic drainage. Variations in normal lymphatic anatomy occur frequently, and assessment of the lymphatic phase is essential in determining the preexisting anomalous channels that will significantly affect the distribution of metastases. Changes at a distance from the primary site without evidence of bypassing channels or lymphatic obstruction with collateral circulation should be viewed with great caution. Carcino-matous spread at the time of most examinations is usually local in contrast to that seen in lymphomas, which is frequently more diffuse by the time the patient reaches the physician.

Tumor emboli from a primary carcinoma travel along the lymphatic channels and gain access to the marginal sinus of the node. At this point their progress is impeded; they enlarge and obstruct the marginal sinus. Lymphatics do not traverse the area replaced by carcinoma but, rather, are obstructed, distorted, and displaced (Fig. 12.2). This may be manifested by stasis of

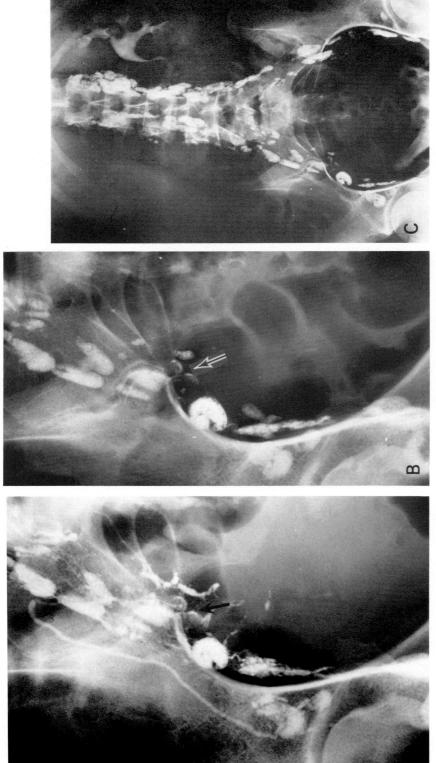

FIGURE 12.5.  METASTATIC CARCINOMA FROM THE UTERINE CERVIX

*A:* Lymphatic phase. Two small nodes in the right iliac chain at the junctional position (*arrow*) demonstrate the failure of the lymphatics to traverse the nodes. *B:* Nodal phase. The two small nodes containing metastatic carcinoma are crescent in configuration (*arrow*). *C:* Intravenous urogram. The right kidney does not visualize. The obstruction of the ureter may be due to other totally replaced nodes not opacified or from extension of the primary carcinoma into the parametrium.

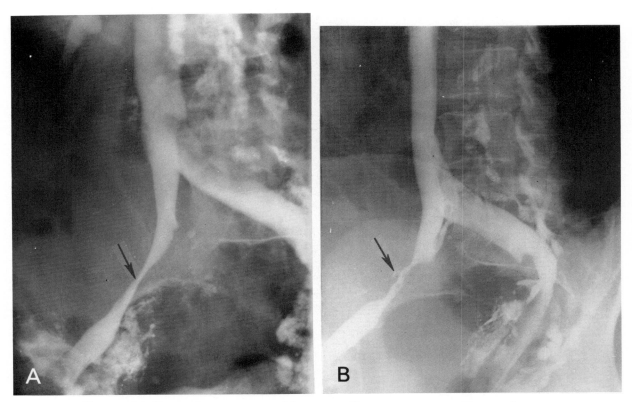

FIGURE 12.6. VENOUS INVOLVEMENT BY METASTATIC CARCINOMA FROM THE UTERINE CERVIX
*A:* Compression of the right external iliac vein (*arrow*) by lymph nodes partially replaced by metastatic carcinoma. Compression can be produced by a mass of any etiology. *B:* Invasion of the right common iliac vein (*arrow*) by metastatic carcinoma totally replacing the lymph nodes.

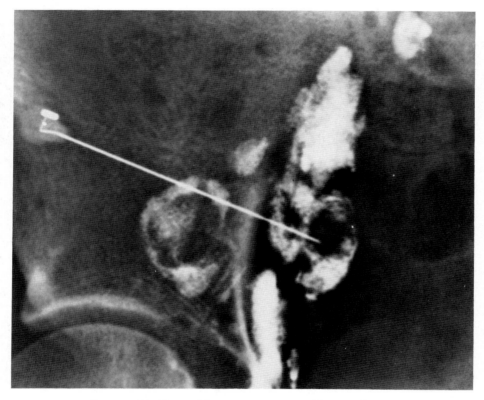

FIGURE 12.7. NODAL METASTASIS FROM THE UTERINE CERVIX

Aspiration biopsy of metastatic carcinoma of right external iliac node. The site of biopsy is within the area of the filling defects of the node.

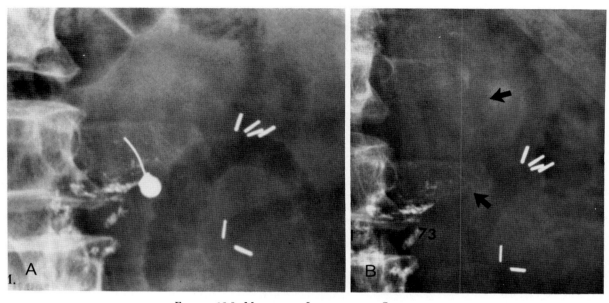

FIGURE 12.8. MALIGNANT LYMPHOMA OR SEMINOMA

*A:* There is a large left retroperitoneal node mass. Only the inferior portion of the lesion is partially opacified by the lymphangiogram. *B:* Aspiration biopsy reveals the lesion to be histiocytic lymphoma.

contrast material in channels on the delayed or 24-hr study. Abnormalities in the lymphatics and in the marginal sinus and, therefore, in the contour of the node usually occur early in carcinomatous appearance. Eventually, alterations also take place in the body of the node. This differs from lymphoma, in which the internal architecture is disrupted early in the course of the disease; marginal defects usually are later manifestations. The major differential diagnosis is not usually between carcinoma and lymphoma but carcinoma versus a false-positive defect produced by fatty replacement, fibrosis, or superimposition of nodes.

The node involved by metastatic carcinoma may be normal in size or enlarged; the shape tends to be more rounded than normal. Metastases most frequently result in a crescent configuration with the lymphatics (during the vascular phase) absent in the sharply defined marginal concavity. The single most reliable criterion for lymphangiographic diagnosis of metastatic carcinoma to a lymph node is *a defect in a node not traversed by lymphatics.* The remaining functioning portion of the node is a crescent shape, the rim sign. The lymphatics leading to the defect are disrupted by the destructive process. It is important to view the lymphatics and nodal defect in multiple projections. If in any one projection the defect is not traversed by the lymphatic channels, the finding is real. This assists in the differentiation from superimposition of vessels.

This appearance can be simulated by abscess formation, caseation necrosis, and fibrosis. In the presence of a known primary malignancy, metastasis is by far the most likely diagnosis.

As the carcinoma progresses, the nodes become totally replaced. The lymphatics may be obstructed or distorted by the carcinomatous focus. Collateral circulation—lymphatic to lymphatic, lymphatic to pre- or paralymphatic, and lymphatic to venous—may be opacified, possibly providing the only evidence of replacement of nodal tissue. Lymphatic obstruction may not be accompanied by collateral channels but may result in a decrease in the number of lymphatics and nodes opacified. Filling of only two of the three major iliac trunks may have great significance (Fig. 12.9).

Interference in lymphatic flow in itself is secondary evidence of metastases. Confirmation is necessary before a conclusive diagnosis can be made. Complete replacement of lymph nodes with associated lymphatic abnormalities must be further evaluated by such complementary procedures as intravenous pyelography, inferior vena cavography, pelvic venography, and notably CT to establish the presence of a mass. Percutaneous fine-needle aspiration biopsy has become essential when a definitive diagnosis is required.

Pelvic and retroperitoneal surgery may interrupt lymphatic trunks and remove lymph nodes. This may result in obstruction of lymphatic

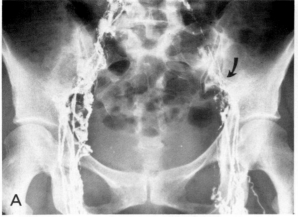

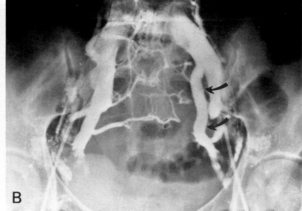

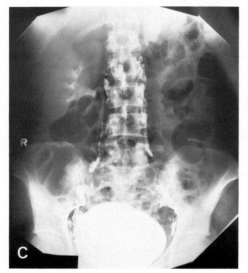

FIGURE 12.9.    METASTATIC CARCINOMA FROM THE UTERINE CERVIX
   *A:* There is a decrease in number of left iliac lymphatics opacified
(*arrow*). *B:* Compression venography demonstrates distortion of the left
internal iliac vein (*arrows*). The changes in the lymphatics and veins are
due to totally replaced lymph nodes. *C:* Intravenous urogram. The left
kidney was not visualized due to obstruction of the ureter by metastatic
disease.

channels or lymphocyst formation. These findings are difficult to differentiate even with venography unless appreciated shortly after the surgical procedure. LAG may assist in the differentiation if the lymphatics opacified from the
lower extremities are in continuity with the lymphocyst (Fig. 12.10). US will define the cystic
structure but may contain internal echoes. CT
usually demonstrates a mass of low attenuation
(Fig. 12.11).

   After radiotherapy and/or chemotherapy the
problem in differentiation becomes more difficult. These therapeutic approaches reduce the
size and number of nodes with usually little effect
on the lymphatic vessels. Irradiation decreases
lymphoid tissue but seldom results in obstruction
unless associated with extensive fibrosis. It may
also decrease the regenerative capacity of lymphatics and nodes. Following radiation therapy,
LAG has been of value in establishing the pres-

ence of metastatic disease (Fig. 12.12). The extent of previous radiotherapy can be accurately
estimated because of the decreased size of the
treated lymph nodes. Under normal circumstances the pelvic nodes are usually larger than
the para-aortic nodes.

   Successful treatment does not necessarily al-
leviate an obstruction secondary to metastatic
disease. The paucity of nodes visualized as the
result of these modes of therapy must be differentiated from total replacement by the malignant disease. CT, US, and venography could
confirm the presence of a mass, which would
probably represent neoplastic disease replacing
the nodes. Needle biopsy can readily establish
the diagnosis; however, when the lymphatics are
normal in number and distribution in the absence of opacified lymphoid tissue, the possibility
of extensive replacement is minimal. This is
readily established by CT. Nodal involvement is

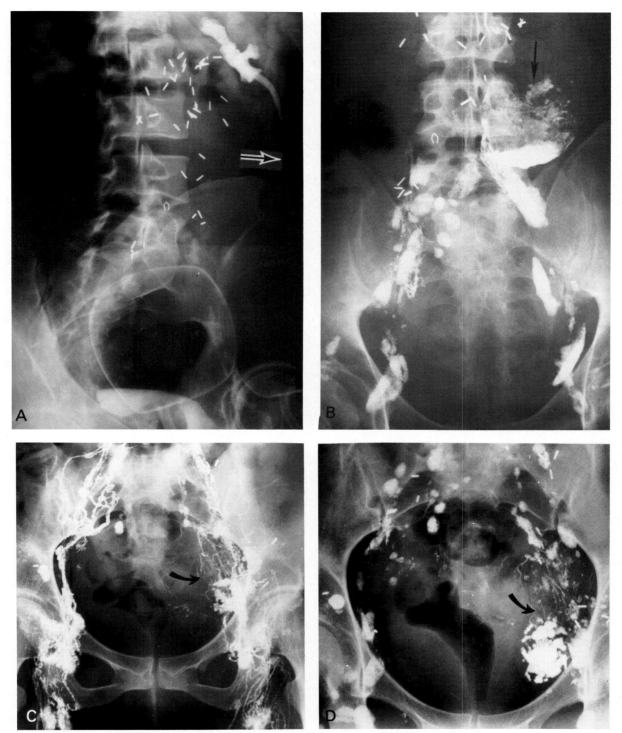

FIGURE 12.10. POSTOPERATIVE LYMPHOCYST VERSUS METASTATIC CARCINOMA

*A:* Intraveous urogram revealed the left ureter displaced by a retroperitoneal mass (*arrow*) in a patient with a left testicular carcinoma previously treated by a retroperitoneal node dissection. *B:* Lymphangiogram opacified the retroperitoneal lymphocyst (*arrow*). *C:* Pelvic lymphocyst in a patient with carcinoma of the cervix. This occurred following node biopsy for staging laparotomy. LAG confirmed the presence of a lymphocyst, a collection of contrast material accumulated in the left iliac area (*arrow*). *D:* Nodal phase demonstrated the collection of contrast in the lymphocyst (*arrow*). When the patient was placed in a dependent position, a fluid level was seen.

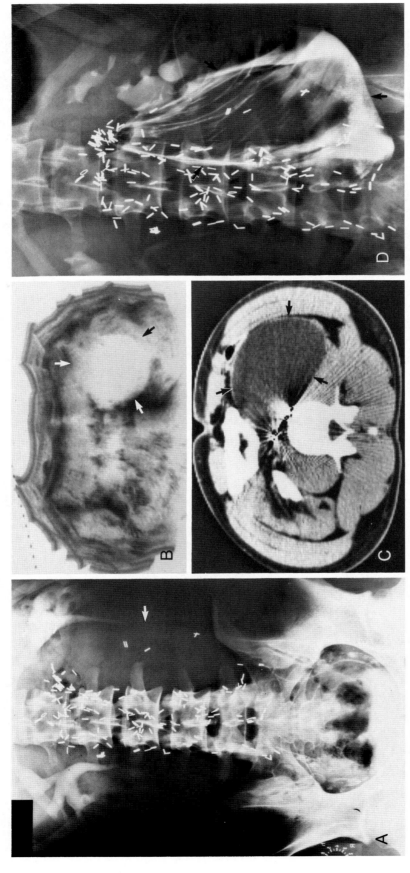

FIGURE 12.11. POSTOPERATIVE LYMPHOCYST FOLLOWING RETROPERITONEAL LYMPH NODE DISSECTION IN A PATIENT WITH CARCINOMA OF THE LEFT TESTICLE

*A:* Intravenous pyelogram. There is postoperative status in retroperitoneal area with multiple surgical clips along the side of the lumbar spine and in the left peritoneal space. There is a large left retroperitoneal soft tissue mass with lateral displacement of left kidney and ureter (*arrow*). *B:* Transverse ultrasonogram of the abdomen. There is a large rounded lympechoic mass along the left side of the aorta (*arrows*). The mass demonstrates some through transmission, compatible with fluid content. The left kidney is displaced laterally and is somewhat hydronephrotic (not well shown on this scan). *C:* CT of the abdomen at the level of L3. There is a large well defined soft tissue mass with low attenuation in the left side of the abdomen with flattening and slight displacement of the psoas muscle. *D:* Cystic puncture with injection of sclerosing solution. There was partial collapse of the cyst after removal of 1200 cc of amber-colored fluid. Sclerosing solution was in the lower part of the cystic cavity.

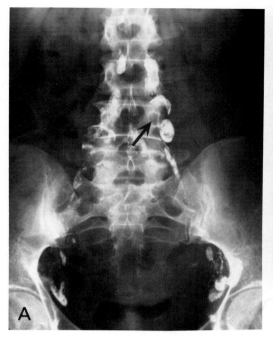
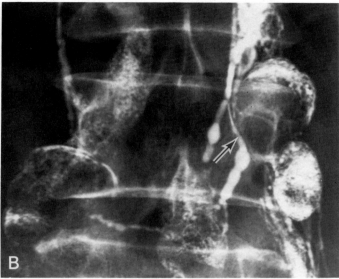

FIGURE 12.12. METASTATIC CARCINOMA OF THE CERVIX FOLLOWING RADIATION THERAPY

*A:* The pelvic nodes are small up to the top of L5. This was the level of the treatment portal. The lymph nodes in the para-aortic area are enlarged and involved by metastatic carcinoma (*arrow*). *B:* The lymphatic phase reveals crescentic configuration of the metastatic nodes and the lymphatics which fail to traverse the defects (*arrow*).

usually associated with distortion or obstruction of lymphatic pathways. Occasionally an apparently normal individual, without any previous therapy, may have relatively few nodes in the retroperitoneal area, but the lymphatic distribution is normal (Fig. 12.13).

## Modes of Metastasis

The modes of lymph node metastasis are in part governed by: (*a*) the normal distribution of lymphatic drainage, (*b*) the variations in normal drainage, and (*c*) the collateral pathways available in the event of obstruction.

In the evaluation of a patient with carcinoma, the nodes involved by metastases should be along the primary and secondary echelons of lymphatic drainage. In interpretation of the lymphangiogram, it is essential to be thoroughly acquainted with the normal lymphatic drainage from the involved viscera. From the pelvic viscera the lymphatic drainage is primarily to the lymph nodes of the internal, external, and common iliac chains as well as to the presacral area. Bilateral pedal LAG opacifies most but not all of these lymph nodes. The external and common iliac pathways consist of three major trunks, the medial, the middle, and the lateral (Fig. 12.14). The

obturator nodes are usually considered to be part of the medial group of the external iliac chain. These nodes are almost invariably opacified. Nodes in the obturator fossa, when present (7%), are seldom visualized. The internal iliac and presacral nodes are not consistently opacified. Changes in lymph nodes at a distance from the sites of usual drainage and in the absence of lymphatic variation or obstruction must be viewed with great caution.

Variations in normal lymphatic anatomy are frequent, and assessment of the lymphatic phase is essential in determining the pre-existing anomalous channels that will significantly affect the distribution (Fig. 12.15). The many variations of normal can be best illustrated by examination of the thoracic duct (Figs. 12.16 and 12.17). The classical distribution of the thoracic duct as described by Bartels (1909) is found in approximately 50% of patients. Opacification of the mediastinal, hilar, paratracheal, and bilateral supraclavicular nodes depends upon the numerous variations of normal (Fig. 12.18). At times lower cervical and axillary node visualization may be a manifestation of these anomalous pathways.

Metastases are usually logical and orderly and are, in part, determined by normal lymphatic

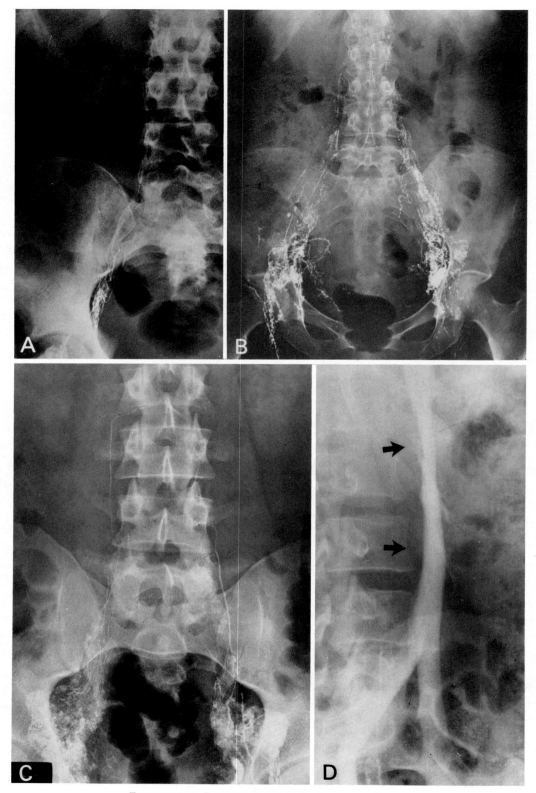

FIGURE 12.13. PAUCITY OF OPACIFIED LYMPHOID TISSUE

A: Postchemotherapy. The number and distribution of channels opacified in the right lumbar area are normal. The absence of nodes is related to treatment for lymphoma. B: The number and distribution of channels in the lumbar region is within the normal range. The lack of lymphoid tissue had no obvious etiology. C: Hodgkin's disease. The number of lymphatics and the distribution of those opacified are abnormal. D: An inferior vena cavogram reveals extrinsic compression by nodes (arrows) totally replaced by Hodgkin's disease.

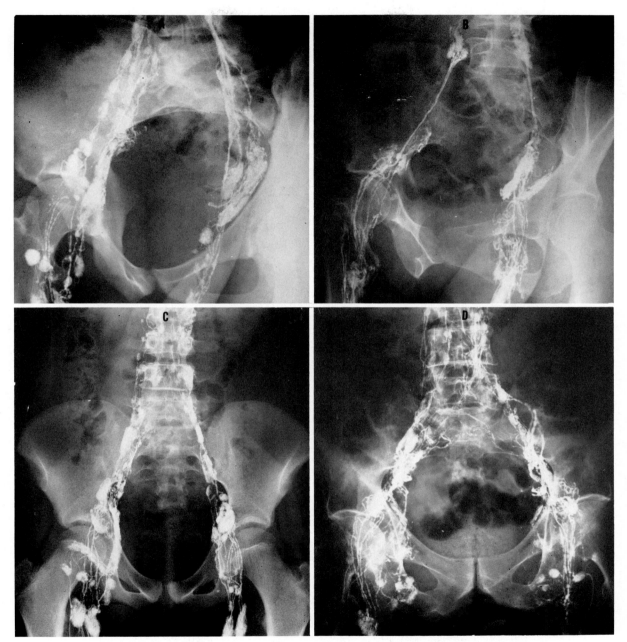

FIGURE 12.14. NORMAL PELVIC LYMPHATICS AND NODES
*A:* Oblique view. Three major trunks, similar bilaterally. *B:* Only one major common iliac trunk opacifies bilaterally as a variation of normal. *C:* Normal distribution of lymphatics and nodes opacified in a child. *D:* Normal distribution in a patient 65 yr of age. The distortion of the left common iliac lymphatics is due to a dilated tortuous iliac artery.

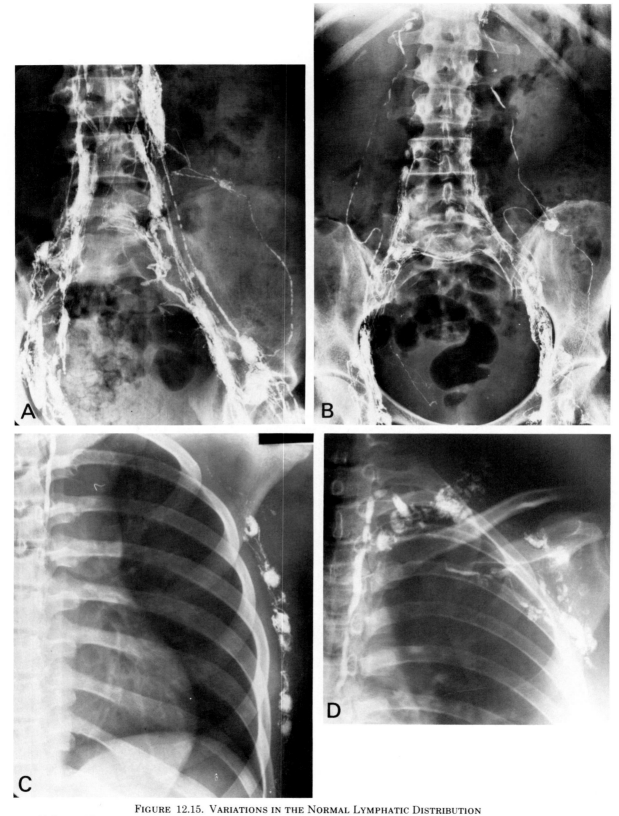

FIGURE 12.15. VARIATIONS IN THE NORMAL LYMPHATIC DISTRIBUTION

*A:* Abdominal lymphatic variations of circumflex iliac lymphatics and nodes. Usually one node is opacified at the iliac: *B:* Retroperitoneal bypass as an unusual variation of the normal. The normal lumbar lymphatics and nodes are also opacified. *C:* Opacification of a bypass from the external iliac lymphatics to the anterior abdominal wall eventually draining into the inferior aspect of the axilla. *D:* Opacification of the lymphatic from the thoracic duct to the superior aspect of the axilla as a variation of the normal.

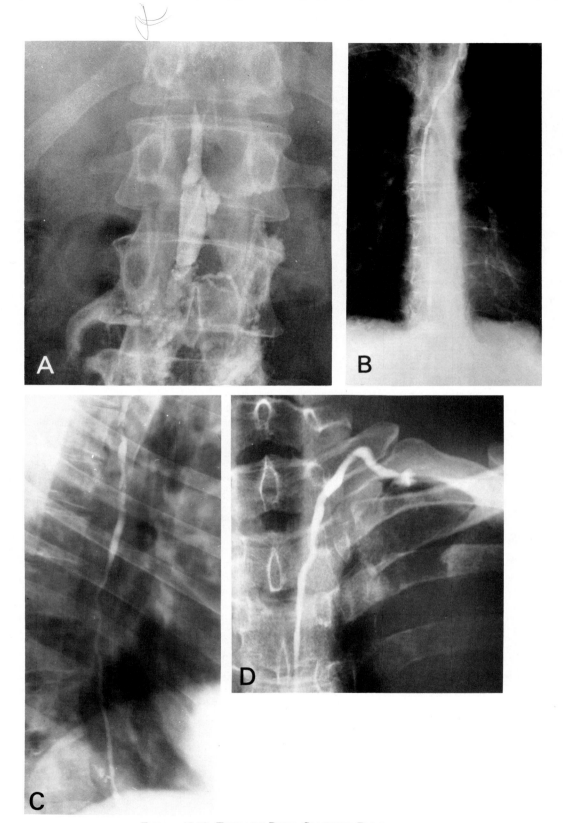

FIGURE 12.16. THORACIC DUCT, CLASSICAL DISTRIBUTION
*A:* Cisterna chyli. *B:* Thoracic duct, anteroposterior view. *C:* Thoracic duct, lateral view. *D:* Terminal portion emptying into the venous angle in the left neck.

drainage and individual variations as long as these vessels are present and patent. Engeset (1959) verified this concept by the injection of tumor cells and mercury into the testicular lymphatics of rats, demonstrating three basic patterns (Fig. 12.19):

1. Metastases to the sentinel node (primary or first echelon draining node frequently at the renal hilar area) preceded lung metastases.
2. Sentinel node and lung metastases occurred simultaneously.
3. Lung metastases existed prior to, or in the absence of, sentinel node metastases.

The alteration in lymphatic dynamics results in utilization of patent collateral pathways that are immediately available at the site of obstruction. The significance of this altered dynamic environment is illustrated by the following case of a patient with melanoma of the right lower extremity treated by local excision and inguinal node dissection (Fig. 12.20). Progressive edema of the right lower extremity ensued. LAG demonstrated an increase in opacified dermal and subcutaneous lymphatic pathways, a manifestation of the obstruction. The normal left inguinal, pelvic, and retroperitoneal areas can be used for comparison. Following the dissection, an entirely new environment was created for subsequent lymphatic flow. The nodes in the right iliac and para-aortic areas were bypassed by collateral channels. Subsequent metastases would progress along these alternate pathways. Any surgical procedures performed in an attempt to eradicate metastases must appreciate this new dynamic environment.

Another case, Figure 12.21, demonstrates the importance of this knowledge prior to the proposed surgical procedure. The patient with a carcinoma of the cervix was to be treated by a pelvic node dissection. The left iliac lymphatic pathways were obstructed by metastases with collateral channels, opacified in the abdominal and chest walls, eventually filling metastatic left axillary nodes. Any attempt to remove the tumor and its metastases surgically would surely fail since the metastases had progressed far beyond the local site. Axillary metastases from a carcinoma of the cervix may also occur if anomalous pathways exist from the thoracic duct to the axillary lymphatics.

Thoracic duct obstruction will also result in the utilization and opacification of collateral channels (Fig. 12.22).

### Paralymphatic Pathways

Pathways, para- or prelymphatic, other than the endothelial-lined lymphatic channels, are available in the event of obstruction. These include the body's potential cavities (pleural, pericardial, and peritoneal), the interstitial spaces, and the perineural and perivascular spaces, which, for the sake of simplicity, can be termed the *pre-* and *paralymphatic system*. These avenues are available for fluid transport and, therefore, could function as routes for dispersion of metastases.

Occasionally, with obstruction of the lymphatic pathways, there is reflux of contrast material into the visceral pathways and eventually into the wall of the viscera (Servelle, 1945). This may explain the mechanism of mural metastases via the lymphatic system (Fig. 12.23). In the presence of obstruction, it is essential to follow the lymphangiographic pattern for days or perhaps weeks by serial roentgenograms to appreciate the complexity of this alternate circulation.

The perineural and perivascular sheaths may also function for lymph flow. The potential space is probably the route of metastasis for perineural spread of carcinoma encircling nerves. A perivascular cuff has been demonstrated as a collateral channel opacified as the result of obstruction of iliac channels by a metastatic carcinoma of the cervix (Fig. 12.23D).

### Lymphaticovenous Anastomosis

Another fascinating alternate pathway available in the event of obstruction is the lymphaticovenous anastomosis, which is a direct communication between these two vascular systems. These communications are best recorded during the injection of the contrast material when there is a forward head of pressure. The difference in velocity of flow makes the event difficult to capture because once the oil droplet enters the venous system, it is caught in the relatively rapid current of venous flow. The transient appearance of radiopaque droplets along the venous distribution is evidence of the presence of these communications (Fig. 12.24A and B). Probably relatively dormant under normal circumstances, these channels can be utilized in the event of an imbalance of pressures in the two systems. This imbalance is most frequently precipitated by malignant involvement or postsurgical obstruction of lymphatic pathways (Jonsson et al., 1982). Opacification of the inferior vena cava was observed in a patient with metastases to the retroperitoneal nodes from a seminoma of the testicle (Fig. 12.24C). The intrahepatic branches of the portal vein were filled during LAG in another patient with obstruction of the major lymphatic pathways (Fig. 24D and E).

In summary, the modes of lymphatic metastases depend upon the normal distribution of

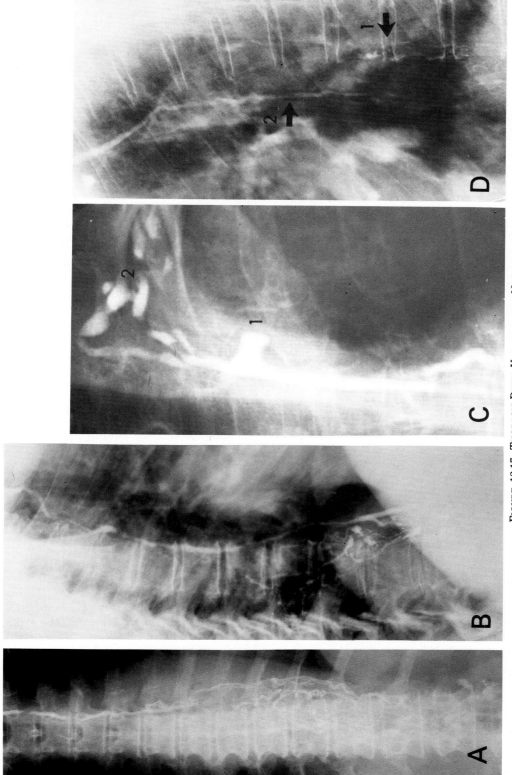

FIGURE 12.17. THORACIC DUCT, VARIATIONS OF NORMAL

*A*: Plexiform origin of the thoracic duct, anteroposterior view. *B*: Plexiform origin of the thoracic duct, lateral view. *C*: Double thoracic duct, lateral view. *D*: Double thoracic duct, lateral view. *E*: Bilateral termination. *F*: Right-sided termination. *G*: Communication with lower cervical lymphatics and nodes.

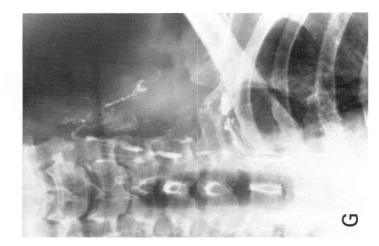

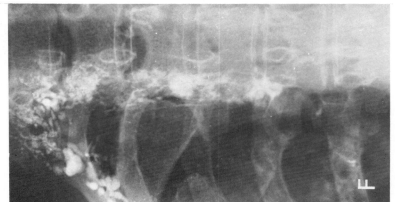

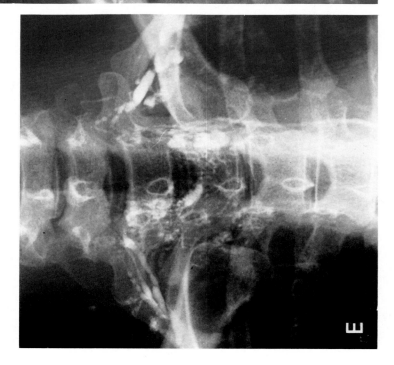

FIGURE 12.17E–G.

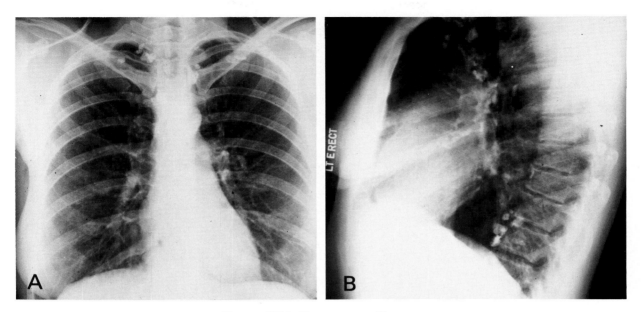

FIGURE 12.18. VARIATIONS OF NORMAL

*A:* Opacification of bilateral supraclavicular and paratracheal nodes. *B:* Mediastinal lymph node opacification as a manifestation of the variations of normal.

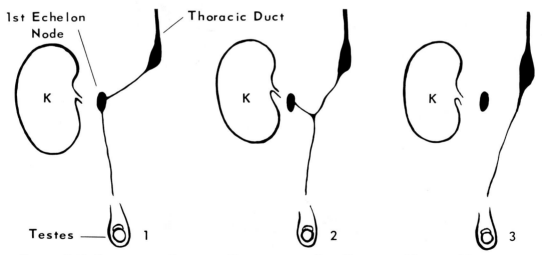

FIGURE 12.19. VARIATIONS IN LYMPHATIC DISTRIBUTION IN PART DETERMINE MODES OF METASTASIS
From Engeset (1959).

FIGURE 12.20. ALTERED LYMPHATIC DYNAMICS INFLUENCE MODES OF METASTASIS (*next page*)

*A:* Edema of the right lower extremity 6 months after a radical inguinal node dissection for melanoma. Opacified dermal and subcutaneous lymphatics are manifestations of lymphatic obstruction. *B:* The right inguinal nodes are still present and are not opacified. The left side can be considered the normal. *C:* The right ascending lumbar nodes were also bypassed as a manifestation of collateral flow (*arrow*).

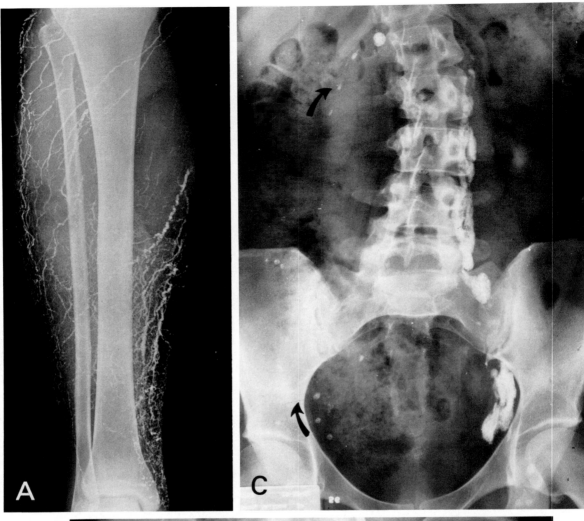

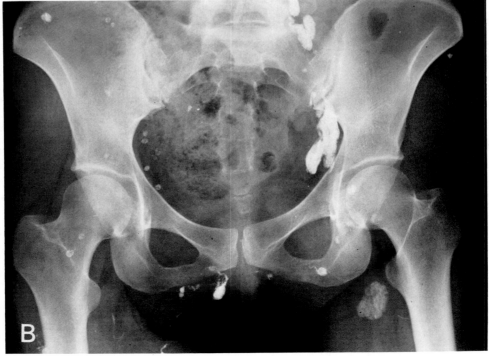

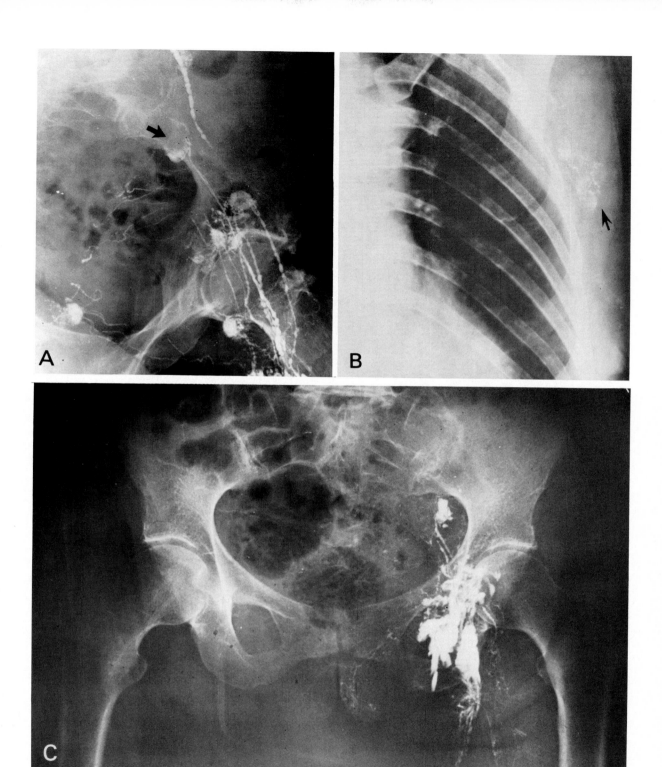

FIGURE 12.21. METASTASIS TO AXILLARY LYMPH NODES FROM CARCINOMA OF THE CERVIX

*A* and *B:* The left iliac nodes show evidence of metastasis. There is obstruction of the iliac lymphatics (*arrow*). The lower axillary nodes are opacified. *C–E:* Another patient with carcinoma of the cervix, with obstruction of the left iliac lymphatics by metastases, demonstrated the lymphatics of the anterior abdominal wall and chest wall (*arrows*) as collateral pathways to the axilla (Wohlgemuth). *F* and *G:* Metastases to axillary nodes were also demonstrated in still another patient with obstruction of the left common iliac lymphatics (*arrows*). Tomograms through the axillary nodes verified the metastasis.

315

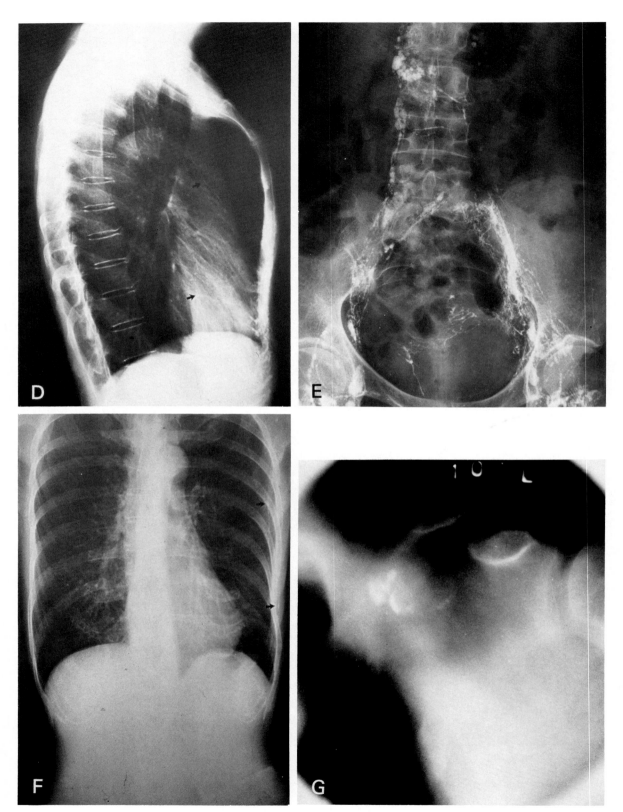

FIGURE 12.21*D–G.*

316

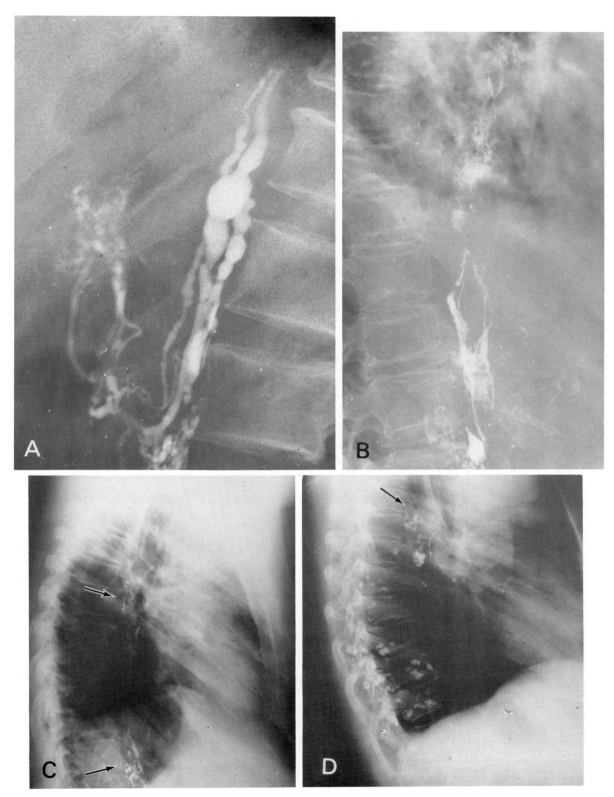

**FIGURE 12.22. THORACIC DUCT OBSTRUCTION**
*A:* Retrograde visualization of the gastrointestinal lymphatics as the result of thoracic duct obstruction. *B:* Carcinoma of the pancreas obstructing the thoracic duct with opacification of collateral channels. *C* and *D:* Obstruction of the thoracic duct by a carcinoma of the lung resulted in opacification of mediastinal lymphatics and nodes (*arrows*).

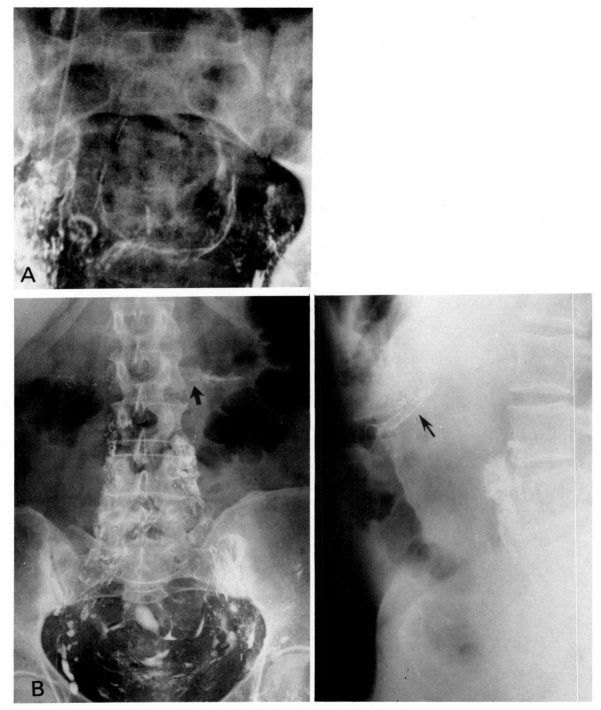

FIGURE 12.23. PARALYMPHATIC PATHWAYS

*A:* Visceral lymphatics opacified in the wall of the rectum. *B:* Contrast material in the wall of the stomach (*arrows*). *C:* The bladder wall lymphatics are delineated (*arrows*). *D:* Perivascular channels demarcate the right iliac artery (*top arrow*). There is apparent continuity with the lymphatics above the kidney (*bottom arrow*).

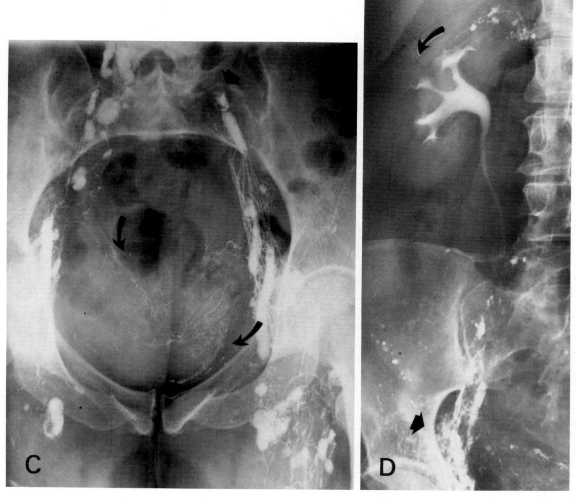

FIGURE 12.23C and D.

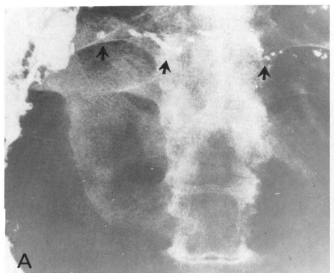

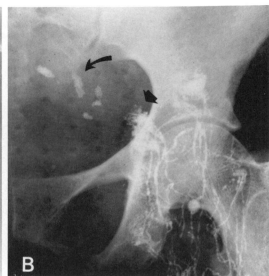

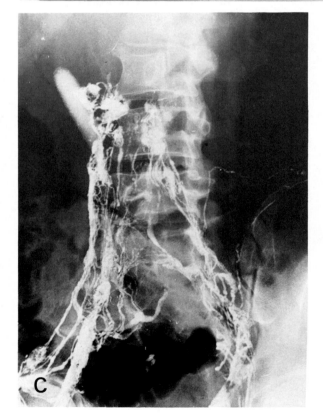

FIGURE 12.24.   LYMPHATICOVENOUS ANASTOMOSES
*A:* Droplets of contrast material in the distribution of sacral veins (*arrows*). *B:* Lymphaticovenous anastomoses secondary to lymphatic obstruction by metastatic carcinoma of the cervix (*arrows*). *C:* Lymphaticoinferior vena caval anastomoses, as described by Wolfel. *D* and *E:* Lymphatico-portal anastomoses (*arrow*) in a patient with carcinoma of the testis with extensive retroperitoneal nodal involvement.

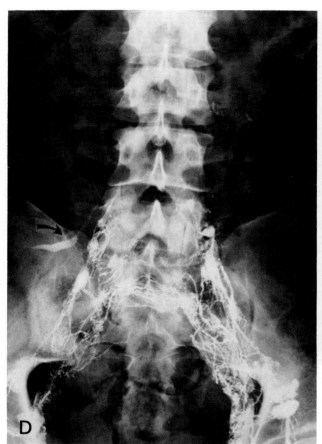
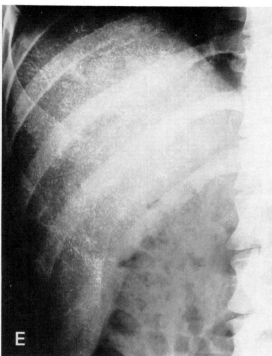

FIGURE 12.24*D* and *E*.

lymphatic drainage, the variations of normal, and the collateral pathways in the event of obstruction of normal channels (which include lymphatic to lymphatic, lymphatic to paralymphatic, and lymphatic to venous).

Utilizing these criteria, the positive diagnosis of nodal metastatic disease by LAG with the assistance of CT, US, venography, pyelography, and percutaneous needle biopsy can yield a positive pathological correlation of 90–95%. Suspicious or negative findings do not influence management of the patient. False-negative exami-

nations are due to (*a*) metastases too small to detect, (*b*) failure of opacification of the involved nodes, and (*c*) disease outside of the lymphatic system. The latter (*b* and *c*) can be documented by CT and US. CT is usually the initial examination followed frequently by LAG to (*a*) define disease in small nodes, (*b*) to confirm the presence of metastases in discrete nodes, and (*c*) at times, to follow the disease. Confirmation can be obtained by percutaneous needle biopsy guided by these modalities.

## TUMORS OF THE FEMALE GENITAL ORGANS

### The Uterine Cervix

Carcinoma of the uterine cervix follows carcinoma of the breast, uterine corpus, and colorectum in incidence of malignant neoplasms of women. The survival rate of patients with advanced carcinoma of the cervix has increased only slightly despite improved control of tumor

in the irradiated area with megavoltage radiotherapy. At M. D. Anderson Hospital the survival rate in stage IIIA cervical carcinoma has improved from 41 to 45% and in stage IIIB from 31 to 36% in the kilovoltage and megavoltage periods, respectively. A prime reason for these changes is the high incidence of lymph node metastases in advanced cervical cancer, many of which are outside the pelvic portals utilized. Improved results with extended radiation fields may be possible with accurate assessment of the extent of disease.

Usually the earlier and smaller the primary neoplasm, the smaller and fewer the metastases. Therefore, the yield of LAG and/or CT in the detection of metastases in patients with carcinoma of the cervix stage I is small. The metastases when present in this group are usually in the pelvis and are most likely included within the usual radiation treatment portal. However, with the more advanced tumors, the bulky or barrel-shaped stage I and above, bilateral pedal LAG and CT offer considerable assistance in determining the extent of involvement because of the relatively high incidence of lymph node metastases.

## Lymphatic Drainage of the Uterine Cervix

The lymphatics of the uterine cervix form a rich plexus. From this plexus, the collecting trunks leave the lateral border of the cervix and gather into three main pedicles: the external iliac, hypogastric, and posterior pedicles (Fig. 12.25).

**External Iliac Pedicle.** This pedicle consists of two to three collecting trunks that follow the course of the uterine artery and pass in front of the uterine artery and in front of the ureter. The trunks then cross the medial aspect of the umbilical artery and terminate in the superior and middle nodes of the middle or medial chain of the external iliac group. This pedicle is designated as the principle chain of the external iliac group.

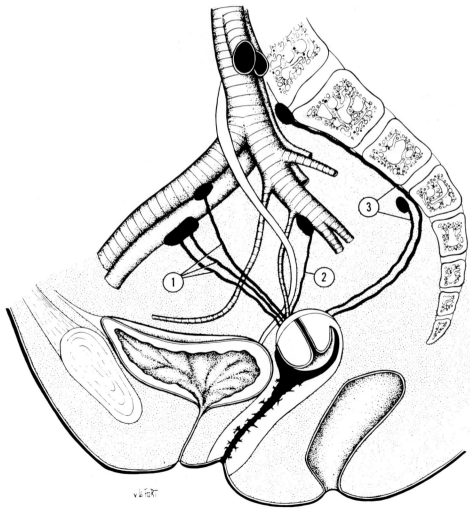

FIGURE 12.25. LYMPHATIC DRAINAGE OF THE UTERINE CERVIX
*1*, External iliac pedicle; *2*, hypogastric pedicle; and *3*, posterior pedicle.

**Hypogastric Pedicle.** This pedicle consists of one to three collecting trunks that follow the course of the uterine vein, pass behind the ureter, and terminate in one of the hypogastric nodes near the uterine artery. Occasionally, a lymphatic trunk passes the hypogastric station and ascends along the common iliac artery to a node of promontory.

**Posterior Pedicle.** The posterior pedicle is formed by two to four collecting trunks which are less rich and less constant than those in the other two pedicles. The trunks run in an antero-posterior direction following the lateral wall of the rectum and later ascend in front of the sacrum; they then terminate in the lateral sacral nodes and in the nodes of the promontory.

**The Intercalating Lymph Nodes.** This group of intercalated nodes includes parametrial nodes and paracervical nodes. In the parametrium, small lymph nodules are often found along the major lymphatic trunks transversing the parametrium. The paracervical nodes are located near the crossing of the uterine artery and the ureter. The collecting trunks of the external iliac pedicle are frequently interrupted by this group of nodes.

In general, the lymphatics of the uterine cervix are drained by the middle and superior nodes of the middle and medial chains of the external iliac group and sometimes also by the hypogastric nodes and the nodes of promontory.

*LAG in Tumors of the Uterine Cervix*

At M. D. Anderson Hospital and Tumor Institute, in the evaluation of 103 patients with advanced cancers of the cervix, including bulky or barrel-shaped stage I lesions and postradiation recurrence, 42 were diagnosed by LAG as having metastasis. Exploratory laparotomy confirmed the presence of metastatic disease in 41 of these 42 patients (sensitivity, 77%). Of the 61 patients considered negative by LAG, 49 were true-negative (specificity, 98%) and 12 were found to have lymph node involvement. The overall accuracy was 87% (Table 12.1). The high

percentage of false-negatives (12%) supports the contention that only a diagnosis of definitely positive disease has any clinical use. This is because microscopic metastases will not cause a significant lymph node defect that can be detected by LAG. Moreover, all of the pelvic and para-aortic lymph nodes are not filled by contrast medium.

Table 12.2 lists the groups of lymph nodes biopsied. In the group with positive roentgenographic and biopsy evidence of malignancy, there were 14 with positive aortic lymph nodes and 10 with disease in the common iliac area. Most of these were beyond the usual field of pelvic irradiation for cervical carcinoma. Only one patient in this series had had a pelvic lymph node biopsy prior to the LAG, but 34 patients had had pelvic irradiation (Table 12.3). It is stressed that, even in the 15 patients with previous irradiation who had both roentgenographic and histological proof of recurrence, previous irradiation did not invalidate interpretation of the subsequent lymphangiograms.

Eight patients were excluded from the study because the abnormal lymph node seen on LAG was still present on follow-up roentgenograms obtained shortly after surgical exploration. This emphasizes the difficulty in lymph node evaluation by laparotomy. Only those easily assessible can be evaluated.

To ensure biopsy of the suspected nodes, radiographs should be taken during and after lap-

TABLE 12.1.
ADVANCED CANCERS OF UTERINE CERVIX—
CORRELATION OF LYMPHANGIOGRAMS AND BIOPSIES

| | |
|---|---|
| Positive | 41 |
| False-negative | 12 |
| Negative | 49 |
| False-positive | 1 |
| Total | 103 |
| Sensitivity | 41 of 53 = 77% |
| Specificity | 49 of 50 = 98% |
| Accuracy | 90 of 103 = 87% |

TABLE 12.2.
ADVANCED TUMORS OF UTERINE CERVIX—GROUPS OF LYMPH NODES BIOPSIED*

| Lymph Node Group | Pos† Pos‡ § | Neg† Neg§ | Neg§ Pos‡ § |
|---|---|---|---|
| Aortic | 14 | 69 | 6 |
| Common iliac | 10 | 41 | 0 |
| External iliac | 20 | 45 | 7 |
| Internal iliac | 1 | 37 | 0 |
| Obturator | 0 | 36 | 3 |
| Inguinal | 2 | 0 | 0 |
| Supraclavicular | 1 | 0 | 0 |

* Does not include actual numbers of lymph nodes, only groups.
† Lymphangiogram diagnosis.
‡ Does not include negative lymph nodes removed at the same time.
§ Biopsy.

TABLE 12.3.
TUMORS OF UTERINE CERVIX—PREVIOUS IRRADIATION

| Pos*-Pos† | Neg*-Neg† | Neg*-Pos† |
|---|---|---|
| 15 | 14 | 5 |

* Lymphangiogram diagnosis.
† Biopsy diagnosis.

arotomy. At times during surgery, nodes are difficult to find or impossible to reach (Fig. 12.26). The removed nodes are placed in the anatomic position on a Plexiglas template that has the outline of the inferior vena cava and the aorta (Fig. 12.27). Specimen radiographs are correlated with the preoperative and postoperative lymphangiogram. The template and specimen radiographs also assist in separating fatty tissue from nonopacified nodes.

LAG and exploratory laparotomy in the staging of patients with carcinoma of the cervix assist in establishing the extent of disease as well as remove large metastatic deposits so that irradiation may be more effective. If metastases were found in the external iliac nodes, the irradiation portals were extended to the level of L4. When disease involved the common iliac nodes and above, treatment was extended to the level of the diaphragm. At present the combination of retroperitoneal node biopsy and extended field irradiation has been frequently associated with severe complications that negate the approach.

Kolbenstvedt (1975), in the evaluation of LAG in 300 patients with carcinoma of the cervix, stages I and II, reported a sensitivity of 29%, a specificity of 96%, and an accuracy of 79%. Lagasse et al. (1979) utilized LAG preoperatively in 95 patients with a sensitivity of 61%, specificity of 78%, and overall accuracy of 73%. Reiffenstuhl (1967) reported a 50% accuracy, Gerteis (1967) a 96% accuracy, and Fuchs and Seiler (1975) an 85% accuracy.

Further application of LAG in the manage-

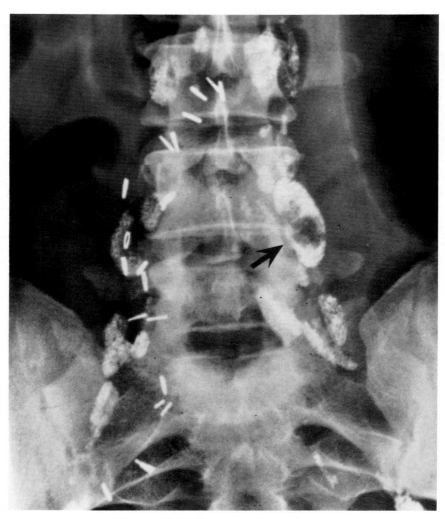

FIGURE 12.26. CARCINOMA OF THE CERVIX

The single metastatic node (*arrow*) was beyond the reach of the surgeon. Postoperative radiographs were necessary to confirm the biopsy of the nodes in question.

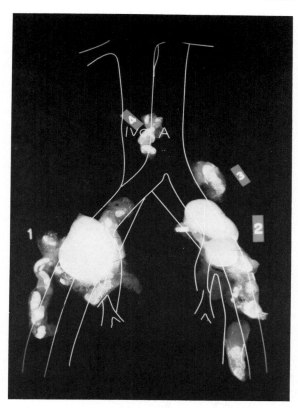

FIGURE 12.27. TEMPLATE UTILIZED FOR SURGICAL
CONFIRMATION

The nodes are specifically labeled, and comparison is made
with the postoperative radiographs. *IVC,* inferior vena cavogram; *A,* aorta; *1,* right external iliac nodes; *2,* left external
iliac nodes; *3,* left common iliac nodes.

### CT in Tumors of the Uterine Cervix

Only a few references regarding CT in the
diagnosis of carcinoma of the uterine cervix have
appeared in radiological literature. Whitley et al.
(1979) reported 17 cases of cervical carcinoma
with preoperative CT scans. The sensitivity was
80% (4 of 5), the specificity was 83% (10 of 12),
and the accuracy was 82% (14 of 17). The false-
positive rate was 11.7% (2 of 17) caused by
lymphoid hyperplasia. The false-negative rate
was 5.8% (1 of 17) due to normal-sized nodes
containing a microscopic lesion. In the Walsh
and Goplerud series (1981) of 75 selected patients with primary untreated cervical carcinoma
evaluated with CT for staging, 19 patients with
pelvic and inguinal node metastases had pathological correlation. CT was true-positive in 7 of
10 patients with pelvic or inguinal lymph node
metastases (sensitivity, 70%). The false-negative
rate was 30% (3 of 10) or 16% (3 of 19). The
results were true-negative in 7 of 9 patients
without metastases (specificity, 78%). The false-
positive rate was 22% (2 of 9) or 11% (2 of 19).
CT was correct in 14 of 19 patients (accuracy,
74%).

### Comparison of LAG and CT in Tumors of the Uterine Cervix

In our institution, 48 patients with carcinoma
of the uterine cervix examined by LAG followed
within a month by CT were reviewed to assess
the findings and their impact on management.
Thirty-five patients were studied as a part of the
primary evaluation and 13 for possible recurrent
disease. At clinical presentation, 7 patients were
stage IB, 14 were IIB, 8 were IIIA, 10 were IIIB,
8 were IVA, and 1 was IVB. Of the 13 patients
with recurrent disease, all had regional radiation
therapy; 2 were also treated by radical hysterec-
tomy.

Of the 48 patients, LAG was negative in 33
patients and positive with lymph node metastases in the remaining 15 patients. The CT scans
were negative in 32 patients and positive in 16
patients. Twenty patients of this group had
pathological correlation by biopsy or surgery.
LAG showed evidence of nodal metastasis in 7,
and overall accuracy was 95%. Six patients had
nodal metastasis on CT, and overall accuracy
was 75% (Fig. 12.28; Tables 12.4 and 12.5). There
were two false-negatives (10%) in CT, one due
to a small lesion less than 1.5–2 cm in diameter
and one caused by obliquity of projection in the
iliac region. One false-negative (5%) by LAG was

ment of carcinoma of the cervix was described
by Hammond et al. (1981). In one study Hammond et al. reviewed 202 patients with carcinoma
of the cervix examined by LAG between 1968–
1970 in an attempt to modify radiotherapy treatment fields, depending upon the extent of disease. An increase in the incidence of positive
LAG was related to an increase in stage, which
in general indicated an increase in the volume of
the primary tumor. In those patients with a
positive LAG, regardless of the stage of the primary lesion, the incidence of distant metastases
was equal, approximately one-third of patients
in each stage. Undoubtedly some patients with
more advanced disease may have died of their
primary malignancy before developing distant
metastases. On the other hand, the incidence of
distant metastases in patients with a negative
LAG was directly related to increasing tumor
stage and bulk.

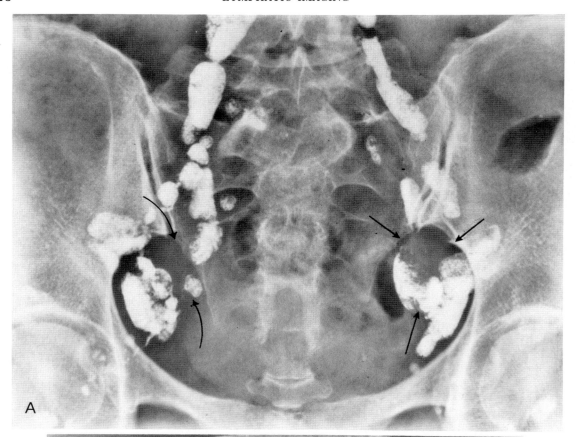

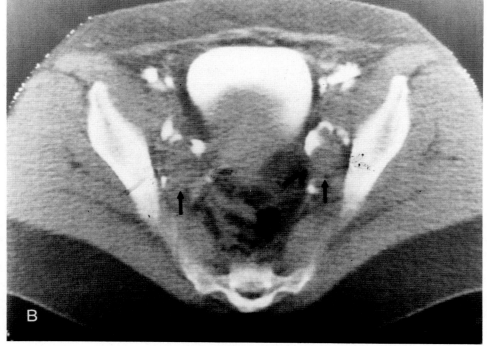

FIGURE 12.28. NODAL METASTASES FROM CARCINOMA OF THE UTERINE CERVIX
*A:* LAG. Abnormal lymph nodes with filling defects in external iliac regions (*arrows*). *B:* CT. Enlarged nodes with filling defects in external iliac areas, similar to those seen on LAG (*arrows*).

TABLE 12.4.
FINDINGS OF LAG AND CT ON 48 PATIENTS WITH
CARCINOMA OF CERVIX

|          | LAG | CT |
|----------|-----|-----|
| Positive | 15  | 16 |
| Negative | 33  | 32 |
| Total    | 48  | 48 |

TABLE 12.5.
PATHOLOGICAL CORRELATIONS OF 20 PATIENTS WITH
CARCINOMA OF CERVIX

|                | LAG | CT |
|----------------|-----|-----|
| Positive       | 7   | 6  |
| False-negative | 1   | 2  |
| Negative       | 12  | 9  |
| False-positive | 0   | 3  |
| Total          | 20  | 20 |

| | LAG | CT |
|-------------|------------------|------------------|
| Sensitivity | 7 of 8 = 87.5%   | 6 of 8 = 75.3%   |
| Specificity | 12 of 12 = 100%  | 9 of 12 = 75%    |
| Accuracy    | 19 of 20 = 95%   | 15 of 20 = 75%   |

caused by postoperative and postirradiation changes with lymphatic obstruction. Three cases showed false-positive findings (13%) on CT resulting from lymphoid hyperplasia and postirradiation fibrosis (Figs. 12.29 and 12.30).

In advanced lesions or postirradiation and postsurgical patients, when LAG shows lymphatic obstruction in the pelvic region with nonopacification of the nodes above the interruption, CT is of value to determine the extent of the disease. It may show normal nodes with no evidence of metastasis or demonstrated nonopacified nodal metastasis in the para-aortic area. In addition to detection of nodal metastasis, the local extension of the lesion of the cervix and extranodal metastases, such as to the urinary tract, liver, and skeleton, can be readily demonstrated by CT (Fig. 12.31).

CT has been applied to mapping the portals for radiation therapy. The detection of pelvic wall and retroperitoneal disease allows the radiotherapist to adjust the treatment to the tumor bulk altering the portals to the change in tumor size. The postirradiation changes are well documented by CT. Residual contrast medium in the lymph nodes from LAG can be used in the follow-up evaluation of a patient at regular intervals. Contrast medium remains in the nodes, yielding diagnostically interpretable information in 75% of the patients for 1 yr and in 35% for 2 yr after the initial LAG. Evaluation of the residual contrast medium-filled nodes by a single roentgenogram of the abdomen every 3–6 months is more feasible, financially more acceptable, and more sensitive than are CT scans done every 3 months (Fig. 12.32). Changes in the nodes, such as localized areas of destruction or enlargement, may indicate disease progression or recurrence. However, if more extensive disease is suspected, especially beyond the lymphatic system, CT becomes essential. Recurrences after surgery or radiation therapy are better detected by CT.

Edeiken-Monroe and Zornoza (1982) described the results of 159 percutaneous transabdominal aspiration needle biopsies on 129 patients with carcinoma of the cervix. The sensitivity was 58%, specificity 100%, predictive value of a positive test 100%, predictive value of a negative test 42%, and the overall accuracy was 68%. Because the predicted value of a negative test was only 42%, a negative biopsy was valueless. Therefore, only positive biopsies should be considered in the management of these patients. One biopsy was complicated by puncture of the left ureter with no subsequent problems found clinically or at exploratory laparotomy. No vascular damage or perforation of a hollow viscus was found in any of the 25 patients who subsequently underwent surgery.

## Uterine Corpus

The most common malignancy of the uterine corpus is adenocarcinoma of the endometrium, the incidence being 95% of the uterine tumors. The majority of pelvic sarcomas arise in the uterus as leiomyosarcoma, endometrial stromal sarcoma, or mixed mesodermal sarcoma. They comprise 3% of all uterine tumors.

### Lymphatic Drainage of the Uterine Corpus

The uterus has four intercommunicating lymphatic networks which run in the mucosa, muscularis, serosa, and subserosal areas. The collecting trunks originate in the lateral borders of the wall as well as in the superior angles of the uterus. They form three main pedicles: the uteroovarian, external iliac, and round ligament pedicles (Fig. 12.33).

**The Principle or Utero-Ovarian Pedicle.** This pedicle is composed of four to six collecting trunks. It leaves the wall below the cornua of the uterus and travels in the broad ligament until it reaches the hilum of the ovary. Here, the trunks anastomose and join with the ovarian lymphatics. Therefore, the uterine trunks ascend with those of the ovary along the ovarian blood vessels, and having arrived at the level of the lower

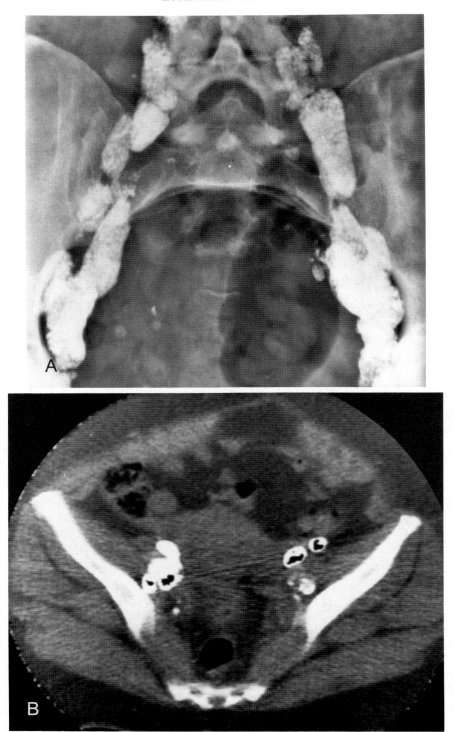

FIGURE 12.29.  LYMPHOID HYPERPLASIA IN A PATIENT WITH CARCINOMA OF THE UTERINE CERVIX
*A:* LAG. Enlarged nodes in external and common iliac regions with normal internal architecture. *B:* CT. Enlarged nodes, greater than 2 cm in diameter, in external iliac regions, considered as abnormal nodes. Computer artifacts are seen in the nodes.

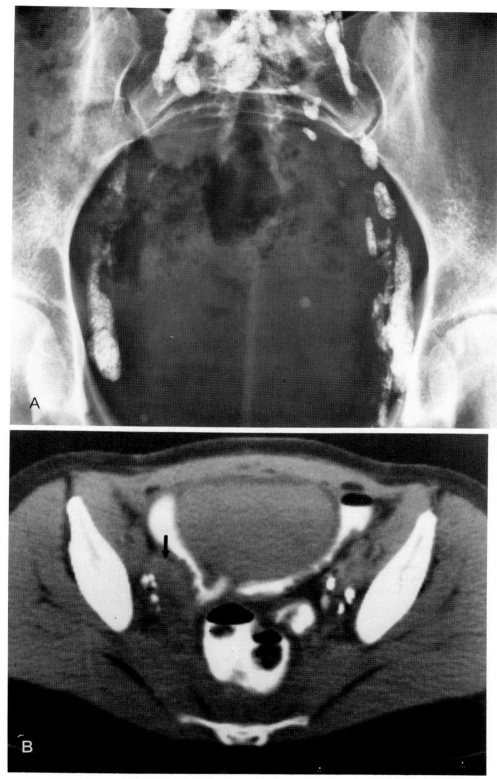

FIGURE 12.30. POSTIRRADIATION FIBROSIS IN RIGHT EXTERNAL ILIAC REGION IN A PATIENT WITH CARCINOMA OF THE
UTERINE CERVIX

*A:* LAG. Postirradiation change in pelvic region with decrease in number and size of the lymph nodes. *B:* CT. An oval-
shaped soft tissue density, medial to the opacified lymph nodes in right external iliac region with a question of tumor mass
(*arrow*). Exploratory laparotomy—postirradiation fibrosis without viable tumor cells.

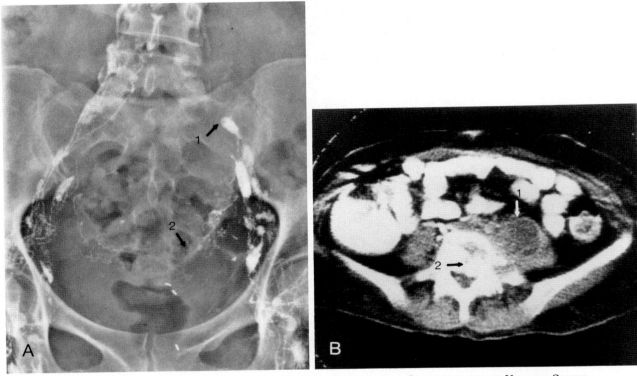

FIGURE 12.31. LYMPH NODE AND BONE METASTASES IN A PATIENT WITH CARCINOMA OF THE UTERINE CERVIX
A: LAG. Complete lymphatic obstruction at the level of the left wing of S1 (1) with retrograde filling of the lymph channels in the floor of the pelvis (2) consistent with nodal metastases in the common iliac region. B: CT of the lower abdomen. A large soft tissue mass from nodal metastases in the left common iliac region with secondary involvement of the vertebral body and left transverse process of L5.

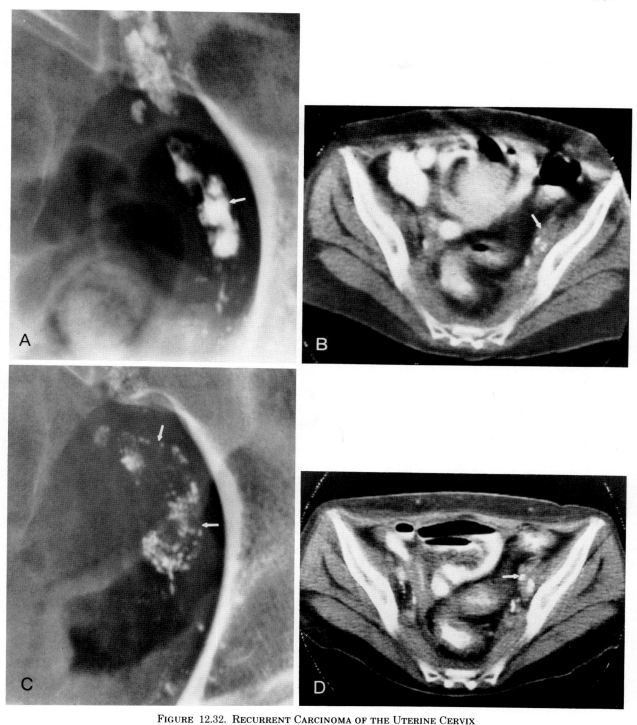

FIGURE 12.32. RECURRENT CARCINOMA OF THE UTERINE CERVIX

*A:* LAG. No evidence of nodal metastases in the left external iliac region (*arrow*). *B:* CT. No definite adenopathy in the left external iliac region (*arrow*). *C:* Plain film of abdomen (5 1/2 months after lymphangiogram) shows considerable enlargement of the nodes with irregular filling defects consistent with metastases in the left external iliac region (*arrows*). *D:* CT (5 1/2 months after initial CT) shows slight enlargement of the partially opacified nodes in the left external iliac region, possibly due to nodal metastasis (*arrow*). The changes in the abnormal nodes on CT are not so pronounced as those seen on LAG. Needle biopsy was positive for nodal metastasis.

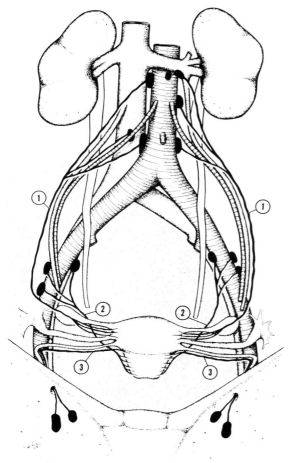

FIGURE 12.33. LYMPHATIC DRAINAGE OF THE UTERINE
CORPUS

*1,* Principal or utero-ovarian trunks; *2,* external iliac
trunks; and *3,* round ligament trunks.

pole of the kidney, they bend medially. On the
right side, they terminate in the precaval and
para-aortic nodes, particularly in the precaval
node near the origin of the inferior vena cava;
on the left side, they terminate in the left para-
aortic and preaortic nodes near the origin of the
inferior mesenteric artery.

**External Iliac Pedicle.** This pedicle contains fewer trunks than the utero-ovarian pedicle. The trunks follow a transverse direction
outward across the medial side of the umbilical
artery and end in the lymph nodes of the middle
chain of the external iliac group, usually in the
uppermost node of this chain.

**Round Ligament Pedicle.** This pedicle is
formed by a single trunk which follows the round
ligament from its insertion in the uterine fundus

to the inguinal canal and ends in the superficial
inguinal nodes.

In summary, the lymphatics of the uterine
corpus terminate in the para-aortic nodes and
the preaortic nodes in the vicinity of the origin
of the inferior mesenteric artery, in the nodes of
the middle group of the external iliac chain, and
sometimes also in the superomedial superficial
inguinal nodes.

### Lymph Node Metastasis in Tumors of the Uterine Corpus

In patients with tumor of the uterine corpus,
metastases to the regional lymph nodes occur
relatively infrequently. In a group of 233 patients
with adenocarcinoma of the uterine corpus
treated at M. D. Anderson Hospital between
1948–1964 with irradiation followed by hyster-
ectomy, only 1 patient was found to have disease
in the pelvic lymph nodes, and 6 patients (3%)
had tumor in the para-aortic nodes. Of 82 patients with adenocarcinoma involving the corpus
and cervix (corpus et collum) treated during the
same period of time, incidence of positive disease
was 6% (5 of 82 patients). Metastasis to the
para-aortic nodes was also seen in 5 patients
(6%).

In employing LAG prior to any treatment of
carcinoma of the uterine corpus in 76 patients
with carcinoma of the uterine corpus, Douglas et
al. (1972) reported an overall incidence of lymph
node metastasis of 19%. The frequency of para-
aortic lymph node metastases in that study was
9%. Kademain et al. (1977) performed lymphangiograms on 108 patients with adenocarcinoma
of the uterine corpus and found lymph node
metastases in 32 patients (29.6%). There was
para-aortic lymph node involvement in 8 patients (7.4%). In their series, histological confirmation was seldom obtained, but short term
follow-up indicated that a positive interpretation
is associated with an extremely poor prognosis.
In view of these statistics, the yield of LAG in
the detection of nodal metastasis in patients with
tumors of the uterine corpus is small but of value
in selected cases, especially in the bulky, more
advanced lesions or those extending to the cervix
(Figs. 12.34–12.36).

The role of CT in the diagnosis of carcinoma
of the uterine corpus is not yet established. Malignant tumors of the uterine corpus confined to
the uterus are often difficult or impossible to
detect unless there is invasion of adjacent structures with a loss of the fat planes. In the advanced lesions of stages III and IV, CT is helpful

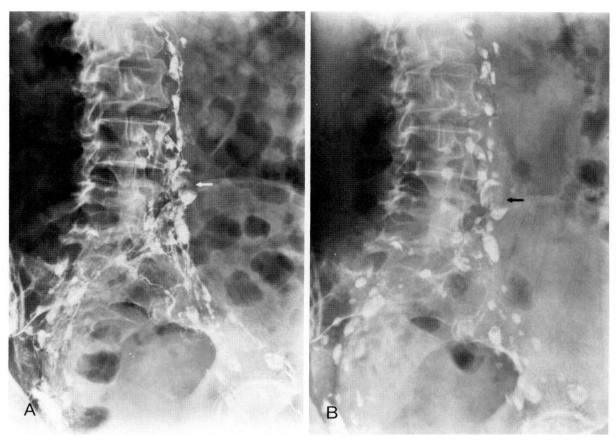

FIGURE 12.34. METASTATIC DISEASE TO THE LEFT LOWER LUMBAR LYMPH NODES FROM ADENOCARCINOMA OF THE
UTERINE CORPUS
A: Lymphatic phase (*arrow*). B: Nodal phase (*arrow*).

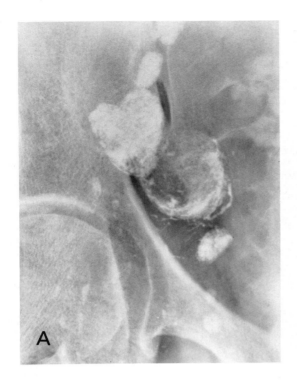

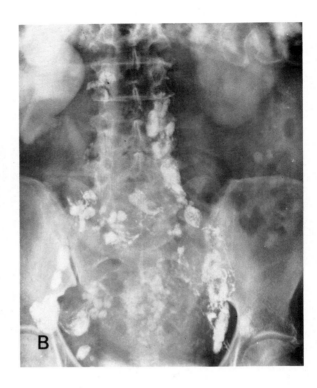

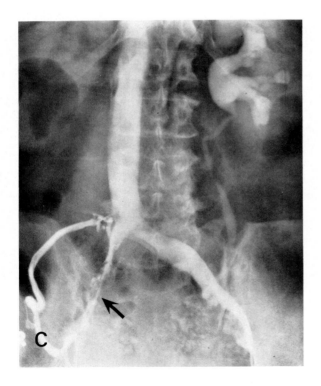

FIGURE 12.35.   METASTASES FROM ADENOCARCINOMA OF
THE UTERINE CORPUS TO THE RIGHT ILIAC LYMPH NODES
    *A:* Crescentic configuration of a right external iliac lymph
node due to metastatic carcinoma. *B:* Obstruction of the right
ureter by metastatic disease. Calcifications are noted in a
uterine leiomyoma. *C:* Compression and invasion into the
right external and common iliac veins (*arrow*) due to the
lymph node metastases. The extent of involvement is more
completely delineated with the help of venography.

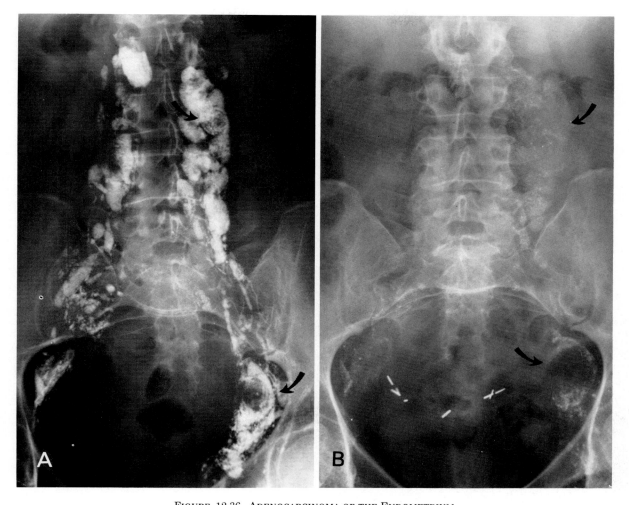

FIGURE 12.36. ADENOCARCINOMA OF THE ENDOMETRIUM

*A:* Metastatic disease (*arrow*) to the external iliac and para-aortic nodes demonstrated in the initial lymphangiogram. *B:* Follow-up roentgenograms 7 months later reveal progression of the disease (*arrows*).

to determine the local pelvic and retroperitoneal extensions (Fig. 12.37).

## The Ovary

Carcinoma of the ovary is the fourth most frequent cause of female cancer deaths in the United States and the leading cause of death among gynecological cancers, accounting for 100,000 deaths in the last 10 yr. The 5-yr survival rates range from 6–51%. These disappointing statistics are in part due to the late stage at which many ovarian cancers are usually discovered. When peritoneal washings are compulsively performed, more than 40% of patients with stage I disease have malignant cells in their washings. Diaphragmatic metastases are also common (44%).

Ovarian tumors have a significant incidence of nodal spread: 12.8% in stage I, 11.8% in stage II, 31.1% in stage III, and 60.0% in stage IV. The importance of lymph node metastases from ovarian neoplasms has been virtually ignored except in the case of dysgerminoma. Little attention is paid to this factor when planning treatment. Bilateral pedal LAG and CT, by demonstrating lymph node and extralymphatic metastases, have value in the more thorough assessment of the extent of disease—a prerequisite for intelligent management of any patient with cancer.

### Lymphatic Drainage from the Ovary

The parenchyma of the ovary contains a rich capillary network of lymphatics, chiefly in the theca externa of the follicles and corpora lutea.

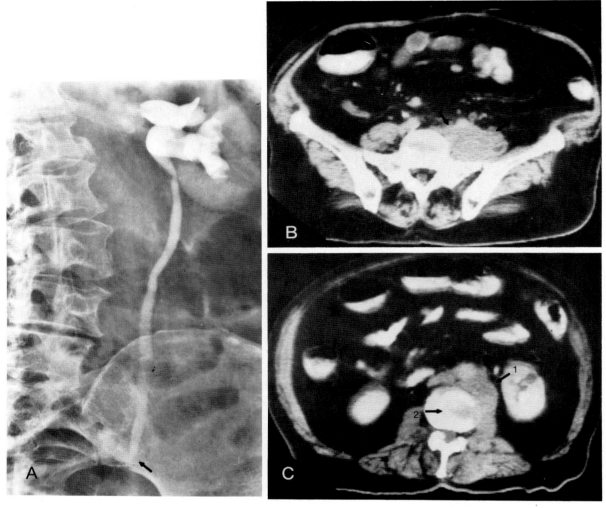

FIGURE 12.37. RECURRENT CARCINOMA OF THE ENDOMETRIUM

*A:* Intravenous pyelogram shows partial obstruction of the left ureter at the level of the pelvic inlet. *B:* CT of the pelvis. A large soft tissue mass from nodal metastasis in the left common iliac region at the level of S1 (*arrows*). *C:* CT of the lower abdomen shows metastatic lesion involving the left para-aortic nodes (*1*). There is secondary involvement of the left side of the vertebral body of L3 (*2*).

Lymphatics are absent in the tunica albugina. Six to eight large lymphatic collecting trunks emerge from the hilum, converging in the mesovarium with the efferent lymph vessels from the uterine fundus and fallopian tube to form the subovarian plexus. In the ovarian suspensory ligament, the lymphatics, with the ovarian blood vessels, cross the ureter and external iliac vessels and travel upward along the lateral aspect of the ureter to the level of the inferior pole of the kidney. Here the lymphatics turn medially, leaving the ovarian blood vessels, and cross the ureter again to reach its medial aspect. This crossing occurs at a higher point on the left than on the right. On the right, the collecting trunks diverge and drain into the precaval and lateral caval nodes, which lie along the inferior vena cava from its bifurcation to the renal pedicle. On the left, these trunks diverge to a lesser extent and at a higher level than on the right and end in the para-aortic and preaortic nodes which are placed one above another below the left renal pedicle (Fig. 12.38).

In 3 of 14 cases, Marcille (1903) discovered an accessory lymphatic pedicle from the ovary. The ovarian collecting trunks traveled in the broad ligament from the hilar plexus and then passed posteriorly under the peritoneum to end in a

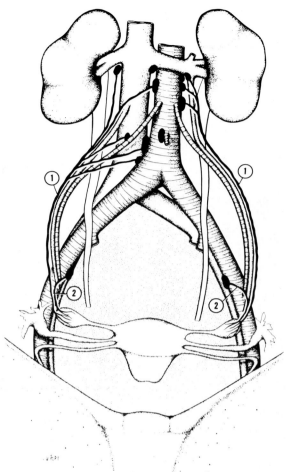

node of the middle chain of the external iliac group (Fig. 12.38). Anastomoses occur between the ovarian lymph vessels and those of the uterus and the fallopian tubes, so that other variations might exist. In addition, the presence of a malignant neoplasm extending beyond the ovary with invasion of adjacent pelvic viscera and peritoneum may allow direct lymphatic continuity with the inguinal nodes and with external and common iliac nodes.

### LAG in Tumors of the Ovary

At M. D. Anderson Hospital, 72 lymphangiograms were performed on 66 patients with 6 patients examined twice. Thirty-three (46%) of these 72 lymphangiograms revealed lymph node metastases, which are presented in Table 12.6. Of the 33 positive examinations, the distribution of lymph node metastases was: para-aortic, 23 (70%); iliac, 19 (58%); inguinal, 9 (27%); and supraclavicular, 2 (6%). Para-aortic nodal involvement alone was seen in 14, and iliac lymph node metastases alone were demonstrated in 4. The combination of iliac and para-aortic nodal metastases was diagnosed by lymphangiography in 9 (Figs. 12.39–12.42). In each of the 9 patients with inguinal node metastases, there was concomitant iliac lymph node involvement. Three of these patients also had para-aortic lymph node metastases. The 2 patients with supraclavicular lymph node metastases also had iliac node involvement (Fig. 12.43).

The relationship between lymph node metastases and histological classification is shown in Table 12.7. Of the 10 patients with nodal metas-

FIGURE 12.38. LYMPHATIC DRAINAGE OF THE OVARY
Normal lymphatic ovarian drainage. *1*, Para-aortic lymphatic pedicle; *2*, external iliac pedicle.

TABLE 12.6.
SUMMARY OF CASES OF CARCINOMA OF THE OVARY

| Histological Classification | Lymphangiogram | | Confirmation of Positive Finding | | |
|---|---|---|---|---|---|
| | Pos | Neg | Surgery | Clinical | None |
| I. Malignant neoplasms, NOS* | 0 | 3 | | | |
| II. Carcinoma, NOS | 4 | 2 | 4 | | |
| III. Müllerian derivative carcinomas | | | | | |
|    A. Serous | 14 | 21 | 10 | 4 | |
|    B. Mucinous | 1 | 1 | | 1 | |
|    C. Endometroid | 3 | 4 | 3 | | |
| IV. Germ cell tumors | | | | | |
|    A. Dysgerminoma | 8 | 3 | 5 | 1 | 2† |
|    B. Embryonal carcinoma | 0 | 2 | | | |
|    C. Teratoma, malignant | 0 | 1 | | | |
|    D. Mixed germ cell tumor | 2 | 0 | 2 | | |
| V. Sex cord tumors | | | | | |
|    A. Granulosa-theca cell | 0 | 0 | | | |
|    B. Sertoli-Leydig | 1 | 2 | 1 | | |
|     Total | 33 | 39 | 24 | 6 | 2 |

* NOS, not otherwise specified.

† In two cases, no laparotomy was performed.

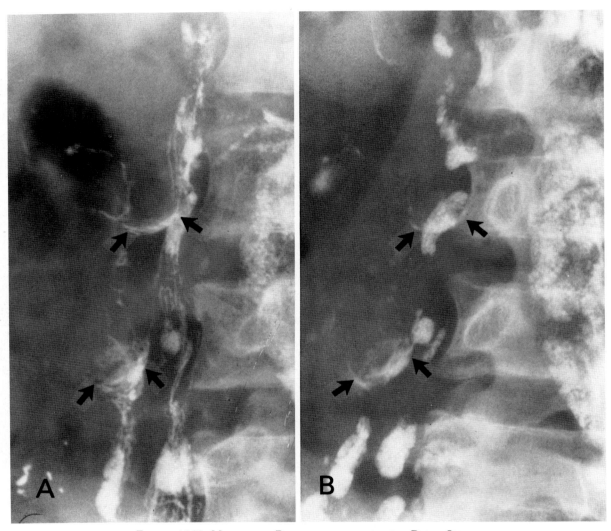

FIGURE 12.39.  METASTATIC DYSGERMINOMA FROM THE RIGHT OVARY

*A:* The lymphatics do not traverse the filling defects in the right lumbar lymph nodes in the lymphatic phase (*arrows*). *B:* Crescent configuration (*arrows*) of the residual functioning portion of these nodes involved by metastases.

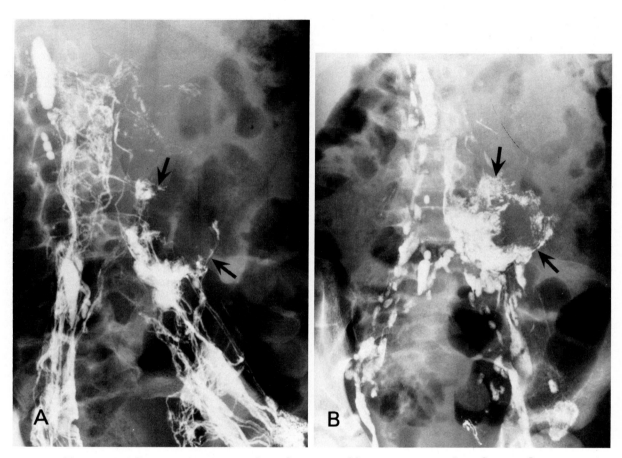

FIGURE 12.40 DYSGERMINOMA OF THE LEFT OVARY WITH METASTASES TO THE LEFT COMMON ILIAC.
A: Lymphatic phase (*arrows*). B: Nodal phase (*arrows*).

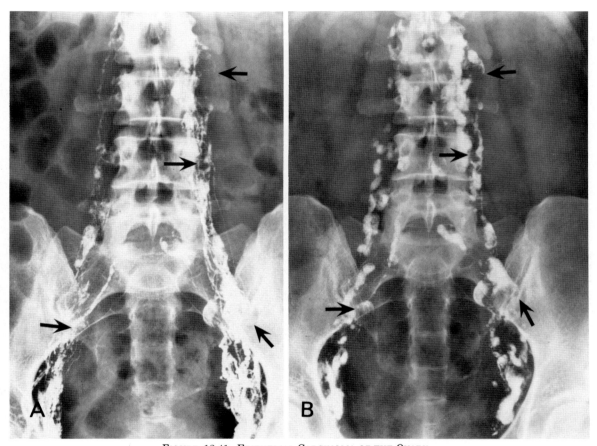

FIGURE 12.41. EPITHELIAL CARCINOMA OF THE OVARY

*A:* Lymphatic phase. The lymphatics do not traverse filling defects in the iliac and para-aortic lymph nodes (*arrows*). *B:* Nodal phase. Note the crescentic configuration of nodes containing metastases (*arrows*).

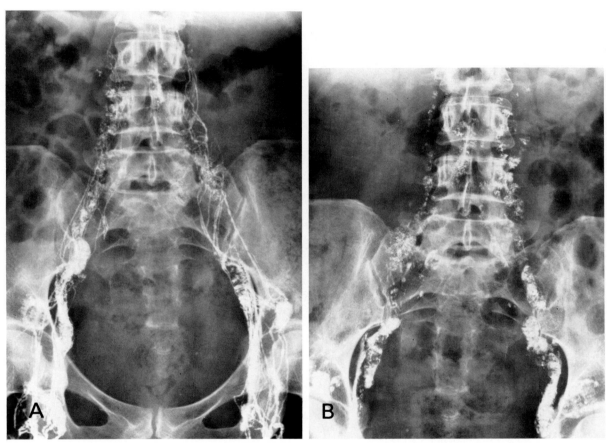

FIGURE 12.42. EPITHELIAL CARCINOMA INVOLVING BOTH OVARIES—SEROUS CYST ADENOCARCINOMA
A: Lymphatic phase. B: Nodal phase; the "lymphoma" pattern in metastatic ovarian carcinoma.

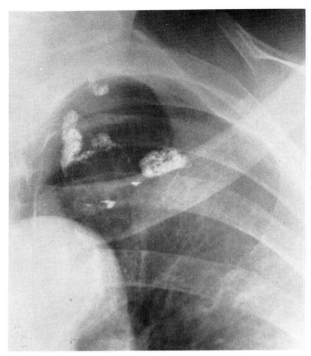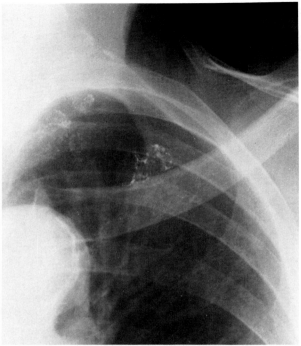

FIGURE 12.43. SUPRACLAVICULAR LYMPH NODE METASTASES FROM OVARIAN CARCINOMA
Progression of supraclavicular metastases over a 6-month period.

TABLE 12.7.
OVARIAN CANCER AND LAG

|  | Distribution of Lymph Node Metastases* | | | | | | |
|---|---|---|---|---|---|---|---|
|  | P | I | P, I | I, In | P,I,In | P,I,S | P,I,In,S |
| Epithelial | 6 | 3 | 3 | 6 | 2 | 1 | 1 |
| Germ cell | 7 | 1 | 2 |  |  |  |  |
| Sex cord tumor | 1 |  |  |  |  |  |  |

* P, para-aortic; I, iliac; In, inguinal; S, supraclavicular.

TABLE 12.8.
STAGE GROUPING FOR PRIMARY CARCINOMA OF THE OVARY

| Stage I | Growth limited to the ovaries |
|---|---|
| Stage II | Growth involving one or both ovaries with pelvic extension |
| Stage III | Growth involving one or both ovaries with widespread intraperitoneal metastases |
| Stage IV | Growth involving one or both ovaries with distant metastases |

tases from cancers of germ cell origin, para-aortic nodal involvement was found in 9 and iliac metastases in 3. Lymph node metastases from ovarian epithelial cancers (Müllerian derivatives and carcinomas not otherwise specified) were found in 22 lymphangiograms; the para-aortic lymph nodes were involved in 13 and the iliac nodes in 16. Of these, para-aortic nodal involvement alone was seen in 6 and combined iliac and para-aortic in 7.

Clinical staging was determined by abdominal exploration. LAG was usually performed following this staging procedure. The distribution of the stages in the 66 patients was: stage I, 5; II, 9; III, 35; and IV, 17 (Table 12.8).

Seven patients with ovarian carcinoma and ascites were studied by LAG to determine whether there was a relationship between lymph node metastases and ascites. Only 1 of these 7 patients had lymph node metastases. Peritoneal implants were found in all 7 patients with ascites. In 1 of these patients, the liver was small with extensive fatty infiltration. Conversely, of the 33 with lymph node metastases, only 1 had ascites. The histological classification of these 7 patients with ovarian carcinoma and ascites was epithelial neoplasm in 6 and germ cell tumors in 1 (a malignant teratoma).

In the literature, lymph node metastases from the ovary have been demonstrated by LAG by Douglas et al. (1971), who found para-aortic nodal metastases in 8 (18%) of 44 patients, by Parker et al. (1974) in 17 (25%) of 69 patients, by Musumeci et al. (1975) in 44 (38%) of 117 patients, and by Fuchs (1969) in 19 (48%) of 39 patients. More recently Musumeci et al. (1980) reported that in carcinoma of the ovary, LAG revealed a sensitivity of 79%, a specificity of 100%, and an accuracy of 92%. The high incidence (46%) of positive lymphangiograms in our series certainly does not reflect the true frequency of nodal metastases in cancer of the ovary. It does emphasize, however, that nodal metastases do occur in both epithelial and germ cell neoplasms of the ovary more frequently than is commonly recognized.

Lymphatic drainage from the ovary is primarily to the para-aortic nodes. This distribution was confirmed by the 70% incidence of para-aortic lymph node metastases in the 33 lymphangiograms with evidence of nodal metastases. However, iliac lymph node metastases were found in 58%, and inguinal node involvement was seen in 27%. This is somewhat higher than might be expected based on Marcille's investigation revealing approximately 20% of 14 cases with an accessory lymphatic pedicle from the ovary which drained to the external iliac lymph nodes. Inguinal lymph node metastases were almost always associated with iliac node disease. This could be due to direct drainage to the inguinal area, as might be expected if the uterus or fallopian tubes were invaded, or to obstruction of iliac lymphatics with retrograde spread.

The distribution of lymph node metastases was further related to the histological types of ovarian neoplasm. The germ cell tumors almost invariably metastasized to the para-aortic nodes (90%) and to a lesser extent to the iliac nodes (30%). On the other hand, the ovarian cancers of epithelial cell origin metastasized to the iliac nodes in 41%. This suggests that the neoplasms of germ cell origin are usually confined to the ovary and spread along the anatomically defined lymphatic drainage. Epithelial cell malignancies are more likely to extend through the capsule to involve adjacent pelvic viscera, which may account for the frequency of pelvic nodal metastases, both to inguinal and iliac lymph nodes. In many instances the ovarian lesion was huge and was described as adhering to the pelvic walls. The iliac nodes may be involved by contiguity. Para-aortic, in addition to iliac and inguinal nodal, metastases in some of these cases may be spread by continuity.

Mediastinal and supraclavicular nodal metastases are most probably a manifestation of variations in normal lymphatic distribution of the thoracic duct. This would explain the apparent continuity of metastases in the pelvic, para-aor-

tic, and supraclavicular lymph nodes in two cases in this series.

Hanks and Bagshaw (1969) have described LAG as an aid in staging and planning the therapy. Para-aortic lymph node metastases were demonstrated in 7 of 20 patients, even though these areas were palpably normal at surgical exploration. As a result of the lymphangiographic findings, the stage was changed in six of these patients, and the therapy was altered.

Ascites, although a frequent finding in patients with ovarian cancer, was found in only seven patients in our series. This may have been a product of the nonrandomized selection. The mechanisms underlying the development of ascites in patients with peritoneal carcinomatosis are still obscure. Ascites may be the result of either an increased inflow or obstruction to outflow of fluid from the peritoneal cavity, especially through the diaphragmatic lymphatics. LAG was performed in these patients to determine if there was a relationship between lymph node metastases producing lymphatic obstruction, lymphatic fistulae, and ascites. Only 1 of 33 patients with lymph node metastases had ascites. On the other hand, each of the 7 patients with ascites was found to have peritoneal implants of ovarian cancer. Increased production of fluid has been attributed to an increased capillary permeability to protein, especially at the peritoneal tumor implants. Perhaps peritoneal implants encroach upon the available surface for fluid absorption by interfering with the lymphatic network draining the peritoneal cavity. Tumor cells were found obstructing diaphragmatic lymphatics in experimentally produced ascites due to peritoneal carcinomatosis. Another etiological agent to be considered in the presence of ascites in patients with ovarian cancer treated by total abdominal irradiation is radiation hepatitis.

## CT in Tumors of the Ovary

With perhaps the exception of dysgerminoma, the importance of lymphatic metastases from carcinoma has been virtually ignored. Perhaps the lack of interest is due to the relatively late stage at which most ovarian carcinomas are discovered. The extent of local and peritoneal spread is usually the dominant factor in determining the treatment plan. At M. D. Anderson Hospital, we performed CT scanning on 23 patients with carcinoma of the ovary, and on 7 of these patients CT was performed following LAG. It is the general feeling that CT is not as useful in detecting early nodal metastases as is the lymphangiogram. However, CT is of value in advanced lesions. Local and extrapelvic extension of disease is appreciated by the invasion of adjacent viscera and pelvic and retroperitoneal lymph nodes (Fig. 12.44). Involvement of para-aortic nodes is more readily identified than that of pelvic nodes because of the surrounding retroperitoneal fat. Large, matted, nodular masses are almost invariable due to metastases in a patient with ovarian carcinoma. Enlargement (1.5 cm or greater) of isolated nodes must be verified by biopsy or LAG (Fig. 12.45). Peritoneal and omental metastases (greater than 2.0 cm) as well as ascites can be demonstrated by CT (Fig. 12.46). With the assistance of the intraperitoneal injection of water-soluble contrast material, smaller peritoneal metastases may be detected. Liver metastases from the ovary are relatively uncommon (10%). In the comparison of scanning techniques, CT is the best single examination to determine the presence and extent of a hepatic mass. In addition to staging by determining the extent of disease, CT is effective in defining radiation therapy fields, monitoring response to treatment, and detecting recurrent tumor.

## The Vulva

The vulva is supplied by a particularly rich capillary network of lymphatics. The collecting trunks are drained into the superficial and deep inguinal nodes. There may be drainage to the hypogastric nodes through the lymphatic network of the urethra and to external iliac nodes. Free anastomoses exist between the lymphatics of both sides of the vulva (Fig. 12.47).

Bilateral pedal LAG opacifies many of these nodes. Although there are added difficulties in the interpretation of changes in the inguinal nodes because of the common occurrence of chronic inflammatory disease, a diagnosis of metastases can be made if the criteria previously discussed are present.

Metastases are frequently observed in the inguinal nodes; one-third of the patients seen with carcinoma of the vulva are found to have metastases. When radical vulvectomy and bilateral inguinal node dissection are planned, preoperative evaluation of the iliac nodes is essential (Figs. 12.48 and 12.49).

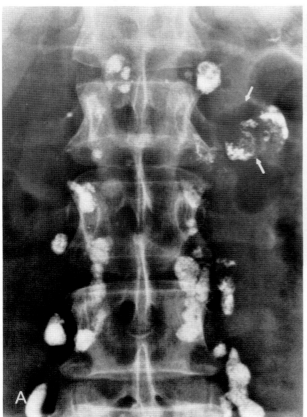

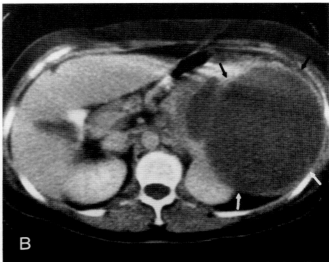

FIGURE 12.44.   LYMPH NODE AND SPLENIC METASTASES FROM CARCINOMA OF THE OVARY

*A:* Lymphangiogram demonstrates nodal metastases in the left para-aortic region (*arrows*). *B:* CT shows large rounded cystic mass in the upper quadrant (*arrows*) with compression of the left kidney. Exploratory laparotomy demonstrated metastases involving most parts of the spleen, left adrenal gland, and para-aortic lymph nodes.

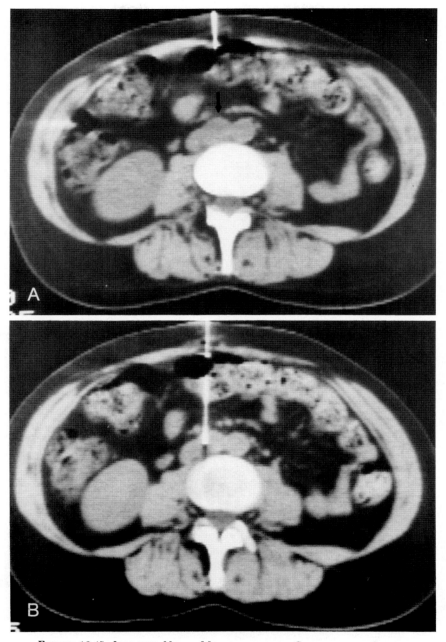

FIGURE 12.45. ISOLATED NODAL METASTASIS FROM CARCINOMA OF OVARY

*A:* CT of the abdomen demonstrates a nodal mass between the aorta and vena cava (*arrow*). *B:* Needle in the nodal mass. The cytological specimen yielded metastatic ovarian carcinoma.

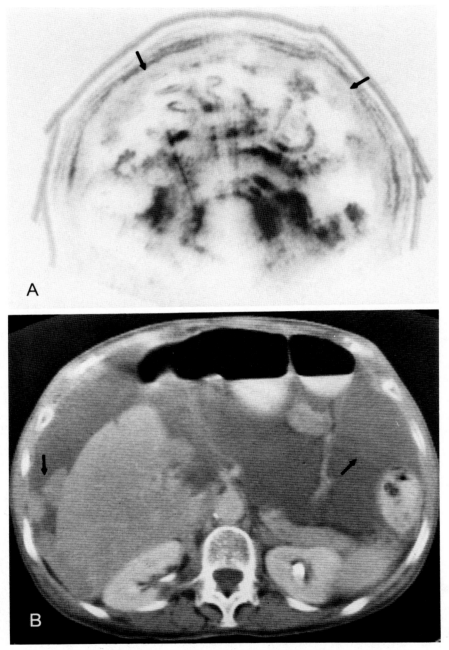

FIGURE 12.46. OVARIAN CARCINOMA WITH OMENTAL METASTASIS AND ASCITES
*A:* Transverse sonogram through the midabdomen shows solid tissue posterior to the anterior abdominal wall consistent with an omental metastasis (omental "cake", *arrows*). There is ascites within the peritoneal cavity. *B:* CT of the abdomen demonstrates ascites and peritoneal metastatic implants (*arrow*).

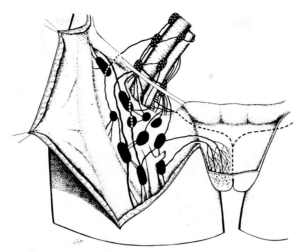

FIGURE 12.47. LYMPHATIC DRAINAGE OF THE VULVA

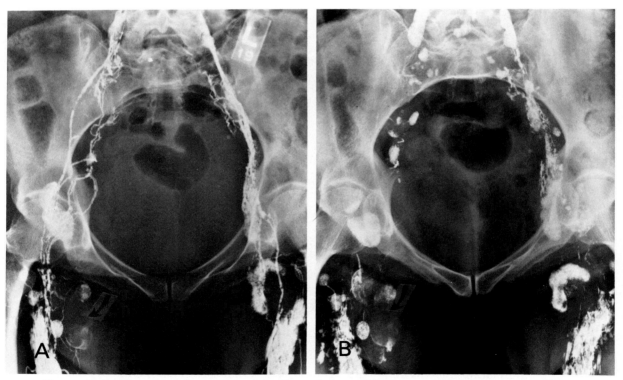

FIGURE 12.48. METASTATIC CARCINOMA TO THE RIGHT INGUINAL NODES FROM A CARCINOMA OF THE VULVA
*A:* Lymphatic phase; the lymphatics do not traverse the defect in the nodes. *B:* Nodal phase, inguinal nodes involved by metastatic disease can be detected by LAG (*arrow*).

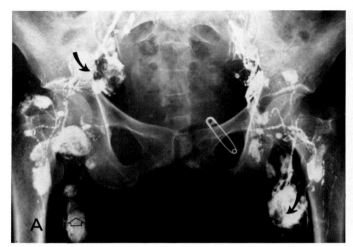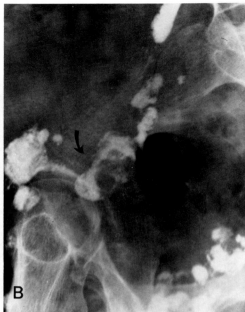

FIGURE 12.49. CARCINOMA OF VULVA

*A:* Metastases in each inguinal area as well as a right external iliac lymph node (*arrows*). *B:* Oblique projection of the right external iliac nodal metastases (*arrows*).

## TUMORS OF THE GENITOURINARY TRACT

### The Testes

Prior to discussion of testicular tumors, a description of the embryology and anatomy of the testicle and its lymphatic drainage is of value.

#### Embryology

The urogenital fold extends from C6 to S2. The ridge divides it into a lateral mesonephric fold and a median genital fold, the analage of the genital gland. The testicle descends from the para-aortic region to the scrotum. Gonadal tissue may exist anywhere along this distribution.

#### Lymphatic Drainage of the Testis

Testicular lymphatics accompany the internal spermatic artery and vein and drain into the lumbar nodes. The right trunks terminate in the right lumbar glands, which lie between the level of the aortic bifurcation and the renal vein. In 10%, these trunks end in a node in the angle between the right renal vein and the inferior vena cava (Rouvière, 1938). The left testicular lymphatics drain into the para-aortic nodes near the left renal vein in approximately two-thirds of the cases. They may also end in glands at the level of the bifurcation of the aorta or drain into the common iliac nodes (Cuneo, 1959) (Fig. 12.50).

Lymphatics from the epididymis may accompany the testicular lymphatics to the lumbar nodes or terminate in the external iliac nodes.

Clinical investigation utilizing direct testicular LAG by Busch et al. (1965), Chiappa et al. (1966), and Cook et al. (1965) have confirmed Rouviere's (1938) findings (Figs. 12.51 and 12.52). They demonstrate testicular lymphatic channels terminating in a sentinel node at the level of L1/L2 on the left and L1/L3 on the right, slightly lateral to the lumbar nodes usually opacified by pedal LAG. From the right testis there may be direct filling of the right lateral nodes, above or below the renal vein, or directly to the left lateral nodes. There may be immediate crossover of the right testicular lymphatics to the contralateral nodes, while the left testicular vessels cross over after permeating the sentinel nodes. From the lumbar nodes, continuity of the lymphatic system is usually maintained through the thoracic duct.

In the final analysis, important nodes are filled by testicular LAG that are not opacified by the pedal route, necessitating the combined approach whenever possible (Figs. 12.53–12.55). Thus far in human testicular LAG with the

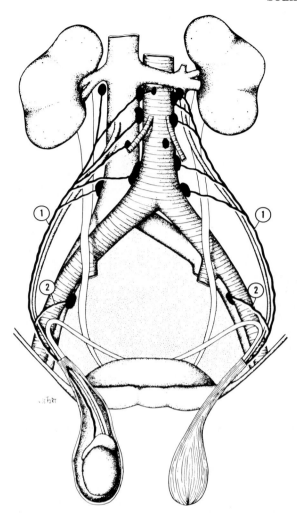

FIGURE 12.50. LYMPHATIC DRAINAGE OF THE TESTICLE
*1,* The major draining trunks empty into the lumbar lymph nodes from the level of the renal hilum to the bifurcation of the aorta. *2,* The external iliac nodes may occasionally drain the testicles.

injection of one or perhaps two testicular lymphatic trunks, analogous categories to those demonstrated by Engeset (1959) in his animal experiments have only in part been found (Fig. 12.19). However, the clinical distribution of metastases from carcinoma of the testicle has paralleled Engeset's findings. On rare occasions pulmonary metastases are discovered in the absence of retroperitoneal disease.

## LAG in Tumors of the Testis

Nodal metastases from testicular malignant disease show several different architectural patterns. Involved nodes are more spherical than

normal and may have a crescent deformity with the lymphatics failing to penetrate the marginal defects (carcinoma pattern) (Figs. 12.56–12.58). Occasionally, they may have an abnormal internal architecture with a relatively intact marginal sinus (lymphoma pattern). The latter picture is more frequently seen in some seminomas, lymphomas, and rhabdomyosarcomas of the testicle (Figs. 12.59–12.61). At times the metastatic nodes show both carcinoma and lymphoma type patterns, a mixed variety. Perhaps this mixed pattern reflects the varied components that are present at times in a testicular neoplasm.

Our experience with 291 cases of testicular malignancies studied by pedal LAG is described in Table 12.9. Patients with seminoma, of whom 24% had abnormal findings by LAG, were treated by radiotherapy alone, making specific nodal correlation impossible. All other testicular malignancies were managed by a combination of surgery and radiotherapy, permitting closer scrutiny of the lymphangiographic findings. A normal lymphangiogram and normal findings at surgical exploration negate the necessity of any radiotherapy.

Surgical or autopsy findings or both were correlated with lymphangiographic findings (Table 12.10). Retroperitoneal node dissections were performed at times following radiation therapy. Of the 50 node dissections in which positive nodes were found, 37 patients were diagnosed preoperatively by pedal LAG (sensitivity, 74%). Positive roentgenographic interpretation had excellent correlation with pathological findings (97%). Surgical exploration was not uniformly undertaken, especially in patients with more advanced disease. Of a total of 83 considered negative by LAG, 70 were negative at surgical exploration (specificity, 98.6%). Of the 13 patients (11%) who exhibited false-negative findings, 4 showed microscopic lesions 3 mm or less in size, 1 had a lesion in the interaorticocaval area, and 8 were found to have metastases in nodes lateral to those usually opacified by pedal LAG. These metastases may have been diagnosed by the testicular route, US, or CT. The overall accuracy was 88.4%.

The lymph nodes removed during the retroperitoneal dissection are placed on a Plexiglas template in their in vivo position, and a radiograph of the nodes is then done (Fig. 12.62). This is compared with the preoperative and postoperative radiographs, especially to verify the presence and removal of abnormal lymph nodes. This is especially important when the node dissection follows the initial course of radiotherapy. At times 2500 rad will produce a dramatic response

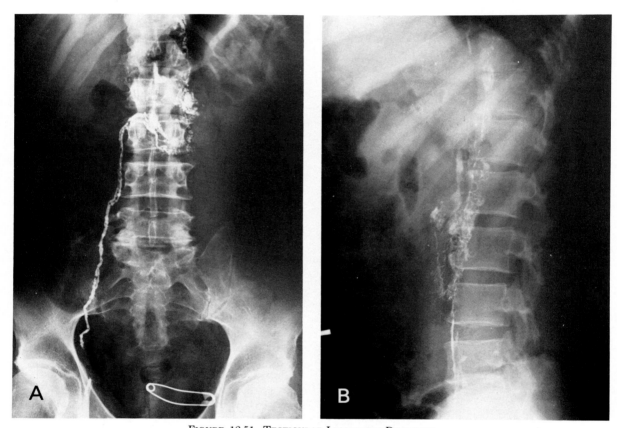

FIGURE 12.51. TESTICULAR LYMPHATIC DRAINAGE

*A:* Right testicular lymphangiogram. Note the para-aortic distribution with crossover to the left side, anteroposterior projection. *B:* Lateral view. (From Busch and Sayegh, 1965.)

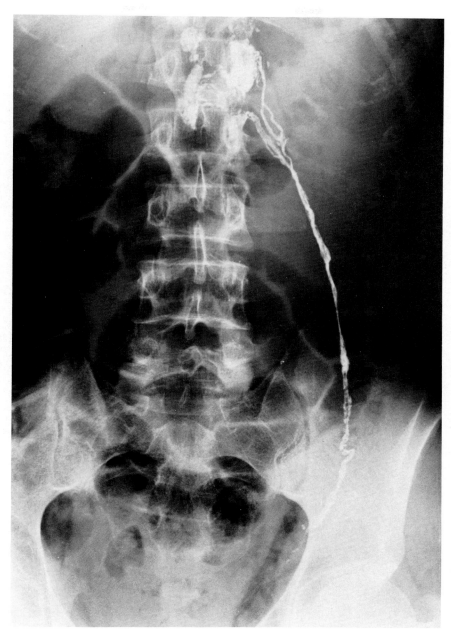

FIGURE 12.52. LEFT TESTICULAR LYMPHANGIOGRAM
Opacification of the left lumbar as well as the nodes between the aorta and inferior vena cava. (From Busch and Sayegh, 1965.)

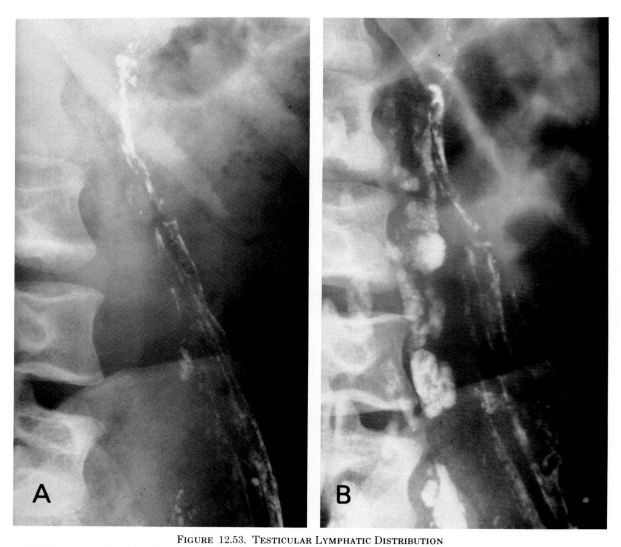

FIGURE 12.53. TESTICULAR LYMPHATIC DISTRIBUTION

*A:* Left testicular lymphangiogram opacifies the first echelon nodes at the level of the renal hilum. These nodes were not visualized by the pedal route, left posterior oblique projection. *B:* Pedal lymphangiogram. The lumbar nodes are opacified, left posterior oblique projection.

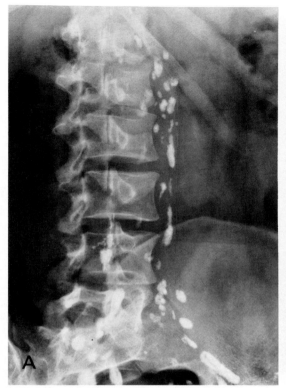

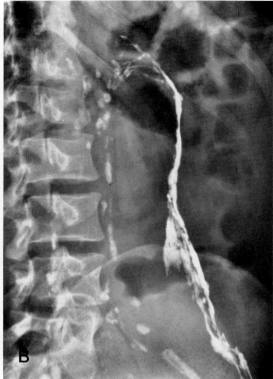

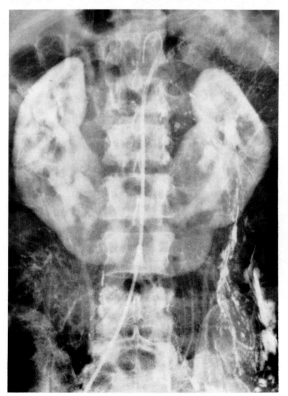

FIGURE 12.54. TESTICULAR LYMPHATIC
DISTRIBUTION IN A PATIENT WITH A HORSESHOE
KIDNEY
*A:* Left oblique projection of the pedal lymphangiogram. *B:* Left testicular lymphangiogram. Nodes that
are not seen via the pedal route are opacified by this
pathway. *C:* Aortogram demonstrates the horseshoe kidney and the location of the lymph nodes opacified by
the left testicular lymphangiogram.

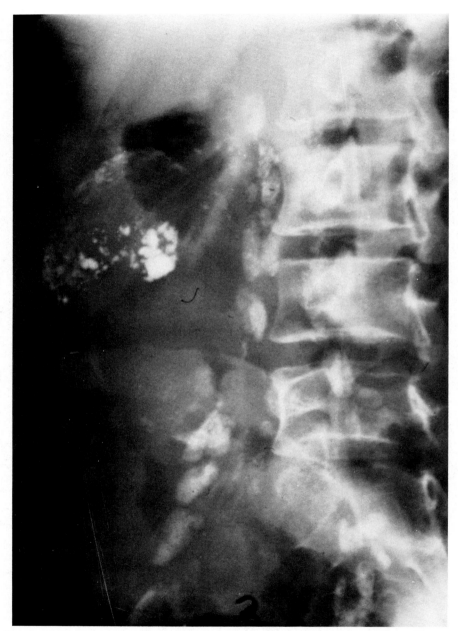

FIGURE 12.55. TESTICULAR LYMPHATIC DISTRIBUTION IN SEMINOMA OF THE RIGHT TESTICLE
Seminomatous metastases to the first echelon node demonstrated by testicular LAG. This involved node was not opacified by pedal LAG. (From Cook et al., 1965.)

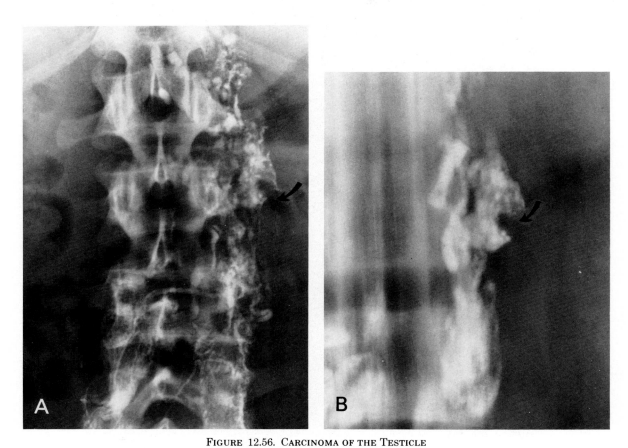

FIGURE 12.56. CARCINOMA OF THE TESTICLE

*A* and *B:* Carcinoma pattern. The lymphatics do not traverse a small defect in the node at the level of L2 on the left (*arrows*). Tomogram through the retroperitoneal nodes enhances the demonstration of the defect and the residual crescentic configuration in metastatic carcinoma from an embryonal carcinoma of the left testicle.

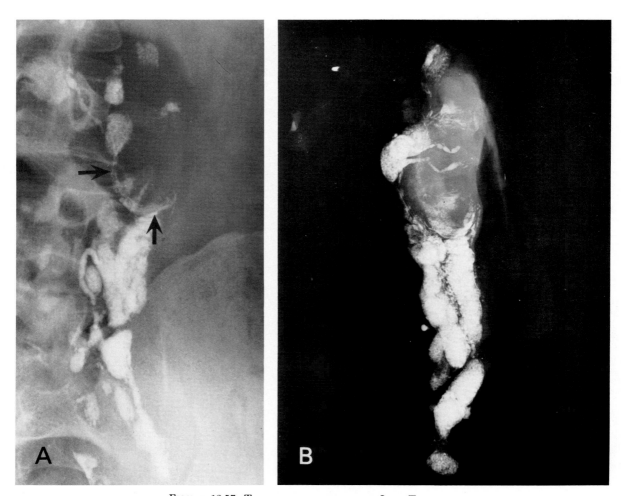

FIGURE 12.57. TERATOCARCINOMA OF THE LEFT TESTICLE

*A:* The crescentic configuration (*arrows*) is the opacification of the residual functioning portion of the node. *B:* The specimen better reveals the extent of the replacement by metastases.

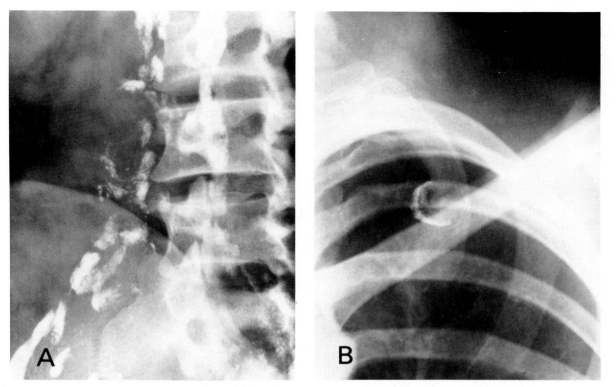

FIGURE 12.58. SEMINOMA OF THE RIGHT TESTICLE WITH LYMPH NODE METASTASES

*A:* The crescent configuration in the retroperitoneal nodes due to metastases. *B:* Supraclavicular metastases in the same patient.

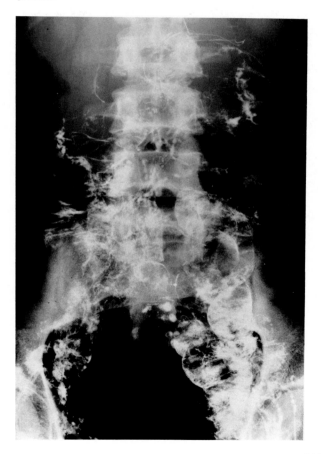

FIGURE 12.59. SEMINOMA OF THE LEFT TESTICLE WITH EXTENSIVE NODAL METASTASES

The lymphangiographic pattern simulates that seen in lymphoma.

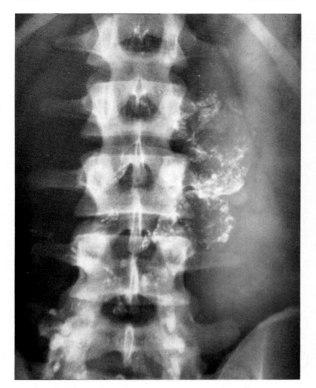

FIGURE 12.60. TERATOCARCINOMA OF THE LEFT TESTIS
   "Lymphomatous" pattern in metastatic carcinoma to the
left para-aortic nodes.

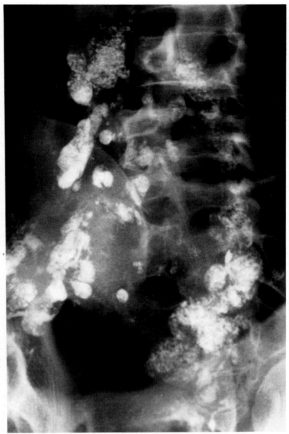

FIGURE 12.61. RHABDOMYOSARCOMA OF THE TESTIS
   The pattern of metastases simulates that seen in lymphoma

in the metastatic disease. In six cases previously
diagnosed as metastatic carcinoma, initial evaluation of the removed retroperitoneal nodes revealed no evidence of neoplasm. However, with
the assistance of specimen radiography to localize the abnormal lymph nodes specifically, re-
evaluation established the presence of necrosis
and radiation effect in areas previously occupied
by metastases or residual neoplasm.

In 11 patients, repeat LAG was performed
following retroperitoneal node dissection. Ligation of lymphatic channels resulted in utilization
of collateral pathways. These collateral pathways
resulted in opacification of nodes beyond the
usual drainage from the testicle. Therefore, any
subsequent metastases might occur along this
new route of lymph flow. In another patient, a
postoperative lymphocyst displaced the ureter
and kidney (Fig. 12.63). Follow-up LAG opacified the large cyst which was treated surgically.
Still another effect of para-aortic node lymphadenectomy was the utilization of lymphaticovenous anastomoses as a collateral pathway in
the face of surgically produced lymphatic obstruction.

The importance of constant monitoring of the
disease by LAG or CT is illustrated in a patient

TABLE 12.9.
LYMPHANGIOGRAMS OF CARCINOMA OF THE TESTICLE
(291 CASES)

|  | Positive | Negative |
|---|---|---|
| Seminoma | 28 | 76 |
| Carcinoma | 76 | 105 |
| Rhabdomyosarcoma | 2 | 4 |
| Total | 106 | 185 |

TABLE 12.10.
LYMPHANGIOGRAPHIC-PATHOLOGICAL CORRELATION IN
121 SURGICAL AND/OR AUTOPSY CASES

| Positive | 37 | Carcinoma | 117 |
|---|---|---|---|
| False-negative | 13 | Rhabdomyosarcoma | 4 |
| Negative | 70 |  |  |
| False-positive† | 1 |  |  |
| Total | 121 |  | 121 |

For the purpose of correlation and patient management, all
equivocal or suspicious readings are considered negative.

| Sensitivity | 37 of 50 = 74% |
|---|---|
| Specificity | 70 of 71 = 98.6% |
| Accuracy | 107 of 121 = 88.4% |

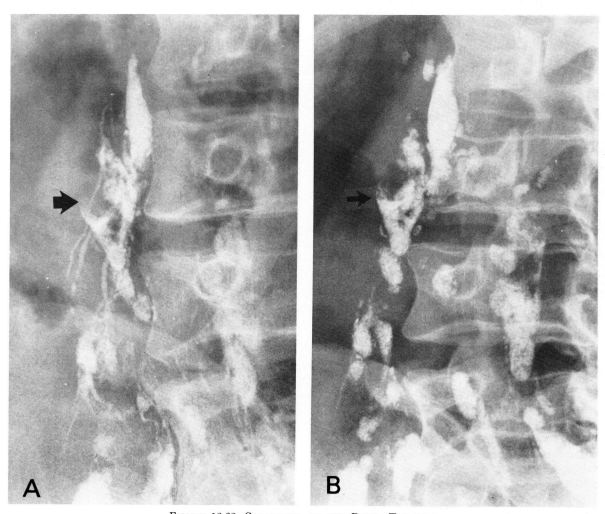

FIGURE 12.62. CARCINOMA OF THE RIGHT TESTICLE

*A:* The single metastatic node is seen in the left para-aortic group of lymph nodes adjacent to the L2 and L3 interspace (*arrow*). The lymphatics do not traverse the defect. *B:* The crescentic configuration (*arrow*) denotes the residual functioning portion of the lymph node. *C:* The Plexiglas template at the time of the dissection. Specimen radiograph confirms the removal of the involved node. The lymph nodes are smaller because of the effect of the radiation therapy. The reduction in size is also due to the magnification caused by the in vivo position of the node. *IVC,* inferior vena cavogram; *A,* aorta; *1,* left para-aortic nodes; *2,* right para-aortic nodes; *3,* common iliac nodes; *arrow,* abnormal node. *D:* The postoperative examination of the abdomen again verifies the removal of the involved nodes.

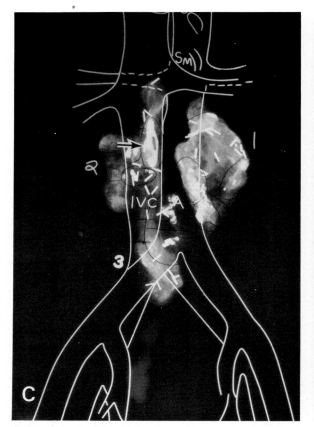
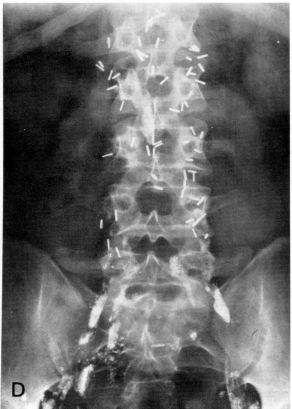

FIGURE 12.62C AND D.

with a seminoma of the right testicle (Fig. 12.64). The right testicular lesion invaded the scrotum. The testicle and a portion of the scrotum were surgically removed, and the right iliac and para-aortic areas were treated by radiation therapy. Follow-up evaluation demonstrated collateral pathways to the lymphatics and nodes in the left inguinal and iliac areas. Metastases subsequently appeared in these nodes.

### CT in Tumors of the Testis

Lee et al. (1979) reported 26 patients with primary testicular tumors studied by CT scan (11 patients had pure seminoma, 5 had embryonal cell carcinoma, 3 had teratocarcinoma, and 7 had mixed cellularity). Of the 10 patients with surgical confirmation of the CT findings, there were 6 true-positives, 2 true-negatives, 1 false-negative, and 1 equivocal. Only 9 patients in this group had LAG. CT and LAG were in agreement in 6, with 1 proven surgically. In 1 case CT was read as equivocal and LAG as negative. No metastases were found at surgery.

Williams et al. (1980) employed US and CT in staging nonseminomatous testicular tumors in 32 patients and reported a sensitivity of 93%, specificity of 82%, and accuracy of 88%.

### Comparison of LAG and CT in Tumors of the Testis

In the Dunnick and Javadpour (1981) series of 63 patients with nonseminomatous testicular carcinoma, 49 patients had surgically proven metastases to the retroperitoneum in the region of para-aortic lymph nodes. CT examinations were performed on 38 of these patients, and tumor was identified in 25 (66%). The overall accuracy was 74%. The false-negative rate was 34% (13 of 38). Forty-four patients with proven metastases underwent LAG, and evidence of lymph node metastases was seen in 34 (77%). The overall accuracy was 82%. The false-negative rate was 23% (10 of 44).

Lackner et al. (1979), in their comparison of LAG and CT in the evaluation of 64 patients with testicular tumors, found with LAG a 73%

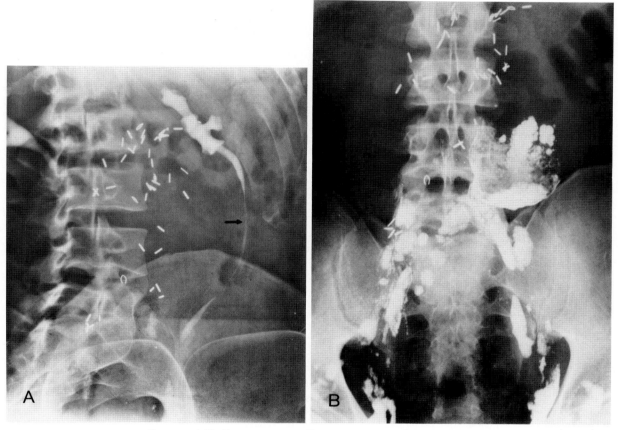

FIGURE 12.63. POSTOPERATIVE RETROPERITONEAL LYMPHOCYST

*A:* The left ureter is displaced anteriorly and laterally (*arrow*). *B:* Repeat lymphangiogram opacifies a large retroperitoneal lymphocyst. The fluid-contrast level is obtained by examining the patient in the erect position.

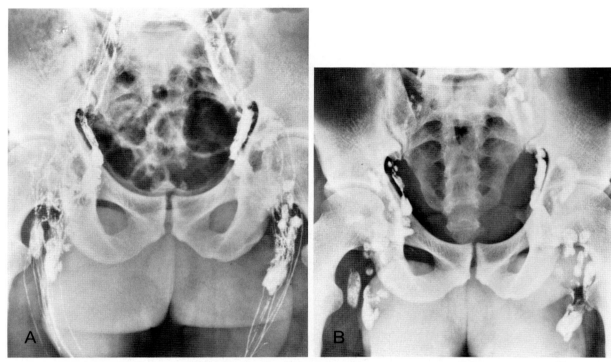

FIGURE 12.64. ALTERATION IN THE DISTRIBUTION OF METASTASES SECONDARY TO THE DISEASE AND THE THERAPY IN A PATIENT WITH SEMINOMA OF THE RIGHT TESTICLE

*A:* The initial study reveals the lymphatics and nodes to be normal. *B:* Nodal phase. *C:* Repeat lymphangiogram 1 yr later following orchiectomy and radiation demonstrates obstruction of the lymphatics in the right inguinal area (*curved arrow*) with collateral circulation to the opposite side (*straight arrow*). *D:* Metastases are noted on the left )(*arrows*), probably due to the alteration in lymphatic flow.

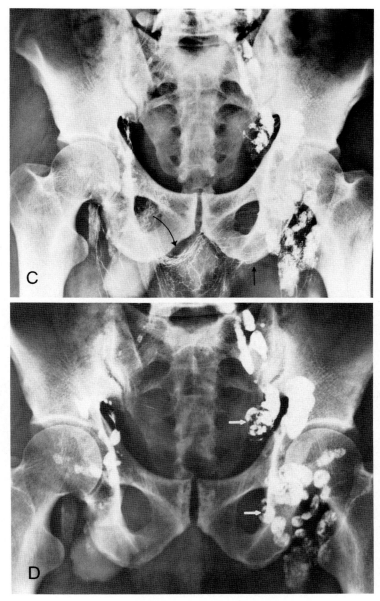

FIGURE 12.64*C* AND *D*.

sensitivity, 79% specificity, and 75% accuracy. Lien et al. (1983) found metastases in 71 of 200 patients with retroperitoneal metastases from testicular tumors. The CT was positive in 66, and LAG was positive in 60.

In our institution, in a comparative study of LAG and CT, CT scans were performed within a month following LAG in 103 patients with carcinoma of the testis (82 with carcinoma and 21 with seminoma). Of these 103 patients, LAG was positive for nodal metastases in 53 patients and was negative in 50. CT detected metastases in 50 patients and no metastases in 53. Thirty-nine of 103 patients had pathological correlation by retroperitoneal lymph node dissection or percutaneous needle biopsy (34 with carcinoma and 5 with seminoma). LAG was proven to be positive in 29 patients, with an overall accuracy of 92.3%. Twenty-six patients were positive on CT, with an overall accuracy of 84.6% (Fig. 12.65; Tables 12.11 and 12.12). The 5 false-negatives in the CT group (12.8%) were due to small lesions less than 1.5–2.0 cm (Fig. 12.66). Two false-negatives in LAG (5.1%) resulted from a micro-

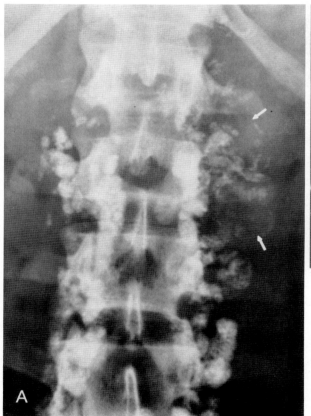

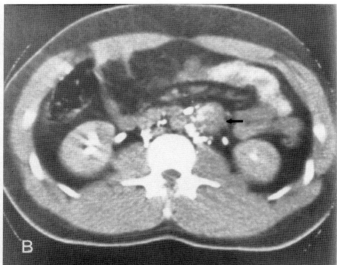

FIGURE 12.65.  CARCINOMA OF THE LEFT TESTIS
*A:* LAG. Nodal metastases with irregular deposition of contrast
medium are seen in left para-aortic area (*arrows*). *B:* CT. Nodal
metastases, partially opacified and partially nonopacified, are shown
to good advantage (*arrow*).

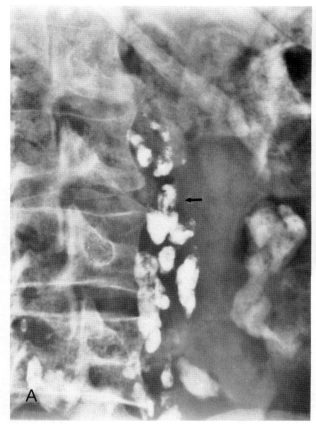

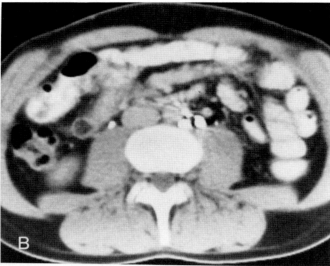

FIGURE 12.66.  CARCINOMA OF THE LEFT TESTIS WITH POST-
THERAPEUTIC CHANGES
*A:* LAG. Slightly enlarged node with filling defects in left upper
para-aortic area (*arrow*). *B:* CT. No measurable adenopathy in
para-aortic areas. At surgery a necrotic tumor mass without viable
tumor cells was found.

scopic lesion in one case, and a lesion in the preaortic and the interaorticocaval regions in another case (Fig. 12.67). One false-positive (2.5%) in the CT group was due to lymphoid hyperplasia, and one false-positive in the LAG group was caused by a benign lesion, sinus histiocytosis. In advanced lesions of carcinoma of the testis, LAG often failed to reveal upper limits of the lesion; however, CT is of definite value in demonstrating the extent of the nodal metastases and the involvement of the adjacent organs. Sometimes when the nodal lesion is high in the renal hilar region, it is often partially visualized by LAG, and CT offers more information to delineate the extent of the lesion (Fig. 12.68).

Given the lack of clear-cut superiority of either CT or LAG in the assessment of nodal metastases from nonseminomatous testicular tumors, it seems reasonable to select the examination with the broadest scope and the greatest patient acceptability. For this reason, Castellino and Marglin (1982) and Lien et al. (1983) recommend CT as the initial imaging procedure. Abnormal results may be confirmed histologically. If cyto-

logical results are negative or if the result of the CT examination itself is negative, LAG is recommended.

At M. D. Anderson Hospital and Tumor Institute, LAG and CT are complementary procedures and have become essential tools in the evaluation as well as the management of patients with testicular malignant disease.

In seminomas, when LAG and CT are positive, radiotherapy is given to the ipsilateral iliac and bilateral retroperitoneal nodes to the diaphragm. The mediastinum and both supraclavicular areas are also treated. In the presence of a negative lymphangiogram and CT, radiotherapy is given only to the level of the diaphragm.

In nonseminomatous malignancies in the past, a patient with a positive lymphangiogram and/or CT was treated by radiotherapy to a tumor dose of 2500 rad to the nodes up to the diaphragm. A retroperitoneal node dissection was then undertaken to remove residual tumor tissue with additional radiotherapy, 2500 rad, following the retroperitoneal node dissection. In the presence of negative lymphangiographic and CT

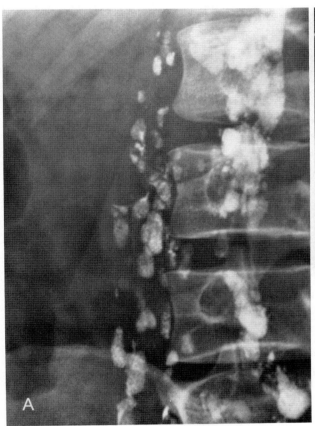

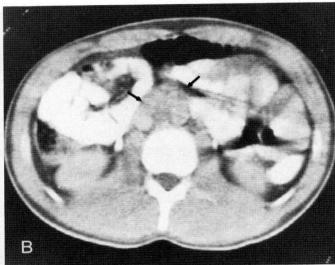

FIGURE 12.67.  CARCINOMA OF THE RIGHT TESTIS
*A:* LAG. No definite evidence of nodal metastasis in right para-aortic area. *B:* CT. Lymphadenopathy in the preaortic and inter-aorticocaval regions with slight separation of the aorta and inferior vena cava (*arrows*). At surgery nodal metastases were found in the para-aortic area.

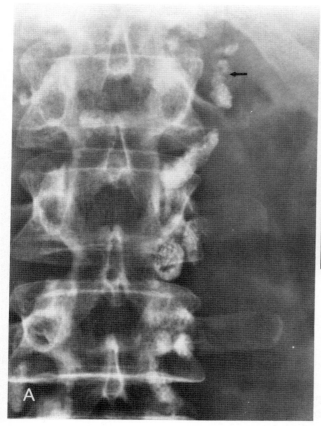

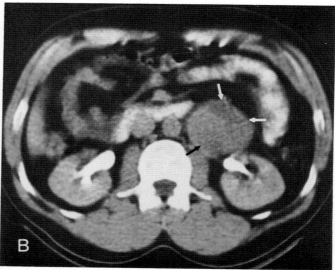

FIGURE 12.68. CARCINOMA OF THE LEFT TESTIS
*A:* LAG. Irregular nodes in left upper para-aortic area (*arrow*).
*B:* CT. Nodal metastases of considerable size in left upper para-aortic area high in the renal pelvis (*arrow*).

TABLE 12.11.
FINDINGS OF LAG AND CT IN 103 PATIENTS WITH
CARCINOMA OF THE TESTIS

|  | LAG | CT |
|---|---|---|
| Positive | 53 | 50 |
| Negative | 50 | 53 |
| Total | 103 | 103 |

TABLE 12.12.
PATHOLOGICAL CORRELATION IN 39 PATIENTS WITH
CARCINOMA OF THE TESTIS

|  | LAG | CT |
|---|---|---|
| Positive | 29 | 26 |
| False-negative | 2 | 5 |
| Negative | 7 | 7 |
| False-positive | 1 | 1 |
| Total | 39 | 39 |
| Sensitivity | 29 of 31 = 93.5% | 26 of 31 = 83.8% |
| Specificity | 7 of 8 = 87.5% | 7 of 8 = 87.5% |
| Accuracy | 36 of 39 = 92.3% | 33 of 39 = 84.6% |

findings, the retroperitoneal node dissection was undertaken initially. If the node dissection was negative, no further treatment was instituted.

By determining the nature, location, and extent of disease in testicular malignancies, LAG and CT facilitate accurate placement of the radiation therapy portal.

Contrast material retained in the lymph nodes can be followed during the course of the disease by roentgenograms of the abdomen to evaluate the effectiveness of the treatment.

At present with stage I disease, normal markers (human chorionic gonadotropin, lactate dehydrogenase, and α-fetoprotein), normal CT, and normal LAG, the patient is observed closely with no further treatment. Markers and follow-up examinations of the abdomen are done every 3 months. CT is performed every 6 months. When there is a change in these parameters, chemotherapy is instituted.

In the presence of more widespread disease, stage II or stage III, where chemotherapy is the initial therapeutic approach, LAG or CT is of assistance in determining the status of the retroperitoneal lymph nodes. After a favorable response to chemotherapy (that is, resolution of pulmonary metastases), the patient is managed by utilizing the markers, CT, and LAG. Surgery is resorted to only when there are persistent defects in nodes or residual tumor. Of 25 patients subjected to surgery with persistent changes on CT and/or LAG, only 1 had residual tumor. Changes in size and architecture of the opacified lymph nodes will assist in determining the response to therapy. If there is inadequate residual contrast material, a repeat lymphangiogram can be performed. We have repeated the study on many patients with a maximum of five lymphangiograms in a patient over a 7-yr period. Under such conditions, instead of a repeat lymphangiogram, CT is of value for follow-up examination.

LAG and CT can also be utilized as a guide to the surgeon if a retroperitonal lymphadenectomy is to be done. Node dissections, regardless of the thoroughness or talents of the surgeon, are seldom complete. Roentgenograms of the abdomen obtained in the operating room during the surgical procedure must be undertaken to ensure the completeness of the dissection. Radioactive and marker substances, such as chlorophyll in Ethiodol, have been utilized in an attempt to achieve a more complete dissection, but they are no longer commercially available. Crossover of the lymphatic drainage between the two sides of the para-aortic region is a normal finding. Contralateral metastases of testicular carcinoma are common; consequently, bilateral node dissection is essential, especially if the neoplasm originates in the right testicle (Fig. 12.69). The extent of the dissection should be determined in part by the lymphatic distribution. This depends upon the level at which the testicular and lumbar lymphatic trunks empty into the thoracic duct. At times this continues above the L2 level to T10 or above. Under such circumstances it is somewhat difficult surgically to remove the complete lymphatic drainage from the testis.

US is less specific than LAG and less sensitive than CT in diagnosis of lymph node metastasis. Because of its ability to differentiate benign cystic lesions from solid or semisolid malignant neoplasm, however, US is useful to diagnose postoperative lymphocyst following retroperitoneal lymph node dissection for carcinoma of the testis (Fig. 12.70).

## The Urinary Bladder

Carcinoma of the bladder is the most common malignancy of the urinary tract. In spite of all modern advances in diagnosis, treatment, and prevention, the mortality from bladder cancer is rising, especially in young men and in industrial centers.

It is often maintained that carcinoma of the bladder tends to remain localized. Metastases from bladder tumor occur relatively late. At first, they appear in the regional lymph nodes; later, they are seen in the para-aortic nodes, liver, lungs, and other organs.

### Lymphatic Drainage of the Bladder

The lymph drainage of the bladder is by three routes (Fig. 12.71):

1. The collecting trunks of the trigone. These trunks emerge from various points of the bladder wall situated medial to the ureters in the female and to the deferent ducts in the male. They follow the uterine or the ductus deferens artery and terminate in the lymph nodes of the middle or medial group of the external iliac chain.
2. The collecting trunks of the posterior wall. The lymphatics arising from these trunks may follow different directions:
   A. They may reach the posterolateral angle of the bladder, cross the umbilical artery, and terminate in one of the nodes of the middle or medial group of the external iliac chain.
   B. Less frequently, they may terminate in the retrocrural nodes.
   C. They may empty into one of the collecting trunks of the trigone.
   D. Occasionally, they may terminate in the hypogastric nodes or in the lateral nodes of the common iliac group.
3. The collecting trunks of the anterior wall. These trunks converge toward the middle third of the lateral border of the bladder, in the region of the middle vesicle artery. They descend toward the origin of the middle vesicle and umbilical arteries, meet the collecting trunks of the posterior wall, merge with them, and share their nodal connections (that is, terminate in the same lymph node).

The course of the collecting trunks is frequently interrupted by small intercalated lymph nodules. In the majority of cases, additional small nodules are found on the wall of the bladder—the paravesicle nodes. The paravesicle nodes can be divided into three groups: anterior, lateral, and posterior. These nodes are situated in the vesicle lodge under the peritoneum posteriorly and under the vesicle fascia anteriorly.

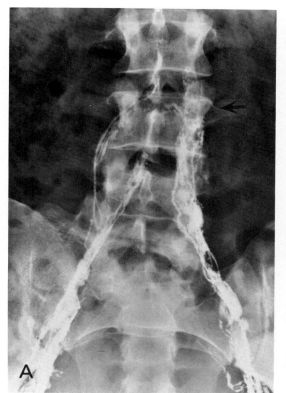

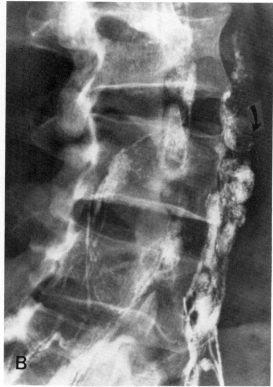

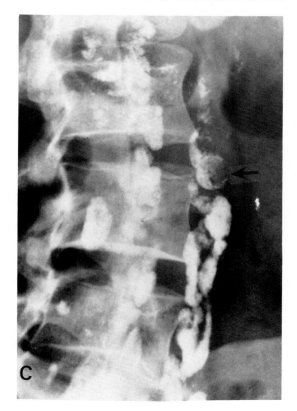

FIGURE 12.69. CROSSOVER METASTASES FROM CARCINOMA OF THE RIGHT TESTICLE TO LEFT PARA-AORTIC LYMPH NODES
*A:* Anteroposterior view, lymphatic phase (*arrow*). *B:* Oblique view, lymphatic phase (*arrow*). *C:* Oblique view, nodal phase (*arrow*).

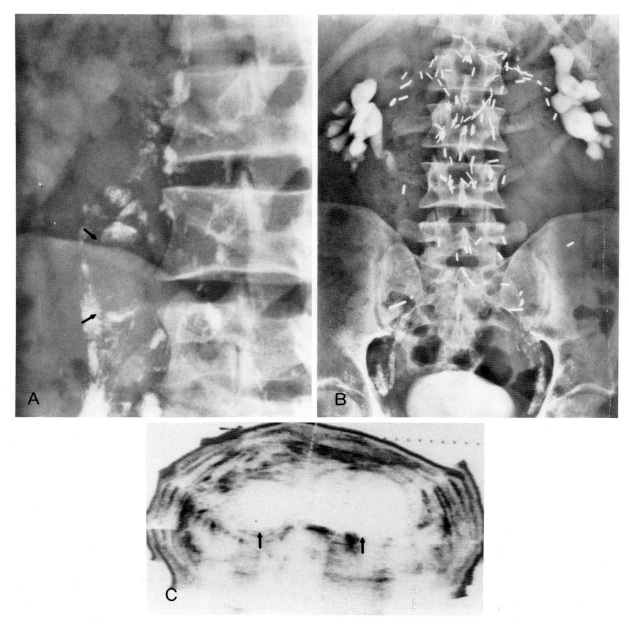

FIGURE 12.70. POSTOPERATIVE LYMPHOCYST

*A:* LAG. Nodal metastases are seen in right lower para-aortic and proximal common iliac regions (*arrows*). *B:* Intravenous pyelogram (postoperative). Multiple surgical clips are seen in the retroperitoneal area resulting from recent lymph node dissection. There is moderate hydronephrosis of both kidneys, more on the left side, with slight ureterectasis and lateral deviation of the proximal portion of the left ureter. *C:* Transverse abdominal ultrasonogram. There is a very large cystic lesion in the midabdomen immediately adjacent to the spine. The lesion has a bilobed appearance and is anechoic with through transmission. Exploratory laparotomy was performed, and two lymphocysts were found. The left one was lateral to the aorta, and the right one was between the aorta and vena cava.

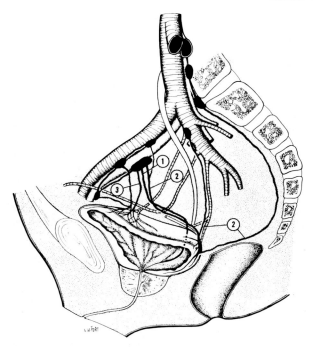

FIGURE 12.71. LYMPHATIC DRAINAGE OF THE BLADDER
*1,* The collecting trunks of the trigone. *2,* The collecting trunks of the posterior wall. *3,* The collecting trunks of the anterior wall.

In summary, if all of the small intercalated nodules and paravesicle nodules are withdrawn from consideration, the first lymphoid echelon for the lymphatics of the bladder is represented by the external iliac lymph nodes, particularly the middle and medial groups, and occasionally by the hypogastric and common iliac nodes.

### LAG in Tumors of the Bladder

LAG will opacify the external and common iliac lymph nodes. In exceptional cases isolated hypogastric nodes (close to the origin of the internal iliac artery) may be demonstrated. Negative findings may result even though the paravesicle or hypogastric nodes and the occasional node in the obturator fossa may be affected by metastases, for these lymph nodes escape visualization.

The indication for LAG in carcinoma of the bladder is the more accurate staging of the disease, which then dictates management. Prognosis is related to the stage of the disease. The modality of treatment also varies with extent of the lesion.

At M. D. Anderson Hospital, staging of a carcinoma of the bladder is clinical and includes cystoscopy and bimanual rectoabdominal pal-

pation of the anesthetized patient. The classification is based upon the system proposed by Jewett and Strong (1946) and modified by Marshall (1956). Allocation to stages O, A, and BI is based entirely on microscopic assessment of the depth of invasion in patients in whom bimanual examination is negative. When bimanual palpation reveals induration or thickening without a definite mass, a stage B2 classification is assigned. If a distinct mass is palpable, the tumor is labeled stage C. Stage DI classification is utilized when there is fixation of the mass to the pelvic or abdominal wall, uterus, or prostate, extension into the vagina, peritoneum or bowel, or microscopic evidence of invasion or prostatic glandular substance. The presence of pelvic lymph node metastases also places the patient in a stage DI classification. Stage D2 is reserved for patients with metastases to lymph nodes at or above the aortic bifurcation or to other sites outside the confines of the true pelvis.

The diagnostic criteria for nodal metastasis in carcinoma of the bladder are the same as those described earlier. The single most reliable criterion is a filling defect in a node not traversed by lymphatics (Figs. 12.72 and 12.73). When the node is completely replaced, the lymphatics may be displaced or obstructed (Fig. 12.74A). Lymphatic obstruction with or without collateral channels may be the sole secondary evidence of nodal replacement. Confirmation by complementary procedures, notably US and CT, is of value to demonstrate the presence of an enlarged replaced node or tumor mass (Fig. 12.74B and C).

In our institution from December 1966–December 1974, 91 patients with carcinoma of the bladder had bilateral pedal lymphangiograms as a part of the assessment of metastatic disease. Sixty of these 91 patients received preoperative irradiation (5000 rad tumor dose in 5 weeks through 10 × 10-cm fields) 6 weeks prior to surgical exploration. In all cases, surgical exploration included careful palpatory scrutiny of the pelvic and para-aortic lymph nodes, and suspicious or enlarged lymph nodes were removed for histological examination. Three patients underwent formal bilateral pelvic lymphadenectomy. The results of lymphangiographic and surgical correlation are shown in Table 12.13. No false-positive lymphangiographic readings were encountered. In nine patients with proven nodal metastases diagnosed by lymphangiogram with excellent correlation of 100%, the sensitivity was 64%. The specific site of the nodal involvement was the common iliac chain in four patients with a concomitant involvement of a para-aortic node

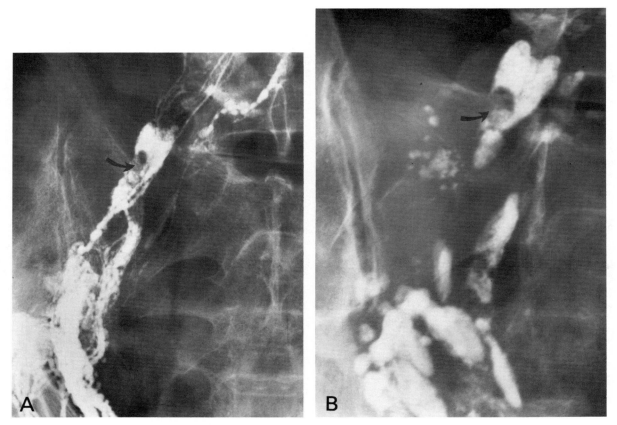

FIGURE 12.72. CARCINOMA OF THE BLADDER
*A:* Metastases to a common iliac node (*arrow*), lymphatic phase. *B:* Nodal phase (*arrow*).

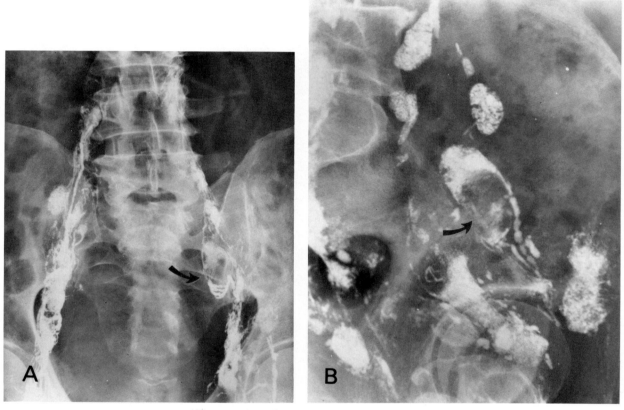

FIGURE 12.73. CARCINOMA OF THE BLADDER
*A:* Metastasis to the left iliac node (*arrow*), lymphatic phase. *B:* Nodal phase (*arrow*).

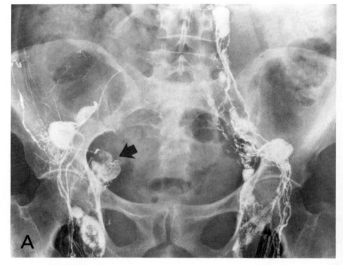

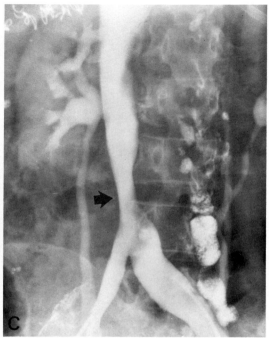

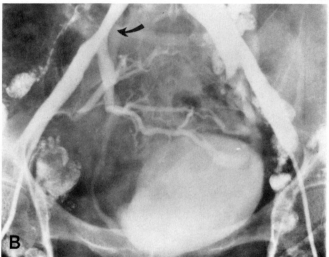

FIGURE 12.74. CARCINOMA OF THE BLADDER
*A:* Primary evidence of metastasis is seen in a right external iliac lymph node, medial chain (*arrow*). Obstruction of lymphatics and collateral pathways are opacified. *B* and *C:* Venography yields complementary information by external compression of the right common iliac vein and inferior vena cava (*arrows*).

TABLE 12.13.
CARCINOMA OF THE BLADDER—LYMPHANGIOGRAPHIC-SURGICAL CORRELATION (60 SURGICAL CASES)

| | |
|---|---|
| Positive | 9 |
| False-negative | 5 |
| Negative | 46 |
| False-positive | 0 |
| Total | 60 |
| Sensitivity | 9 of 14 = 64% |
| Specificity | 46 of 46 = 100% |
| Accuracy | 55 of 60 = 91.6% |

in one. The external chain was exclusively involved in two patients, and in two others both the common and external chains were involved. The remaining one patient had both lympho-

matous and carcinomatous disease in the same lymph nodes with extensive involvement of the pelvic and para-aortic nodes (Fig. 12.75).

As might be expected, lymphangiograms positive for metastatic disease were encountered more frequently with the more advanced clinical stages as shown in Table 12.14. The true-negative readings were found in 46 patients, and the specificity was 100%. False-negative interpretations were encountered in five instances (9.8%). The sites of tumor involvement not diagnosed by lymphangiograms included the external iliac chains in two instances: one of these two patients had microscopic foci of metastasis, and the other patient had lymphatic obstruction with incomplete filling of the external iliac nodes. An un-

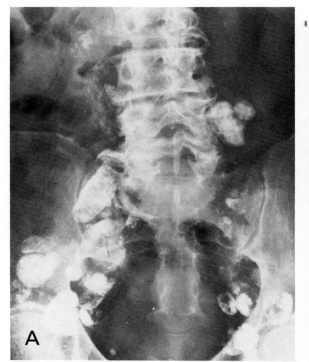

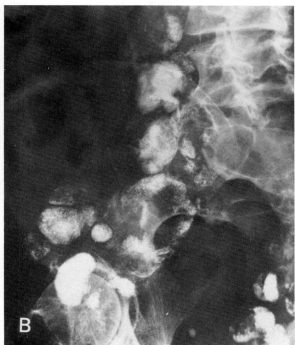

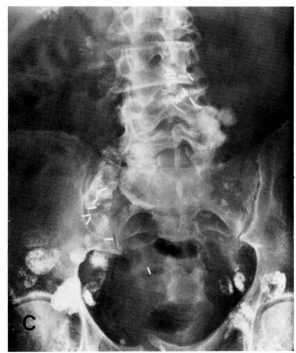

FIGURE 12.75.  CARCINOMA OF BLADDER AND
LYMPHOMA

*A:* Diffuse nodal involvement is due to nodular lymphoma.
Metastatic carcinoma from the bladder is seen in a right
external iliac node, medial chain, anteroposterior view. *B:*
Oblique view. *C:* Following therapy. The clips are at the sites
of biopsy. The patient was treated by radiotherapy and
chemotherapy.

TABLE 12.14.

CARCINOMA OF THE BLADDER—LYMPHANGIOGRAPHIC-SURGICAL CORRELATION ACCORDING TO CLINICAL STAGE OF DISEASE

| Interpretation | Clinical Stage | | | | Total No. of Patients |
|---|---|---|---|---|---|
| | B1 | B2 | C | D | |
| Positive | 1 | 1 | 3 | 4 | 9 |
| False-positive | 0 | 0 | 0 | 0 | 0 |
| Negative* | 14 | 12 | 16 | 4 | 46 |
| False-negative | 1 | 0 | 2 | 2 | 5 |

* For the purpose of correlation and patient management, all equivocal or suspicious readings were considered negative.

expected metastatic focus was encountered in the obturator nodes near the obturator foramen in three cases. The overall accuracy was 92%.

Our findings of positive lymphangiograms in 7% of patients with stages B1 and B2 disease, 14% of patients with stage C disease, and 40% of patients with fixation of the tumor to the pelvis or abdominal wall (stage D1) underscore the value of this procedure in reducing the number of patients subjected to unnecessary and futile surgical exploration. Surgical treatment for patients with stage D1 lesions has proven highly unsatisfactory. Laplante and Brice (1973)treated 97 consecutive patients with pathologically demonstrated stage D vesical carcinoma with only 5 patients free of neoplasm 5 yr after radical cystectomy. Only 6 of 35 patients with stage D1 lesions (17%) undergoing radical cystectomy by Dretler and associates (1980) survived 5 yr without evidence of recurrent disease. Our experience suggests that equal or better results can be achieved with the use of radiotherapy alone or, more recently, intra-arterial cis platinum, cytoxan, and adriamycin (CISCA) (Wallace et al., 1982), obviating the unnecessary risks and morbidity associated with radical surgery.

## CT in Tumors of the Bladder

In the Koss et al. (1981) series, CT staging was performed in 49 patients with known carcinoma of the bladder. The overall accuracy of CT staging in 25 patients (15 stage B or less, 4 stage C, and 6 stage D) with surgically confirmed disease stage was 16 (64%). The overall accuracy of CT in predicting lymph node metastases was 92% (23 of 25). The sensitivity was 60% (3 of 5), and the specificity was 100% (20 of 20). The false-negative rate was 8% (2 of 25) due to small nodes, 1.5 cm or less, and there was no false-positive.

Walsh et al. (1980) detected enlarged pelvic nodes by CT in 32 of 127 patients (25%) (15 with

carcinoma of the cervix, 13 with bladder carcinoma, and 7 with carcinoma of the prostate). Pelvic or inguinal lymph nodes were confirmed pathologically in 35 patients. CT detected a true-positive in 17 of 20 patients with lymph node metastases (sensitivity, 85%), false-negative in 3 of 20 patients with lymph node metastases, 15% (or 3 of 35, 9%), true-negative in 10 of 15 patients without metastases (specificity, 67%), and false-positive of lymph node metastasis in 5 of 15 patients, 33% (or 5 of 35, 14%). CT was correct in 27 of 35 patients (accuracy, 77%).

Morgan et al. (1981) reported CT scanning of 24 patients with bladder carcinoma and surgical confirmation in 18 of these patients. The sensitivity was 75% (3 of 4), specificity was 86% (12 of 14), and overall accuracy was 83% (15 of 18). The false-negative rate was 6% (1 of 18) due to a microscopic tumor deposit in a normal-sized node. The false-positive rate was 11% (2 of 18) caused by benign changes in nodes.

## Comparison of LAG and CT in Tumors of the Bladder

In our series, 67 patients with carcinoma of the bladder had lymphangiograms, followed within a month by CT scans (Tables 12.15 and 12.16). Thirty-seven had pathological correlation with cystectomy or lymph node biopsy. LAG was proved to be positive in 10, with an overall accuracy of 97.2%. On CT scanning, there were eight patients found to have nodal metastasis with an overall accuracy of 91.8%. One false-negative (2.7%) in the LAG group was due to a

TABLE 12.15.

FINDINGS OF LAG AND CT IN 67 PATIENTS WITH CARCINOMA OF THE BLADDER

| | LAG | CT |
|---|---|---|
| Positive | 20 | 15 |
| Negative | 47 | 52 |
| Total | 67 | 67 |

TABLE 12.16.

PATHOLOGICAL CORRELATION IN 37 PATIENTS WITH CARCINOMA OF THE BLADDER

| | LAG | CT |
|---|---|---|
| Positive | 10 | 8 |
| False-negative | 1 | 3 |
| Negative | 26 | 26 |
| False-positive | 0 | 0 |
| Total | 37 | 37 |
| | | |
| Sensitivity | 10 of 11 = 91% | 8 of 11 = 72.7% |
| Specificity | 26 of 26 = 100% | 26 of 26 = 100% |
| Accuracy | 36 of 37 = 97.3% | 34 of 37 = 91.9% |

microscopic metastatic lesion. There were three false-negatives (8.1%) on CT scans; two were due to small lesions less than 1.5–2.0 cm in diameter, and one was missed in the common iliac region due to obliquity of the projection (Fig. 12.76).

In a series (Lee et al., 1978) of 26 patients with pelvic tumor (8 with carcinoma of the prostate, 6 with bladder carcinoma, 6 with carcinoma of the testis, 5 with gynecological tumors, and 1 with spermatic cord tumor) studied with CT scanning, 14 of them also had LAG as part of the staging procedure. The two studies were each correct in 57% of all cases (8 of 14). The false-negative rate of CT was 41% (5 of 12) or 36% (5 of 14); the false-negative rate for LAG was 37% (3 of 8) or 21% (3 of 14), with a 40% false-positive rate (2 of 5) or 14% (2 of 14).

It is axiomatic that staging is the single most important factor in deciding upon therapy and determining the prognosis for carcinoma of the bladder. The accuracy of the commonly employed clinical methods for staging ranges from 50–81%. These methods are unable accurately to assess lymph node metastases in patients with clinically localized bladder carcinoma. When strict criteria are used for interpretation of the roentgenographic findings, LAG complemented by CT becomes a simple, direct, highly reliable method of demonstrating clinically unsuspected metastases in the lymph nodes. It is the policy of this institution for all patients presenting with carcinoma of the bladder to have a complete routine examination for staging. Biopsies are taken to estimate the extent of the disease histologically, and, if there is an invasive bladder carcinoma present (stage B1–D), the patient is examined by bilateral pedal LAG complemented by CT as indicated. If the lymphangiogram and CT are negative for nodal metastasis and the patient has an invasive bladder carcinoma, preoperative external irradiation, 5500 rad with a four-field box technique, is followed 6 weeks after completion of radiotherapy by a total cystectomy, prostatectomy, and ileal conduit urinary diversion procedure. If the lymphangiogram is positive for metastatic disease in the pelvic lymph nodes, the patient is randomized with half the patients receiving banjo or extended field radiotherapy and the other half of the group receiving pelvis irradiation. If the para-aortic nodes are involved, the patient is treated with

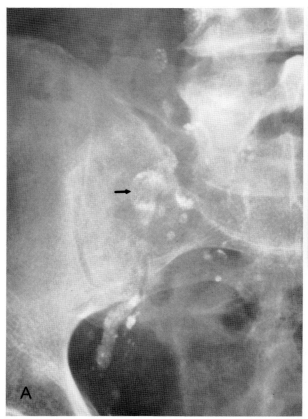

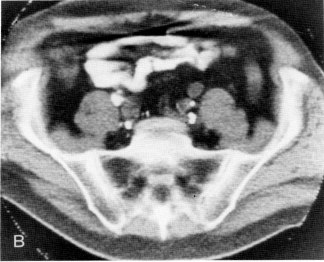

FIGURE 12.76. RECURRENT CARCINOMA OF THE URINARY BLADDER

*A:* Radiograph of the abdomen, 3 months after LAG, showing an enlarged node with filling defects consistent with metastasis in the right common iliac region (*arrow*). *B:* CT. No definite adenopathy in pelvic or para-aortic region. Needle biopsy disclosed nodal metastasis in the right iliac region.

chemotherapy. More recently, patients with stage D2 carcinoma of the bladder are treated by chemotherapy, utilizing CISCA. If the disease is predominantly in the pelvis, cisplatinum is delivered intra-arterially.

## The Prostate

Carcinoma of the prostate is the most prevalent neoplasm of the male genital organs. This tumor has gained increasing clinical importance because of the greater number of men who are reaching later decades of life. Metastasis is predominantly through hematogenous routes, although lymphatic metastasis is common even in the early stage of the disease. The incidence of lymph node metastases is related to the size of the primary neoplasm as well as the presence of extraprostatic invasion (Tables 12.17–12.19).

### Lymphatic Drainage of the Prostate

The lymphatic networks of the prostate are drained by four collecting trunks (Fig. 12.77): the external iliac, hypogastric, posterior, and inferior pedicles.

**The External Iliac Pedicle.** It is formed by a single trunk of the lymphatics which arises from the superior surface and upper part of the posterior surface of the prostate. This trunk ascends along the medial border of the seminal vesicle and passes above the terminal segment of the ureter to terminate in one of the nodes of the middle group of the external iliac chain.

**The Hypogastric Pedicle.** It is formed by a single trunk and arises from the inferior part of the prostate. It ascends on its posterior surface toward the superior surface of the gland and then turns outward along the prostatic artery to terminate in one of the hypogastric nodes.

**The Posterior Pedicle.** It is composed of two or three trunks and arises from the posterior

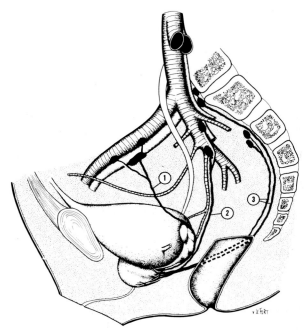

FIGURE 12.77. LYMPHATIC DRAINAGE OF THE PROSTATE
*1*, External iliac pedicle. *2*, Hypogastric pedicle. *3*, Posterior pedicle.

TABLE 12.17.
CARCINOMA OF PROSTATE

| | |
|---|---|
| Stage A | Two or less microscopic foci of cancer in a specimen obtained in the course of treatment of benign disease |
| Stage B | Palpable tumor confined within the capsule of the prostate |
| Stage C | Locally invasive (pelvic wall, base of bladder, etc.) |
| Stage D | Distant metastases |

TABLE 12.18.
RELATIONSHIP OF RECTAL SIZE OF PROSTATIC CANCER TO INCIDENCE OF LYMPH NODE METASTASES*

| Size of Local Lesion | No. of Cases | No. with Positive Nodes | Percentage with Positive nodes |
|---|---|---|---|
| Nodule | 29 | 2 | 7 |
| <35 g | 132 | 26 | 20 |
| 35–80 g | 185 | 81 | 44 |
| 80–150 g | 55 | 28 | 51 |
| >150 g | 12 | 11 | 92 |
| Total | 413 | 148 | 36 |

* From Flocks et al. (1959).

TABLE 12.19.
INCIDENCE OF LYMPH NODE METASTASES IN PATIENTS WITH DISEASE LIMITED TO PROSTATE AND WITH EXTRAPROSTATIC INVASION

| | Disease Limited to Prostate | Lymph Nodes Positive | Extra-prostatic Invasion | Lymph Nodes Positive |
|---|---|---|---|---|
| Whitmore and MacKenzie (1959) | 2 | 0 | 18 | 9 |
| Arduino and Glucksman (1962) | 54 | 5 | 17 | 14 |
| Flocks et al. (1959) | 29 | 2 | 384 | 146 |
| Total | 85 | 7 | 419 | 169 |

surface of the prostate. It is directed posteriorly in the medial aspect of the rectovesical fascia toward the sacrum and then terminates in lymph nodes located on the medial side of the second sacral foramen or in the nodes in the region of the promontory of the sacrum.

**The Inferior Pedicle.** It is usually formed by a single trunk and descends from the anterior border of the prostate to the floor of the perineum. There it follows the internal pudendal artery around the ischial spine into the pelvis and terminates in one of the hypogastric nodes near the origin of the internal iliac artery.

In summary, the first lymphoid echelon for the lymphatics of the prostate is represented by the entire lymphoid girdle at the superior strait of the pelvis, via the external iliac, the hypogastric, and the promontory nodes. The lymphatics of the prostate are in communication with those of the bladder, the seminal vesicle, and the rectum.

### LAG in Tumors of the Prostate

Of the regional lymph nodes, only the external iliac nodes can be demonstrated on the lymphangiogram. Occasionally, the hypogastric nodes near the origin of the internal iliac artery may be visualized. Opacification of the promontory node is usually uncertain. The indications for LAG in carcinoma of the prostate are suspicion of nodal metastasis and uncertainty about operability or further therapeutic measures.

The lymphangiographic findings in nodal metastases from carcinoma of the prostate are varied and show different architectural patterns. The lymph node may be enlarged with marginal filling defects or with partial replacement having crescentic appearance similar to that usually seen in classical carcinoma of epithelial origin (Figs. 12.78 and 12.79). The involved node may appear moderately enlarged with irregular internal architecture and fairly well circumscribed filling defects simulating malignant lymphoma (Fig. 12.80). Fragmented nodes with multiple filling defects may also be seen. Lymphatic obstruction with or without collateral lymph channels is often associated with these abnormal nodes (Fig. 12.81). When lymph node is completely replaced by tumor tissue with collateral lymphatic pathways, the presence of a mass may be detected or confirmed by CT.

In our institute from August of 1967–February of 1975, 59 patients with carcinoma of the prostate had pedal lymphangiograms. Fourteen (24%) of these patients had nodal metastases with positive lymphangiograms, one in stage B,

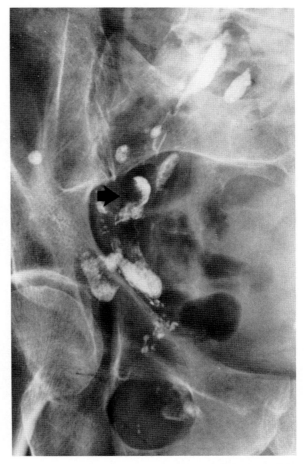

FIGURE 12.78. CARCINOMA OF THE PROSTATE
Nodal phase demonstrates the crescentic configuration denoting metastatic carcinoma (*arrow*). Lymphatics failed to traverse this defect.

seven in stage C, and seven in stage D. The sites of nodal involvement were the common iliac and para-aortic nodes in one patient of stage B, the external iliac nodes in seven patients of stage C, and both iliac and para-aortic nodes in five patients of stage D. One patient of stage D had metastasis in the inguinal and external iliac nodes with lymphatic obstruction in the pelvic region and showed poor opacification of para-aortic nodes, which was inadequate for proper interpretation. Two patients with pelvic and para-aortic metastases had supraclavicular nodal involvement. It should be emphasized that in one patient of stage B the lymphangiogram showed a positive finding in common iliac and para-aortic nodes. It can probably be explained by the fact that the lymphatic spread in the patient is most likely through the hypogastric pedicle of the lymphatic drainage of the prostate.

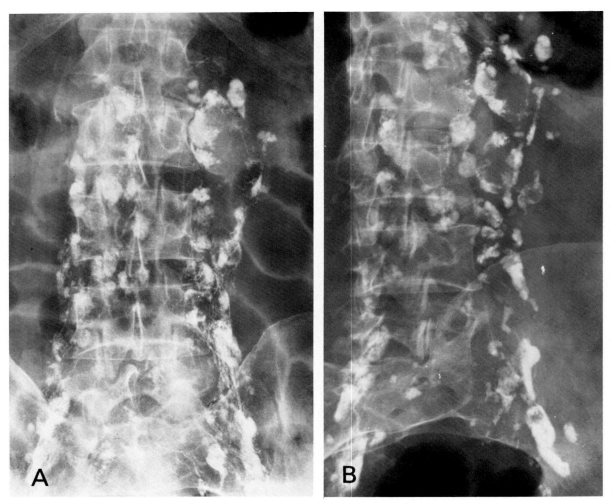

FIGURE 12.79. CARCINOMA OF THE PROSTATE
Involvement of common iliac and para-aortic nodes on the left. *A:* Lymphatic phase. *B:* Nodal phase.

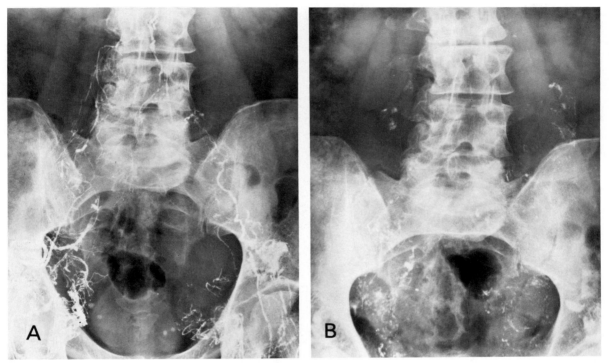

FIGURE 12.80. CARCINOMA OF THE PROSTATE
Extensive involvement yields fragmented nodes at times simulating lymphoma. *A:* Lymphatic phase. *B:* Nodal phase.

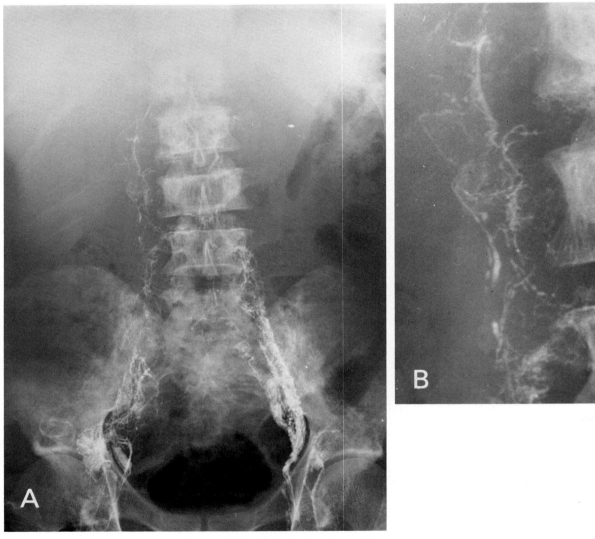

FIGURE 12.81. CARCINOMA OF THE PROSTATE

*A:* Complete replacement of nodes by metastatic carcinoma produces distortion of the lymphatics which circumvent the totally replaced nodes. *B:* Magnified view of distorted para-aortic lymphatics. The bones are involved by osteoblastic metastases. Original magnification ×2.

Generally speaking, as the clinical stage increases from A to D, there is a progressive increase in the incidence of positive para-aortic lymph node involvement so that almost all stage D patients show positive para-aortic lymph node involvement as well as positive pelvic nodes. None of the 14 patients with positive lymphangiograms had an exploratory laparotomy. With strict diagnostic criteria, interpretation of the lymphangiograms in carcinoma of the testicle, bladder, and cervix generally has excellent surgical correlation. Therefore, a positive lymphangiogram in a patient with carcinoma of the pros-

tate was considered definite evidence of metastasis, and the patient was treated accordingly.

In another series, from March of 1975–February of 1978, 208 patients with carcinoma of the prostate had pedal lymphangiograms. Forty-seven (23%) of these patients had nodal metastases with positive lymphangiograms, 40 in stage C and seven in stage D. Four of these 47 had nodal architectural changes most compatible with configuration seen in lymphoma due to metastatic carcinoma, confirmed histologically by percutaneous needle biopsy in 3. Of the 40 patients with stage C disease and positive lymphangiograms, lymph node biopsy confirmed the findings in 20. Percutaneous aspiration biopsy of the lymph nodes established metastatic disease in 11, while pelvic lymphadenectomy confirmed the presence of metastases in 9. Lymphangiographic appreciation of para-aortic nodal metastases in the absence of iliac involvement is unusual but does occur (Fig. 12.82). This distribution could still be in continuity if the metastases in the pelvis are not opacified (i.e., metastases in the hypogastric or presacral areas or in nodes completely replaced by tumor).

Lymph node metastases from carcinoma of the prostate have been demonstrated by LAG in recent literature. LAG has been reported to be 78–89% accurate in the detection of lymph node metastases from carcinoma of the prostate. Rummelhardt and Fussek (1970) performed lymphangiograms on 102 patients with carcinoma of the prostate and found an 80.1% diagnostic accuracy of the abnormal lymphangiograms when correlated with nodes obtained at surgery or autopsy. Castellino et al. (1973) reported 89% accuracy in nine patients with nodal metastases when correlated with excised lymph nodes. Correlating LAG with pelvic lymphadenectomy in 67 patients with carcinoma of the prostate, Spellman et al. (1977) obtained an overall accuracy of 78% (52 of 67), sensitivity of 57% (16 of 28), and specificity of 92% (36 of 39).

### CT in Tumors of the Prostate

In the evaluation of the lymph node metastasis from carcinoma of the prostate by CT, there were a few small series reported in the literature. Morgan et al. (1981) performed CT scanning in 29 patients with carcinoma of the prostate, and there was surgical confirmation in 16 of these patients. The sensitivity was 33% (2 of 6), specificity was 100% (10 of 10), the false-negative readings were 25% (4 of 16), and the overall accuracy was 75% (12 of 16). Benson et al. (1981) used CT to study 23 patients with carcinoma of the prostate and reported a sensitivity of 13%, specificity of 93%, and accuracy of 65%. Levine et al. (1981) found in 15 patients a sensitivity of 100%, specificity of 88%, and accuracy of 93%. In 46 patients with carcinoma of the prostate, Golimbu et al. (1980) used CT to detect metastases with a sensitivity of 29%, specificity of 93%, and overall accuracy of 70%. The advantage of CT is its ability to detect abnormal nodes in hypogastric and presacral areas (Fig. 12.83). Totally replaced nodes suggested by lymphatic obstruction with or without collateral circulation can be well delineated by CT. In advanced lesions with lymphatic obstruction in the pelvic region and nonopacification of the node in the para-aortic area, CT has definite value in revealing the size and extent of the lesion.

Depending primarily upon the stage of carcinoma of the prostate, various therapeutic modalities have been used for its treatment. The ability to define the exact extent of the disease accurately would be highly beneficial in the decision as to the choice of modality of treatment. Nodal metastases have been observed in early operable carcinoma of the prostate (Flocks et al., 1959). When the seminal vesicle is involved, there is a high incidence (at least 82.4%) of pelvic lymph node metastases (Arduino and Glucksman, 1962). The various clinical classifications are mainly based upon clinical methods and serum phosphatase levels and are often inaccurate. LAG and CT are of great benefit in revealing lymph node metastases and in assessing the exact extent of disease, especially in patients with apparently localized disease.

As to the management of carcinoma of the prostate at M. D. Anderson Hospital and Tumor Institute, lymphangiograms, complemented by CT if indicated, are routinely obtained in patients with stage C, that is, locally invasive prostatic carcinoma with involvement of the base of the bladder and/or seminal vesicle or fixation of the prostate to the pelvic wall. If the lymphangiogram is positive, radiation therapy is not considered, and the patient is treated with hormonal manipulation, usually orchiectomy and estrogens. If the lymphangiogram and CT are negative, the patient either receives radiation therapy to the prostate or open surgical staging with lymphadenectomy. Chemotherapy is now the preferred approach in advanced prostatic carcinoma. Systemic FAM (5-fluorouracil, adriamycin, and mitomycin-C) or vincristine has been effective. Intra-arterial chemotherapy is used if the pelvic disease is the predominant manifestation.

### The Penis

Carcinoma of the penis is an uncommon malignant disease accounting for less than 1% of all deaths from cancer in men in the United States. The disease occurs predominantly between the ages of 50–80 yr with an average of 65 yr. Although no specific etiological factors have been demonstrated, squamous cell carcinoma of the penis appears to be related to poor personal and sexual hygiene.

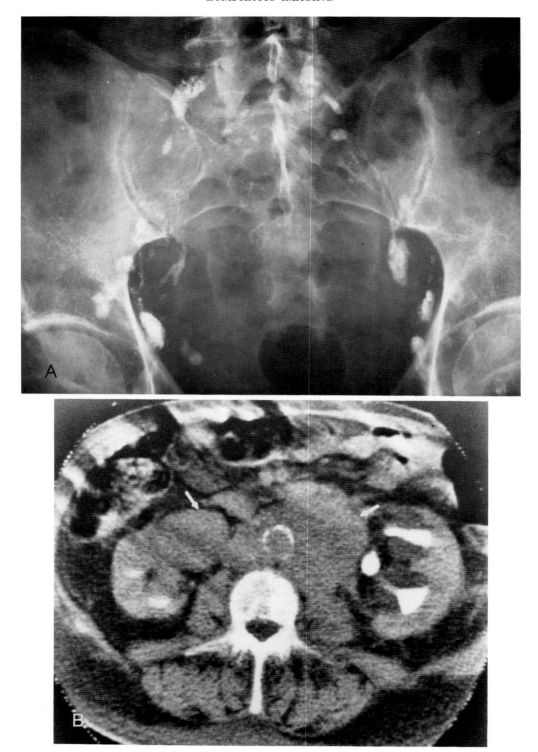

FIGURE 12.82. CARCINOMA OF THE PROSTATE WITH PARA-AORTIC NODAL METASTASIS
*A:* LAG. No evidence of nodal metastasis in the pelvic region. *B:* CT. Extensive nodal metastasis in para-aortic areas, mainly on the left side (*arrows*) with bilateral hydronephroses.

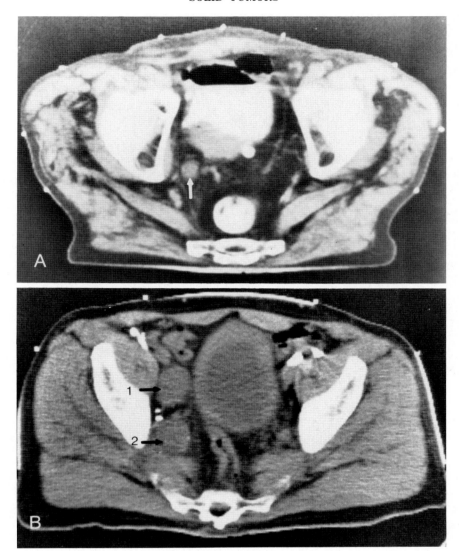

FIGURE 12.83. HYPOGASTRIC NODE METASTASES
*A:* Metastatic lesion to the right hypogastric node in a patient with carcinoma of the bladder (*arrow*). *B:* Metastatic lesion in right external iliac and hypogastric nodes (*1* and *2*) in another patient with carcinoma of the prostate.

### Lymphatic Drainage of the Penis

The lymphatics of the prepuce drain to the superior and medial group of the superficial inguinal nodes. The lymphatics of the glans penis join those of the urethra and prepuce and proceed in two groups: those that follow the femoral canal terminating in the deep inguinal nodes, including the node of Cloquet and the medial retrocrural lymph nodes; and those that follow the inguinal canal and drain into the lateral retrocrural lymph nodes. The lymphatics of the corpora cavernosa penis end in the superior and medial group of the superficial inguinal nodes and sometimes in the deep inguinal nodes or the retrocrural external iliac nodes (Fig. 12.84). The right and left inguinal lymph nodes have a rich communication with each other through subcutaneous lymphatics.

### Lymph Node Metastasis in Carcinoma of the Penis

Carcinoma of the penis may arise on the glans, the retroglandular sulcus, the prepuce, and rarely from the skin of the shaft. The gross appearance of the lesion, usually squamous type, may be either proliferative or ulceroinfiltrative. The pro-

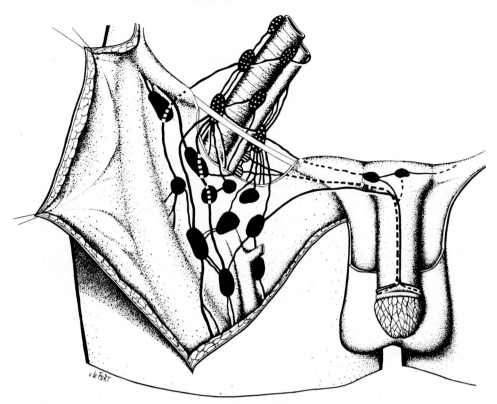

FIGURE 12.84. LYMPHATIC DRAINAGE OF THE PENIS

liferative type often is very well differentiated, and the ulceroinfiltrative type tends to be more undifferentiated.

Nodal metastases from carcinoma of the penis are rarely found in the proliferative type of lesion. The ulceroinfiltrative lesion metastasizes more readily. Metastasis from carcinoma of the penis is usually to the inguinal and external iliac nodes. Distant metastases to abdominal nodes, liver, and lung can occur.

LAG by both penile and pedal routes has been utilized to define lymph node involvement from carcinoma of the penis. For the most part, the pedal approach is more universally performed. Only a portion of the inguinal nodes are opacified by this technique. Although the inguinal lymph nodes are frequently involved by chronic inflammatory disease, the information obtained by pedal LAG is still valid and useful. Again, the single most reliable criterion representing metastasis is a defect in a node not traversed by lymphatics (Figs. 12.85 and 12.86). The other criteria enumerated previously are also operative here.

CT is not as useful in detecting early nodal metastasis as is LAG. However, in advanced lesions, CT is of definite value in detecting pelvic extension of the lesion and defining distant metastases.

## The Large Intestine

Seventy-five percent of all intestinal cancers arise in the colon, rectum, and anus. At the time of the initial surgical procedure, venous invasion and region lymph node metastases are found frequently. Blood vessel invasion has been reported in 36–41%, depending upon the site of the primary (Grinnell, 1942). This incidence correlated with subsequent metastasis to liver, lungs, or other viscera. When liver metastases were found, lymph node involvement was invariably present. Regional lymph node metastases noted during curative resection have been seen in one-half to two-thirds of the patients (Gilchrist, 1959, Keynes, 1961). Dukes and Bussey (1958) reported that an overall 5-yr survival rate with nodal metastases without vein invasion was 57.7%, while with venous invasion it was 20%. Copeland et al. (1968) suggested that the survival rate varied inversely with the number of metastatic nodes: no nodes, 48%; one node, 26.8%; and five or more nodes, 9.1%. Crile et al. (1971)

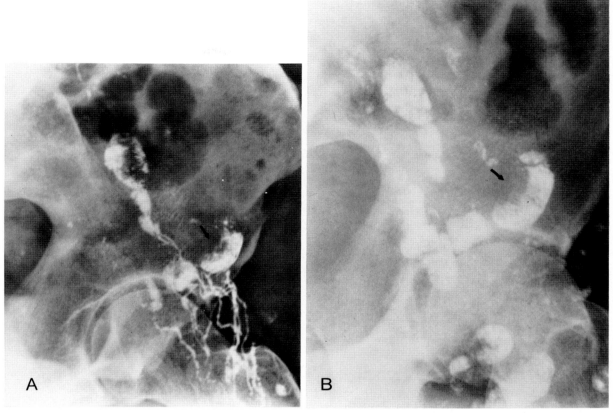

FIGURE 12.85. CARCINOMA OF THE PENIS WITH METASTASIS TO A RETROCRURAL NODE
*A:* Lymphatic phase. *B:* Nodal phase.

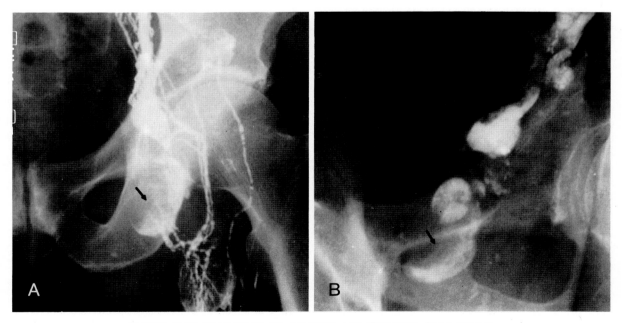

FIGURE 12.86. METASTASIS TO INGUINAL AND EXTERNAL ILIAC NODES
*A:* Lymphatic phase. *B:* Nodal phase.

postulated that at one point in the growth of metastases in lymph nodes they begin to act as primary tumors and shed tumor cells into the blood. Such a period does not begin until a nodal metastasis is large and penetrates the capsule. Therefore, lymph node involvement in carcinoma of the large intestine is a most important prognostic factor. The relative position and extent of lymph node metastasis determine the outcome far more than the size of the primary lesion or its penetration through the wall of the colon and rectum (Dukes and Bussey, 1958).

*Lymphatic Drainage of the Large Intestine*

Lymphatics of the large intestine arise from the rich lymphatic plexuses of the wall and drain eventually to the central nodes of the superior mesenteric chain, the central nodes of the inferior mesenteric chain, or the para- and preaortic nodes. Between the gut and terminal nodes are several sets of additional nodes, called the paracolic, the intermediate, and the principal nodes. The principal node is located near the root of the mesenteric vessels. The lymph vessels may pass through all of these sets of nodes in succession, or they may run directly to the principal nodes. There are important differences in the drainage of the right and left halves of the colon. The lymphatics of the ascending colon and proximal two-thirds of the transverse colon drain to the central nodes of the superior mesenteric chain. The remaining one-third of the distal transverse colon and the superior extremity of the descending colon are drained by the lymphatics that accompany the inferior mesenteric veins and terminate in the central nodes of the superior mesenteric chain. The greater part of the descending colon is drained to the nodes which accompany the left colic artery and then the nodes of the inferior mesenteric chain. The collecting trunks of the sigmoid colon are emptied into the central nodes of the inferior mesenteric chain. The central group of the inferior mesenteric chain is drained in turn by the left para- and preaortic nodes, while the central group of the superior mesenteric chain is drained by the intestinal lymphatic trunk which usually anastomoses with one of the lumbar trunks above the renal artery, generally with the left of the initial part of the thoracic duct. Sometimes, as a normal variation, the efferent trunks from the central group of the superior mesenteric chain terminate in the left para- and preaortic nodes immediately adjacent to the renal artery (Fig. 12.87A).

The lymphatics of the rectum and anal canal have numerous anastomoses with those of the prostate, seminal vesicle, vagina, and bladder. The collecting trunks are divided into three groups: inferior, middle, and superior. The inferior collecting trunks originate in the cutaneous part of the anus. They run forward and outward in the subcutaneous tissue of the perineum and the medial aspect of the thigh and drain into the superficial inguinal nodes. The middle collecting trunks, which arise from the anal canal and the inferior extremity of the rectum, usually follow the middle hemorrhoidal vessels and terminate in the hypogastric nodes. They may accompany the middle sacral and lateral sacral arteries and drain to the nodes of the promontory and to the lateral sacral nodes.

The superior collecting trunks spring from the anal canal and extend through the entire length of the rectum and traverse one or several intercalating nodes along the course of the superior hemorrhoidal blood vessels. They finally terminate as follows. The short trunks, which come from every region of the rectum, terminate in the nodes situated at the level of the bifurcation of the superior hemorrhoidal artery. These are the most important lymph nodes draining the rectum. The middle trunks ascend, without stopping at the nodes of the bifurcation, to a node placed along the inferior mesenteric artery near the origin of its lowest sigmoid branch. The long trunks, which spring from the lower portion of the rectum, terminate in the nodes placed at the summit of the pelvic mesocolon near the origin of the left colic artery. By means of the efferent trunks of the inferior mesenteric chain, the rectal lymph is finally poured into the preaortic and left para-aortic nodes (Fig. 12.87B).

*LAG in Carcinoma of the Large Intestine*

The lymph nodes initially involved in carcinoma of the large intestine are usually in the first echelon distribution and out of the scope of LAG except possibly in carcinoma of the anus. Despite the frequency of regional lymph node metastases at the time of the curative bowel resection, LAG has not as yet been utilized routinely in carcinoma of the large intestine. By pedal LAG the lymph nodes which can be demonstrated are the second echelon distribution of the nodes from the large intestine to the iliac and para-aortic regions. Nodal metastases from the right side of the colon are only rarely demonstrated. Metastasis from the left side of the colon and rectum can be delineated but occurs later in the course of the disease. Preliminary investigation of the value of this examination in

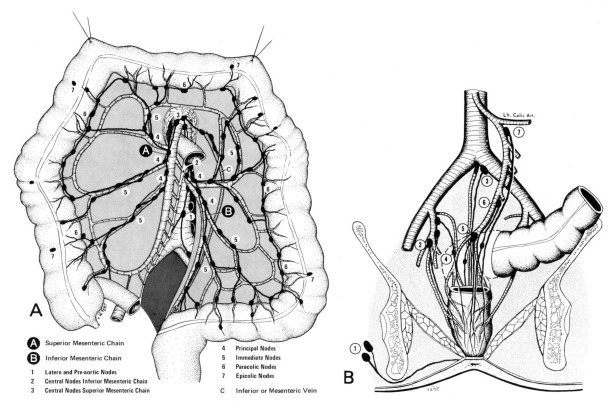

A
B
A  Superior Mesenteric Chain
B  Inferior Mesenteric Chain

1  Latero and Pre-aortic Nodes
2  Central Nodes Inferior Mesenteric Chain
3  Central Nodes Superior Mesenteric Chain

4  Principal Nodes
5  Immediate Nodes
6  Paracolic Nodes
7  Epicolic Nodes

C  Inferior or Mesenteric Vein

FIGURE 12.87. LYMPHATIC DRAINAGE OF THE COLON
*A:* Schematic drawing of the lymphatics of the colon and the sigmoid. *B:* Schematic drawing of the sigmoid and rectum. *1– 7* are as in *A.*

patients with carcinoma of the colon and rectum was done at Thomas Jefferson University Hospital. Fifty-five patients who returned at varying intervals after the initial resection with complaints suggesting recurrence or metastases were studied by LAG. Slightly more than 50% of these patients were found to have metastases as detected by this examination (Figs. 12.88–12.90).

### CT in Tumors of the Large Intestine

Ellert and Kreel (1980) described CT changes in 55 patients with malignant colonic tumors. A local recurrence alone was found in 44%, distant metastases alone in 10%, and the combination in 46%. Pelvic or para-aortic lymphadenopathy was noted in 8 (80%) of 10 patients with pulmonary metastases compared with 5 (42%) of 12 of those with hepatic metastases. Of the 10 patients with hydronephrosis, 5 showed regional lymphadenopathy.

At M. D. Anderson Hospital, Mayes and Zornoza (1980) reviewed CT examinations of 80 cases of carcinoma of the colon. Fifty-two CT examinations demonstrated evidence of disease in the pelvis and abdomen. The most common finding was a pelvic mass (22 patients). Retroperitoneal adenopathy was present in 12 patients. Liver metastases were identified in 20 patients. Adrenal metastases were demonstrated in 8 patients.

CT is a sensitive tool for determining the extent of disease in the pelvis or the abdomen (Figs. 12.91 and 12.92). It allows the visualization of the many potential areas of metastases (Fig. 12.93).

### The Breast

Carcinoma of the breast is the most common type of malignant neoplasm occurring in females over 40 yr of age. Prognosis depends upon the size of the primary carcinoma as well as the presence of lymph node metastasis. Despite all recent efforts in management, survival rates have not changed significantly. Earlier detection of the primary lesion will probably influence survival. The place of LAG of the upper extremity in the diagnosis and management of patients with carcinoma of the breast has still not been

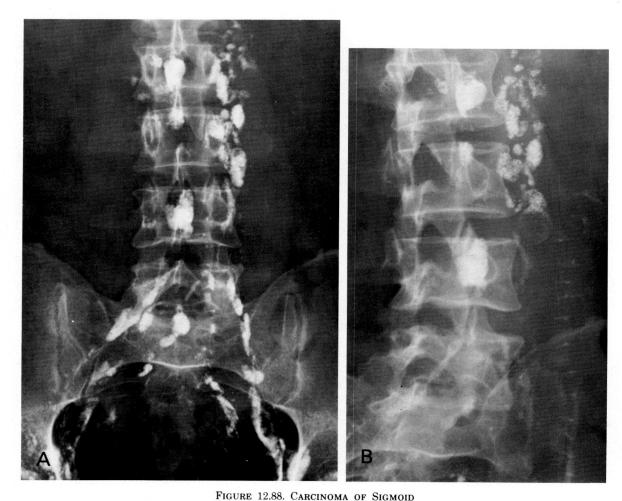

FIGURE 12.88. CARCINOMA OF SIGMOID
*A:* Nodal phase of lymphangiogram performed just prior to resection of the sigmoid neoplasm. *B:* Five months after surgery a left para-aortic node is obviously involved by metastasis. *C:* Nodal phase of lymphangiogram performed just prior to resection of the sigmoid neoplasm in another patient. *D:* After 1½ yr left para-aortic nodes are involved by metastases.

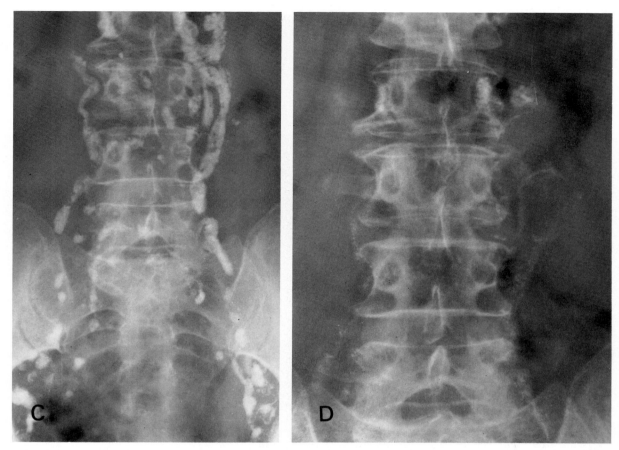

FIGURE 12.88C AND D.

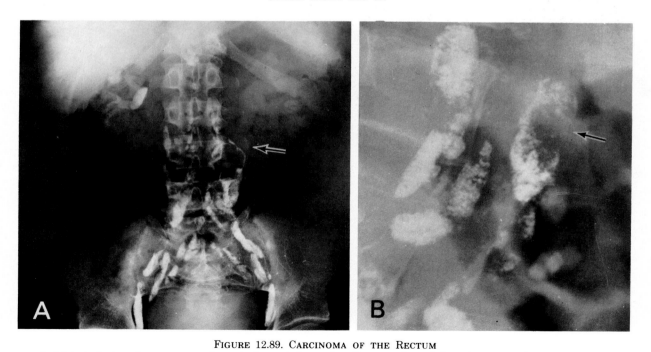

FIGURE 12.89. CARCINOMA OF THE RECTUM

*A:* Metastasis to a lower para-aortic node (*arrow*) 6 months after resection of the primary neoplasm. *B:* Para-aortic metastases obstructing the left kidney (*arrow*) from a carcinoma of the rectum in another patient.

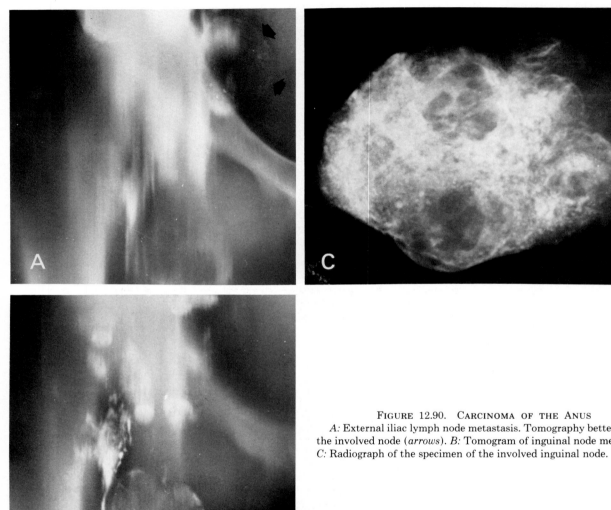

FIGURE 12.90.  CARCINOMA OF THE ANUS
*A:* External iliac lymph node metastasis. Tomography better defines
the involved node (*arrows*). *B:* Tomogram of inguinal node metastasis.
*C:* Radiograph of the specimen of the involved inguinal node.

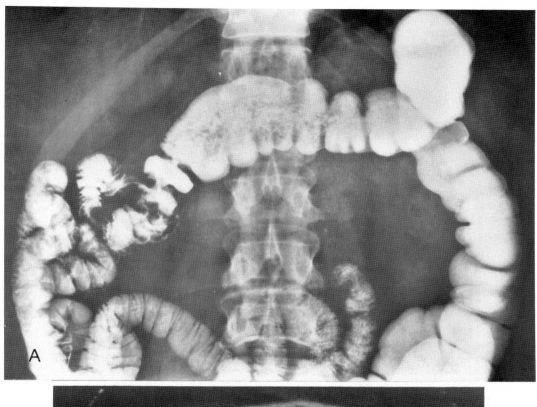

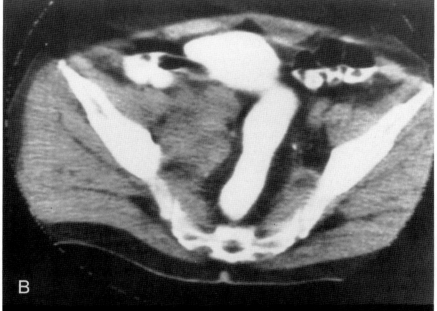

FIGURE 12.91. RECURRENT CARCINOMA OF THE CECUM WITH METASTASES TO PARA-AORTIC AND ADRENAL NODES
A: Barium enema (18 months postoperatively). Status post-right hemicolectomy with ileotransverse anastomosis. There is no evidence of recurrence. B: CT of the pelvis (18 months postoperatively). A large pelvic mass is displacing the rectosigmoid to the left. C: CT of the middle abdomen (18 months postoperatively). Nodal metastases in the para-aortic area (*arrows*). D: CT of the upper abdomen (18 months postoperatively). Adrenal metastasis on the right (*arrow*).

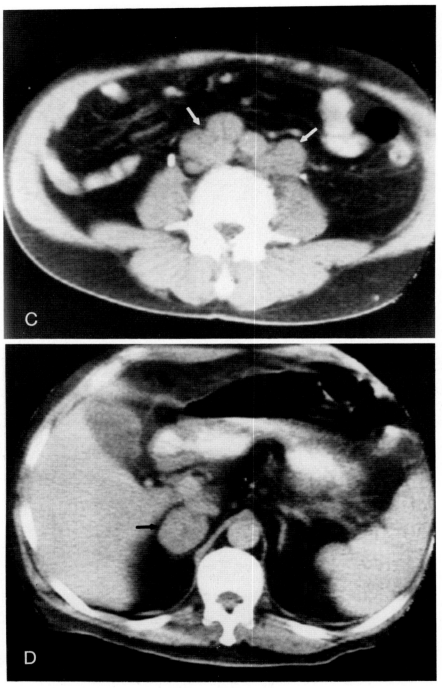

FIGURE 12.91C AND D.

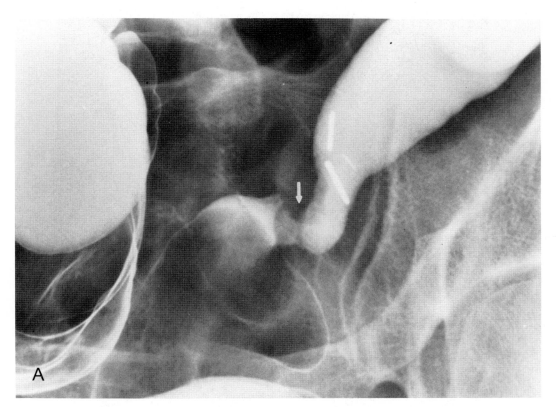

FIGURE 12.92. RECURRENT CARCINOMA OF THE SIGMOID WITH PARA-AORTIC LYMPHADENOPATHY AND LIVER
METASTASES

*A:* Barium enema. There is postoperative status of the sigmoid. Narrowing of the lumen with irregular contour is noted in the region of the anastomosis due to recurrence (*arrow*). *B:* CT of the upper abdomen. There is ascites (*1*) and liver metastasis (*2*). *C:* CT of the middle abdomen. There are calcified nodal metastases in the left para-aortic area (*arrow*).

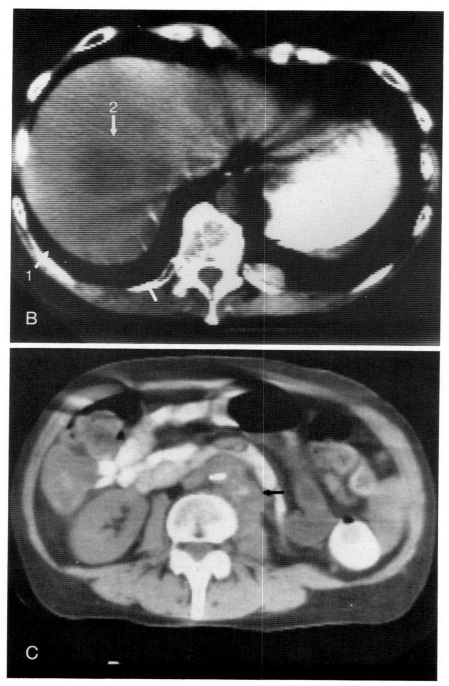

FIGURE 12.92*B* AND *C*.

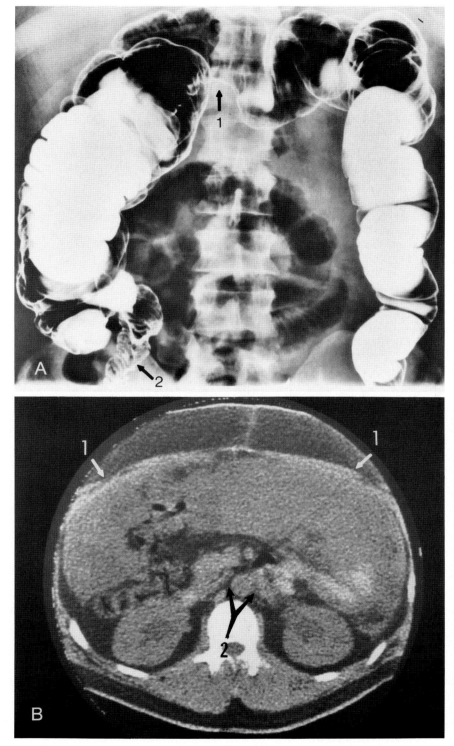

FIGURE 12.93. CARCINOMA OF THE SIGMOID WITH OMENTAL METASTASIS

*A:* Barium enema. There is an indentation in the inferior aspect of the midtransverse colon with slight mucosal pleating (*1*). The distal ileum also shows an indentation and mucosal tethering (*2*). These changes are consistent with secondary involvement. *B:* CT of the abdomen. There is an extensive omental metastasis (*1*) associated with ascites. Nodular metastases are also noted in the periaortic area (*2*).

established. Perhaps the more limited surgical approach of simple mastectomy or local excision of the breast mass plus radiotherapy may find new application for this procedure.

### Lymphatic Drainage of the Breast

**Lymphatics of the Skin of the Breast.** The lymphatics of the skin of the breast have a particular arrangement at the level of the nipple and areola. In this region, they form a dense areolar network with subareolar lymphatic plexuses. To the outer side of the subareolar plexus, the lymphatic network has the same arrangement as the lymphatic network of the skin of the anterior chest wall and is continuous with the lymphatics of the skin of the surrounding region, forming an uninterrupted network over the entire surface of the chest, neck, and abdomen. By this mechanism, the lymphatics of the skin of one breast communicate with those of the opposite breast. Collecting trunks of the skin of the breast may cross the midline and drain into the axillary nodes of the opposite side.

**Lymphatics of the Breast Proper (Mammary Gland).** The lymphatic network of the breast arises from the inter- or perilobular spaces. A few of the collecting trunks follow the lactiferous ducts and end in the subareolar plexuses of the lymphatics of the skin of the breast, but most of these trunks terminate in the axillary nodes. Some end in the internal mammary chain, and, rarely, others empty into the supraclavicular nodes. The lymphatics of the breast may be grouped into the following pathway (Fig. 12.94):

PRINCIPAL AXILLARY PATHWAYS. The axillary pathways are formed by the lateral and medial trunks. The lateral trunk receives a principal tributary from the superior part of the breast. The medial trunk passes below the areola and receives a principal tributary from the inferior part of the breast. After winding around the anterior border of the base of the axilla, the lateral and medial trunks traverse the axillary fascia of the base of the axilla and terminate in the nodes of the external mammary chain situated at the level of the second and third intercostal spaces. Some of the collecting trunks do not stop at the external mammary nodes but run directly into the nodes of the axillary vein group or to those of the central group. The efferent vessels of the axillary lymphatics unite to form the subclavian lymphatic trunks, which may terminate in three ways: (*a*) They may empty directly into the jugulosubclavian confluence. (*b*) They may join the jugular and bronchomediastinal lymphatic trunks to form a common lym-

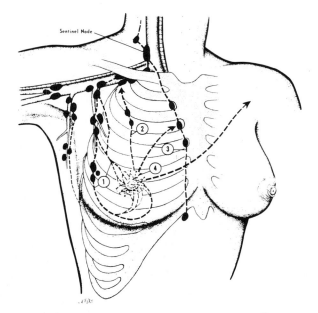

FIGURE 12.94. LYMPHATIC DRAINAGE OF THE BREAST
*1*, Principal axillary pathways. *2*, Accessory axillary pathways. *3*, Internal mammary pathways. *4*, Subareolar lymphatic plexus.

phatic duct and empty into the jugulosubclavian confluence. (*c*) They may empty into the jugular lymphatic trunk.

ACCESSORY AXILLARY PATHWAYS. The accessory axillary pathways drain the upper medial region of the breast and are of two kinds: (*a*) Transpectoral lymph pathways consist of lymphatics which emerge from the periphery of the breast and pass across the pectoralis major. Some of these traverse the pectoralis major with the pectoral branches of the superior thoracic and thoracoacromial arteries and terminate in subclavicular nodes. Others accompany the arterial rami, which perforates the pectoralis major below the inferior border of the pectoralis minor and terminates in several axillary nodes. (*b*) Retropectoral lymph pathways consist of one or two lymph vessels which wind around the inferior border of the pectoralis major and ascend directly toward the subclavicular nodes by passing either behind the pectoralis minor, along the axillary vein, or between both pectoral muscles.

INTERNAL MAMMARY LYMPH PATHWAYS. The internal mammary pathways drain the central and medial regions of the breast. The collecting trunks run along the perforating branches of the internal mammary blood vessels. They traverse the pectoralis major and the intercostal muscles and empty into the nodes of the internal mammary chain situated in the intercostal spaces at the sternal border. The internal mammary lymphatic trunks may terminate in: (*a*) the thoracic duct (left) or the lymphatic duct (right), (*b*) the lowest lymph node (sentinel node) of the supraclavicular group, or (*c*) directly into the jugulosubclavian vein confluence.

SUPRACLAVICULAR LYMPH PATHWAYS. Although the lymphatic trunks coming from the superomedial part of the breast may terminate in some supraclavicular nodes as reported in 3 of 100 cases by Mornard (cited by Rouvière, 1938), it is generally believed that the supraclavicular lymph nodes do not have direct connection with the breast but, rather, are involved by a retrograde permeation of the lymphatics which connect them with the deeply placed sentinel nodes. Sentinel nodes lie close to the confluence of the internal jugular and subclavian vein and are first to be involved by metastasis from the breast which reaches them by way of the subclavian or internal mammary lymphatic trunks.

### LAG in Carcinoma of the Breast

In regional lymph node metastasis, the axillary nodes are often involved, probably because the upper outer quadrant of the breast is the common site of disease. In relatively few cases, the axillary nodes are bypassed, and the first nodes involved are those of the subclavian and supraclavicular groups. The internal mammary nodes are involved especially from the tumors of the inner quadrant of the breast. Nodes of the anterior mediastinum or even the opposite axilla may be involved. These metastatic lesions are derived particularly from tumor located in the inner quadrant of the breast.

Lymphangiographic demonstration of lymph node metastasis from the breast is deficient in that upper limb LAG does not opacify all of the axillary nodes. In addition, the supraclavicular nodes are not constantly opacified, and the internal mammary nodes are not demonstrated (Fig. 12.95).

Currently, the indications for upper limb LAG for carcinoma of the breast are detection of axillary nodal metastasis and evaluation of postmastectomy and postirradiation edema of the upper extremity.

Opacification of the lymphatic drainage has been reported after the injection of contrast material directly into the breast. This is not consistent and has never received adequate clinical trial. Experimental opacification of internal mammary nodes has been accomplished by the intraperitoneal injection of contrast material. This same pathway has been appreciated in a patient with a carcinoma of the cervix staged by

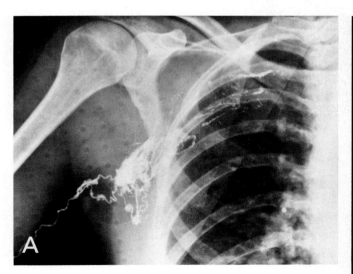
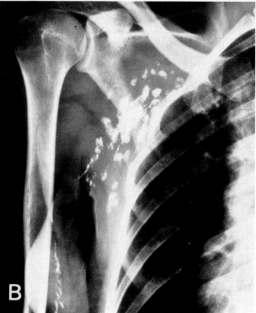

FIGURE 12.95. NORMAL AXILLARY LYMPHATICS AND NODES

pelvic node biopsy. A lymphatic fistula into the peritoneal cavity was visualized during lower extremity LAG. The contrast material outlined the small bowel. Eventually internal mammary lymph nodes were opacified (Fig. 12.96).

The diagnosis of metastatic carcinoma to the axillary lymph nodes can be established when the criteria previously described are employed (Fig. 12.97). This procedure has received adverse criticism because of the incomplete demonstration of all of the axillary nodes (Kendall et al., 1963; Shibata et al., 1966; Kitt et al., 1972). When positive, however, the information has a high degree of pathological correlation.

### CT in Carcinoma of the Breast

The internal mammary lymph pathways drain the central region and inner quadrant of the breast. In carcinoma of the breast, especially medial in location, the internal mammary nodes may be involved. Internal mammary adenopathy may be visualized on lateral chest roentgenogram as a retrosternal soft tissue mass. Internal mammary lymphoscintigraphy can be used as a rational adjunct to identify the nodal involvement (Ege, 1978). Accurate assessment of the presence of internal mammary lymphadenopathy relies upon CT (Meyer and Munzenrider, 1981). In addition, CT can evaluate the adjacent mediastinal extension and the regional bony involvement.

In advanced carcinoma of the breast with intra-abdominal metastases, involvement of retroperitoneal lymph nodes does occur. Figure 12.98 is of a case of carcinoma of the breast with metastases to the stomach, mesentery, and para-aortic lymph nodes.

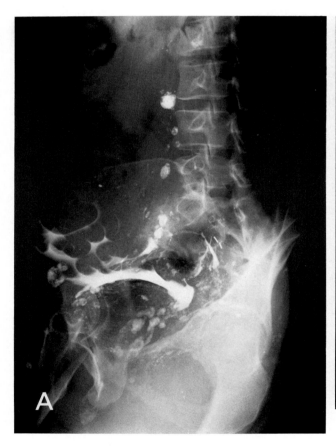 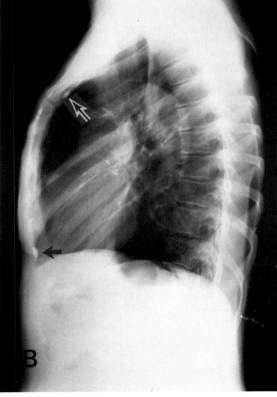

FIGURE 12.96. OPACIFICATION OF INTERNAL MAMMARY NODES VIA PERITONEAL ROUTES
*A:* Fistulous tract into peritoneal cavity with contrast material outlining small bowel loops. *B:* Opacification of internal mammary nodes (*arrows*).

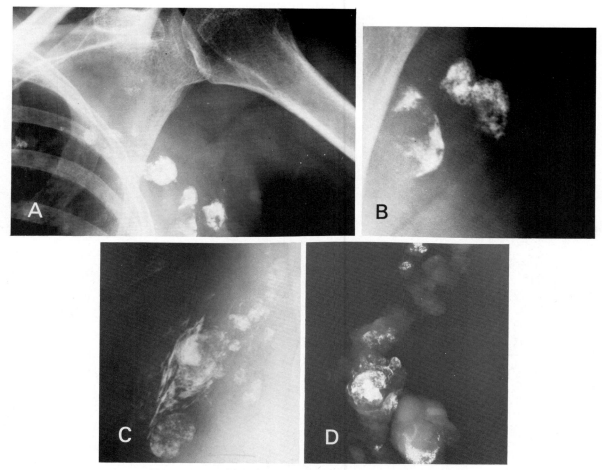

FIGURE 12.97. METASTATIC CARCINOMA FROM THE BREAST

*A:* Metastasis to the left axillary nodes from carcinoma of the breast. B: Magnification of nodes in *A*. Original magnification ×2. *C:* Metastatic carcinoma to the right axillary nodes from carcinoma of the breast in another patient. *D:* Radiograph of specimen.

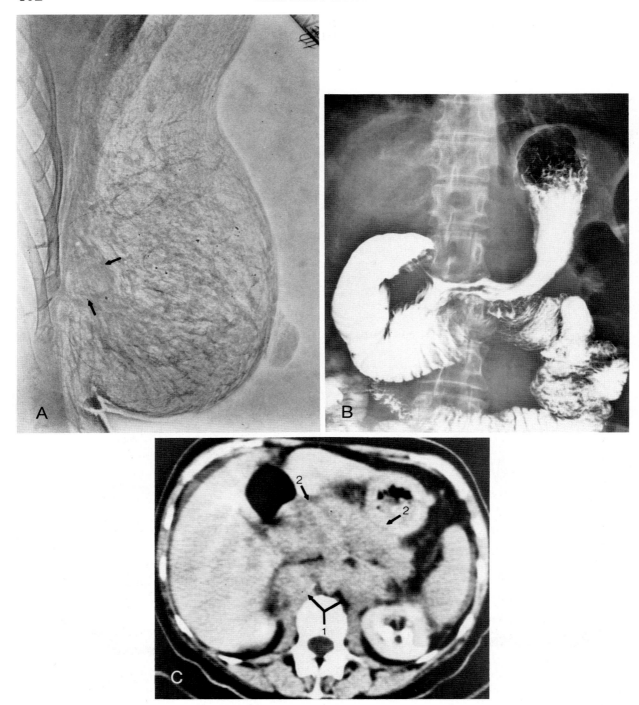

FIGURE 12.98. CARCINOMA OF THE BREAST WITH METASTASES TO THE STOMACH, THE MESENTERY, AND THE PARA-
AORTIC LYMPH NODES

*A:* Xeromammogram. A tumor mass is situated quite deep and close to the chest wall in the lower portion of the right breast
(*arrows*). *B:* Upper gastrointestinal study. The stomach is of markedly reduced volume, having a linitis plastica appearance.
This is secondary to submucosal metastasis. In addition, there is an extrinsic pressure defect involving the lesser curvature
side of the stomach which represents mass effect. There is rather marked dilatation of the duodenal bulb and loop which
resembles a mesenteric drag syndrome, probably due to retroperitoneal lymphadenopathy. *C:* CT of upper abdomen. There is
an extensive lymphadenopathy in the para-aortic and mesenteric areas (*1* and *2*). Needle biopsy under ultrasonic guidance
was performed in the retroperitoneal area. The pathological diagnosis was adenocarcinoma.

# UPPER EXTREMITY EDEMA, INCLUDING POSTMASTECTOMY AND POSTIRRADIATION EDEMA

In edema, lymphatic dynamics frequently depend on lymphatic-venous interplay. The etiology of many forms of secondary edema lies in the upset of balance that normally prevails between the two compartments. This is best presented by an analysis of the dynamics associated with the production of edema of an extremity. Differentiation of the mechanisms can be made by performing both LAG and venography. Our findings can be classified as follows: lymphatic obstruction; venous occlusion—intrinsic and extrinsic; and combined lymphatic and venous disease. These classifications are most dramatically illustrated in the variety of mechanisms seen in postmastectomy edema.

Radical mastectomy involves extensive dissection of the regional lymph nodes at the axilla which, in most instances, is beyond the regenerative power of the lymphatics to restore. Reestablishment of satisfactory lymphatic drainage depends on the existence of lymphatic vessels which are not resected at operation and the development of collateral lymph channels with rerouting of lymph flow. Following radical mastectomy, obstruction of the lymph flow is usually seen in the axillary region. The collateral channels may be seen in the anterior chest wall to the internal mammary and mediastinal lymph nodes and not infrequently to the opposite axillary nodes (Fig. 12.99). The cephalic (radial) lymphatic trunk is also a major pathway through which the collateral channels drain into the supraclavicular nodes. Collateral channels through the lymphatics in the posterior chest wall to the paravertebral nodes and the opposite axillary nodes may be observed.

## Lymphatic Obstruction

The sequelae of lymphatic obstruction have been described previously. Figure 12.100A shows

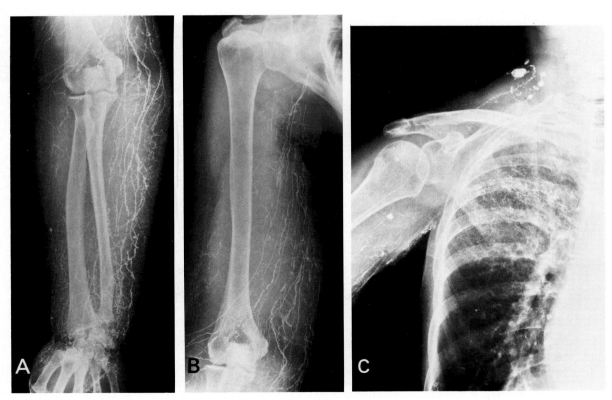

FIGURE 12.99. LYMPHATIC OBSTRUCTION WITH COLLATERAL CIRCULATION POSTMASTECTOMY
A: Edematous forearm showing lymphatic obstruction. Opacification of multiple channels are a manifestation of obstruction. B: Edematous arm from obstruction in the axilla. Increase in the number of channels opacified. C: Collateral circulation of chest wall. D: Opacification of supraclavicular lymph nodes bilaterally, internal mammary nodes bilaterally, and left axillary lymph nodes due to collateral pathways. Anteroposterior projection. E: Lateral projection (*arrows*, opacified internal mammary nodes). F: Venogram. Patent axillary vein.

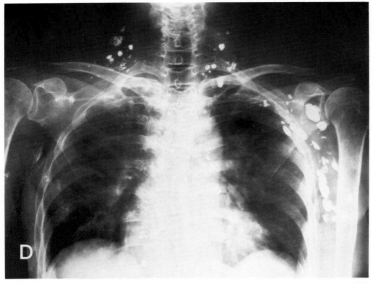

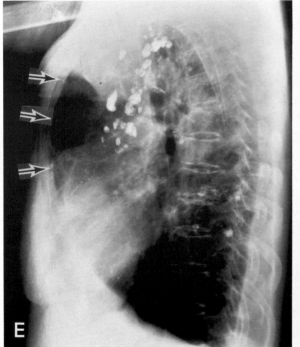

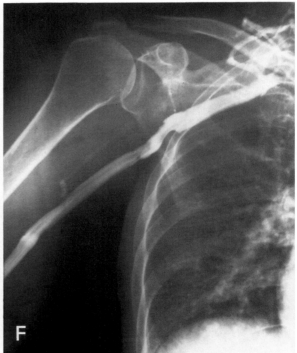

FIGURE 12.99*D–F*.

a case of postmastectomy edema following radical mastectomy and axillary lymph node dissection; the lymphangiographic picture is that usually seen in patients with lymphatic obstruction. The site of obstruction was in the axilla. Multiple collateral channels are clearly seen attempting to circumvent the obstruction. The lymphatics are dilated and tortuous with associated dermal backflow. The venogram (Fig. 12.100*B*) was normal.

## Venous Occlusion

Venous occlusion may be either intrinsic (thrombophlebitis) or extrinsic (vascular compression) in origin. The patient shown in Figure 12.101*A* and *B* had carcinoma of the breast which was treated by radical mastectomy and axillary dissection followed by radiation therapy. Postmastectomy edema gradually developed. The venogram revealed intrinsic disease, chronic

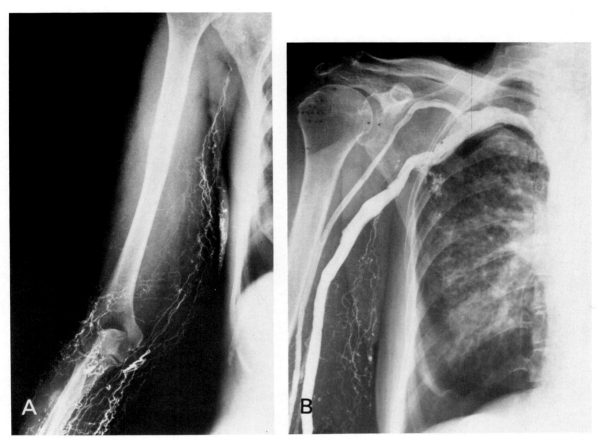

FIGURE 12.100. POSTMASTECTOMY EDEMA
*A:* Lymphatic obstruction. *B:* Normal axillary vein.

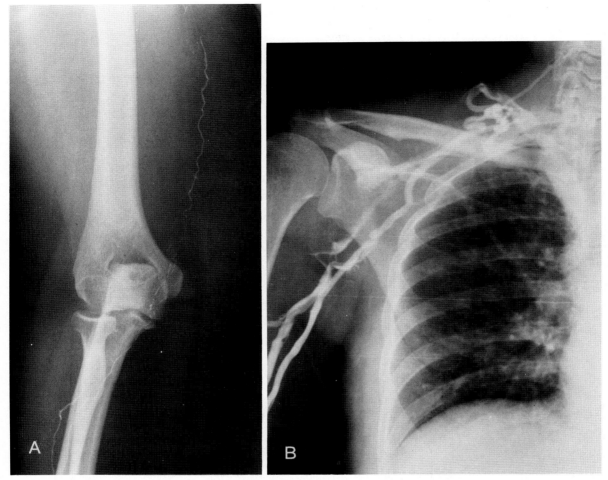

FIGURE 12.101. POSTMASTECTOMY EDEMA—THROMBOPHLEBITIS
*A:* Normal lymphatics. *B:* Thrombophlebitis of axillary vein.

thrombophlebitis. Lymphangiograms showed also a decrease in the caliber and number of the lymphatics opacified. It is believed by many that chronic thrombophlebitis is usually coupled with perivascular lymphangitis. In an attempt to explain our findings, it is postulated that there is stasis in the lymphatics of the extremity, thereby making fewer channels available for active flow. On the other hand, perhaps the decrease in caliber is secondary to the increase in interstitial tissue pressure, stasis, or spasm.

Extrinsic venous disease may be due to enlarged lymph nodes, inflammatory or neoplastic in origin, compressing the veins. It may also be produced by fibrotic or inflammatory changes in the perivascular tissues secondary to surgery or radiation therapy and may eventuate in an occlusion of the vein. Figure 12.102*A* and *B* shows extrinsic venous disease in a patient with a car-

cinoma of the breast. There was edema of the arm prior to any form of therapy. The lymph nodes compressing the vein proved to be inflamed.

## Combined Lymphatic and Venous Disease

Most frequently encountered is a combination of these two entities. In such situations the vein is involved either by intrinsic or extrinsic disease. Lymphangiograms show lymphatic obstruction. There is usually an associated soft tissue suffusion of contrast material.

Obstruction of the superior vena cava and right subclavian vein by carcinoma of the lung may also occlude lymphatic flow (Fig. 12.103*A* and *B*). The increased venous pressure inhibits normal flow of lymph into the subclavian vein at the venous angle. The lymphangiogram shows

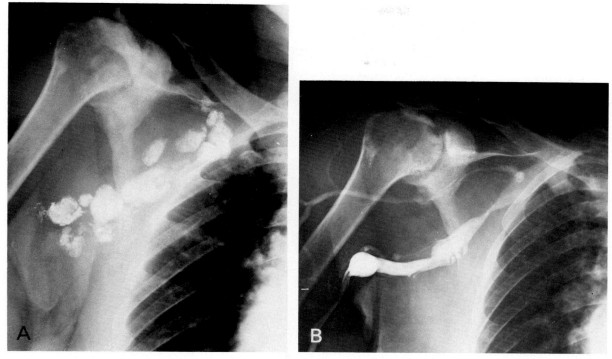

FIGURE 12.102. EDEMA—EXTRINSIC VENOUS COMPRESSION
*A:* Enlarged nodes compressing the axillary vein. *B:* Venogram. Compression of axillary vein.

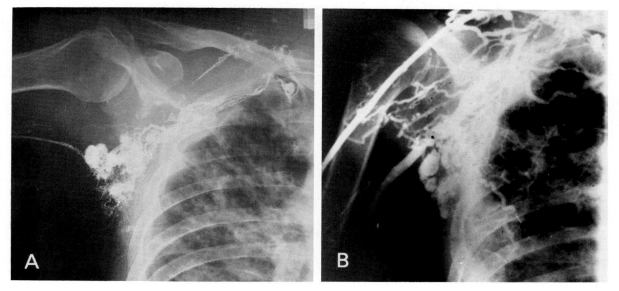

FIGURE 12.103. EDEMA—LYMPHATIC AND VENOUS DISEASE IN CARCINOMA OF THE LUNG
*A:* Lymphatic obstruction with collateral circulation. *B:* Venous obstruction with collateral circulation.

marked collateral lymphatic circulation in the axillary and supraclavicular areas and in the lateral chest wall. There are irregular supraclavicular lymph nodes demonstrated which are diagnostic of metastatic disease. Venograms demonstrate filling of accessory venous channels bypassing the occlusion.

Figure 12.104*A* and *B* shows a patient with Hodgkin's disease and extensive axillary lymph node involvement. The diagnosis was established

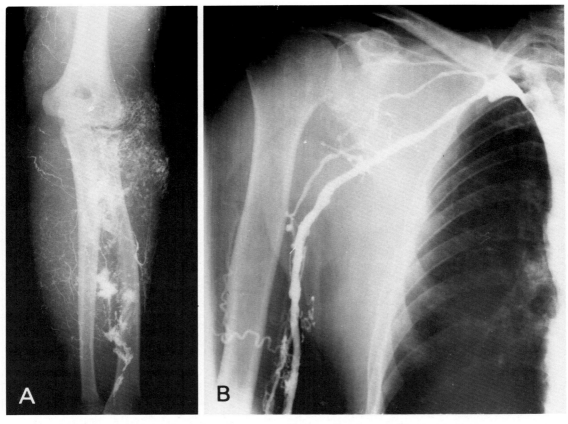

FIGURE 12.104. EDEMA—LYMPHATIC AND VENOUS DISEASE IN HODGKIN'S DISEASE
After lymph node biopsy and radiation therapy. *A:* Lymphatic obstruction. *B:* Venous disease, thrombophlebitis.

by axillary lymph node biopsy and followed by radiation therapy to the axilla. There was progressive edema of the arm. The lymphangiogram shows an extensive collateral lymphatic network; these vessels are, in general, fine in caliber, and there is soft tissue suffusion of the radiopaque material. The venogram demonstrates an irregular axillary vein, suggesting thrombophlebitis.

Another patient with extrinsic venous disease in combination with lymphatic obstruction is shown in Figure 12.105*A* and *B*. This patient developed edema of the arm following a radical mastectomy and radiation therapy. The axillary and cephalic veins are tapered in the axilla, suggesting extrinsic compression. The lymphangiogram reveals extensive collateral circulation through lymphatics of fine caliber and slight soft tissue suffusion of the contrast material. The lymphangiographic picture in such instances has been consistent.

## MALIGNANT TUMORS OF THE SKIN

### Lymphatic Drainage of the Skin

*Lymphatics of the Extremity*

The skin of the upper extremity, including the hand, is drained by cutaneous lymphatics which follow a long course to the epitrochlear and axillary nodes. Most of thse lymphatics go directly to the axillary nodes.

The skin of the lower extremity is drained almost entirely by cutaneous lymphatics which empty into the inguinal nodes. Only a small area of the skin of the heel is drained by the popliteal nodes (Fig. 12.106*A*).

*Lymphatics of the Trunk*

The skin of the anterior and posterior chest walls is drained by the axillary and supraclavicular nodes. The lymphatics of the lumbar region and of the anterior abdominal wall empty into the inguinal nodes (Fig. 12.106*B*).

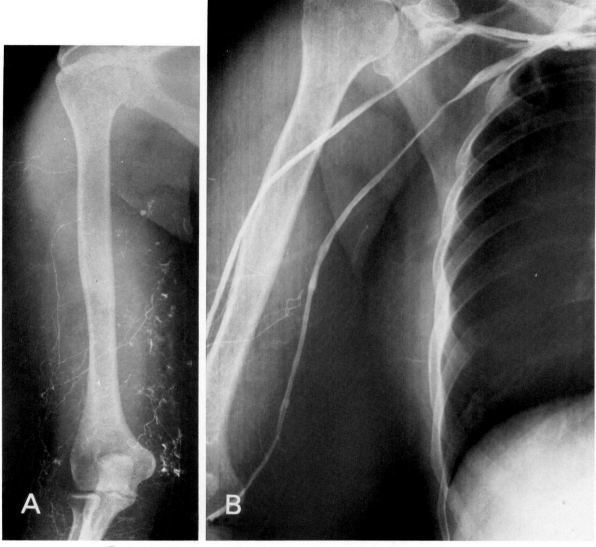

FIGURE 12.105. EDEMA—POSTMASTECTOMY AND POSTRADIATION THERAPY
*A:* Lymphatic obstruction. *B:* Extrinsic compression of axillary and cephalic veins.

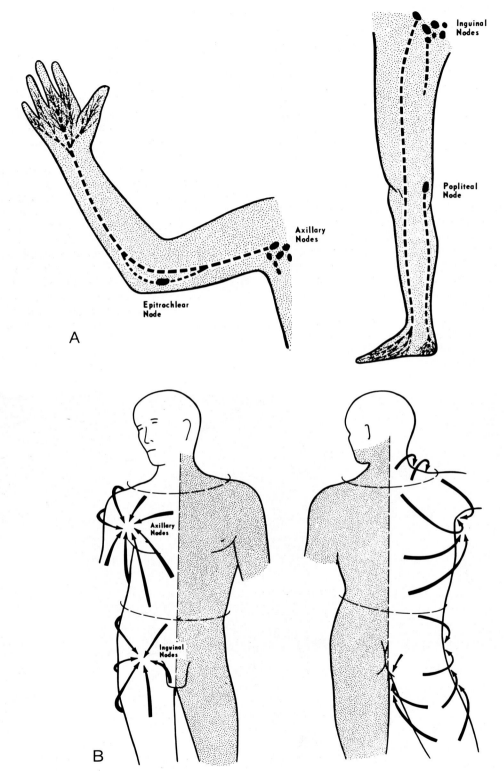

FIGURE 12.106. LYMPHATIC DRAINAGE OF THE SKIN
*A:* Lymphatics of the skin of the extremities. *B:* Lymphatics of the skin of the trunk.

## Carcinoma of the Skin

Carcinoma of the skin is one of the most frequent forms of cancer and is mostly squamous cell. Basal cell carcinoma is rare. Lymphatic spreading is practically unknown in basal cell carcinoma. Lymphatic metastasis does occur in about 10–20% of all cases of squamous cell carcinoma, but it usually occurs late. An example of squamous cell carcinoma of the hand, with axillary metastasis, is presented in the Figure 12.107.

## Malignant Melanoma of the Skin

Malignant melanoma is one of the most malignant tumors of the skin. It invades the blood and the lymphatics early and metastasizes widely. There is no tumor which disseminates more widely or involves more organs than malignant melanoma. It tends to enlarge the organs it invades; often its metastases are pigmented. The first metastasis is often seen in the skin around the periphery of the tumor, and regional lymph nodes are involved early. The tumor frequently spreads to organs not usually the site of metastases, such as the spleen and heart.

*LAG in Malignant Melanoma*

**Diagnosis of Lymph Node Metastasis.** The mechanism of metastasis to the lymph nodes from malignant melanoma is similar to that of carcinoma. In some cases, the metastases lodge at the periphery of the node as marginal filling defects and mimic those of metastatic carcinoma (Fig. 12.108). In other cases, there is enlargement of the node with rounded appearance and large central filling defects (Cox et al., 1966). The central position of the defects may be explained by the fact that the number of tumor emboli is particularly large. Few of the tumor cells deposit in the marginal sinuses, and most invade the inner structure of the node with formation of large central filling defects. The capsule of the node usually is well preserved, and there is little interference of the afferent lymph vessels. This change is not commonly seen in other types of metastases. The node sometimes becomes significantly enlarged with large central filling defects and puddling of the contrast medium at one place (Fig. 12.109).

The presence of the nodes not visualized by LAG because of complete replacement by tumor

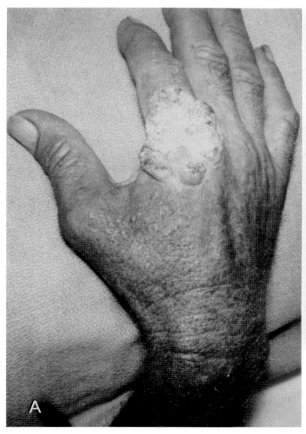

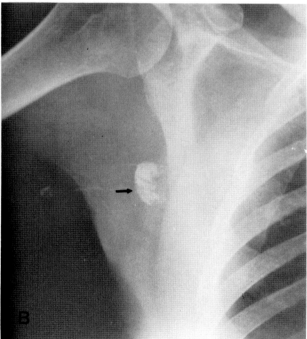

FIGURE 12.107. LYMPHANGIOGRAM SHOWING METASTATIC LESION IN THE RIGHT AXILLA FROM CARCINOMA OF THE RIGHT HAND
*A:* Photograph of the right hand showing carcinoma of the hand. *B:* Right upper limb lymphangiogram showing nodal metastasis in right axilla.

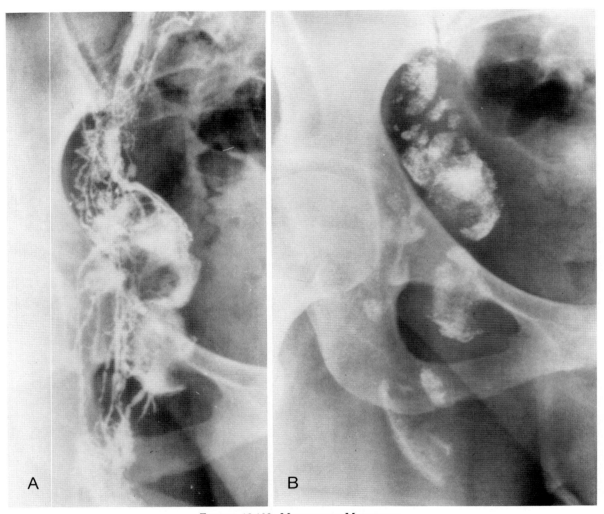

FIGURE 12.108. MALIGNANT MELANOMA

Lymphangiogram showing metastatic melanoma involving the right inguinal and external iliac nodes. The nodes are enlarged with filling defects. *A:* Vascular phase. *B:* Nodal phase.

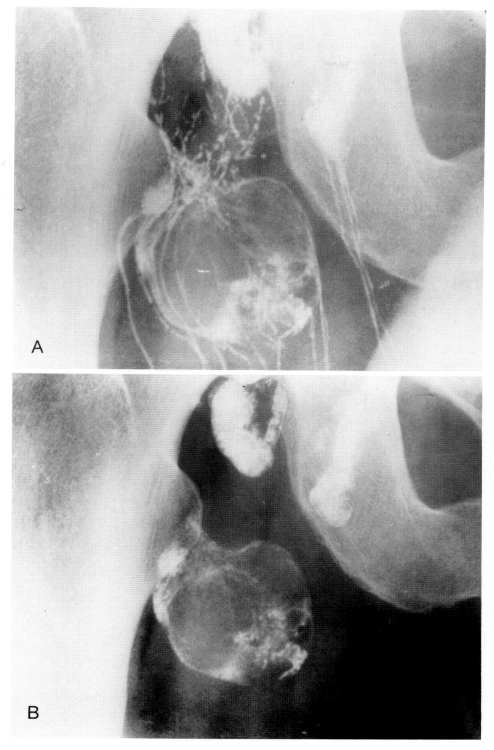

**FIGURE 12.109. MALIGNANT MELANOMA**
Lymphangiogram showing metastatic lesion in the right inguinal region. The node is significantly enlarged with a large spherical filling defect and puddling of contrast medium at one place. *A:* Vascular phase. *B:* Nodal phase.

can be inferred from secondary changes in the lymph vessels, as in carcinoma, or more accurately by CT. In advanced cases, when the most of lymph nodes are replaced by tumor cells, the lymph nodes may show marked disruption of the nodal architecture with irregular deposition of contrast medium in the nodal areas and beyond the normal pathway (Fig. 12.110).

**Detection of In-transit Metastasis.** In-transit metastases are deposits which have lodged in the superficial lymph channels between the primary tumor or its excision site and the regional lymph nodes. The precise mechanism whereby in-transit metastases are formed is unknown. They are seldom, if ever, found in association with any other type of cancer of the skin. Most investigators believe that aggregates of melanoma cells metastasize as emboli from primary lesions to the regional lymph nodes.

The principal contributing factor in the formation of the in-transit metastasis is lymphatic obstruction. In a patient with a normal lower extremity, the contrast medium passes quickly through the lymph vessels of the foot to the regional inguinal lymph nodes in an average time of 7 min. In the presence of enlarged metastatic nodes in the inguinal region, the lymphatic circulation time from foot to groin becomes more than 10 min (Stehlin et al., 1966). If the lymph channels become obstructed, lymph stasis ensues and may be manifested by the presence of lymphedema; however, stagnation of lymph flow can occur without resultant lymphedema. Lymph stasis facilitates the entrapment of melanoma emboli within the lumen of the lymph channels where they remain and grow. When the lymphatic collateral pathway is inadequate or not established in lymphatic obstruction, a reversal of lymph flow with development of dermal backflow occurs. This manifestation further enhances implantation of the melanoma emboli in a retrograde fashion within the skin and subcutaneous tissue via dermal backflow.

The lymphatic obstruction with stasis is most often produced by regional radical lymph node dissection. Figure 12.111 shows the lymphangio-

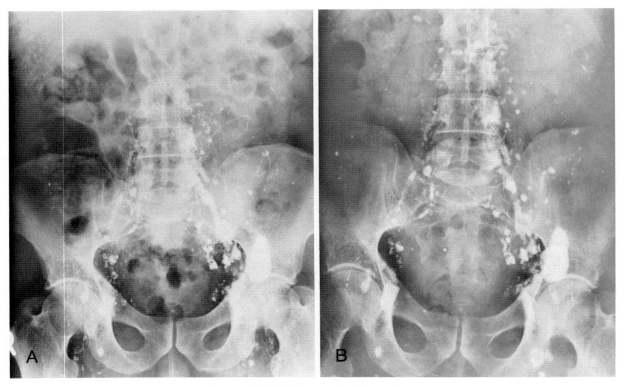

FIGURE 12.110. MALIGNANT MELANOMA

Lymphangiogram showing advanced metastatic melanoma in the pelvic and para-aortic areas with irregular deposition of contrast medium in nodal areas and extensive collateral lymph channels in pelvic and retroperitoneal areas. *A:* Vascular phase. *B:* Nodal phase.

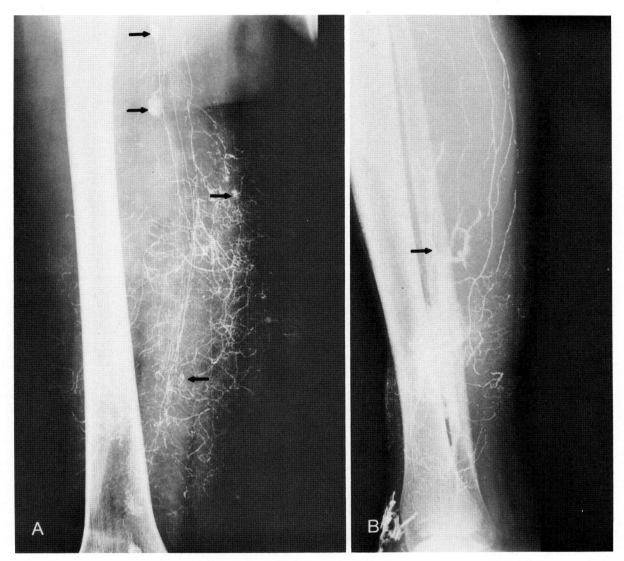

FIGURE 12.111. IN-TRANSIT METASTASES FOLLOWING RADICAL GROIN LYMPH NODE DISSECTION
*A* and *B:* Lymphangiogram demonstrating lymphatic obstruction in lower extremity following radical groin node dissection and extensive secondary lymphedema with collateral lymph channels and dermal backflow. *Arrows* in the thigh point to in-transit metastasis. Note extensive pooling of the dye in lower leg. Perivascular lymphatics in the leg are indicated by an *arrow*. *C* and *D:* Clinical photographs showing scar in the upper medial aspect of right thigh resulting from groin dissection. In-transit metastases are seen in the medial aspect of the thigh and proximal medial aspect of the leg. Lymphedema is present.

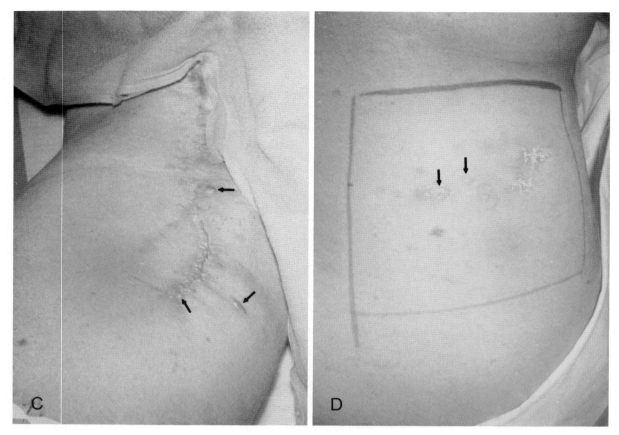

FIGURE 12.111C AND D.

gram of a patient with secondary lymphedema and in-transit metastasis following radical groin lymph node dissection. Partial lymphatic obstruction may or may not cause clinically obvious lymphedema or stasis; this depends upon the number of regional lymph nodes involved and the extent of replacement by metastasis as well as upon formation or function of the collateral lymph channels. This obstruction leads to a selective type of lymph stasis or partial obstruction. Figure 12.112 shows inguinal metastases associated with partial lymphatic obstruction and in-transit metastasis. An extensive vein stripping operation and wide deep excisional de-

fects in the region of the primary melanoma may produce partial obstruction in a local area. Figure 12.113 demonstrates in-transit metastasis in a patient with a deep and wide excisional defect from a vein stripping operation in the region of the primary melanoma.

*CT in Malignant Melanoma*

The findings of CT in nodal involvement in malignant melanoma are not as characteristic as that of LAG. However, it can delineate the extent of the lesion, particularly in the abdomen with extranodal involvement (Figs. 12.114 and 12.115).

## SARCOMAS OF THE SOFT TISSUE

Soft tissue sarcomas are a small and exclusive group of tumors of mesodermal origin (smooth muscle, striated muscle, fat, connective tissue, and blood vessel). Fibrosarcoma, liposarcoma, or malignant fibrohistiocytoma occur most fre-

quently. They appear at any site where the parent tissue is present. Other lesions include leiomyosarcoma, rhabdomyosarcoma, angiosarcoma (hemangioendothelioma, hemangiopericytoma, and Kaposi's sarcoma), and synovial sarcoma.

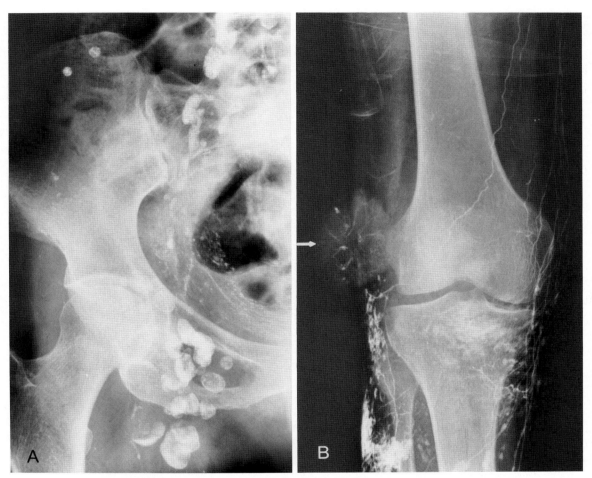

FIGURE 12.112. IN-TRANSIT METASTASES FOLLOWING PARTIAL LYMPHATIC OBSTRUCTION FROM INGUINAL NODE METASTASES

A–C: Lymphangiograms showing partial lymphatic obstruction produced by enlarged metastatic nodes in the right inguinal region and by primary melanoma on the lateral aspect of the right knee. The lymph channels are numerous and tortuous. Extensive pooling of the contrast medium below the knee is seen. Note the lymphatic pattern within the primary melanoma (B, arrow). There is no obvious lymphedema of the lower extremity. D: Clinical photograph showing large primary melanoma on the lateral aspect of the right knee and cutaneous and subcutaneous in-transit metastases in thigh and leg (arrows). There is no apparent lymphedema.

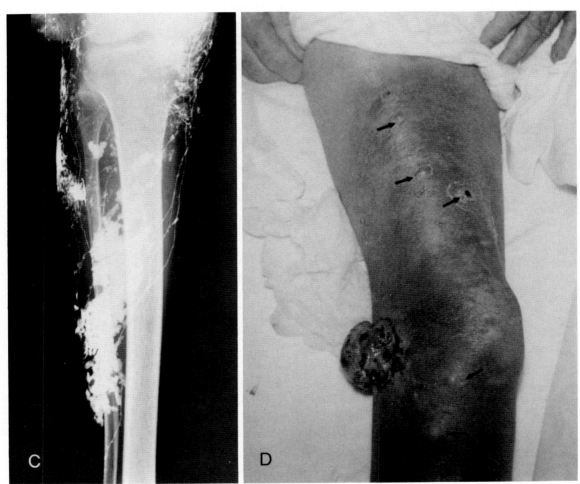

FIGURE 12.112*C* AND *D*.

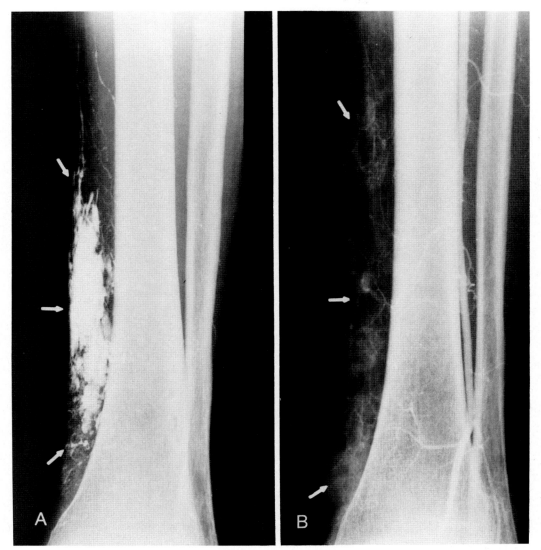

FIGURE 12.113. IN-TRANSIT METASTASES FOLLOWING PARTIAL LYMPHATIC OBSTRUCTION FROM VEIN STRIPPING OPERATION

*A:* Lymphangiogram demonstrating partial lymphatic obstruction produced by surgical defect from extensive vein stripping operation in the lower medial aspect of the leg. Dilatation of the lymph channels and pooling of the contrast medium are seen in the lower medial third of the leg corresponding to the location of in-transit metastasis. Lymph channels proximal to this region are relatively normal. *B:* Arteriogram showing abnormal vessels in the region of in-transit metastasis. *C:* Clinical photograph showing cutaneous and subcutaneous in-transit metastasis in the medial aspect of the leg (*1*). Visible scar from extensive vein stripping operation (*2*). No lymphedema. Primary melanoma on sole of foot.

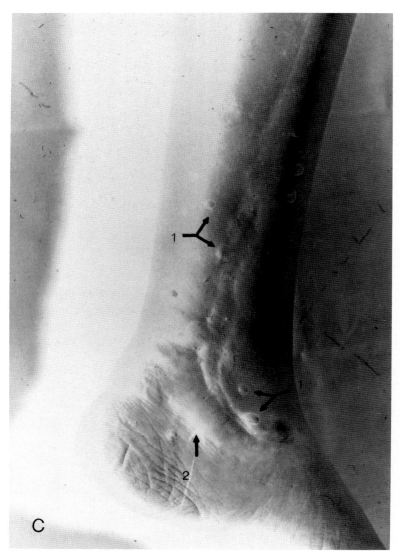

FIGURE 12.113C.

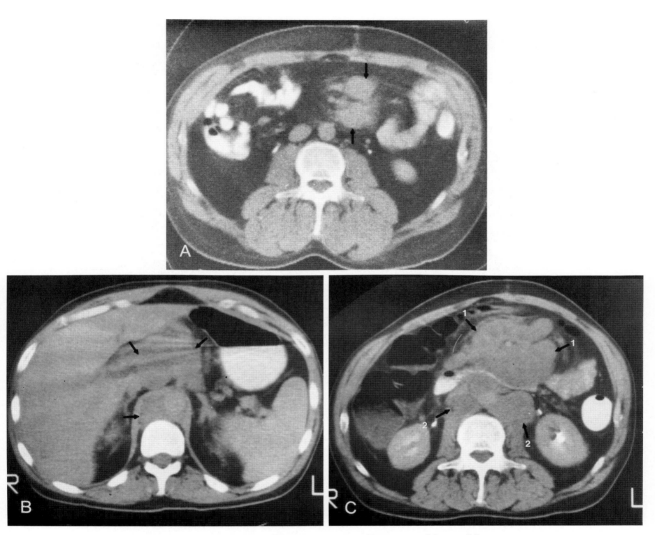

FIGURE 12.114. MALIGNANT MELANOMA WITH EXTENSIVE NODAL METASTASES
*A:* CT of the abdomen. Two small mesenteric lymph nodes are seen in the middle abdomen just to the left of midline (*arrows*). CT guided biopsy of mass was positive for malignant melanoma. *B:* CT of the upper abdomen (6 months later). There is rapid progression of the lesion with retrocrural and celiac nodal metastases (*1* and *2*). *C:* CT of the lower abdomen (6 months later). There are extensive mesenteric metastases (*1*) and periaortic lymphadenopathy (*2*).

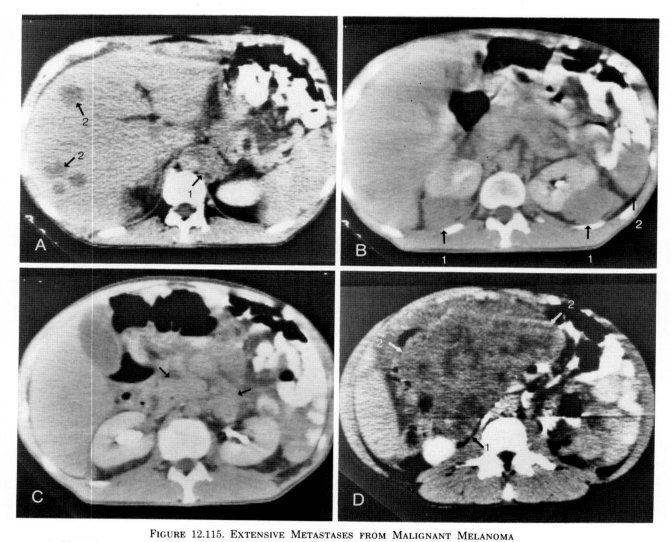

FIGURE 12.115. EXTENSIVE METASTASES FROM MALIGNANT MELANOMA
*A:* CT of the upper abdomen. Retrocrural and liver metastases (*1* and *2*). *B:* CT of the upper abdomen, 2 cm inferior to *A.*
Retrorenal mass (*1*) and mass in left side of the abdomen with anterior displacement of the small intestine (*2*). *C:* CT of the
middle abdomen. Nodal metastases in periaortic areas (*arrows*). *D:* CT of the lower abdomen. Right para-aortic and mesenteric
metastases with areas of necrosis (*1* and *2*).

## Lymphatic Drainage of the Soft Tissue

The soft tissue of the upper extremity is drained by the deep lymph vessels which follow the main neurovascular bundles (radial, ulnar, interosseous, and brachial). They are less numerous than the superficial lymph vessels with which they communicate at intervals. Along their course a few lymph nodes occur. Most deep lymph vessels terminate in the lateral group and sometimes in the central group of the axillary nodes.

The soft tissue of the lower extremity is drained by the deep lymphatics which accompany the main blood vessels of the extremity and so comprise anterior tibial, posterior tibial, peroneal, popliteal, and femoral sets. The deep lymph vessels of the foot and leg are interrupted by the popliteal nodes, but those from the thigh pass directly to the deep inguinal nodes. The efferent vessels of the popliteal nodes follow the route of the femoral vessels to the deep inguinal nodes almost entirely, but a few may accompany the great saphenous vein and end in the superficial inguinal nodes.

## Lymph Node Metastasis

All of the soft tissue sarcomas tend to appear pseudoencapsulated, spread locally, and have a decided tendency to recur. They have certain common characteristics in their metastases which are very frequently carried by hematogenous routes to the lungs, liver, and various other organs. Metastases to regional lymph nodes are uncommon in fibrosarcomas and liposarcomas but may be encountered in about half of the patients with rhabdomyosarcomas and synovial, clear cell, and epithelioid sarcomas (del Regato and Spjut, 1977). Kaposi's sarcoma is a neoplasm that commonly causes multiple nodular or plaque-like hemorrhagic skin lesions. They are usually located on the extremities but may occur anywhere on the skin or mucous membranes. Lymphatic and other visceral involvement is common. The disease is common among African blacks and individuals of Mediterranean origin. Recently the relationship between male homosexuals and the development of Kaposi's sarcoma has been documented (Hymes et al., 1981).

Tallroth (1976) investigated the incidence of lymph node metastases by lymphography in 71 patients with soft tissue sarcomas. There was a marked difference in the incidence of recurrences and metastases as well as in the tendency to disseminate through the lymphatics (Table 12.20). The soft tissue sarcomas differ in their propensity to spread in accordance with the degree of malignancy of the tumor. A total of 24 of 71 soft tissue sarcomas (33.8%) had lymphatic dissemination to the regional lymph nodes, and in 8 of these (3 rhabdomyosarcoma, 2 synovial, and 3 neurogenic sarcoma), there was further spread to distant lymph nodes (11.2%). The tendency to metastasize first via the lymphatics or via the blood vessels is variable. The time relation between lymphatic and hematogenous dissemination is shown in Table 12.21.

TABLE 12.21.
TIME RELATION BETWEEN LYMPHATIC AND HEMATOGENIC DISSEMINATION IN 40 PATIENTS WITH SOFT TISSUE CARCINOMA AND METASTASES*

| Diagnosis | No. of Cases | Lymphatic Dissemination before Hematogenic | Hematogenic Dissemination before Lymphatic |
|---|---|---|---|
| Fibrosarcoma | 9 | | 9 |
| Liposarcoma | 2 | | 2 |
| Leiomyosarcoma | 2 | 1 | 1 |
| Rhabdomyosarcoma | 8 | 6 | 2 |
| Synovial sarcoma | 5 | 4 | 1 |
| Neurogenic sarcoma | 9 | 6 | 3 |
| Miscellaneous sarcomas | 5 | 3 | 2 |
| Total | 40 | 20 | 20 |

* From Tallroth (1976).

TABLE 12.20.
INCIDENCE OF RECURRENCE, METASTASIS, AND LYMPHATIC DISSEMINATION IN 71 PATIENTS WITH SOFT TISSUE SARCOMAS*

| Diagnosis | No. of Cases | Recurrence or metastasis | Metastasis | Lymphatic Dissemination | First Metastasis In Lymphatics |
|---|---|---|---|---|---|
| Fibrosarcoma | 19 | 15 | 9 | | |
| Liposarcoma | 10 | 5 | 2 | | |
| Leiomyosarcoma | 5 | 3 | 2 | 2 | 1 |
| Rhabdomyosarcoma | 9 | 8 | 8 | 8 | 6 |
| Synovial sarcoma | 7 | 5 | 5 | 4 | 2 |
| Neurogenic sarcoma | 12 | 9 | 9 | 7 | 4 |
| Miscellaneous sarcomas | 9 | 5 | 5 | 3 | 2 |
| Total | 71 | 48 | 40 | 24 | 15 |

* From Tallroth (1976).

The lymphangiographic patterns of the soft tissue sarcomas have no specific features. In rhabdomyosarcoma the appearance may mimic malignant lymphoma. In general, the findings are similar to that of carcinoma, ranging from nodal filling defects with lymphatic stasis through complete replacement of the node by tumor with development of collateral lymphatic channels. This is illustrated by a patient with fibrosarcoma of the knee with metastasis to the inguinal lymph node (Fig. 12.116) and another patient with liposarcoma of the leg with pelvic nodal metastases (Fig. 12.117). Figure 12.118 shows a case of synovial sarcoma of the left thigh with metastasis to the left external iliac node, which is well shown on CT image. Figures 12.119 and 12.120 illustrate lymphangiographic findings in two homosexual males.

## MALIGNANT TUMORS OF BONE

### Lymphatic Drainage of Bone

The lymphatics of the bones of the upper and lower extremities leave by the nutrient foramina, traverse the periosteum, and empty into the nearby deep collecting trunks. They finally drain into the axillary nodes in the upper extremity and into the inguinal nodes in the lower extremity. The lymphatics of the periosteum of the upper end of the tibia usually terminate in the popliteal nodes; however, some of the lymphatics which originate from the medial aspect of the upper end of the tibia empty into the superficial inguinal lymph nodes.

### Malignant Tumors of Bone

Metastases from malignant bone tumors vary with the type of tumors. In sarcomas of the bone, Ewing's sarcoma metastasizes early and widely. Its spread by the blood stream is common. Lymph node metastasis also occurs and has a high incidence of distant dissemination. Osteogenic sarcoma primarily spreads by the blood stream and metastasizes most often to the lungs. About 5% may metastasize to regional lymph nodes. The lymph node involvement is a sign of late metastasizing. Chondrosarcoma very characteristically grows into the large veins with

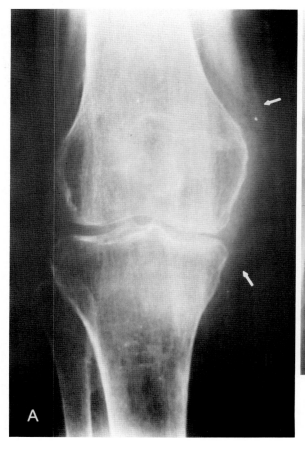

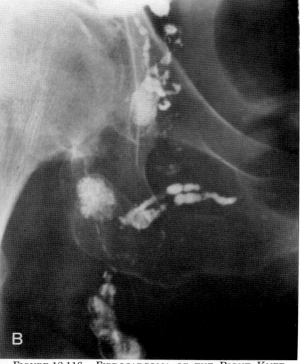

FIGURE 12.116.   FIBROSARCOMA OF THE RIGHT KNEE
*A:* Roentgenogram of the right knee showing a large soft tissue mass in the anteromedial aspect of the right knee. *B:* Lymphangiogram demonstrating metastatic lesion involving the right superficial and deep inguinal nodes.

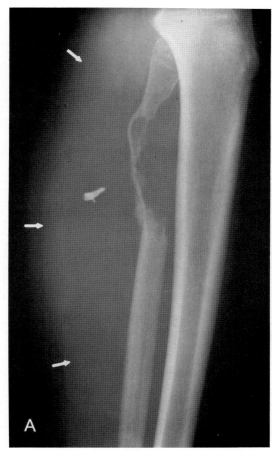

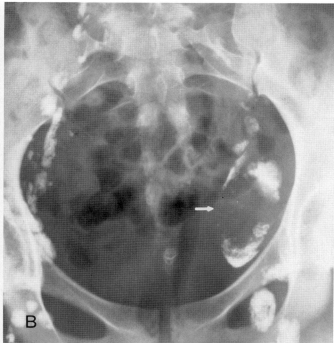

FIGURE 12.117. LIPOSARCOMA OF LEFT LEG WITH NODAL
METASTASIS

*A:* Roentgenogram of left leg shows a soft tissue mass of considerable size in the posterior aspect of the upper two-thirds of the left
leg (*arrows*). There is an osteolytic lesion involving the proximal
fibula due to secondary invasion. *B:* Lymphangiogram shows a
metastatic lesion with a large filling defect in the left external iliac
region (*arrow*).

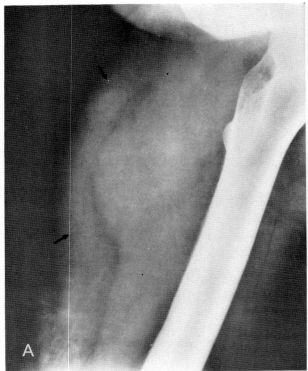

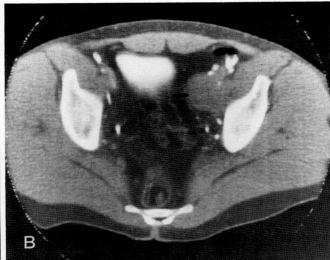

FIGURE 12.118. NODAL METASTASIS FROM SYNOVIAL SARCOMA

*A:* Roentgenogram of the left femur shows a soft tissue mass in the medial aspect of the proximal part of the left thigh with loss of fat plane and extension to the subcutaneous tissue (*arrows*). There is no evidence of bony invasion. *B:* CT of the pelvis shows a nonopacified metastatic lesion involving the left external iliac node (*arrow*). There are opacified lymph nodes from lymphangiogram in external iliac regions on both sides.

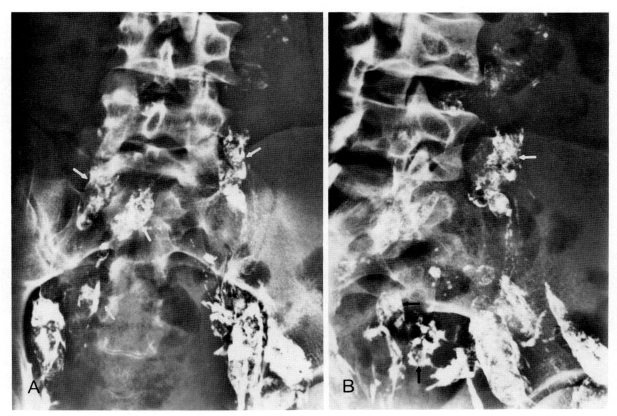

FIGURE 12.119. KAPOSI'S SARCOMA
*A:* Anteroposterior view of nodal phase of LAG demonstrates enlarged nodes with multiple filling defects in the external iliac and common iliac regions on both sides (*arrows*). There is poor opacification of the nodes in para-aortic areas. *B:* Left oblique view of nodal phase of LAG. Abnormal nodes with filling defects are shown to good advantage (*arrows*).

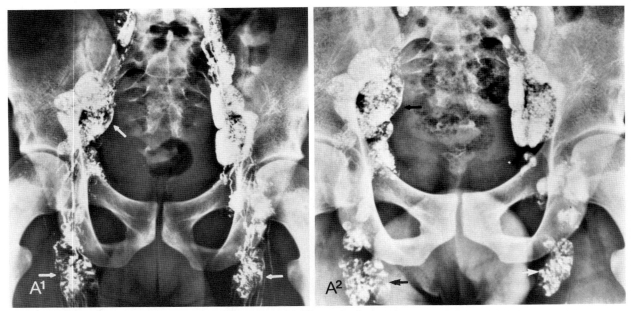

FIGURE 12.120. KAPOSI'S SARCOMA

*A:* Pelvic region. *A1:* Lymphatic phase. Enlarged nodes with irregular distribution of the contrast medium within the nodes in the inguinal and right external iliac regions (*arrows*). *A2:* Nodal phase. Enlarged nodes with multiple filling defects in the inguinal and right external iliac regions (*arrows*). *B:* Pelvic and abdominal region. *B1:* Right oblique view of lymphatic phase. Enlarged nodes with irregular distribution of contrast medium within the nodes in the external iliac and common iliac region (*arrows*). *B2:* Right oblique view of nodal phase. Enlarged nodes with filling defects in the external iliac and common iliac region. Biopsy of the right inguinal nodes yielded microscopic findings consistent with Kaposi's sarcoma.

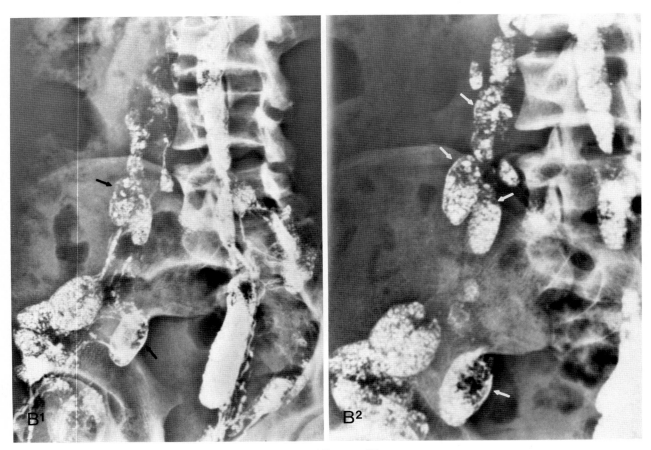

FIGURE 12.120*B1* AND *B2.*

metastasis to the lungs and occasionally to other organs and only rarely metastasizes to regional lymph nodes. Malignant fibrous histiocytomas have a tendency to metastasize to the lungs by a hematogenous route. Lymph node involvement may occur in advanced cases. Multiple myeloma invariably is discovered only after it has spread to many bones. Later in the course of the disease, lymph nodes, spleen, liver, and other organs may be involved. Pulmonary metastasis is rare. Occasionally, in some instances of malignant tumor of the bone, the lymph nodes become involved by direct extension from the neighboring bone lesion (del Regato and Spjut, 1977).

Tallroth (1976) evaluated the incidence of recurrence, metastasis, and lymph node dissemination by lymphography in 56 patients with bone sarcomas (Table 12.22). Of all of the 56 bone sarcomas, 16 (28.6%) had lymph node metastases; 13 were to regional lymph nodes (5 osteosarcoma, 1 chondrosarcoma, 3 Ewing's sarcoma, and 4 reticulosarcoma), 8 to distant nodes (5 osteosarcoma, 1 Ewing's sarcoma, and 2 reticulosarcoma), and 5 to both (3 osteosarcoma and 2 reticulosarcoma). The time relation between lymphatic and hematogenous dissemination varies, and early lymphatic dissemination occurs (Table 12.23).

Lymphangiographic findings in malignant tumors of the bone are generally similar to those of carcinoma (Figs. 12.121–12.123). Multiple myeloma invading the lymph nodes is rare. In the early case, the findings are small, irregularly distributed filling defects in the involved nodes. Figure 12.124 shows an advanced multiple myeloma with extensive involvement of the lymph nodes in the pelvic and para-aortic areas. CT is of value to delineate the extent of the lesion and the involvement of other structures (Fig. 12.125).

## Malignant Lymphoma of Bone

In generalized malignant lymphoma, the bones usually become involved either by direct extension from the affected neighboring lymph nodes or by metastatic spread through the blood stream. Direct invasion of the bone most likely occurs in areas where the bones stand close by the affected chains of the lymph nodes. These areas are the vertebral bodies, vertebral ends of the ribs, sternum, and ilium along its crest and near the sacroiliac joint (Fig. 12.126). Metastasis by way of the blood stream results in scattered seeding of the marrow of various bones with lymphomatous tissue. In some instances of generalized malignant lymphoma, attention is first called to the complaints arising from the skeletal lesion. This happens most often in connection with Hodgkin's disease. As a rule, in such cases, the skeletal complaints merely happen to occupy the foreground of the clinical picture. A study of the patients invariably reveals generalized lymphoma with indubitable involvement of the lymph nodes. Such cases do not represent instances of primary lymphoma of the bone since the skeletal involvement is secondary to that of the lymphatic system.

Primary lymphoma of the bone is meant to refer to cases in which a lymphoma starts in a bone. While it is true that any of the malignant lymphomas may appear primarily in the bone, by abundant experience the occurrence of primary lymphoma of the bone has been established only in connection with reticulum cell sarcoma (histiocytic lymphoma). The course pursued by

TABLE 12.23.
TIME RELATION BETWEEN LYMPHATIC AND HEMATOGENIC DISSEMINATION IN 28 PATIENTS WITH BONE SARCOMAS AND METASTASES*

| Diagnosis | No. of Cases | Lymphatic Dissemination before Hematogenic | Hematogenic Dissemination before Lymphatic |
|---|---|---|---|
| Osteosarcoma | 15 | | 15 |
| Chondrosarcoma | 1 | 1 | |
| Ewing's sarcoma | 8 | 4 | 4 |
| Reticulosarcoma | 4 | 2 | 2 |
| Total | 28 | 7 | 21 |

* From Tallroth (1976).

TABLE 12.22.
INCIDENCE OF RECURRENCE, METASTASIS, AND LYMPHATIC DISSEMINATION IN 56 PATIENTS WITH BONE SARCOMAS*

| Diagnosis | No. of Cases | Recurrence or Metastasis | Metastasis | Lymphatic Dissemination | First Metastasis in Lymphatics |
|---|---|---|---|---|---|
| Osteosarcoma | 17 | 15 | 15 | 7 | – |
| Chondrosarcoma | 21 | 5 | 1 | 1 | 1 |
| Ewing's sarcoma | 9 | 8 | 8 | 4 | 4 |
| Reticulosarcoma | 4 | 4 | 4 | 4 | 2 |
| Total | 56 | 30 | 28 | 16 | 7 |

* Modified from Tallroth (1976).

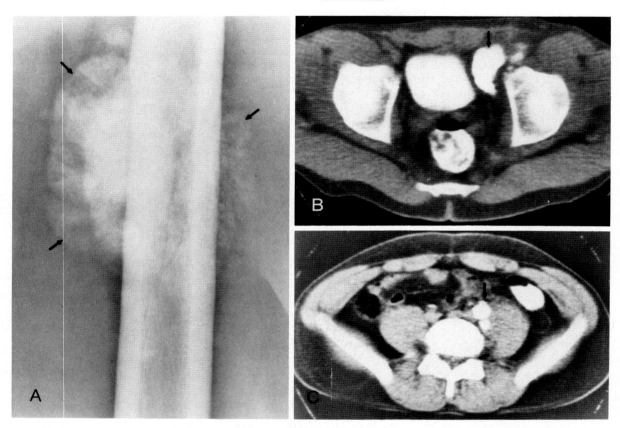

FIGURE 12.121. OSTEOSARCOMA OF THE LEFT FEMUR WITH INGUINAL AND ILIAC NODAL METASTASES
*A:* Roentgenogram of left femur. Cortical osteosarcoma of the midportion of the left femur (*arrows*). *B:* CT scan at the level of the external iliac region. Calcified and ossified nodal metastases in left inguinal region (*arrow*). *C:* CT scan at the level of L5. Calcified and ossified metastases in the nodes in left common iliac region (*arrow*).

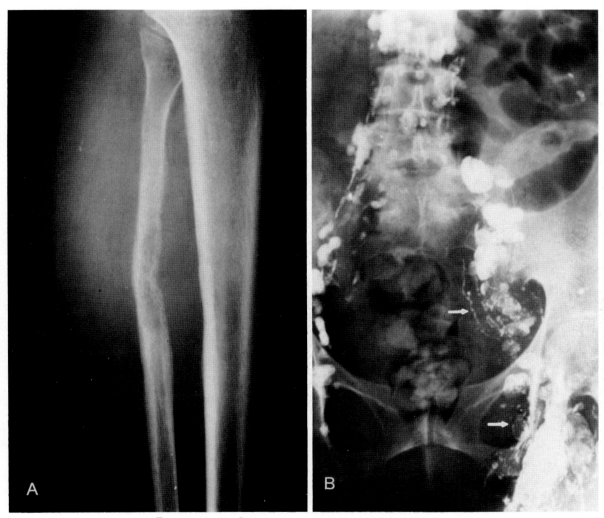

FIGURE 12.122. CHONDROSARCOMA OF THE LEFT FIBULA
*A:* Roentgenogram of the left leg showing destructive lesion involving the proximal fibula. *B:* Lymphangiogram demonstrating metastatic lesion involving the left inguinal and external iliac nodes (*arrows*).

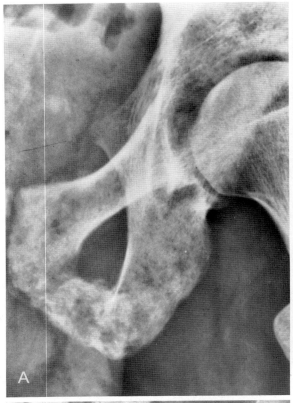

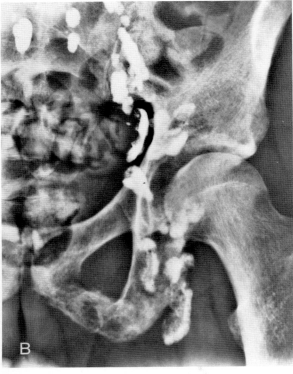

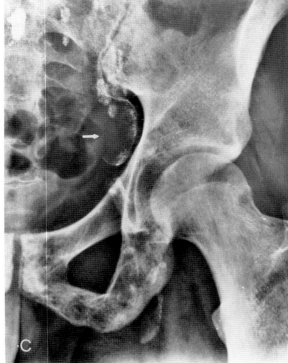

FIGURE 12.123.  NODAL METASTASIS FROM EWING'S
SARCOMA

*A:* Roentgenogram of the pelvis. Mixed osteolytic and
osteoblastic lesion involving left ischium and pubic ramus.
*B:* LAG (initial examination). No definite evidence of
nodal metastasis in the pelvic region. *C:* LAG (4 months
later). Metastatic lesion involving left external iliac node
with large filling defect (*arrow*).

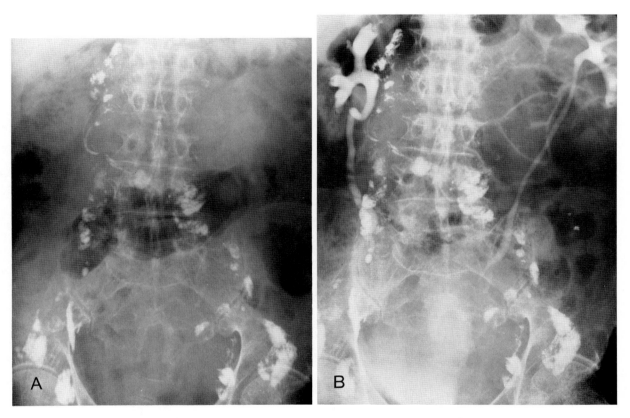

FIGURE 12.124. MULTIPLE MYELOMA WITH INVOLVEMENT OF THE LYMPH NODES
*A:* LAG. Extensive nodal involvement in right para-aortic and proximal common regions and left external iliac and common iliac areas. There is a large nonopacified soft tissue mass in the left para-aortic. *B:* Intravenous pyelogram. There is marked lateral displacement of the left kidney and abdominal segment of the ureter. Slight lateral displacement of the abdominal segment of the right ureter is also noted. Aspiration biopsy was performed under fluoroscopy. The histopathological diagnosis was myeloma.

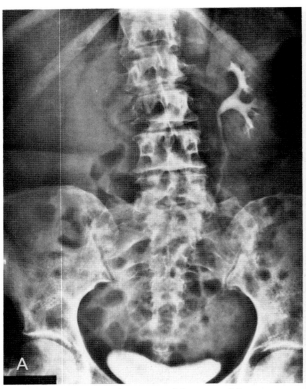

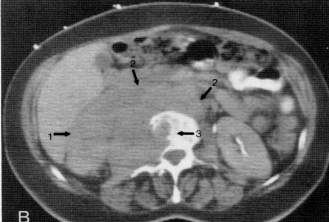

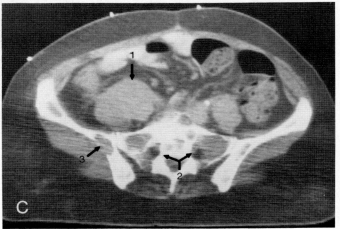

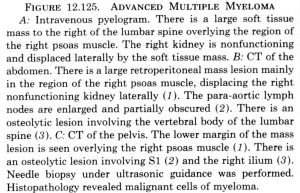

FIGURE 12.125. ADVANCED MULTIPLE MYELOMA
*A:* Intravenous pyelogram. There is a large soft tissue
mass to the right of the lumbar spine overlying the region of
the right psoas muscle. The right kidney is nonfunctioning
and displaced laterally by the soft tissue mass. *B:* CT of the
abdomen. There is a large retroperitoneal mass lesion mainly
in the region of the right psoas muscle, displacing the right
nonfunctioning kidney laterally (*1*). The para-aortic lymph
nodes are enlarged and partially obscured (*2*). There is an
osteolytic lesion involving the vertebral body of the lumbar
spine (*3*). *C:* CT of the pelvis. The lower margin of the mass
lesion is seen overlying the right psoas muscle (*1*). There is
an osteolytic lesion involving S1 (*2*) and the right ilium (*3*).
Needle biopsy under ultrasonic guidance was performed.
Histopathology revealed malignant cells of myeloma.

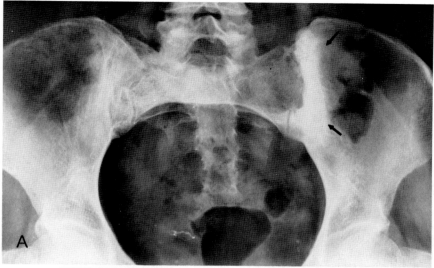

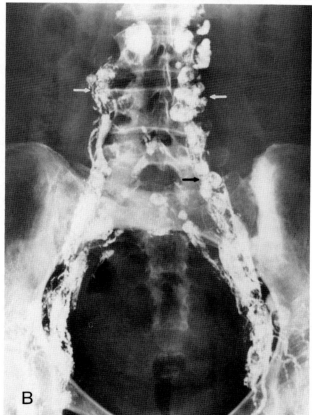

FIGURE 12.126. HODGKIN'S DISEASE OF THE LEFT ILIUM
*A:* Roentgenogram of the pelvis showing osteoblastic lesion involving the medial aspect of the left ilium (*arrows*). *B:* Lymphangiogram demonstrating extensive nodal lesion in the common iliac and para-aortic areas.

reticulum cell sarcomas of the bone is variable. In some cases, the lesion may remain localized to the affected bone without involvement of the regional lymph nodes. In others, the lesion may still show a tendency to remain localized, but it does spread to the regional lymph nodes (Fig. 12.127). In still other cases, reticulum cell sarcoma of bone may heal after radiation therapy,

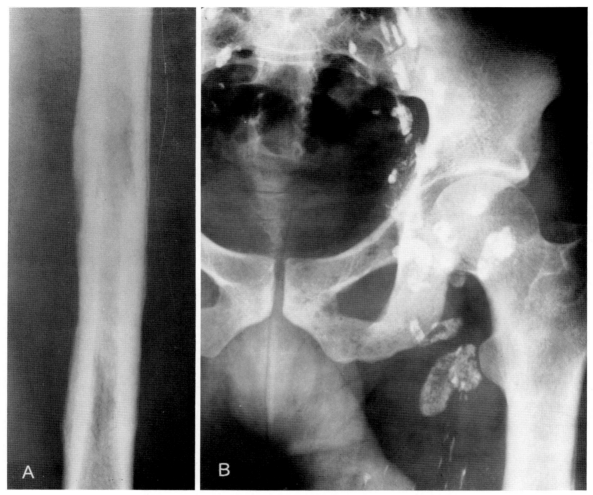

FIGURE 12.127. RETICULUM CELL SARCOMA OF THE LEFT FEMUR

*A:* Roentgenogram of the left femur showing destructive lesion involving the proximal part of the left femur. *B:* Lymphangiogram demonstrating lymphomatous lesion involving the nodes in the left inguinal and distal external iliac regions. There is osteolytic lesion in the inferior ramus of the left pubis and ischium.

but some years later the patient may develop similar lesions in other bones. Even though some lymph nodes may also be involved, the disease remains one which centers in the skeleton. Finally, one may encounter cases in which reticulum cell sarcoma presents as a primary lesion of the bone and even yields to radiation therapy, but the disease eventually becomes generalized with involvement of the lymph nodes. Such dissemination may appear within a year or two after the presenting bone lesion has been discovered, or it may occur years later.

## Lymphangiomatosis of Bone

Lymphangiomatosis of the bone is a rare disease entity. The pathogenesis of the disease is poorly understood. Various etiologies have been suggested, and a congenital malformation is the most likely cause. The bone changes are radiolucent in nature and usually finely etched by a thin sclerotic margin. A portion of the lesion may be quite ill defined; however, the lesions affect both the cortex and the spongiosa of the medullary cavity and are widespread in distribution. The medullary lesion may be quite large with mild expansion of the bone and thinning of the cortex. The skull, flat bones, and ribs, as well as the long bones, are usually involved. Bone defects have been noted less frequently in the spine and scapula. The small bones of the extremities have been spared. Characteristically, the radiolucent areas in the bone apparently result from pressure atrophy from ectatic endothelium-lined channels of the lymphatic tissue. Microscopic differentiation of the lesion from hemangiomatosis is difficult and often impossible.

The condition is usually discovered during childhood or adolescence, either accidentally or because of a pathological fracture. Most reported cases are in the 10–15-yr age group, although a few are seen in early childhood.

The diagnosis can be made radiographically without the need for biopsy. The radiographic features are as follows: (*a*) There is widespread osteolytic lesion of the bone, occasionally with pathological fracture. The lesion affects both the cortex and the spongiosa of the involved bone.

(*b*) The lesion is avascular. (*c*) There is usually soft tissue swelling, without venous involvement, due to soft tissue lymphangiomas and lymphatic stasis.

The pertinent lymphangiographic findings are stasis and collateral circulation with complete or partial lymphatic obstruction. There is a paucity of normal lymph nodes in the involved areas with multiple large dilated lymphatic plexus within the associated soft tissues. Contrast medium can be seen within the bone lesions for many months (Fig. 12.128).

## MISCELLANEOUS CONDITIONS

### Carcinoma of the Nasopharynx

Regional metastatic lymphadenopathy is usually present with every malignant tumor of the nasopharynx. In advanced carcinoma of the nasopharynx, distant nodal metastasis may involve the retroperitoneal lymph nodes (Fig. 12.129).

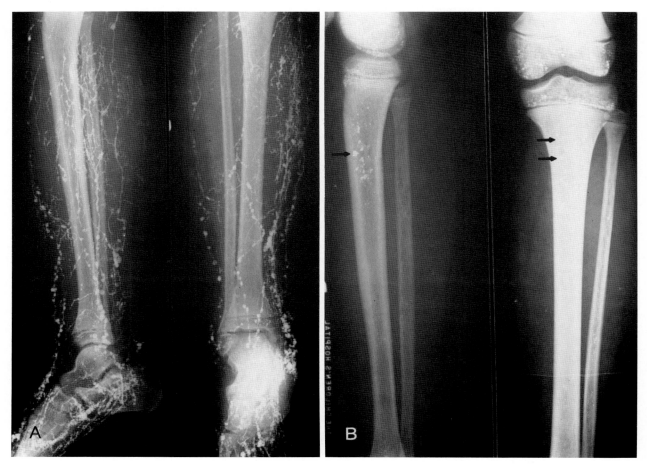

FIGURE 12.128. LYMPHANGIOMATOSIS
Lymphangiomatosis in a child with lower extremity edema. *A:* Lymphatic phase. Numerous dilated tortuous lymphatics in the involved leg. *B:* Nodal phase. Opacification of the lacunae in the bone (*arrows*) suggests communication with skeletal lymphatics.

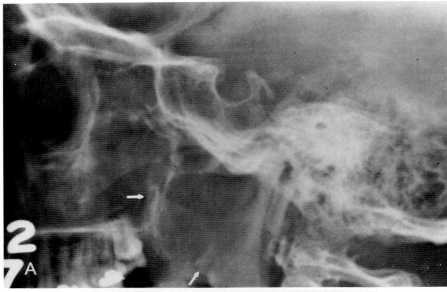

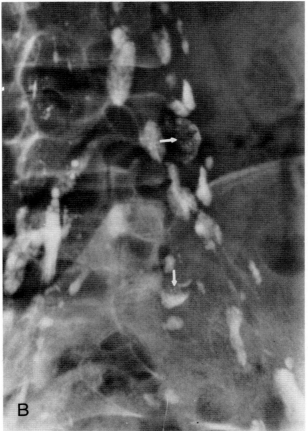

FIGURE 12.129. LYMPHOEPITHELIOMA OF THE NASOPHARYNX WITH NODAL METASTASES TO THE RETROPERITONEAL AREA

*A:* Lateral soft tissue roentgenogram of the nasopharynx. A large soft tissue mass occupies almost the entire nasopharynx (*arrows*). There is no evidence of regional bony destruction. *B:* LAG. Metastatic lesion in the lymph nodes in the left lower para-aortic and common iliac regions (*arrows*).

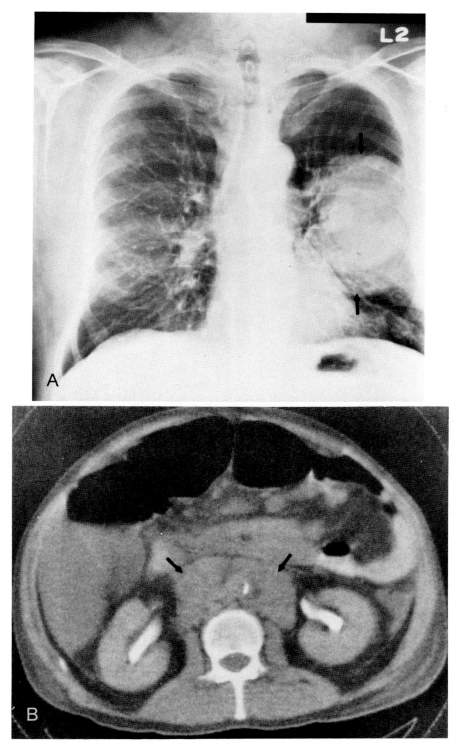

FIGURE 12.130. ADENOCARCINOMA OF THE LUNG WITH RETROPERITONEAL NODAL METASTASIS
*A:* Chest roentgenogram showing a large soft tissue mass in left middle lung field (*arrows*). *B:* CT of the abdomen revealing extensive periaortic lymphadenopathy surrounding the aorta and vena cava (*arrows*).

## Carcinoma of the Lung

The lymphatics of the lungs form a rich net-work. The superficial lymphatics of the visceral pleura and the deep lymphatics accompanying the bronchi and pulmonary veins are the most important. Lymphatic spread of carcinoma of the lung is the most common, and the hilar, mediastinal, and paratracheal lymph nodes almost always are involved. The disease can travel via the lymphatics through the diaphragm and involves the retroperitoneal lymph nodes in the region of the kidney and along the aorta (Rouviere, 1938) (Figs. 12.130 and 12.131).

## Carcinoma of the Esophagus

The lymph-capillary networks of the mucosa and the muscular layers of the esophagus gather on the external surface in three groups of col-

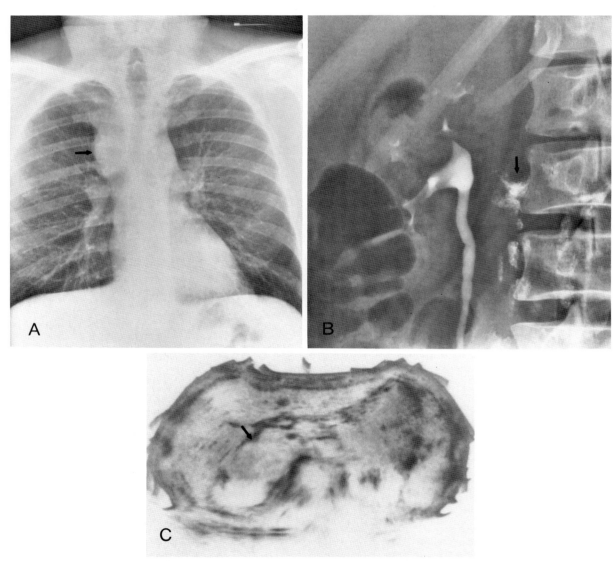

FIGURE 12.131. ADENOCARCINOMA OF THE LUNG WITH METASTASES TO PARA-AORTIC LYMPH NODES AND ADRENAL GLAND

*A:* Posteroanterior chest roentgenogram. A tumor mass is in the right superior mediastinum (*arrow*). *B:* Intravenous pyelogram (3 months after LAG). There is a nodal metastasis with crescent filling defect in right para-aortic area (*arrow*). *C:* Transverse ultrasonogram of the upper abdomen. Enlargement of the right adrenal with posterior and lateral displacement of the right kidney is due to metastasis (*arrow*).

lecting trunks: (*a*) the upper trunks, which end in the cervical lymph node along the internal jugular vein and in the supraclavicular lymph nodes; (*b*) the middle trunks, which end in the posterior mediastinal lymph nodes and in the retrotracheal lymph nodes; and (*c*) the lower trunks, which drain to the abdominal lymph nodes, especially those of the cardia and of the lesser curvature of the stomach. The lymphatic vessels from any one segment of the esophagus may drain directly into the closest node or empty into nodes at considerable distance, either above or below the lesion (Rouvière, 1938).

The route of lymph node metastasis in carcinoma of the esophagus varies with the location of the lesion. In carcinoma of the upper third of the esophagus, lymphatic spread may involve lymph nodes of the lower jugular chain or of the supraclavicular group. Tumor of the middle third of the esophagus may metastasize to the mediastinum and to the abdominal lymph nodes. Tumors of the lower third of the esophagus usually metastasize predominantly to the abdominal

nodes, including para-aortic nodes (Dormanns, 1939).

Routine upper gastrointestinal examination occasionally may demonstrate evidence of abdominal metastasis (Fig. 12.132). However, CT is the most efficient modality and the method of choice for evaluation of the intra-abdominal metastases to the lymph nodes, liver, and adrenal gland (Daffner et al., 1979) (Fig. 12.133).

**Neuroblastoma**

This sarcoma of nervous system origin is composed chiefly of neuroblasts and affects mostly infants and children up to 10 yr of age. Most such tumors arise in the autonomic nervous system or in the adrenal medulla. It occasionally metastasizes to the lymph nodes.

The lymphangiographic appearance either is similar to that of carcinoma or mimics lymphocytic lymphoma (Fig. 12.134). CT is of value to delineate the extent of nodal lesion and the involvement of extranodal structures (Fig. 12.135).

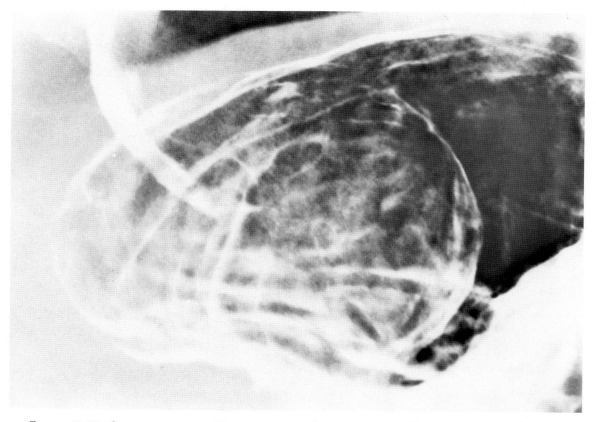

FIGURE 12.132. CARCINOMA OF THE ESOPHAGUS WITH INTRA-ABDOMINAL METASTASIS TO THE STOMACH
Spot film of fundus of the stomach. There is a large submucosal metastasis involving the fundus of the stomach in a patient with treated squamous carcinoma of the midthoracic esophagus.

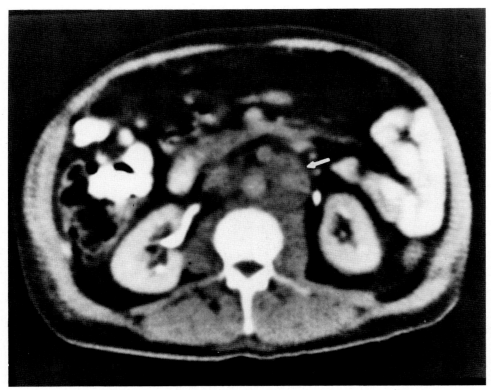

FIGURE 12.133. CARCINOMA OF THE ESOPHAGUS WITH METASTASIS TO THE PARA-AORTIC LYMPH NODES
CT of the abdomen. Metastatic lymphadenopathy is noted in the left para-aortic area from a patient with carcinoma of the distal esophagus.

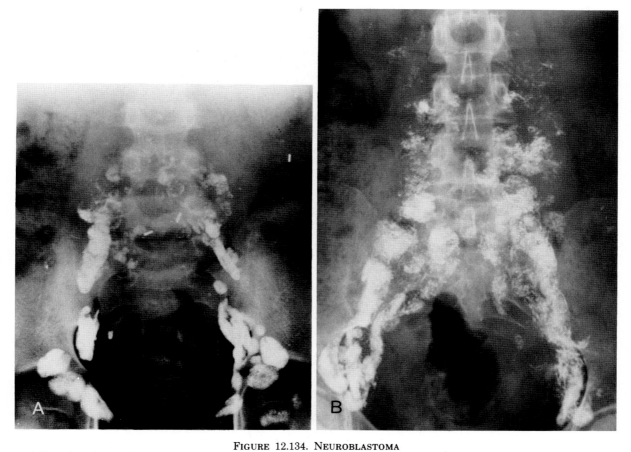

FIGURE 12.134. NEUROBLASTOMA

*A:* Lymphangiogram showing extensive metastatic lesion simulating carcinoma involving the common iliac and para-aortic nodes on both sides. *B:* Lymphangiogram showing extensive metastatic lesion mimicking malignant lymphoma in the pelvic and para-aortic areas.

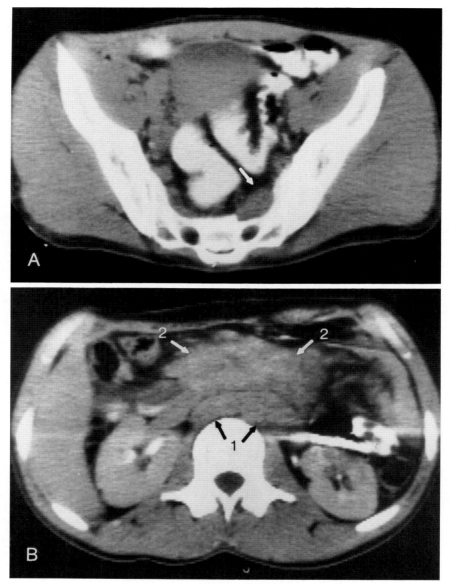

FIGURE 12.135. NODAL METASTASES FROM NEUROBLASTOMA OF AN UNKNOWN PRIMARY

*A:* CT of the pelvis showing a soft tissue mass in left presacral region and near the left piriformis muscle (*arrow*). *B:* CT of the abdomen revealing para-aortic lymphadenopathy (*1*) and a mesenteric mass (*2*).

## REFERENCES

Arduino LJ, Glucksman MA: Lymphatic spread from prostatic cancer. *J Urol* 88:91, 1962.

Bartels P: Das Lymphgefassystem. In: *Handbuch d. Anatomie d. Menschen.* Jena, G. Fischer, 1909.

Benson KH, Watson RA, Spring B, Agee RE: The value of computerized tomography in evaluation of pelvic lymph nodes. *J Urol* 126:63, 1981.

Busch FM, Sayegh ES, Shenault OW: Some uses of lymphangiography in the management of testicular tumors. *J Urol* 93:490, 1965.

Castellino RA, Marglin SI: Imaging of abdominal and pelvic lymph nodes: lymphography or computed tomography? *Invest Radiol* 17:433, 1982.

Castellino RA, Ray G, Blank N, Govan D, Bagshaw M: Lymphangiography in prostatic carcinoma; preliminary observations. *JAMA* 223:877, 1973.

Chiappa S, Uslenghi C, Bonadonna G: Combined testicular and foot lymphangiography in testicular carcinoma. *Surg Gynecol Obstet* 123:104, 1966.

Cook FE, Lawrence DD, Smith JR, Gritti EJ: Testicular

carcinoma and lymphangiography. *Radiology* 84:420, 1965.

Copeland EM, Miller LD, Jones ES: Prognostic factors in carcinoma of the colon and rectum. *Am J Surg* 116:875, 1968.

Cox KR, Hare WSC, Bruce PT: Lymphography in melanoma: correlation of radiology with pathology. *Cancer* 19:637, 1966.

Crile G Jr, Isbister W, Deodhar SD: Demonstration that large metastases in lymph nodes disseminate cancer cells to blood and lungs. *Cancer* 28:657, 1971.

Cuneo B: Note pur les lymphatiques du testicle. *Bull Mem Soc* 46:574, 1959.

Daffner RH, Halber MD, Postlethwait RW, Korobkin M, Thompson WM: Carcinoma of the esophagus. II. Carcinoma. *AJR* 133:1051, 1979.

del Regato JA, Spjut HJ: *Ackerman and del Regato's Cancer: Diagnosis, Treatment & Prognosis*, ed 5. St Louis, CV Mosby, 1977.

Dormanns E: Das Oesophaguscarcinom: Ergebnisse der unter mitarbeit von 39 pathologischen Instituten Deutschlands durchgefuhrten Erhebung uber das oesophaguscarcinom (1925–1933). *Z Krebsforsch* 49:86, 1939.

Douglas B, MacDonald JS, Baker JW: Lymphography in carcinoma of ovary. *Proc R Soc Med* 54:400, 1971.

Douglas B, MacDonald JS, Baker JW: Lymphography in carcinoma of the uterus. *Clin Radiol* 23:286, 1972.

Dukes CE, Bussey HJR: The spread of rectal cancer and its effect on prognosis. *Br J Cancer* 12:309, 1958.

Dunnick NR, Javadpour N: Value of CT and lymphography: distinguishing retroperitoneal metastases from non-seminomatous testicular tumors. *AJR* 136:1093, 1981.

Edeiken-Monroe B, Zornoza J: Carcinoma of the cervix: percutaneous lymph node aspiration biopsy. *AJR* 138:655, 1982.

Ege GN: Internal mammary lymphoscintigraphy: a rational adjunct to the staging and management of breast carcinoma. *Clin Radiol* 29:453, 1978.

Ellert J, Kreel L: The value of CT in malignant colonic tumors. *J Comput Tomogr* 4:225, 1980.

Engeset A: An experimental study of the lymph node barrier—injection of Walker carcinoma 256 in the lymph vessels. *Extrait Acta Union Int Centre Cancer* 15: nos 3–4, 1959.

Engeset A: Irradiation of lymph nodes and vessels. *Acta Radiol Suppl* 229:1, 1964.

Flocks RH, Culp D, Porto R: Lymphatic spread from prostatic cancer. *J Urol* 81:194, 1959.

Fuchs WA: Malignant tumors of the ovary. In Fuchs WA, Davidson JW, Fischer HW (eds): *Recent Results in Cancer Research—Lymphography in Cancer*. New York, Springer, 1969.

Fuchs WA, Seller RG: Lymphography in carcinoma of the uterine cervix. *Acta Radiol* 16:353, 1975.

Gerteis W: The frequency of metastases in carcinoma of the cervic and corpus. In Ruttimann A (ed): *Progress in Lymphology*. Stuttgart, George Thieme Verlag, 1967.

Gilchrist RK: Lymphatic spread of carcinoma of the colon. *Dis Colon Rectum* 2:69, 1959.

Golimbu M, Morales P: Extended pelvic lymphadenectomy. *Urology* 15:298, 1980.

Grinnell RS: The lymphatic and venous spread of carcinoma of the rectum. *Ann Surg* 116:200, 1942.

Hammond JA, Herson J. Freedman RS, Hamberger AD, Wharton JT, Wallace S, Rutledge FN: The impact of lymph node status on survival in cervical carcinoma. *Int J Radiat Oncol Biol Physics* 7:1713, 1981.

Hanks GE, Bagshaw MA: Megavoltage radiation therapy and lymphangiography in ovarian cancer. *Radiology* 93:649, 1969.

Henriksen E: Distribution of metastases in stage I carcinoma of the cervix; study of 66 autopsied cases. *Am J Obstet Gynecol* 80:919, 1960.

Hymes KB, Cheung T, Greene JB, Prose NS, Marcus A, Ballard H, William DC, Laubenstein LJ: Kaposi sarcoma in homosexual men. A report of eight cases. *Lancet* 2:598, 1981.

Jewett HJ, Strong GH: Infiltrating carcinoma of the bladder: relation of depth of penetration of the bladder wall to incidence of local extension and metastases. *J Urol* 55:366, 1946.

Jonsson K, Wallace S, Jing BS: The clinical significance of lymphovenous anastomoses in malignant disease. *Lymphology* 15:95, 1982.

Kademain MT, Buchler DA, Wartanen GW: Bipedal lymphangiography in malignancies of the uterine corpus. *AJR* 129:903, 1977.

Kendall BE, Arthur JP, Patey OH: Lymphangiography in carcinoma of the breast. *Cancer* 16:1233d, 1963.

Keynes WM: Implication from the bowel lumen in cancer of the large bowel. *Ann Surg* 153:357, 1961.

Kitt K, Lukacs L, Varga G: Diagnostic value of lymphography of the arm in the preoperative diagnosis of early metastases in breast cancer. *Am J Surg* 123:712, 1972.

Kolbenstvedt S: Lymphography in the diagnosis of metastases from carcinoma of the uterine cervix, stage I and II. *Acta Radiol (Suppl)* 16:81, 1975.

Koss JC, Arger PH, Coleman BG, Mulhern CB Jr, Pollack HM, Wein AJ: CT staging of bladder carcinoma. *AJR* 137:359, 1981.

Lackner K, Weissbach L, Bolt I, Scherholz K, Brecht G: Computertomographischer nachweis von lymphknotenmetastasen bei malignen hodentumoren. Ein vergleich der ergebnisse von lymphographie und computertomographie. *ROEFO* 130:636, 1979 (German, English abstr).

Lagasse LD, Ballon SC, Berman M, Watring WG: Pretreatment lymphangiography and operative evaluation in carcinoma of the cervix. *Am J Obstet Gynecol* 134:219, 1979.

Laplante M, Brice M II: The upper limits of hopeful application of radical cystectomy for visical carcinoma: does nodal metastasis always indicate incurability. *J Urol* 109:261, 1973.

Lee JK, Stanley RJ, Sagel SS, McClennan BL: Accuracy of CT in detecting intraabdominal and pelvic lymph node metastases from pelvic cancers. *AJR* 131:675, 1978.

Lee JK, McClennan BL, Stanley RJ, Sabel SS: Computed tomography in the staging of testicular neoplasms. *Radiology* 130:387, 1979.

Levine MS, Arger PH, Coleman BG, Mulhern CB Jr, Pollack AM, Wein AJ: Detecting lymphatic metastases from prostatic carcinoma: superiority of CT. *AJR* 137:207, 1981.

Lien HH, Kolbenstvedt A, Talle K, Fossa SD, Klepp O, Ous S: Comparison of computed tomography, lymphography, and phlebography in 200 consecutive patients with regard to retroperitoneal metastases from testicular tumor. *Radiology* 146:129, 1983.

Marcille M: Lymphatiques et ganglions ilio-pelviens. *Tribune Medicale*, pp 165–170, 1903.

Marshall VF: Current clinical problems regarding bladder tumors. In Marshall VF (ed): *Bladder Tumors: A Symposium*. Philadelphia, JB Lippincott, 1956, pp 1–8.

Mayes GB, Zornoza J: Computed tomography of colon carcinoma. *AJR* 135:43, 1980.

Meyer JE, Munzenrider J: Computed tomographic demonstration of internal mammary node metastases in patients with locally recurrent breast carcinoma. *Radiology* 139:661, 1981.

Morgan CL, Calkins RF, Cavalcantl EJ: Computed tomography in the evaluation, staging and therapy of carcinoma of the bladder and prostate. *Radiology* 140:751, 1981.

Musumeci R, Banfi A, Candiani GB, De Palo GM, Di Re F, Lattuada A, Luciani L, Mangioni C, Mattioli G, Natale N, Pizzetti F: Lymphographic evaluation in ovarian carcinoma of epithelial origin (in Italian). *Tumori* 61:151, 1975.

Musumeci R, De Palo G, Kenda R, Tesoro-Tess JD, De Re F, Petrillo R, Rilke F: Retroperitoneal metastases from ovarian carcinoma: reassessment of 365 patients studied with lymphography. *AJR* 134:449, 1980.

Parker BR, Castellino RA, Fuks ZY, Bagshan MA: The role of lymphography in patients with ovarian cancer. *Cancer* 34:100, 1974.

Plentl A, Friedman E: Lymphatic System of the Female Genitalia. Philadelphia, WB Saunders, 1971, vol II.

Reiffenstuhl G: The prognostic value of lymphography in carcinoma of the uterine cervix. In Ruttimann A (ed): *Progress in Lymphology*. Stuttgart, George Thieme Verlag, 1967.

Rouvière H: *Anatomy of the Human Lymphatic System* (translated by Tobias JM). Ann Arbor MI, Edwards, 1938.

Rummelhardt H, Fussek H: Lymphangioadenographie in der urologie. Erfahrungen und Ergebrisse (in German). *Urologe* 9:333, 1970.

Servelle M: A propos de lymphographie experimental et clinique. *J Radiol Electrol* 26:165, 1945.

Shibata HR, McLena P, Vezina JL, Inglis FG, Tabah EJ; Axillary lymphography in carcinoma of the breast. *Surgery* 60:329, 1966.

Shipley WU, Kopelson G, Novack BH, Ling GG, Dretler SP, Prout GR Jr: Preoperative irradiation, lymphadenec-

tomy and [125]iodine implant for patients with localized prostatic carcinoma: a correlation of implant dosimetry with clinical results. *J Urol* 124:639, 1980.

Spellman MC, Castellino RA, Ray GR, Pistenma DA, Bagshaw MA: An evaluation of lymphology in localized carcinoma of the prostate. *Radiology* 125:637, 1977.

Stehlin JS Jr, Smith JL, Jing BS, Sherrin D: Melanoma of the extremities complicated by in-transit metastasis. *Surg Gynecol Obstet* 122:3, 1966.

Tallroth K: Lymphatic dissemination of bone and soft tissue sarcomas—a lymphographic investigation. *Acta Radiol* (Suppl 349), 1976.

Wallace S, Chuang VP, Samuels M, Johnson D: Transcatheter intraarterial infusion of chemotherapy in advanced bladder cancer. *Cancer* 49:640, 1982.

Walsh JW, Goplerud DR: Prospective comparison between clinical and CT staging in primary cervical carcinoma. *AJR* 137:997, 1981.

Walsh JW, Amendala MA, Konerding KF, Tisnado J, Hazra TA: Computed tomographic detection of pelvic and inguinal lymph-node metastases from primary and recurrent pelvic malignant disease. *Radiology* 137:157, 1980.

Whitley NO, Brenner DE, Aisner J, et al: Computed tomography in the preoperative evaluation of cervical carcinoma. Scientific Exhibit, Radiological Society of North American, Atlanta, 1979.

Whitmore WF Jr, Mackenzie AR: Experiences with various operative procedures for the total excision of prostatic cancer. *Cancer* 12:396, 1959.

Williams RD, Feinberg SB, Knight LC, Fraley EE: Abdominal staging of testicular tumors using ultrasonography and computed tomography. *J Urol* 123:872, 1980.

## SUGGESTED READINGS

Abbes M: Experience with lymphangiography in the surgical management of breast cancer. *Int Surg* 47:243, 1967.

Ackerman LV, and del Regato JA: *Cancer; Diagnosis, Treatment and Prognosis*. ed 4 St Louis, CV Mosby, 1970.

Aegerter EE, Peale AR. Kaposi's sarcoma, a critical survey. *Arch Pathol* 34:413, 1942.

Alcorn FS, Mategrano VC, Petasnick JP, Clark JW: Contributions of computed tomography in the staging and management of malignant lymphoma. *Radiology* 125:71, 1977.

Amendola MA, Walsh JW, Amendola BE, Tishado J, Hall DJ, Goplerud DR: Computed tomography in evaluation of carcinoma of the ovary. *J Comput Assist Tomogr* 5:179, 1981.

Ariel IM, Resnick M: Altered lymphatic dynamics caused by cancer metastases. *Arch Surg* 94:117, 1967a.

Ariel IM, Resnick MI: Altered lymphatic dynamics following groin and axillary dissection: its relationship to treatment policies for malignant melanoma. *Surgery* 61:210, 1967b.

Askar O, Kassem KA: The lymphatics of the leg in deep venous thrombosis. *Br J Radiol* 42:122, 1969.

Athey PA, Wallace S, Jing BS, Gallager HS, Smith JP: Lymphangiography in ovarian cancer. *AJR* 123:106, 1975.

Baddeley H, Bhana D: Lymphography in Kaposi's sarcoma. *Clin Radiol* 22:391, 1971.

Baltaxe HA, Meade JW, Temes GD: Lymphatic and venous examination of the postphlebitic extremity. *Radiology* 91:478, 1968.

Bell RD, Keyl MJ, Shrader FR: Renal lymphatics: the internal distribution. *Nephron* 5:454, 1968.

Bellman S, Oden B: Regeneration of surgically divided lymph vessels. *Acta Chir Scand* 116:99, 1957.

Benninghoff DL, Herman PG, Nelson JH Jr: Clinicopathologic correlation of lymphography and lymph node metastases in gynecological neoplasms. *Cancer* 19:885, 1966.

Berdon WE, Baker DH, Poznanski A: Opacification of retrosternal lymph nodes following barium peritonitis. Report of two cases. *Radiology* 106:171, 1973.

Biggs JS: Lymphography in carcinoma of the cervix. *Aust N Z J Obstet Gynaecol* 5:147, 1965.

Biggs JS, Mackay EV: Pelvic lymphocysts displayed by lymphography. *J Obstet Gynaecol Br Commonw* 73:264, 1966.

Bodie JF, Linton DS Jr: Hepatic oil embolization as a complication of lymphangiography. *Radiology* 99:317, 1971.

Boyd AD, Altemeier WA: Lymphangiography in management of malignant neoplasms of lower extremities. *Arch Surg* 86:911, 1963.

Brizel HE, Livingston PA, Grayson EV: Radiotherapeutic applications of pelvic computed tomography. *J Comput Assist Tomogr* 3:453, 1979.

Burney BT, Klatte EC: Ultrasound and computed tomography of the abdomen in the staging and management of testicular carcinoma. *Radiology* 132:415, 1979.

Calnan J, Kountz SL: Effect of venous obtruction on lymphatics. *Br J Surg* 52:800, 1965.

Carlson V, Delclos L, Fletcher GH: Distant metastases in squamous cell carcinoma of the uterine cervix. *Radiology* 88:961, 1967.

Castellino RA: The role of lymphography in "apparently localized" prostatic carcinoma. *Lymphology* 8:16, 1975.

Celis A, Kuthy J, Del Castillo E: Importance of the thoracic duct in spread of malignant diseases. *Acta Radiol* 45:169, 1956.

Chavez CM: The clinical significance of lymphaticovenous anastomosis. Its implications in lymphangiography. *Vasc Dis* 5:35, 1968.

Chavez CM, Picard JD, Davis D: Liver opacification following lymphangiography: pathogenesis and clinical significance. *Sugery* 63:564, 1968.

Chiappa S, Bonadonna G, Uslenghi C, Veronesi U: Lymphangiography in the diagnosis of retroperitoneal node metastases in rectal cancer. *Br J Radiol* 45:584, 1967.

Cochrane WJ: Ultrasound in gynecology. *Radiol Clin North Am* 13:457, 1975.

Cohn I: Cause and prevention of recurrence following surgery for colon cancer. *Cancer* 28:183, 1971.

Cole WH, Roberts SS, Webb RS, Strehl FW, Oates GD: Dissemination of cancer with special emphasis on vascular spread and implantation. *Ann Surg* 161:753, 1965.

Comas MR, Morris CH, Averette HE: Lymphography and vulvar carcinoma. *Obstet Gynecol* 33:177, 1969.

Conrad J, Elkin M, Romney SL: Pelvic angiography and lymphangiography in the evaluation of the patient with carcinoma of the cervix. *Surg Gynecol Obstet* 122:983, 1966.

Danese C, Howard JM: Postmastectomy lymphedema. *Surg Gynecol Obstet* 120:797, 1965.

Delclos L, Fletcher GH, Gutierrez AE, Rutledge FN: Adenocarcinoma of the uterus. *AJR* 105:603, 1969.

de Roo T, Van Minden SH: Lymphographic findings in a series of 258 patients with tumors of the testes. *Lymphology* 6:97, 1973.

Dolan PA, Hughes RR: Lymphography in genital cancer. *Surg Gynecol Obstet* 118:1286, 1964.

Doppman JL, Chretien P: Visceral pelvic venography in carcinoma of the cervix. *Radiology* 98:405, 1971

Dunnick NR, Jones RB, Doppman JL, Speyer J, Myers CE: Intraperitoneal contrast infusion for assessment of intraperitoneal fluid dynamics. *AJR* 133:221, 1979.

Edwards JM, Kinmont JB: Lymphovenous shunts in man. *Br J Surg* 56:699, 1969.

Farrell J: Lymphangiographic demonstration of lymphovenous communication after radiotherapy in Hodgkin's disease. *Radiology* 87:630, 1966.

Fein RL, Taber DO: Foot lymphography in the testis tumor patient; a review of fifty cases. *Cancer* 24:248, 1969.

Feldman GB, Knapp RC, Order SE, Hellman S: Role of lymphatic obstruction in formation of ascites in murine ovarian carcinoma. *Cancer Res* 32:2663, 1972.

Feldman MG, Kohan P, Edelman S: Lymphangiographic studies in obstructive lymphedema of the upper extremity. *Surgery* 59:935, 1966.

Fisher EP, Fisher B: Experimental studies of factors influencing hepatic metastases. I. The effect of number of tumor cells injected and time of growth. *Cancer* 12:926, 1959a.

Fisher B, Fisher EP: Experimental studies of factors influencing hepatic metastases. II. Effect of partial hepatectomy. *Cancer* 12:929, 1959b.

Fisher B, Fisher EP: Experimental studies of factors influencing hepatic metastases. III. Effect of surgical trauma with special reference to liver injury. *Ann Surg* 150:731, 1959c.

Fisher EP, Turnbull RB: The cytologic demonstration and significance of tumor cells in the mesenteric venous blood in patients with colorectal carcinoma. *Surg Gynecol Obstet* 100:102, 1955.

Fletcher GH, Rutledge FN: Carcinoma of uterine cervix. in Deeley TJ (ed): *Modern Radiotherapy: Gynaecological Cancer*. London, Butterworths, 1971.

Fred HL, Eiband JM, Collins LC: Calcifications in intraabdominal and retroperitoneal metastases. *AJR* 91:138, 1964.

Freimanis AS: Echographic diagnosis of lesions of the abdominal aorta and lymph nodes. *Radiol Clin North Am* 13:557, 1975.

Fuchs WA, Girod M: Lymphography as a guide to prognosis in malignant testicular tumors. *Acta Radiol* 16:305, 1975.

Galesanu MR, Rosenbaum S: Diagnosis of lymph node invasion of bladder and prostatic cancer by lympho- and pelvic phlebography. *Int Urol Nephrol* 5:163, 1973.

Ganon JH, Mount BM, Khonsari H, MacKinnon KJ: Lymphography in germinal tumors of the testis. *Br J Urol* 44:136, 1972.

Ghahremani GG, Straua FH: Calcification of distant lymph node metastases from cancer of the colon. *Radiology* 99:65, 1971.

Ginaldi S, Wallace S, Jing BS, Bernardino ME: Carcinoma of the cervix: lymphangiography and computed tomography. *AJR* 136:1087, 1981.

Gottesfeld KR: Ultrasound in obstetrics and gynecology. *Semin Roentgenol* 10:305, 1975.

Gray SH, Cohen RA: Lymphaticovenous anastomoses involving the portal system: report of a case with metastatic carcinoma of vagina. *Am Surg* 32:410, 1966.

Grossman I, Von Phul R, Fitzgerald JP, Nash S, Turner AF, Kurohara SS, George F III: The early lymphatic spread of manifest prostatic adenocarcinoma. *AJR* 120:673, 1974.

Guernsey JM, Doggett RLS III, Mason GR, Kohatsu S, Obeaheiman HA: Combined treatment of cancer of the esophagus. *Am J Surg* 117:157, 1969.

Hagen S, Bjorn-Hansen R: Lymphography in the treatment of carcinoma of the vulva. *Acta Radiol (Diagn)* 11:609, 1971.

Harell GS, Breiman RS, Glatstein EJ, Marshall WH Jr, Castellino RA: Computed tomography of the abdomen in the malignant lymphomas. *Radiol Clin North Am* 15:391, 1977.

Hartgill JC: Lymphogram control during pelvic lymphadenectomy. *Proc R Soc Med* 64:401, 1971.

Havrilla TR, Reich NE, Haaga JR: The floating aorta in computerized tomography: a sign of retroperitoneal pathology. *Computed Axial Tomogr* 1:107, 1977.

Henriksen E: Lymphatic spread of carcinoma of cervix and body of uterus: study of 420 necropsies. *Am J Obstet Gynecol* 58:924, 1949.

Herman P, Beninghoff D, Schwartz J: A physiological approach to lymph flow in lymphography. *AJR* 91:1207, 1964.

Hill DR, Quintous EC, Walsh PC: Prostate carcinoma; radiation treatment of the primary and regional lymphatics. *Cancer* 34:156, 1974.

Hirabayashi K, Graham J: Genesis of ascites in ovarian cancer. *Am J Obstet Gynecol* 106:492, 1970.

Hliniak I, Vorbrodt J: The use of lymphangiography in cervical cancer. *Radiol Diagn* 13:655, 1972.

Hodari AA, Hodgkinson CP: Lymphography as a diagnostic aid in female genital malignancy. *Obstet Gynecol* 29:34, 1967.

Hreshchychyn MM, Sheehan RR: Collateral lymphatics in patients with gynecologic carcinoma. *Am J Obstet Gynecol* 91:118, 1965.

Hughes JH, Patel AR: Swelling of the arm following radical mastectomy. *Br J Surg* 53:4, 1966.

Hulten L, Ahren C, Rosencrantz M: Lymphangio-adenography in carcinoma of the breast. Comparative clinical, roentgen, and histologic appraisal of the method for the demonstration of the lymph node metastases. *Acta Chir Scand* 132:261, 1966.

Husband JE, Peckham MJ, MacDonald JS, Hendry WF:

The role of computed tomography in the management of testicular teratoma. *Clin Radiol* 30:243, 1979.

Jackson RJ: Lymphographic studies related to the problem of metastatic spread from carcinoma of the female genital tract. *J. Obstet Gynaecol Br Commonw* 74:339, 1967.

Jackson RJ: Topography of the iliopelvic lymph nodes. Consideration relating to the treatment of carcinoma of the cervix. *Am J Obstet Gynecol* 104:1118, 1969.

Jacobs JB: Selective gonadal venography. *Radiology* 92:885, 1960.

Jaffe HL *Tumors and Tumorous Conditions of the Bone and Joints*. Philadelphia, Lea and Febiger, 1958.

Janca K, Popovic L, Dimovic D: Lymphography in disease of the penis. *Int Urol Nephrol* 4:59, 1972.

Jing BS, McGraw JP, Rutledge, F: Gynecologic applications of lymphangiography. *Surg Gynecol Obstet* 119:763, 1964.

Jing BS, Wallace S, Zornoza J: Metastases to retroperitoneal and pelvic lymph nodes: computed tomography and lymphangiography. *Radiol Clin North Am* 20:511, 1982.

Job TT: Lymphaticovenous communications in common rats and their significance. *Am J Anat* 24:467, 1918.

Johnson DE, Kaesler KE, Kaminsky S, Jing BS, Wallace S: Lymphangiography as an aid in staging bladder carcinoma. *South Med J* 69:28, 1976.

Jonsson K, Ingemansson S, Ling L: Lymphography in patients with testicular tumors. *Br J Urol* 45:548, 1973.

Keating GM: Lymphangioadenography in the study of malignant disease in gynecology. *J Med Soc N J* 63:89, 1966.

Kilcheski TS, Arger PH, Mulhern CB, Coleman BG, Kressel HY, Mikuta JI: Role of computed tomography in the presurgical evaluation of carcinoma of the cervix. *J Comput Assist Tomogr* 5:378, 1981.

Kitchen G: Lymphangiographic studies in a case of postmastectomy lymphangiosarcoma. *Br J Radiol* 45:388, 1972.

Kittridge RD, Burger R, Finby N, Draper JW: An illustration of an approach to the diagnosis of pelvic disease. *J Urol* 89:607, 1963.

Koehler PR, Schaffer B: Peripheral lymphaticovenous anastomoses. Report of two cases. *Circulation* 35:401, 1967.

Korobkin M: Computed tomography of the retroperitoneal vasculature in lymph nodes. *Semin Roentgenol* 16:251, 1981.

Kreel L: The EMI whole body scanner in the demonstration of lymph node enlargement. *Clin Radiol* 27:421, 1976.

Kreel L, George P: Postmastectomy lymphangiography detection of metastases and edema. *Ann Surg* 163:470, 1964.

Lang EK, Simon KJ, Cummings DH, Byrd EH Jr, Moore HE, Tannehill RH, West WC Jr, Tate WB, Brooks GG, Dilworth EE: Arteriography, pelvic pneumography and lymphangiography augmenting assessment and staging of carcinoma of the cervix. *South Med J* 63:1249, 1970.

Lawson TL, Albarelli JN: Diagnosis of gynecologic pelvic masses by gray scale ultrasonography: analysis of specificity and accuracy. *AJR* 128:1003, 1977.

Lecart C, Lenfant P: Critical appraisal of lymphangiography in cancer of the female genital tract. *Lymphology* 4:100, 1971.

Lee KF, Greening R, Kramer S, Hahn GA, Kuroda K, Lin SR, Koslow WW: The value of pelvic venography and lymphography in the clinical staging of carcinoma of the uterine cervix. *AJR* 111:284, 1971.

MacDonald JS: Lymphography in renal tumors. *Br J Radiol* 42:959, 1969.

MacDonald JS: Lymphography in malignant disease of the urinary tract. *Proc R Soc Med* 63:1237, 1970.

Maier JG, Schamber DT: The role of lymphography in the diagnosis and treatment of malignant testicular tumors. *AJR* 114:482, 1972.

Malek P: Some questions of the pathophysiology of the lymphatic system. *Rev Czech Med* 5:153, 1959.

Marshall WH Jr, Breiman RS, Harell GS, Glatstein E, Kaplan HS: Computed tomography of abdominal para-aortic lymph node disease: preliminary observations with a 6 second scanner. *AJR* 128:759, 1977.

Marsili E, Manfredi L, Borreani B: Lymphography in the study of cancer of the rectum. *Panninerva Med* 9:62, 1967.

McCarthy WD, Pack GT: Malignant blood vessel tumors. A report of 56 cases of angiosarcoma and Kaposi's sarcoma. *Surg Gynecol Obstet* 91:465, 1950.

McLand TC, Kalisher L, Stark P, Greene R: Intrathoracic lymph node metastases from extrathoracic neoplasms. *AJR* 131:403, 1978.

McNeer G, Das Gupta T: Routes of lymphatic spread of malignant melanoma. *Cancer* 15:168, 1965.

McPeak CJ, Constantinides SG: Lymphangiography in malignant melanoma: a comparison of clinicopathological and lymphangiographic findings in 21 cases. *Cancer* 17:1586, 1964.

Messinger NH, Beneventano TC, Siegelman SS: Intraflexural cancer of the colon: clinical-radiologic-pathologic correlations. *Dis Colon Rectum* 14:255, 1971.

Mitchell N, Feder IA: Kaposi's sarcoma with secondary involvement of the jejunum, perforation and peritonitis. *Ann Intern Med* 31:324, 1949.

Musumeci R, Bombarda A, Cataldo I, Fontana F, Petrillo R, Zanini M: Lymphographic evaluation in bone and soft tissue sarcomas. *Tumori* 63:283, 1977.

Nair MK: The diagnostic value of lymphangiography in the study of female genital cancer. *Indian J Cancer* 4:275, 1967.

Neyazaki E, Kupic EA, Marshall WH: Collateral lymphaticovenous communications after experimental obstruction of the thoracic duct. *Radiology* 85:423, 1965.

Nielubowicz J, Olszewski W: Surgical lymphaticovenous shunts in patients with secondary lymphedema. *Br J Surg* 55:440, 1968a.

Nielubowicz J, Olszewski W: Experimental lymphovenous anastomosis. *Br J Surg* 55:449, 1968b.

Nixon GW: Lymphangiomatosis of bone demonstrated by lymphangiography. *AJR* 110:582, 1970.

Phillips JH: The lymphatic system with particular reference to cardiac edema. *Bull Tulane Med Fac* 14:187, 1957.

Picard J: Lymphography in cancer of the ovary. *Gynecol Obstet (Paris)* 63:585, 1964.

Piver SM, Barlow JJ: Para-aortic lymphadenectomy in staging patients with advanced local cervical cancer. *Obstet Gynecol* 43:544, 1974.

Piver SM, Wallace S, Castro JR: The accuracy of lymphangiography in carcinoma of the uterine cervix. *AJR* 111:278, 1971.

Pollard W: Lymphangiography in the surgical treatment of carcinoma of the cervix. *Clin Radiol* 20:463, 1969.

Prando A, Wallace S, Von Eschenbach AC, Ting BS, Rosengren JE, Hussey DH; Lymphangiography in staging of carcinoma of the prostate. *Radiology* 131:641, 1979.

Raskin M: Combination of CT and ultrasound in the retroperitoneal and pelvic examination. *Crit Rev Diagn Imaging* 13:173, 1980.

Redman HC: Computed tomography of the pelvis. *Radiol Clin North Am* 15:441, 1977.

Redman HC, Glatstein E, Castellino RA, Federal WA: Computed tomography as an adjunct in the staging of Hodgkin's disease and non-Hodgkin's lymphoma. *Radiology* 124:381, 1977.

Reichert FL: The regeneration of the lymphatics. *Arch Surg* 13:871, 1926.

Reiffenstuhl G: *The Lymphatics of the Female Genital Organs.*

Philadelphia, JB Lippincott, 1964.

Riveros M, Garcia R, Cabanas R: Lymphadenography of the dorsal lymphatics of the penis. Techniques and results. *Cancer* 20:2026, 1967.

Rockoff SD, Lipsit ER, Nolan NG: Advances in the diagnostic imaging of cancer. *Curr Probl Cancer* 5:4, 1980.

Roddenberry H, Allen L: Observations on the abdominal lymphaticovenous communications of the squirrel monkey (*Saimire sciures*). *Anat Rec* 159:147, 1967.

Rosenquist CJ, Wolfe DC: Lymphangioma of bone. *J Bone Joint Surg* 50A:158, 1968.

Roxin T, Bujar H: Lymphographic visualization of lymphaticovenous communications and their significance in malignant hemolymphopathies. *Lymphology* 3:127, 1970.

Rutledge F, Dodd GD, Kasilag FB: Lymphocysts: a complication of radical pelvic surgery. *Am J Obstet Gynecol* 77:1165, 1959.

Safai B, Good R: A review and recent developments. *CA* 31:2, 1981.

Schaffer B, Koehler PR, Daniel CR, Wohl GT, Rivera E, Meyers WA, Skelley JT: A critical evaluation of lymphangiography. *Radiology* 80:917, 1963.

Schaner EG, Head GL, Doppman JL, Young RC: Computed tomography in the diagnosis, staging and management of abdominal lymphoma. *J Comput Assist Tomogr* 1:176, 1977.

Servelle M: Pathology of the thoracic duct. *J Cardiovasc Surg* 4:702, 1963.

Servelle M: *Pathologie Vasculaire.* Paris, Masson et Cie, 1975.

Servelle M, Deysson G: Reflux of intestinal chyle in lymphatics of the leg. *Ann Surg* 133:324, 1951.

Servelle M, Nogues C: *The Chyliferous Vessels.* Paris, Expansion Scientifique Francaise, 1981.

Smedal MI, Evans JA: Cause and treatment of edema of arm following radical mastectomy. *Surg Gynecol Obstet* 111:29, 1960.

Snow JH, Goldstein HM, Wallace S: Comparison of scintigraphy, sonography and computed tomography in evaluation of hepatic neoplasms. *AJR* 132:915, 1979.

Steidl RA: Extensive calcified retroperitoneal lymph node metastases from a primary carcinoma of the cecum. *Radiology* 89:263, 1967.

Steinberg AO, Madayag MA, Bosniak MA, Morales PA: Demonstration of two unusually large pelvic lymphocyts by lymphangiography. *J Urol* 109:477, 1973.

Stephens DH, Williamson B Jr, Sheedy PF, Hattery RR, Miller WE: Computed tomography of the retroperitoneal space. *Radiol Clin North Am* 15:377, 1977.

Sukov RJ, Scardino PT, Sample WF, Winter J, Confer DJ: Computed tomography and transabdominal ultrasound in the evaluation of the prostate. *J Comput Assist Tomogr* 1:281, 1977.

Takashima T, Benninghoff DL: Lymphaticovenous communications and lymph reflux after thoracic duct obstruction. An experimental study in the dog. *Invest Radiol* 1:188, 1966.

Tashibana S: Lymph node metastases in cancer of the uterine cervix. *J Jpn Obstet Gynecol Soc* 3:71, 1956.

Tawil W, Belanger R: Prognostic value of the lymphangiogram in carcinoma of the uterine cervix. *Radiology* 109:597, 1973.

Terry LN Jr, Piver SM, Hanks GE: The value of lymphangiography in malignant disease of the uterine cervix. *Radiology* 103:175, 1972.

Thomas JL, Bernardino ME, Bracken RB: Staging of testicular carcinoma: comparison of CT and lymphangiography. *AJR* 137:991, 1981.

Threefoot SA: Gross and microscopic anatomy of the lymphatic vessels and lymphaticovenous communications. *Cancer Chemother Rep* 52:1, 1968.

Threefoot SA, Kossover MF: Lymphaticovenous communications in man. *Arch Intern Med* 117:213, 1966.

Tsangaris NT, Yutzy CV: A lymphangiographic study of postmastectomy lymphedema. *Surg Gynecol Obstet* 123:1228, 1966.

Turner-Warwick RT: The lymphatics of the breast. *Br J Surg* 574, 1957.

Van Den Brenk HAS: Effects of ionizing radiations on regeneration and behavior of mammalian lymphatics; in vivo studies of Sandison Clark chambers. *AJR* 78:837, 1957.

Van Engelshoven JMA, Kreel L: Computed tomography of the prostate. *J Comput Assist Tomogr* 3:45, 1979.

Van Minden SH: The value of lymphography in tumors of the testes. *Radiol Clin Biol* 40:274, 1971.

Vincent CC: Pelvic lymphangiography. The method, its diagnostic and therapeutic aid in female genital malignancies. *J Natl Med Assoc* 58:28, 1966.

Wahlqvist L, Hulten L, Rosencrantz M: Normal lymphatic drainage of the testis studied by funicular lymphography. *Acta Chir Scand* 132:454, 1966.

Wajsman Z, Baumgartner G, Murphy GP, Merrin C: Evaluation of lymphangiography for clinical staging of bladder tumors. *J Urol* 114:712, 1975.

Wallace N: Lymphography in the management of testicular tumors. *Clin Radiol* 20:453, 1969.

Wallace S, Jackson L: Diagnostic criteria for lymphangiographic interpretation of malignant neoplasia. *Cancer Chemother Rep* 52:125, 1968.

Wallace S, Jing BS: Lymphangiography; diagnosis of nodal metastases from testicular malignancies. *JAMA* 213:94, 1970.

Wallace S, Jing BS: Lymphangiography in tumors of the female genital system. *Radiol Clin North Am* 12:79, 1974.

Wallace S, Jing BS: Testicular malignancies and the lymphatic system. In Johnson DE (ed): *Testicular tumors,* ed 2. Flushing, NY, Medical Examination Publishing Co, 1976.

Wallace S, Jing BS: Carcinoma. In Clouse ME (ed): *Clinical Lymphography (Golden's Diagnostic Radiology).* Baltimore, Williams & Wilkins, 1977.

Wallace S, Jing BS: Disorders of the lymphatic system. In Teplick JG, Haskin ME (eds): *Surgical Radiology: A Complement in Radiology and Imaging to the Sabiston-Davis-Christopher Textbook of Surgery.* Philadelphia, WB Saunders, 1981, Vol II.

Wallace S, Jackson L, Dodd GD: Lymphangiographic interpretation. *Radiol Clin North Am* 3:467, 1965.

Wallace S, Jackson L, Dodd GD: Radiographic demonstration of lymphatic dynamics. *Prog Clin Cancer* 3:157, 1967.

Wallace S, Jing BS, Medellin H: Endometrial carcinoma: radiologic assistance in diagnosis, staging, and management. *J Gynecol Oncol* 2:287, 1974.

Wallace S, Jing BS, Zornoza J: Lymphangiography in the determination of the extent of metastatic carcinoma; the potential value of percutaneous lymph node biopsy. *Cancer* 39:706, 1977.

Wallace S, Jing BS, Bernardino ME, Thomas J: Lymphadenopathy. In Margulis AR, Gooding CA (eds): *Diagnostic Radiology 1980.* New York, Academic Press, 1981.

Walsh JW, Rosenfield AT, Jaffe CC, Schwartz PE, Simeone J, Dembner AG, Taylor KJW: Prospective comparison of ultrasound and computed tomography in the evaluation of gynecologic pelvic mass. *AJR* 131:955, 1978.

Walsh JW, Taylor KJW, Wasson JF, Schwartz PE, Kosenfield AT: Gray-scale ultrasound in 204 proved gynecologic masses: accuracy and specific diagnostic criteria. *Radiology* 130:391, 1979.

Weinerman PM, Arger PH, Coleman BG, Pollack HM, Banner MP, Wein AJ: Pelvic adenopathy from bladder and prostate carcinoma: detection by rapid-sequence computed tomography. *AJR* 140:95, 1983.

Wharton JT, Smith JP, Delclos L, Fletcher GH: Tumors of ovary. In *Gynecology and Obstetrics*. Philadelphia, FA Davis, 1945.

Wheeler JS: Lymphography in early prostatic cancer. *Urology* 3:444, 1974.

Winterberger AR: Radiographic diagnosis of lymphangiomatosis of bone. *Radiology* 102:321, 1972.

Wirtanen GW, Miller RC: Bladder lymphatics and tumor dissemination. *J Urol* 109:58, 1973.

Wolfel DA: Lymphaticovenous communications, a clinical reality. *AJR* 95:766, 1965.

Yune HY, Klatte EC: Lymphography in lymphatic obstruction. *Radiology* 92:824, 1969.

Zelch MG, Haaga JR: Clinical comparison of computed tomography and lymphangiography for detection of retroperitoneal lymphadenopathy. *Radiol Clin North Am* 17:157, 1979.

Zornoza J, Wallace S, Goldstein HM, Lukeman JM, Jing BS: Transperitoneal percutaneous retroperitoneal lymph node aspiration biopsy. *Radiology* 122:111, 1977.

# 13

# *Lymph Node Imaging of the Thorax*

THERESA C. McLOUD, M.D., AND JACK E. MEYER, M.D.

Lymphadenopathy in the thorax may be associated with a variety of diseases both benign and malignant. Lymph node enlargement is a frequent feature of such unrelated disorders as granulomatous infections (tuberculosis and fungal disease), occupational diseases (silicosis, coal worker's pneumoconiosis), sarcoidosis, and malignancy (lymphoma, bronchogenic carcinoma, and metastases from extrathoracic tumors). Improvements in technology, particularly the advent of computed tomography (CT), have permitted earlier and more accurate detection of enlarged mediastinal and hilar lymph nodes. CT is now used extensively in staging bronchogenic carcinoma and lymphoma and in detection of mediastinal and hilar metastases.

## BRONCHOGENIC CARCINOMA

Development of a comprehensive and accepted system for staging carcinoma of the lung has made evaluation of mediastinal lymph node metastases of utmost importance (Carr and Mountain, 1974; Mountain et al., 1974; Armstrong and Bragg, 1975). The presence of lymph node spread has long been known to affect prognosis significantly. Complete resections in patients without mediastinal nodal metastases produce 5-yr survival in 30–45% of patients, depending on the cell type; if mediastinal nodes are involved, fewer than 10% of patients live 5 yr (Mountain, 1974). The presence of isolated positive hilar nodes does not appear to affect prognosis (Bergh and Schersten, 1965; TNM Classification, 1972), but mediastinal lymph node metastases contraindicate surgery. A bronchogenic carcinoma is considered unresectable when contralateral lymph node or high ipsilateral lymph node involvement is present. Occasionally, radical pneumonectomy may be performed with lymph node dissection when low ipsilateral or subcarinal nodes are present, especially if the tumor is squamous cell carcinoma (Mountain, 1974). Thus the radiological diagnosis of mediastinal lymphadenopathy influences both the selection of patients for surgery and the preoperative staging of bronchogenic carcinoma.

In recent years the TNM (tumor-nodes-metastasis) staging system for cancers of the lung has been widely accepted and implemented (TNM Classification, 1972; Carr and Mountain, 1974; Mountain et al., 1974; Armstrong and Bragg, 1975). T characterizes the size, location, and gross features of the primary tumor; N is the extent of regional lymph node metastases; and M is the presence or absence of distant metastases. The staging of regional lymph nodes is listed as follows:

$N_0$ No demonstrable metastases to regional lymph nodes

$N_1$ Metastases to lymph nodes in the ipsilateral hilar region including direct extension

$N_2$ Metastases to lymph nodes in the mediastinum

$N_1$ involvement places the patient in stage I or stage II depending on other factors, whereas $N_2$ involvement requires placement in stage III. The main objective of the TNM staging of lung cancer is to aid in treatment planning and to assess prognosis (Mountain, 1974).

Early studies indicate that the extent of regional lymph node metastases does correlate with prognosis. Among 1568 cases of bronchogenic carcinoma staged by the TNM system, those categorized as $N_0$ had a 25–30% 5-yr survival; $N_1$ cases had a 10–15% 5-yr survival; and $N_2$ cases had a 2–4% 5-yr survival (Mountain et al., 1974).

The patterns of metastatic spread to the mediastinum from various lung lobes have been clearly described by Rouviere (1938). Briefly, the anatomic pathways may be summarized as follows. Right upper lobe tumors spread directly to right paratracheal nodes; lesions in the right middle lobe either metastasize directly to the right paratracheal chain or via subcarinal nodes. Spread to subcarinal or periesophageal nodes may occur from right lower lobe cancers with later extension into the paratracheal area on the right. As expected, cancers on the left metastasize to the left paratracheal chain, but they may involve the right paratracheal nodes by direct extension from subcarinal metastases, particularly if the primary lesion is in the left lower lobe. This concept of spread of tumor may be overly simplified because drainage does occur from right to left as well as left to right (Goldberg et al., 1974; Murray, 1976; Heitzman, 1977), but as a general rule, contralateral metastasis without ipsilateral metastasis is more common with left lung neoplasms (Goldberg et al., 1974; Heitzman, 1977).

# LYMPHOMA

The histological and staging classifications of malignant lymphomas are reviewed in other chapters. The diagnostic assessment of extent of involvement is a critical component in clinical staging of patients with this disease, and roentgenological techniques play an essential role in this assessment, particularly in the thorax.

Mediastinal lymphadenopathy is extremely common in Hodgkin's disease and is often accompanied by unilateral or bilateral hilar adenopathy (Kaplan, 1980). In a study of 164 patients with newly diagnosed Hodgkin's disease, 67% had radiographic evidence of intrathoracic disease, and 99% of this subgroup had lymphadenopathy; the most frequent sites of nodal involvement were the anterior mediastinal, tracheobronchial, and paratracheal groups (Filly et al., 1976). The mediastinum is also involved in an appreciable proportion of patients with non-Hodgkin's lymphoma, especially diffuse histiocytic and lymphoblastic lymphomas (Kaplan, 1980). Among 136 patients with non-Hodgkin's lymphoma, 43% showed evidence of intrathoracic disease at diagnosis; 83% of them had evidence of intrathoracic adenopathy (Filly et al., 1976). Involvement of only one lymph node group was more common in patients with non-Hodgkin's lymphoma (40%) than in those with Hodgkin's disease (15%) (Filly et al., 1976; Blank and Castellino, 1980).

# EXTRATHORACIC MALIGNANCIES

Metastatic disease from extrathoracic neoplasms occasionally causes mediastinal and hilar lymph node enlargement. In a study of 1071 cases of extrathoracic malignant neoplasms, only 25 (2.3%) had evidence of hilar or mediastinal lymph node metastases on serial chest roentgenograms (McLoud et al., 1978). In contrast, hematogenous or lymphangitic metastases were present in the lungs in almost one-half (40%) of the 25 cases.

The primary malignancies likely to metastasize to the mediastinum include tumors of the head and neck (for example, upper respiratory passage, oral cavity, and neck), genitourinary malignancies, breast carcinomas, and malignant melanomas (McLoud et al., 1978). The route and mechanism of extension of lymph node metastases into the thorax from these sites are not completely understood.

In genitourinary neoplasms, spread of tumor occurs from the lymphatics draining the pelvis and abdomen into the thoracic duct. Absence or incompetence of valves in the ducts may result in reflux of tumor emboli into the bronchomediastinal trunks. Retrograde flow into the mediastinal nodes and interlobular lymphatics may then ensue (Baltaxe and Constable, 1968; Grant and Levin, 1974). Reflux into mediastinal nodes during lymphangiography normally occurs in 5–14% of patients, presumably owing to incompetent valves (Rosenberger et al., 1972).

Cancers of the nasal and oral cavities and neck primarily metastasize to regional lymphatics (i.e., one of the three lymphatic chains in the neck). Communication between the anterior cervical chain and anterior mediastinal lymph nodes has been described by Rouvière (1938); this route is presumed to be the course by which mediastinal lymph node metastases occur.

In breast carcinoma, inner quadrant lesions are drained by lymphatics that terminate in the internal mammary nodes (Handley and Thackray, 1949). Communications between the upper parasternal and anterior mediastinal nodes have been noted, suggesting a direct route by which mediastinal metastases occur (Rouvière, 1938).

Finally, metastases to the mediastinum from malignant melanoma probably spread through many lymphatic groups. Although melanoma disseminates widely to many organs, it initially spreads to regional lymph nodes.

## RADIOLOGICAL ANATOMY OF MEDIASTINAL LYMPH NODES

The anatomy of mediastinal lymph nodes has been described by Rouvière (1938). He divided the visceral intrathoracic lymph nodes into (*a*) intrapulmonary, (*b*) peritracheobronchial (right and left paratracheal chains), (*c*) bifurcation or subcarinal nodes, (*d*) posterior mediastinal, and (*e*) anterior mediastinal or prevascular nodes. We use Rouvière's nomenclature with some minor modifications. Nodes of the pulmonary root, proximal intrapulmonary nodes, and nodes of the aorticopulmonary window are included within the group of anterior mediastinal nodes. Figure 13.1 is a schematic diagram of some of the mediastinal lymph node chains.

Mediastinal lymphadenopathy is usually recognized on the standard chest roentgenogram by lobulation or other changes in mediastinal contour, sometimes accompanied by increased density. Contour changes are often subtle, and their recognition requires a clear understanding of radiographic and mediastinal anatomy (Heitzman, 1977; Blank and Castellino, 1980). Several imaging procedures may be used to evaluate mediastinal lymphadenopathy either due to metastases from bronchogenic carcinoma, extrathoracic neoplasms, or intrathoracic lymphoma. In addition to the standard posteroanterior and lateral chest roentgenograms, these include conventional tomography, barium esophagography, CT, and, in the lymphomas and bronchogenic carcinoma, gallium-67 citrate scanning. CT scanning represents a major advance in detection of mediastinal lymphadenopathy. Because of the cross-sectional display and the abundant fat in the mediastinum, enlarged lymph nodes can be identified as discrete densities in most instances rather than as secondary alterations in mediastinal contour. In this chapter the radiographic findings produced by lymph node enlargement are described for each of the anatomic groups mentioned previously along with the distribution of adenopathy that can be expected in lymphoma, bronchogenic carcinoma, and metastatic disease. Finally, the various modalities used in imaging intrathoracic lymph nodes are reviewed.

### Anterior Mediastinum

Anterior mediastinal adenopathy produces increased density anterior to the great vessels that can be seen retrosternally on the lateral chest roentgenogram (Fig. 13.2) (McCort and Robbins,

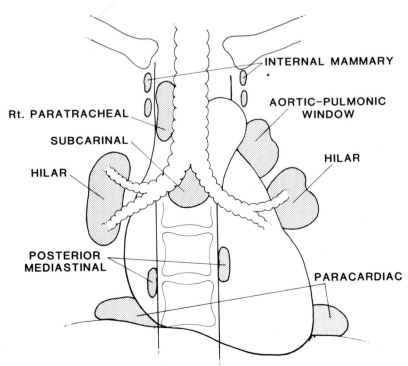

FIGURE 13.1. SCHEMATIC DIAGRAM OF LYMPH NODES OF THE MEDIASTINUM
(From McLoud TC, Meyer JE: Mediastinal metastases. *Radiol Clin North Am* 20:453–467, 1982.)

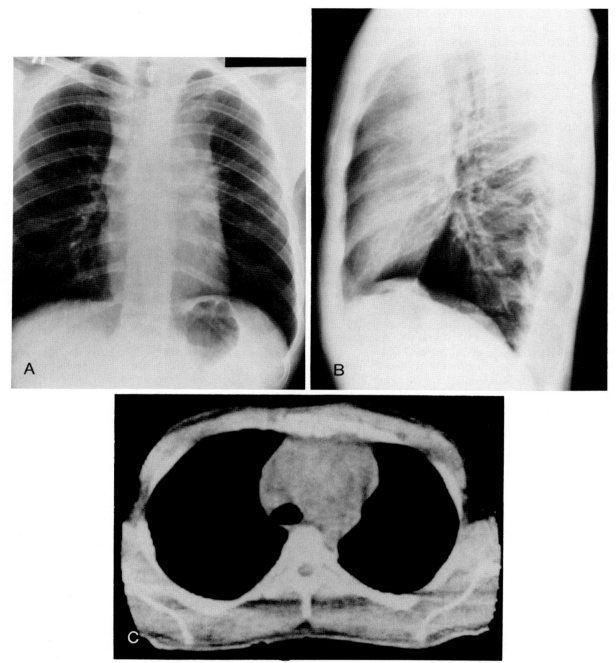

FIGURE 13.2. BILATERAL PREVASCULAR OR ANTERIOR MEDIASTINAL ADENOPATHY IN A 26-YR-OLD PATIENT WITH
HODGKIN'S DISEASE
*A*: Posteroanterior film. The widened mediastinal interface on the right extends below the tracheobronchial angle. The left
paratracheal nodes are probably enlarged also because the trachea is shifted to the right. *B*: Lateral film. Note obliteration of
the retrosternal clear space. *C*: CT at the level of the aortic arch. Large anterior mediastinal mass has obliterated normal fat
planes. (From McLoud TC, Meyer JE: Mediastinal metastases. *Radiol Clin North Am* 20:453–467, 1982.)

1951). On the posteroanterior view, enlargement
of the right prevascular group can be recognized
by mediastinal widening located more laterally
than the pretracheal nodes and more inferiorly

than the tracheobronchial angle (Fig. 13.2) (Bein
et al., 1978). On the left side, prevascular lymphadenopathy above the aortic arch produces similar widening of the mediastinum. Differentia-

tion from enlarged left paratracheal nodes is difficult, but lateral mediastinal tomograms may aid in differentiating the two groups (Blank and Castellino, 1972; Berkmen and Javors, 1976; Bein et al., 1978).

Enlargement of prevascular lymph nodes can readily be identified on CT. Normal nodes are usually less than 1 cm in diameter and are defined by surrounding mediastinal fat (Schnyder and Gamsu, 1981). Since these nodes are located near the great vessels, infusion of contrast material can help distinguish lymphadenopathy from normal vascular structures. More frequently, however, particularly in patients with lymphoma, a large single continuous mass is observed in the anterior mediastinum (Fig. 13.2). Often, the caudal extent of such lesions is underestimated on plain films because they tend to blend with the cardiac silhouette. The cross-sectional display of CT with the administration of contrast material allows ready separation of the heart from anterior adenopathy above the diaphragm.

The aorticopulmonary window is that portion of the mediastinum encompassed by the aortic arch above and the left pulmonary artery below (Heitzman, 1977). This area contains the so-called ductus lymph nodes (lowest of the prevascular chain), usually one or two in number, which lie transversely along the superior margin of the pulmonary artery. Normally the pleural reflection between the aortic arch and left pulmonary artery is either slightly concave or relatively straight toward the left lung, or it is invisible (Blank and Castellino, 1980). A convex margin indicates lymphadenopathy involving either the ductus nodes or occasionally the inferior nodes of the left tracheobronchial chain (Blank and Castellino, 1972, 1980; Heitzman et al., 1975) (Fig. 13.3). On CT, this area normally contains only areolar tissue and fat. Therefore, any rounded soft tissue density greater than 1 cm within the aorticopulmonary window indicates an enlarged lymph node (Fig. 13.4).

In bronchogenic carcinoma, metastases to lymph nodes in the anterior mediastinum are rather uncommon (McCort and Robbins, 1951), but lymph nodes on the left side in the aorticopulmonary window are often involved when spread comes from left upper lobe cancers (Fig. 13.4). Such patients may present with hoarseness due to recurrent laryngeal nerve paralysis. Identification of such involvement is important because this area is inaccessible during mediastinoscopy. In metastatic disease from extrathoracic tumors, only one-fourth of the cases in McLoud et al.'s (1978) series showed involvement of anterior mediastinal lymph nodes, usually in association with enlargement of other lymph node groups. Involvement of anterior mediastinal nodes occurs more frequently in Hodgkin's than in non-Hodgkin's lymphoma (Filly et al., 1976). In Filly et al.'s (1976) study of 164 patients with Hodgkin's disease, 67% had radiographic evidence of intrathoracic disease, and 46% had anterior mediastinal lymphadenopathy. The anterior compartment was the most frequently noted area of single lymph node group involvement. Among the 136 patients with non-Hodgkin's lymphoma, 43% showed evidence of intrathoracic involvement; only 13% had enlargement of anterior mediastinal nodes.

## Paratracheal Lymph Nodes

The right paratracheal lymph nodes are in contact with the right mediastinal pleura. If enlarged, they are easily seen projecting into the air-filled medial margin of the right upper lobe on a standard posteroanterior chest roentgenogram (McCort and Robbins, 1951; Heitzman et al., 1971; Heitzman, 1977) (Fig. 13.5). The nodal mass may be smooth or lobulated and may be associated with distortion of the trachea. Normally, a line of soft tissue density, the right paratracheal stripe, is produced by contact of the lung with the right lateral wall of the trachea. The width of the paratracheal line should not exceed 4 mm (Savoca et al., 1977). In the presence of adenopathy, this stripe may be widened or obliterated.

The azygos node is the lowest member of the right paratracheal chain. The position of this node varies somewhat with the azygos vein, which lies in the angle formed by the trachea and the right main bronchus (Heitzman et al., 1971; Heitzman, 1977; Blank and Castellino, 1980). Any density in that angle greater than 10 mm should be considered abnormal (Fraser and Pare, 1978) (Fig. 13.6). Distinction between an enlarged azygos vein and azygos adenopathy is not difficult. This vein responds to changes in posture and intrathoracic pressure. On fluoroscopic examination, an enlarged azygos vein will decrease in size during a sustained Valsalva maneuver.

The left paratracheal group of lymph nodes is difficult to delineate on standard radiographs because this chain lies medially and posteriorly to the aortic arch and the left subclavian artery (McCort and Robbins, 1951). These nodes are smaller and fewer than those in the right paratracheal chain (Rouviere, 1938; McCort and Robbins, 1951). Widening of the superior me-

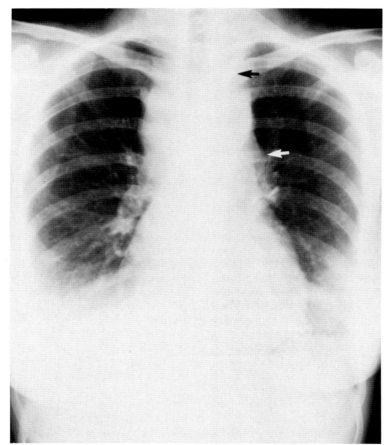

FIGURE 13.3. FIFTY-YEAR-OLD WOMAN WITH CHRONIC LYMPHOCYTIC LEUKEMIA AND BILATERAL MEDIASTINAL
ADENOPATHY
   Enlarged nodes in the aorticopulmonary window produce convexity of the pleural reflection between the aortic arch and
the left pulmonary artery (*lower arrow*). *Upper arrow* points to enlarged left prevascular nodes widening the pleural reflection
over the left subclavian artery. (From McLoud TC, Meyer JE: Mediastinal metastases. *Radiol Clin North Am* 20:453–467,
1982.)

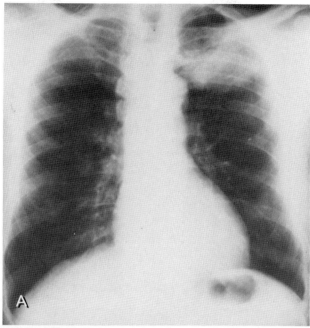

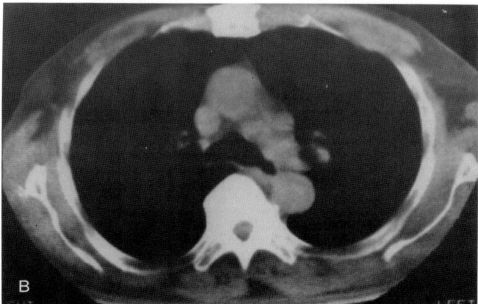

FIGURE 13.4. LARGE MASS IN THE LEFT UPPER LOBE

*A*: Posteroanterior radiograph shows no evidence of enlarged nodes. *B*: CT scan shows two enlarged lymph nodes in the aorticopulmonary window. Metastatic tumor from the primary bronchogenic carcinoma in the left upper lobe was proven at surgery.

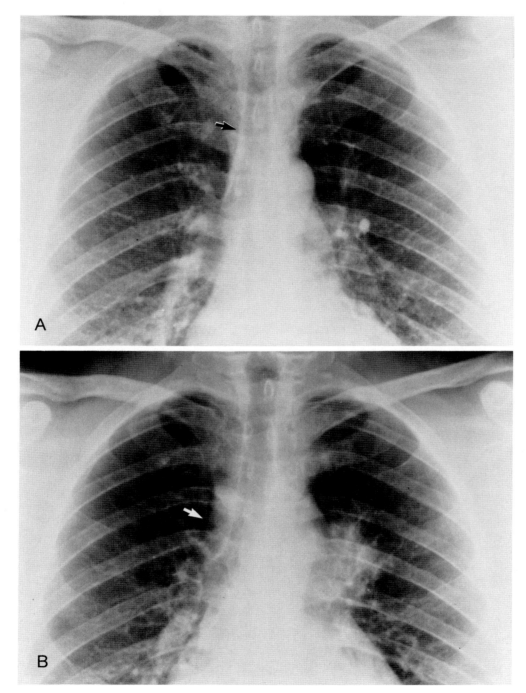

FIGURE 13.5. RIGHT PARATRACHEAL ADENOPATHY IN A 40-YR-OLD MAN WITH HODGKIN'S DISEASE DEMONSTRATED BY PROGRESSIVE ALTERATION IN THE RIGHT PARATRACHEAL PLEURAL REFLECTION

*A*: The right paratracheal stripe is of normal width (*arrow*). *B*: One year later it is markedly widened (*arrow*). There is also left hilar adenopathy.

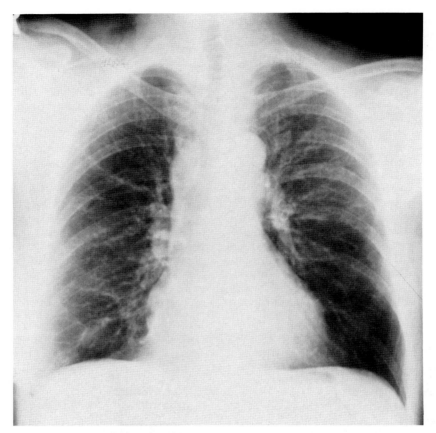

FIGURE 13.6. THIS 59-YR-OLD WOMAN HAD UNDERGONE LEFT RADICAL MASTECTOMY FOR BREAST CARCINOMA 7 YR PREVIOUSLY

Enlarged azygos node. Proven metastatic lesion from the breast at mediastinoscopy. (From McLoud et al., 1978.)

diastinum on the left on the posteroanterior view or on anteroposterior tomography is usually secondary to left prevascular adenopathy because these nodes lie more laterally than the left paratracheal group and will, therefore, become visible at an earlier stage of enlargement. Barium esophagrams may aid differentiation of the two groups. When sufficiently enlarged, left paratracheal lymph nodes will indent the left lateral margin of the esophagus or the trachea (Fig. 13.2) (McCort and Robbins, 1951).

CT is particularly useful in detection of paratracheal lymphadenopathy, especially in the azygos area. Schnyder and Gamsu (1981) reported that normal lymph nodes in the pretracheal retrocaval space can be seen on CT examination in 80% of subjects. They found CT to be useful (*a*) in clarifying the nature of an abnormality in the azygos region identified on chest radiographs and (*b*) in detecting subtle but significant azygos node enlargement not evident on plain films.

The paratracheal chains on both sides are common sites of metastatic spread from bronchogenic carcinoma. Lesions in the right upper, right middle, and superior segment of the right lower lobe commonly drain to the right paratracheal chain. Similarly, on the left side, left upper lobe tumors and those arising from the superior region of the left lower lobe drain into the left paratracheal area. Crossover may occur via the subcarinal nodes to the right paratracheal chain from left lower lobe cancers (McCort and Robbins, 1951). Among patients with metastatic disease to mediastinal lymph nodes from extrathoracic neoplasms, the right paratracheal chain was the most frequently involved lymph node group (60%) (McLoud et al., 1978). Bilateral paratracheal adenopathy was noted in 25%. Paratracheal adenopathy is commonly identified in patients with lymphoma, particularly Hodgkin's disease. In Filly et al.'s (1976) series, 40% of the 164 patients with newly diagnosed Hodgkin's disease had adenopathy in this region; only 13% of those with non-Hodgkin's lymphoma had similar involvement.

## Subcarinal Adenopathy

Subcarinal or bifurcation nodes are often difficult to detect until they are moderately enlarged. Widening of the carinal angle is not considered a reliable index of the presence of adenopathy in this area unless the adenopathy is massive (Fig. 13.7) (McCort and Robbins, 1951). Enlarged subcarinal nodes do intrude into the cephalad portion of the azygoesophageal recess, however, and displace it posteriorly and to the right. Such a finding can occasionally be identified on a well penetrated posteroanterior roentgenogram, but tomography is usually required for confirmation (Fig. 13.8). A normal configuration of the azygoesophageal line does not exclude subcarinal adenopathy because nodal masses 1–2 cm in diameter may fail to alter the configuration of the recess (Heitzman et al., 1971). Esophagography is particularly useful in establishing enlargement of the posterior group of subcarinal nodes. A smooth impression on the anterior wall of the middle third of the barium-filled esophagus is diagnostic (McCort and Robbins, 1951; Fleischner and Sachesse, 1963).

Detection of subcarinal adenopathy has been greatly facilitated by CT. Demonstration of the mediastinum in transverse projection allows easy recognition of enlarged nodes as they encroach on the lung in the upper portion of the azygoesophageal recess, under and behind the right main and intermediate bronchus (Heitzman et al., 1977) (Fig. 13.9). The subcarinal lymph nodes are frequently involved in patients with bronchogenic carcinoma, particularly those arising in the lower lobes of both lungs. The posterior group of subcarinal lymph nodes is not accessible during staging mediastinoscopy. Therefore, radiological recognition of nodal enlargement in this area

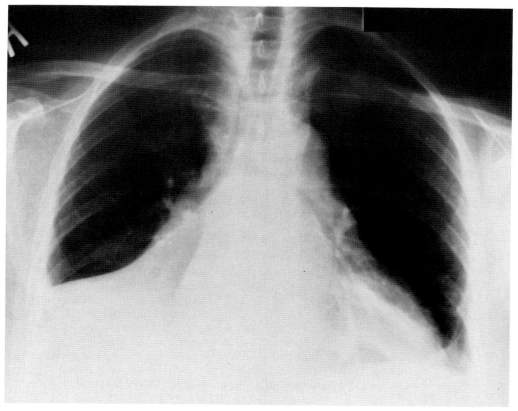

FIGURE 13.7. MALIGNANT MELANOMA METASTATIC TO THE MEDIASTINUM IN A 45-YR-OLD MAN
Massive subcarinal adenopathy with splaying and elevation of the carina is evident. Combined right middle and lower lobe atelectasis resulted from compression of the intermediate bronchus. (From McLoud TC, Meyer JE: Mediastinal metastases. *Radiol Clin North Am* 20:453–467, 1982.)

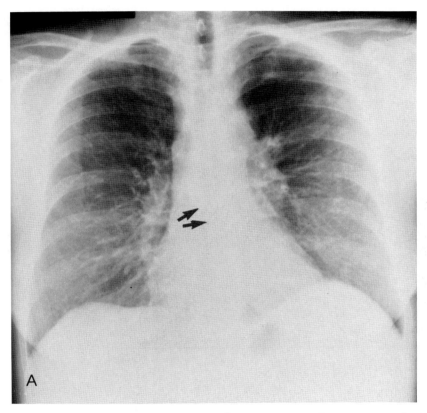

FIGURE 13.8. SUBCARINAL ADENOPATHY IN A 54-YR-OLD WOMAN WITH BRONCHOGENIC CARCINOMA
*A*: There is a left hilar mass. In addition, there is loss of the cephalad portion of the azygoesophageal recess (*arrows*). *B*: Overpenetrated view after mediastinoscopy more clearly delineates subcarinal nodes intruding into the azygoesophageal recess (*arrows*). *C*: Barium swallow in the right anterior oblique projection. There is a smooth extrinsic impression on the anterior wall of the esophagus. (From McLoud TC, Meyer JE: Mediastinal metastases. *Radiol Clin North Am* 20:453–467, 1982.)

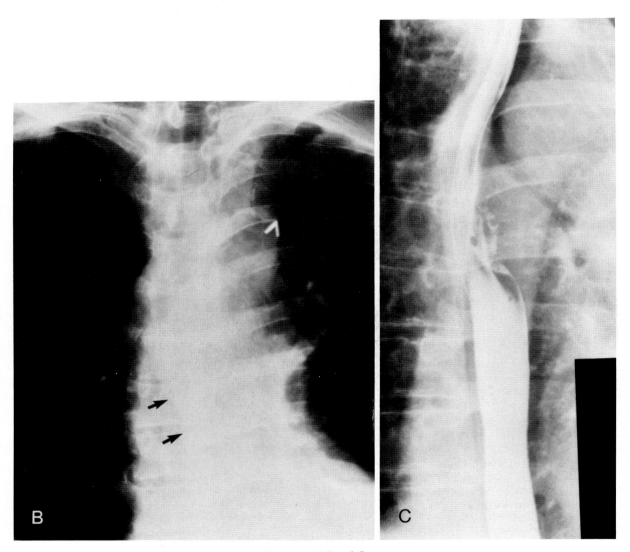

FIGURE 13.8*B* and *C*.

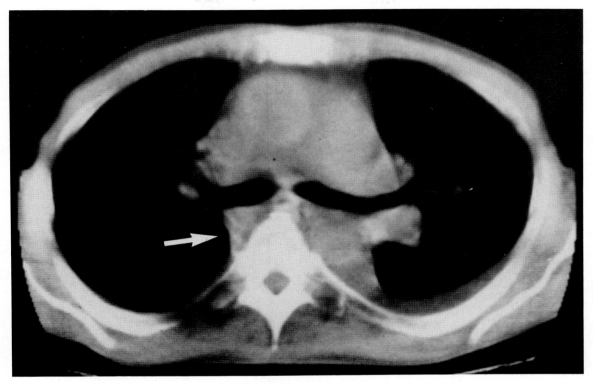

FIGURE 13.9. WIDESPREAD METASTATIC THYROID CARCINOMA IN A 54-YR-OLD MAN
CT scan shows subcarinal (*arrow*) and left hilar adenopathy. There is also a left pleural effusion.

either on barium esophagram or CT scanning is extremely important. These nodes are infrequently involved in patients with metastatic disease to the mediastinum and also in patients with thoracic lymphoma (Filly et al., 1976; McLoud et al., 1978). The prevalence of adenopathy in this area is probably underestimated, however, because subcarinal nodes are not clearly visible on the standard posteroanterior and lateral chest films.

## Posterior Mediastinal Lymph Nodes

These nodes extend caudally adjacent to the esophagus from the level of the inferior pulmonary veins to the diaphragmatic hiatus (Rouviere, 1938). Lymphadenopathy is manifest on the posteroanterior roentgenogram of the chest by subtle or gross widening and lobulation in the normally straight contours of the paramediastinal reflection adjacent to the dorsal spine (Blank and Castellino, 1980). Subtle lobulations in the contour of the pleural reflections in the posterior mediastinum are visible on adequately positioned and penetrated roentgenograms (Fig. 13.10).

CT scans of the lower thorax and upper abdomen are particularly useful in assessment of

paraspinal lymph node enlargement. The cross-sectional display allows demonstration of the diaphragmatic crura as they pass from the lateral aspects of the vertebral bodies to the adjacent surface of the aorta. Normal retrocrural structures include the aorta, nerves, azygos vein, thoracic duct, and lymph nodes. Any structure other than the aorta that is 6 mm or greater in diameter should be considered an enlarged lymph node (Callen et al., 1977) (Fig. 13.10).

Posterior mediastinal lymphadenopathy is rare in patients with bronchogenic carcinoma (McCort and Robbins, 1951) and uncommon in patients with mediastinal metastases (4% in McLoud's series) (Filly et al., 1976). In non-Hodgkin's lymphoma and Hodgkin's disease, the incidences are reported to be 10% and 5%, respectively (Filly et al., 1976; Blank and Castellino, 1980). Retrocrural lymphadenopathy in the lymphomas is often associated with para-aortic lymphadenopathy in the upper and middle abdomen (Callen et al., 1977).

## Diaphragmatic Lymph Nodes

These aggregates of lymphoid tissue are located either anterior or lateral to the pericardium and drain into the internal mammary lymph

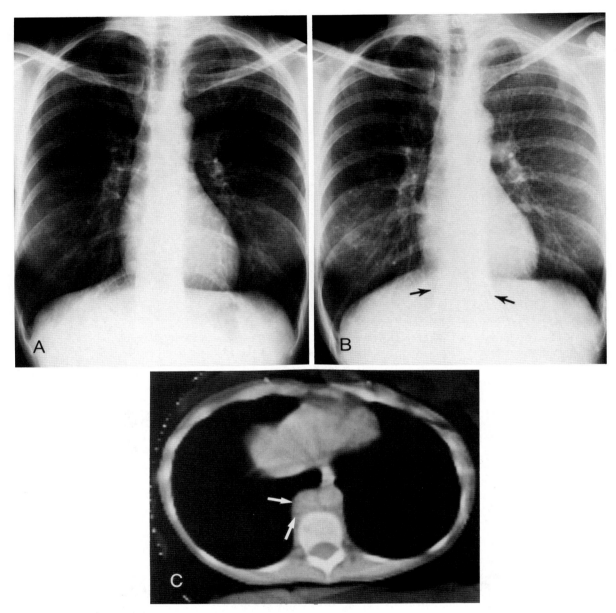

FIGURE 13.10. POSTERIOR MEDIASTINAL ADENOPATHY IN A PATIENT WITH CERVICAL CARCINOMA
*A*: Normal posteroanterior roentgenogram. *B*: One year later. Widening and lateral displacement of both paraspinal lines.
*C*: CT confirms the presence of retrocrural lymphadenopathy. Nodal metastases were also observed in the upper abdomen.
(From McLoud TC, Meyer JE: Mediastinal metastases. *Radiol Clin North Am* 20:453–467, 1982.)

node chain. When enlarged, they produce abnormalities visible on posteroanterior roentgenograms of the chest as convex bulges at the cardiophrenic angles (Castellino and Blank, 1972) (Fig. 13.11). Normal fat deposits cause considerable anatomic variation in this area and obscure the etiology of roentgenographic abnormalities. In this setting, when either lymphadenopathy is suspected or a baseline examination is desired, lymphadenopathy can be discriminated from lipomatous tissue with CT.

Primary bronchogenic carcinoma and extrathoracic metastases involving diaphragmatic lymph nodes are extremely rare. In patients with

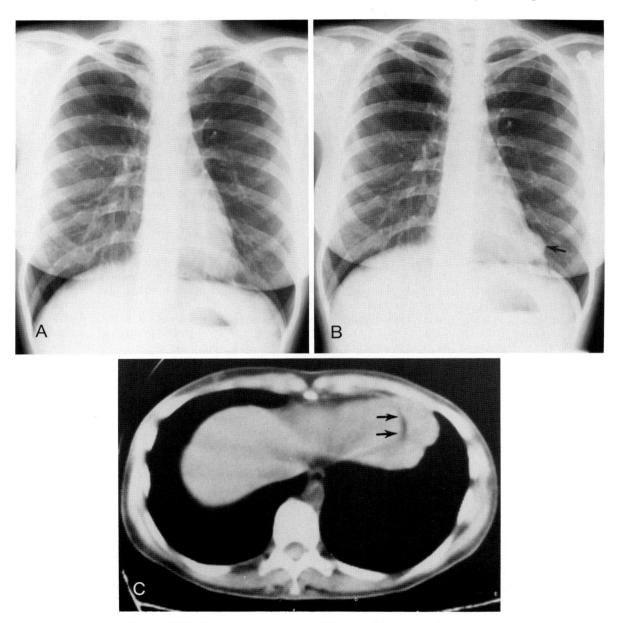

FIGURE 13.11. DIAPHRAGMATIC LYMPH NODES IN MALIGNANT LYMPHOMA
*A*: Posteroanterior chest roentgenogram shows that the left cardiac border is slightly irregular. *B*: One year later, there is a nodular bulge in the left cardiophrenic angle (*arrow*). *C*: CT scan at this time confirms the presence of enlarged paracardiac nodes (*arrows*). The mass is larger than expected from the chest radiograph. (From McLoud TC, Meyer JE: Mediastinal metastases. *Radiol Clin North Am* 20:453–467, 1982.)

Hodgkin's disease enlargement of cardiophrenic nodes is often noted during relapse of the disease (Castellino and Blank, 1972). One possible explanation is that these regions are not included in the radiotherapy field or that they do not receive the maximum dose due to marginal location in the treatment field (Castellino and Blank, 1972).

## Internal Mammary Lymph Nodes

Autopsy studies have shown the presence of three to five lymph nodes on either side of the sternum; the highest concentration is in the first three intercostal spaces located within 3 cm of the lateral sternal margin (Haagensen, 1971). Internal lymphadenopathy is seen most commonly in breast carcinoma and may be visible on the lateral roentgenogram as a retrosternal mass (Fig. 13.12). Delineation of these nodes on frontal radiographs, even when supplemented with tomography, is quite unusual.

Accurate assessment of the presence of internal mammary lymphadenopathy requires CT (Fig. 13.12). Besides being more sensitive in detection of these abnormalities, CT can reliably demonstrate the size, contour, bilaterality, adjacent anatomic contours, and any accompanying bone destruction (Meyer and Muzenrider, 1981). This information is quite useful in planning radiation therapy.

Except in patients with breast carcinoma, metastases to internal mammary nodes are extremely rare (McLoud et al., 1978). Adenopathy in this area occurs in fewer than 10% of patients with lymphoma (Filly et al., 1976; Blank and Castellino, 1980) and is extremely rare in bronchogenic carcinoma.

## Hilar Lymph Nodes

Enlarged hilar lymph nodes, which occur at the points of bifurcation of the lobar and segmental bronchi, may produce a so-called potato-like configuration of mild to moderate lobulation of the hilar structures (Fig. 13.13). Less frequently, adenopathy produces a nonspecific hilar prominence on standard posteroanterior and lateral chest roentgenograms and may be difficult to distinguish from prominent pulmonary arteries. Linear tomography may be quite helpful in this situation. Specifically, 55° oblique tomography of the hilus has been recommended (Favez et al., 1975; McLeod et al., 1976). This projection reveals the bronchi in profile and permits distinction between vascular shadows and adenopathy by demonstrating enlarged nodes and their characteristic location in the bronchial angles. Enlargement of hilar nodes can also be assessed with CT. Usually thin sections are required, and contrast may be necessary to differentiate enlarged nodes from vascular structures.

Metastasis to hilar nodes occurs frequently in bronchogenic carcinoma. The hilar nodes are usually the first site of involvement, particularly in tumors arising in the middle portions of the lungs. Metastasis to hilar nodes from extrathoracic neoplasms may be either bilateral and symmetrical or unilateral with or without mediastinal adenopathy (McLoud et al., 1978).

Hilar adenopathy is frequently noted in patients with lymphoma, particularly Hodgkin's disease, in which 45% of patients may show hilar involvement at initial diagnosis (Filly et al., 1976; Blank and Castellino, 1980). Hilar involvement is unusual in these patients, however, in the absence of detectable mediastinal adenopathy.

# DIAGNOSTIC WORK-UP AND IMAGING PROCEDURES

## Bronchogenic Carcinoma

As mentioned previously, preoperative assessment of mediastinal and hilar metastases is important in the determination of resectability of bronchogenic carcinoma, but nodal enlargement can be malignant or benign, as in reactive hyperplasia. Therefore, mediastinal exploration usually must be performed for precise histological diagnosis. The radiologist's role, as a general rule, is limited to determining the location of suspected lymphadenopathy so that the appropriate surgical approach (i.e., cervical mediasti-

noscopy or anterior mediastinotomy) for mediastinal biopsy can be chosen.

Multiple imaging methods may be used to detect mediastinal lymphadenopathy. Standard chest radiographs are diagnostic in 50–75% of patients (Baker et al., 1974). Conventional tomography is more sensitive than standard films, particularly for demonstrating right paratracheal, left aorticopulmonary, and subcarinal adenopathy, regions outlined by contiguous aerated lung. A negative mediastinum on tomography does not exclude the presence of lymph node metastases, however, and false-negative rates as

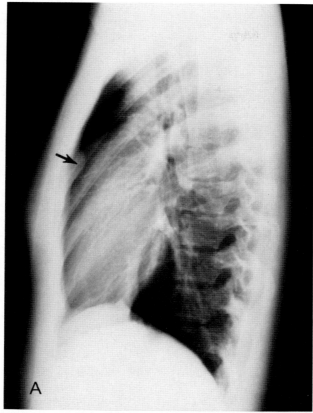

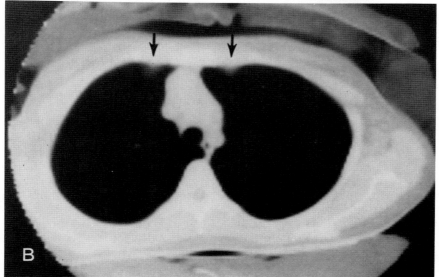

FIGURE 13.12. INTERNAL MAMMARY LYMPHADENOPATHY

*A*: The 3-cm oval retrosternal mass is secondary to a metastasis from known breast carcinoma (*arrow*). *B*: CT confirms the presence of internal mammary adenopathy (*arrows*). (From McLoud TC, Meyer JE: Mediastinal metastases. *Radiol Clin North Am* 20:453–467, 1982.)

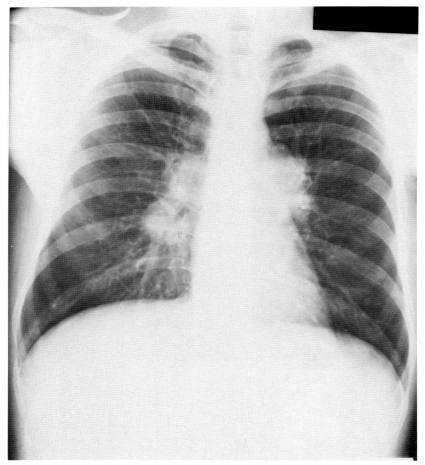

FIGURE 13.13. BILATERAL SYMMETRICAL HILAR ADENOPATHY PRODUCING ENLARGEMENT AND LOBULATION OF HILAR DENSITIES
Biopsy proved metastatic melanoma. (From McLoud et al., 1978.)

high as 30% have been reported (Mintzer et al., 1979). Barium esophagrams have been used to demonstrate mediastinal lymphadenopathy, particularly in the subcarinal region. Enlarged posterior subcarinal nodes create a smooth extrinsic compression on the anterior wall of the esophagus. Detection of such nodes is important because they are beyond the reach of the mediastinoscope.

Because of its cross-sectional imaging and improved contrast resolution between different tissues, CT has advantages over conventional techniques in the detection of mediastinal adenopathy. CT now appears to be the imaging method of choice for radiological staging of bronchogenic carcinoma, although some controversy still exists. One major problem has been definition of the size of abnormal lymph nodes (Faling et al., 1981; Osborne et al., 1982). Nodes greater than

2 cm are invariably abnormal, while nodes 1 cm or less are considered to be of normal size. The intermediate range of 1–2 cm is often indeterminate. Secondly, like other radiological techniques, CT lacks tissue specificity. It cannot distinguish lymph node enlargement due to a reactive process from that due to tumor metastasis. CT will also fail to detect intracapsular spread of metastatic disease in lymph nodes of normal size.

Several studies have addressed the role of CT in the detection of mediastinal metastases from bronchogenic carcinoma. Shevland et al. (1978) compared CT to conventional tomography in the assessment of resectability in 37 patients with suspected bronchogenic carcinoma. They found 16 correct positives and 18 correct negatives on CT compared with 13 correct positives and 18 correct negatives on conventional tomography.

However, there were also one false-positive and two false-negatives on CT. In addition, only 5 of the 16 correct positives were proven by mediastinoscopy and biopsy. Osborne et al. (1982) evaluated 42 patients with $T_2$ bronchogenic carcinoma by means of plain radiography, conventional tomography, and CT scans to compare their accuracy in assessing mediastinal and hilar nodal metastases. Definitive staging was achieved by thoracotomy. In the 25 patients with hilar or mediastinal adenopathy, CT of the mediastinum was more sensitive (94% true-positive ratio) but not more specific than the other two, and conventional tomography was no more accurate for hilar evaluation. The authors concluded that CT was not accurate enough for routine staging, and, therefore, surgical staging is still necessary. Faling et al. (1981) found that CT scans accurately predicted mediastinal neoplastic adenopathy in 15 of 17 patients with bronchogenic carcinoma who had surgically proven mediastinal metastases, yielding a sensitivity of 88%; their specificity was also high at 94% with a true-negative scan in 32 of 34 instances.

Because of the ambiguity of these results and the known lack of specificity of CT, it is reasonable to conclude that a patient should not be denied surgery without microscopic demonstration of tumor within nodes shown to be enlarged by CT. In most patients, this determination can be made by mediastinoscopy. In view of the high sensitivity of CT, however, the argument can be made that the absence of enlarged nodes precludes the need for staging mediastinoscopy. In such patients, even if microscopic metastases are detected in normal-sized nodes at the time of thoracotomy, resection in many instances can still be accomplished.

The choice of an ideal imaging modality for the detection of lymph node metastases in the hilus is also somewhat controversial. Some consider conventional tomography using 55° posterior angulation to be superior to CT (McLeod et al., 1976; Heitzman, 1981). Naidich et al. (1981) have reported, however, that CT can be extremely accurate in detection of hilar lymphadenopathy, particularly if thin sections and rapid scanning times are used. Contrast material may be necessary to differentiate enlarged pulmonary arteries from hilar nodes. Ipsilateral hilar lymph node involvement places the patient in an $N_1$ category in the staging of bronchogenic carcinoma. Such patients may be resectable, particularly if the tumor is squamous cell carcinoma.

There has been considerable interest in the use of gallium-67 citrate for imaging of mediastinal and hilar lymph nodes in the staging of pulmonary malignancies and lymphoma. The affinity of gallium-67 for both inflammatory and tumor lesions is well known. Uptake of $^{67}$Ga in primary bronchogenic carcinoma is reported to occur in 64–100% of patients (Grebe et al., 1971; Ito et al., 1971). In a review by Larson et al. (1975) of 280 reported cases of lung carcinoma, the prevalence of positive scans was 85%. Use of the $^{67}$Ga scan for assessing mediastinal and hilar metastases has been the subject of several recent reports. Fosburg et al. (1979) compared 70 positive $^{67}$Ga lung scans with chest roentgenograms, mediastinal tomograms, and endoscopic findings. Gallium-67 was more sensitive (88%) than mediastinal tomography (81%) and chest roentgenography (75%) in assessing mediastinal metastases. Citing this study, several authors have suggested that the $^{67}$Ga scan can be used to determine which patients should undergo mediastinoscopy (Peters, 1977; Alazraki et al., 1978; Fosburg et al., 1979). If the primary tumor concentrates gallium and the mediastinum does not, the patient may be spared a staging mediastinoscopy and be referred directly for thoracotomy; if both the primary lesion and the mediastinum take up gallium or if the primary lesion does not concentrate gallium, the patient should undergo a staging mediastinoscopy. However, this approach is still debatable (Bekerman et al., 1980). More recent reports have been unable to duplicate these initial results: Gallium scanning had a sensitivity of 60% or less when compared to pathological findings obtained at thoracotomy or mediastinoscopy (DeMeester et al., 1979; Hirleman et al., 1980).

## Thoracic Lymphoma

CT is the method of choice in the diagnostic work-up of patients with lymphoma whenever mediastinal adenopathy is suspected on the chest roentgenogram. Experience has demonstrated that CT permits more precise localization of disease as well as more accurate determination of extent of involvement. Extension of lymphoma into the pulmonary parenchyma can also be detected.

Several studies have documented the impact of CT in planning radiation treatment of lymphoma and bronchogenic carcinoma in the thorax (Goitein et al., 1979; Hobday et al., 1979; Muzenrider et al., 1979). CT more clearly delineates tumor extent, changing the assessment of the size of lesions and, thus, the volume of tissue irradiated (Emami et al., 1978). One of the most striking examples of this application is the presence of subtle lateral soft tissue extension from the mediastinum, which is not discernible by any other diagnostic method and is probably the cause for local failure in some patients treated primarily with radiotherapy.

Posteroanterior and lateral chest roentgenograms should be taken every 3–6 months for follow-up of patients with lymphoma. Again, CT is recommended for monitoring the initial response to radiation therapy.

In lymphoma, gallium-67 citrate scans have proved useful in the detection of sites of involvement above the diaphragm (Larson et al., 1973). Studies already performed and in progress show that gallium is a sensitive but nonspecific indicator of hilar and mediastinal involvement in such patients (Bekerman et al., 1980). Accordingly, routine gallium scans are not recommended; instead they should be used selectively to elucidate special problems in the mediastinum.

## Metastasis from Extrathoracic Neoplasms

Because metastases to mediastinal lymph nodes from extrathoracic neoplasms are relatively rare, screening posteroanterior and lateral chest roentgenograms are probably sufficient in patients with tumors with a propensity to metastasize to this area. Follow-up films should be obtained at regular intervals, preferably every 6 months. Alterations in mediastinal contour by comparison with old films require attention. If an abnormality is suspected, other imaging procedures may be required. Although CT is the method of choice in the evaluation of suspected mediastinal adenopathy, it is not recommended as a screening procedure in the search for mediastinal metastases. In many such patients with extrathoracic neoplasms, however, it will be used to search for parenchymal lung metastases. In such instances, the mediastinum should be carefully evaluated at the same sitting.

# REFERENCES

Alazraki NP, Ramsdell JW, Taylor A, Friedman PJ, Peters RM, Tisi GM: Reliability of gallium scan, chest radiography compared with mediastinoscopy for evaluating mediastinal spread in lung cancer. *Am Rev Resp Dis* 117:415–420, 1978.

Armstrong JD, Bragg DG: Radiology in lung cancer: problems and prospects. *Cancer* 25:246–263, 1975.

Baker RR, Stitik FP, Summer WR: Preoperative evaluation in patients with suspected bronchogenic carcinoma. *Curr Probl Surg* 1–48, December 1974.

Baltaxe HA, Constable WC: Mediastinal lymph node visualization in the absence of intrathoracic disease. *Radiology* 90:94–99, 1968.

Bein ME, Putman CE, McLoud TC, Mink JH: A reevaluation of intrathoracic lymphadenopathy in sarcoidosis. *AJR* 131:409–415, 1978.

Bekerman C, Hoffer PB, Bitran JD, Gupta RG: Gallium-67 citrate imaging studies of the lung. *Semin Nucl Med* 10:286–301, 1980.

Bergh NP, Schersten T: Bronchogenic carcinoma: a follow-up study of a surgically treated series with special reference to the prognostic significance of lymph node metastasis. *Acta Chir Scand (Suppl)* 347:1–42, 1965.

Berkmen YM, Javors BR: Anterior mediastinal adenopathy in sarcoidosis. *AJR* 127:983–987, 1976.

Blank N, Castellino RA: Patterns of pleural reflections of the left superior mediastinum. *Radiology* 102:585–589, 1972.

Blank N, Castellino R: The intrathoracic manifestations of the malignant lymphomas and leukemias. *Semin Roentgenol* 15:227–245, 1980.

Callen PW, Korobkin M, Isherwood I: Computed tomographic evaluation of the retrocrural prevertebral space. *AJR* 129:907–910, 1977.

Carr DT, Mountain CF: The staging of lung cancer. *Semin Oncol* 1:229–234, 1974.

Castellino R, Blank N: Adenopathy of the cardiophrenic angle (diaphragmatic) lymph nodes. *AJR* 114:509–515, 1972.

DeMeester TR, Golomb HM, Kirchner P, Rezai-Zadeh K, Bitran JD, Streeter DL, Hoffman PC, Cooper M: The role of gallium-67 scanning in the clinical staging and preoperative evaluation of patients with carcinoma of the lung. *Ann Thorac Surg* 28:451–464, 1979.

Emami B, Melo A, Carter BL, Munzenrider JE, Piro AJ: The value of computed tomography in radiotherapy of lung cancer. *AJR* 131:63–68, 1978.

Faling LJ, Pugatch RD, Jung-Legg Y, Daly BD Jr, Hong WK, Robbins AH, Snider GL: Computed tomographic scanning of the mediastinum in the staging of bronchogenic carcinoma. *Am Rev Respir Dis* 124:690–695, 1981.

Favez G, Willa C, Heinzer F: Posterior oblique tomography at an angle of 55 degrees in chest roentgenology. *AJR* 120:907–915, 1975.

Filly R, Blank N, Castellino RA: Radiographic distribution of intrathoracic disease in previously untreated patients with Hodgkin's disease and non-Hodgkin's lymphoma. *Radiology* 120:277–281, 1976.

Fleischner FG, Sachesse E: Retrotracheal lymphadenopathy in bronchial carcinoma revealed by the barium filled esophagus. *AJR* 90:792–798, 1963.

Fosburg RG, Hopkins GB, Kan MK: Evaluation of the mediastinum by gallium-67 scintigraphy in lung cancer. *J Thorac Cardiovasc Surg* 77:76–82, 1979.

Fraser RG, Pare JAP: *Diagnoses of Diseases of the Chest*, ed 2. Philadelphia, WB Saunders, 1978.

Goitein M, Wittenberg J, Mendiondo M, Doucette J, Friedberg C, Ferrucci J, Gunderson L, Linggood R, Shepley WU, Fineberg HV: The value of CT scanning in radiation therapy treatment planning: a prospective study. *Int J Radiat Oncol Biol Phys* 5:1787–1798, 1979.

Goldberg EM, Shapiro CM, Glicksman HS: Mediastinoscopy for assessing mediastinal spread in clinical staging of lung carcinoma. *Semin Oncol* 1:205–215, 1974.

Grant T, Levin B: Lymphangiographic visualization of pleural and pulmonary lymphatics in a patient without chylothorax. *Radiology* 113:49–50, 1974.

Grebe SF, Steckenmeser R, Romer M: Radioaktive gallium-

67 in der nuklearmedizinischen Tumordiagnostik. *Munch Med Wochenschr* 113:238–244, 1971.

Haagensen CD: *Diseases of the Breast*. Philadelphia, WB Saunders, 1971.

Handley RS, Thackray AC: The internal mammary lymph chain in carcinoma of the breast: a study of 50 cases. *Lancet* 2:276–278, 1949.

Heitzman ER: *The Mediastinum*. St Louis, CV Mosby, 1977.

Heitzman ER: Computed tomography of the thorax. Current perspectives. *AJR* 136:2–12, 1981.

Heitzman ER, Scrivani JV, Martino J, Moro J: The azygos vein and its pleural reflections. *Radiology* 101:259–266, 1971.

Heitzman ER, Lane EJ, Hammack DB, Rimmier LJ: Radiological evaluation of the aortic-pulmonic window. *Radiology* 116:513–518, 1975.

Heitzman ER, Goldwin RL, Proto AV: Radiologic analysis of the mediastinum utilizing computed tomography. *Radiol Clin North Am* 15:309–329, 1977.

Hirleman MT, Yiu-Chiu VS, Chiu LC, Schapiro RL: The resectability of primary lung carcinoma: a diagnostic staging review. *CT* 4:146–163, 1980.

Hobday P, Hodson NJ, Husband J, Parker RP, Macdonald JS: Computed tomography applied to radiotherapy treatment planning: techniques and results. *Radiology* 133:477–482, 1979.

Ito Y, Okuyama S, Awano T, Takahashi K, Sato T, Kanno I: Diagnostic evaluation of [67]Ga scanning in lung cancer and other diseases. *Radiology* 101:355–362, 1971.

Kaplan HS: Essentials of staging and management of malignant lymphomas. *Semin Roentgenol* 15:219–226, 1980.

Larson SM, Milder MS, Johnston GS: Interpretation of [67]Ga photoscan. *J. Nucl Med* 14:208–214, 1973.

Larson SM, Milder MS, Johnston GS: Tumor-seeking radiopharmaceuticals: gallium-67. In Subramanian G, Rhodes BA, Cooper JF (eds): *Radiopharmaceuticals*. New York, Society of Nuclear Medicine, 1975, pp 413–432.

McCort JJ, Robbins LL: Roentgen diagnosis of intrathoracic lymph node metastases in carcinoma of the lung. *Radiology* 57:339–359, 1951.

McLeod RA, Brown LR, Miller WE, DeRenee RA: Evaluation of the pulmonary hila by tomography. *Radiol Clin North Am* 14:51–84, 1976.

McLoud TC, Kalisher L, Stark P, Greene R: Intrathoracic lymph node metastases from extrathoracic neoplasms. *AJR* 131:403–407, 1978.

Meyer JE, Muzenrider J: Computed tomographic demonstration of internal mammary node metastases in patients with locally recurrent breast carcinoma. *Radiology* 139:661–663, 1981.

Mintzer RA, Malave SR, Neiman HL, Michaels LL, Vanecko RM, Sanders JH: Computed vs. conventional tomography in evaluation of primary and secondary pulmonary neoplasms. *Radiology* 132:653–659, 1979.

Mountain CF: Surgical therapy in lung cancer: biologic, physiologic, and technical determinants. *Semin Oncol* 1:253–258, 1974.

Mountain CF, Carr DT, Anderson WAD: Clinical staging of lung cancer. *AJR* 120:130–138, 1974.

Murray JF: *The Normal Lung: The Basis for Diagnosis and Treatment of Disease*. Philadelphia, WB Saunders, 1976.

Muzenrider JE, Pilepich M, Rene-Ferrero JB, Tchakarova I, Carter BL: Use of body scanner in radiotherapy treatment planning. *Cancer* 40:170–179, 1979.

Naidich DP, Khouri NF, Stitik FP, McCauley DI, Siegelman SS: Computed tomography of the pulmonary hila. Abnormal anatomy. *J Comput Assist Tomogr* 5:468–475, 1981.

Osborne DR, Korobkin M, Ravin CE, Putnam CE, Wolfe NG, Sealy WC, Young WG, Breiman R, Heaston D, Ram P, Halber M: Comparison of plain radiography, conventional tomography and computed tomography in detecting intrathoracic lymph node metastases from lung carcinoma. *Radiology* 142:157–161, 1982.

Peters R: Staging of lung cancer. *Chest* 71:633–634, 1977.

Rosenberger A, Haler O, Abrams HL: The thoracic duct: structural, functional and radiology aspects. *CRC Crit Rev Clin Radiol Nucl Med* 3:523–541, 1972.

Rouviere H: *Anatomy of the Human Lymphatic System* (translated by Tobias MJ). Ann Arbor, MI, Edwards Brothers, 1938.

Savoca CJ, Austin JHM, Golderg H: The right paratracheal stripe. *Radiology* 122:295–301, 1977.

Schnyder PA, Gamsu G: CT of the pretracheal retrocaval space. *AJR* 136:303–308, 1981.

Shevland JE, Chiu LC, Schapiro RL, Young JA, Rossi NP: The role of conventional tomography and computed tomography in assessing the resectability of primary lung cancer: a preliminary report. *CT* 2:1–19, 1978.

*TNM Classification of Malignant Tumors*. Geneva, International Union against Cancer and American Joint Committee on Cancer Staging and End Results Reporting, 1972.

# 14

# *Computed Tomography of Cervical Lymph Nodes*

DEBORAH L. REEDE, M.D., AND R. THOMAS BERGERON, M.D.

Prior to the era of computed tomography (CT), lymphangiography was used in attempts to visualize cervical lymph nodes. Lymphangiography can be performed either by directly instilling contrast medium into the lymphatics (Fisch and Sigel, 1964; Sigel, 1980) or by injecting contrast medium into the perilymphatic tissues (Gruart et al., 1967; Matoba and Kikuchi, 1969; Sachdeva et al., 1974). Although direct instillation provides clearer images than does indirect injection, the technique is difficult and this method still has limitations. In essence, filling defects in cervical lymph nodes may be seen in reactive as well as malignant nodes; thus, the lymphangiographic criteria used for assessment of lymph node disease in the abdomen (which are highly specific) are not directly applicable to cervical lymph node disease. In addition, large groups of metastatic or hyperplastic nodes proximal to the area of interest may prevent contrast agent from filling distal nodes or entire nodal groups, thus precluding a satisfactory study or even causing a false-negative interpretation. Radiation therapy, surgery, or inflammatory disease may alter or create new pathways by lymphaticolymphatic or lymphaticovenous shunts (Johner, 1970; Sigel, 1980). In sum, cervical lymphangiography for detection of occult cervical metastases has not gained acceptance because the procedure is both technically difficult and not always reliable.

As in the abdomen and chest, cervical nodes can be demonstrated with CT. Mancuso et al. (1981) were the first to report on the use of CT in evaluation of cervical lymph node metastases. They showed that CT could be used to detect clinically palpable nodes as well as to locate occult regional node metastases. Reede and Bergeron (1982) and Reede et al. (1982c) have reported the usefulness of CT in detecting regional metastatic disease and in staging head and neck tumors.

High resolution CT has dramatically improved the accuracy of staging head and neck tumors by providing a definition of the location and extent of the primary lesion with a single imaging modality. Additionally, CT scanning is capable of detecting clinically occult regional node metastasis.

Knowledge of the location of various cervical lymph node chains and the modes of disease spread in head and neck neoplasms is essential in evaluation of patients with head and neck tumors. A review of cervical nodal anatomy follows. Normal cervical lymph nodes are frequently not identifiable on CT; therefore, scans of diseased nodes are used to demonstrate the CT locations of the major cervical lymph node chains.

## NORMAL ANATOMY

The French anatomist, Rouvière (1938), divided lymph nodes of the head and neck into 10 principal groups (Fig. 14.1): occipital, mastoid, parotid, submandibular, facial, submental, sublingual, retropharyngeal, anterior cervical, and lateral cervical. The first six groups form a so-called pericervical lymph node ring at the junction between the head and neck (Fig. 14.2) (Rouviere, 1938). Sublingual and retropharyngeal nodes are located within this lymphoid ring. The anterior and lateral cervical nodes descend anteriorly and laterally in the neck.

### Occipital Nodes

These nodes are located at the junction between the neck and cranial wall. Their three groups are named according to their location: superficial (Fig. 14.3), subfascial, and submuscular or subsplenius (deep occipital nodes). The

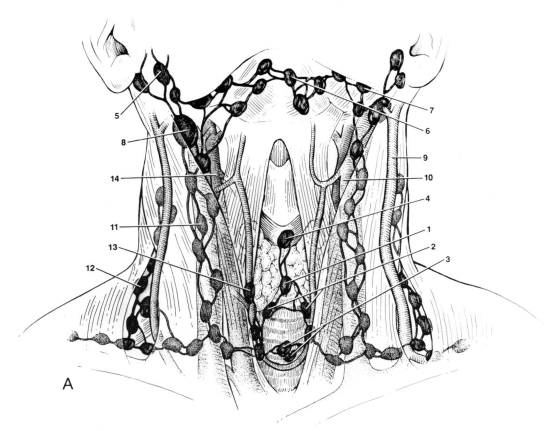

FIGURE 14.1. LYMPH NODE CHAINS IN THE HEAD AND NECK

*A*: Frontal view. *B*: Lateral view. *1*, Pretracheal nodes; *2*, paratracheal nodes; *3*, infraglandular nodes; *4*, prelaryngeal (Delphian) nodes; *5*, parotid nodes; *6*, submental nodes; *7*, submandibular nodes; *8*, jugulodigastric node; *9*, external jugular vein; *10*, internal jugular vein; *11*, internal jugular node; *12*, spinal accessory nodes; *13*, anterior jugular nodes; *14*, common carotid artery; *15*, transverse cervical nodes. *16*, mastoid nodes; *17*, occipital nodes; *18*, spinal accessory nerve; *19*, facial nodes. (From Reede DL, Bergeron RT, Whelan MA, Cohen NL, Persky MS: Computed tomography of cervical lymph nodes. *RadioGraphics* 3:339–351, 1983.)

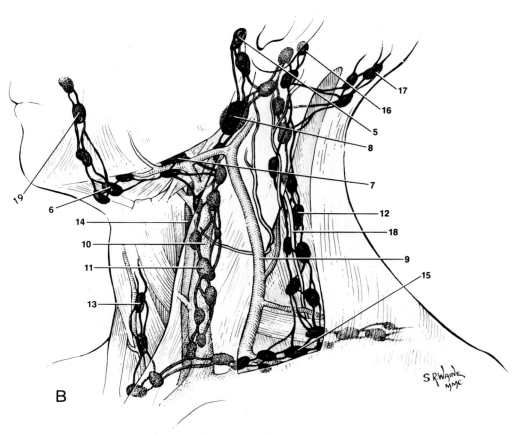

FIGURE 14.1*B*

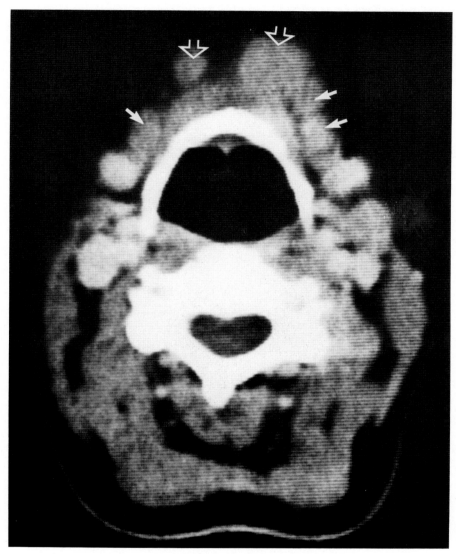

FIGURE 14.2. SUBMENTAL AND SUBMANDIBULAR NODES

Submental (*open arrows*) and submandibular nodes (*closed arrows*) forming a partial ring of enlarged lymphoid tissue around the anterior aspect of the neck. (Reactive nodes.)

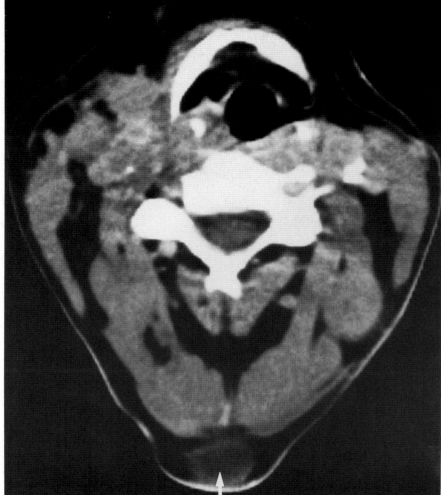

FIGURE 14.3. OCCIPITAL NODE

A low density node with rim enhancement (*arrow*) is visible just below the skin in the posterior aspect of the neck. Also note the multiple bilateral enlarged internal jugular nodes with rim enhancement. The carotid sheath structures cannot be identified. (Metastatic squamous cell carcinoma.)

afferent vessels drain lymph from the occipital region, and the efferent vessels direct flow primarily to the spinal accessory chain (Montgomery, 1971).

**Mastoid Nodes**

These nodes are located behind the ear. Their afferent vessels drain the parotid region and a portion of the auricular skin. Their efferent vessels travel to the intra-auricular parotid nodes and superior internal jugular nodes (Montgomery, 1971).

**Parotid Nodes**

Nodes in this group may be located either superficial to or within the gland itself and, thus, are termed *extraglandular* or *intraglandular* nodes (Feind, 1972). These nodes may be enlarged in benign processes, such as granulomatous disease (sarcoid and tuberculosis), as well as neoplastic processes, such as metastatic disease (Fig. 14.4) and lymphoma. Both intra- and extraglandular nodes are common sites for metastases from malignancies of the temple, scalp, ear, and, occasionally, the face, neck, and palate. The most common neoplasms to metastasize to this area are melanomas and squamous cell carcinomas (Cornog and Gray, 1976).

The afferent vessels for this group drain lymph from the midline, anteriorly over the forehead and upper face to the postauricular region. The efferent vessels drain directly or indirectly into the jugular chain (Montgomery, 1971).

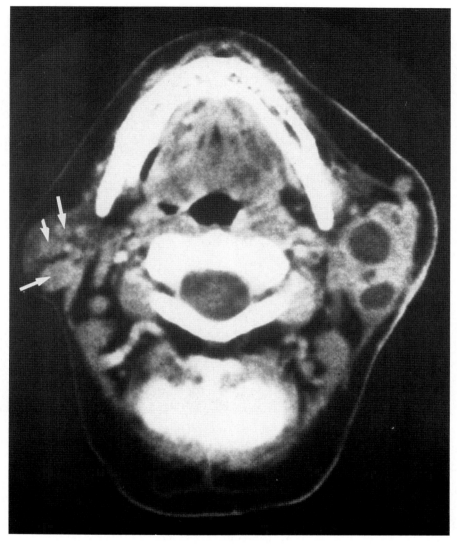

FIGURE 14.4. PAROTID NODES
Contrast CT scan demonstrating multiple low density nodes with rim enhancement in the region of the left parotid gland.
Several nonenhancing nodes are present in the region of the right parotid gland (*arrows*). (Metastatic squamous cell carcinoma.)

## Submandibular Nodes

These nodes are located in the submandibular (digastric) triangle along the inferior border of the mandible. They can be situated anywhere laterally, from insertion of the anterior belly of the digastric anteriorly and to the angle of the mandible posteriorly (Fig. 14.5) (Montgomery, 1981). On the basis of their location, these nodes can be divided into three groups: preglandular, prevascular, and retrovascular. Their afferent vessels drain the lateral chin, lower lip, cheeks, nose, mucosa of the anterior part of the nasal fossa, gums, teeth, soft and hard palate, tongue anterior to the lingual vein, submandibular gland, sublingual gland, and floor of the mouth. Their efferent vessels carry lymph to the internal jugular chain.

## Facial Nodes

These nodes lie in the subcutaneous tissues of the face and generally follow the course of the facial artery and vein. Their afferent vessels drain the upper and lower lids, nose, upper and lower lip, entire cheek, and, rarely, the gums and palate. Their efferent vessels drain to the submandibular nodes.

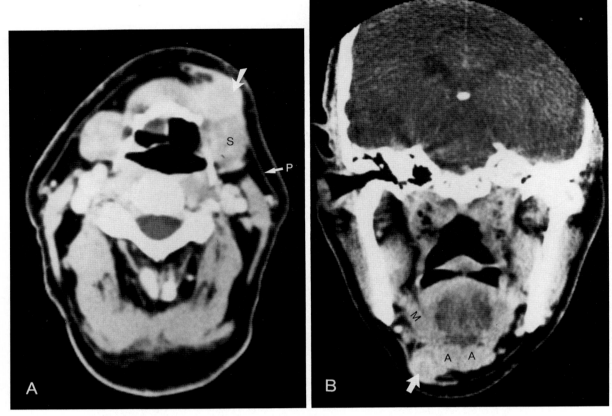

FIGURE 14.5. SUBMANDIBULAR NODES

Axial (*A*) and coronal (*B*) views demonstrate an enhancing left submandibular node (*large arrows*). This node is located lateral to the anterior belly of the digastric muscle (*A*) and mylohyoid muscle (*M*). The fascial planes between this node and the submandibular gland (*S*) and platysma (*P*) are obliterated. (Metastatic squamous cell carcinoma.)

## Submental Nodes

These nodes are positioned below the mylohyoid muscle in the submental triangle between the anterior bellies of the digastric muscles (Fig. 14.6). Small, clinically insignificant nodes are often seen in this area on CT scans. Their afferent vessels drain the chin, middle lower lip, cheeks, incisor region of the gums, anterior floor of the mouth, and tip of the tongue. Their efferent vessels carry lymph to the submandibular nodes and internal jugular chains. These vessels may cross to the opposite side (Montgomery, 1971).

## Sublingual Nodes

These nodes have two components, the lateral and median groups. The lateral nodes follow the course of the lingual vessels, and the median nodes are located between the genioglossus mus-

cles. Enlargement of these nodes is rarely appreciated on CT scans.

## Retropharyngeal Nodes

This chain consists of the median and lateral groups. The median group is located in the midline in direct continuity with the posterior wall of the nasopharynx. These nodes are positioned at about the level of the lateral masses of the second cervical vertebra.

In contradistinction to the median group, the lateral group runs the length of the pharynx. These nodes are lateral to the longus capitus and longus coli muscles (Fig. 14.7*A*) and, therefore, are in close proximity to the extracranial portions of cranial nerves IX, X, XI, and XII (Fig. 14.7*B*). Pathology in this area can produce cranial nerve palsies in any one of these nerves.

The afferent vessels to these nodes drain the

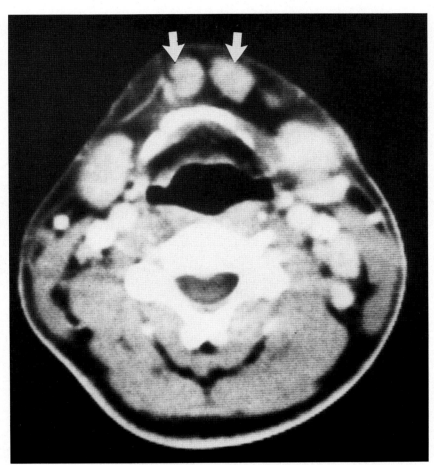

FIGURE 14.6. SUBMENTAL NODES
Nonenhancing submental nodes (*arrows*) are visible anterior to the hyoid bone. Several enhancing nodes are visible in the lateral cervical chains bilaterally. (Tuberculous adenitis.)

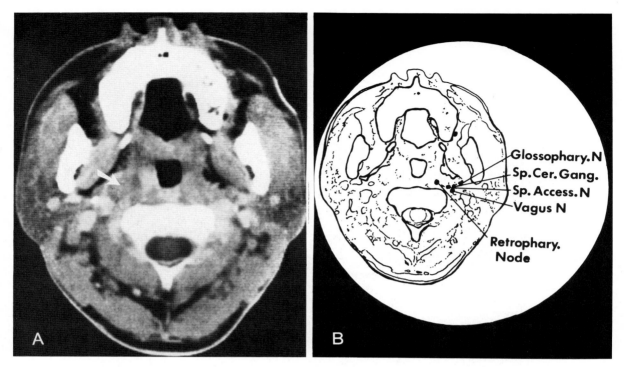

FIGURE 14.7. RETROPHARYNGEAL NODES

*A*: A low density lesion with rim enhancement (*arrow*) is visible in the right prevertebral area. This is a lateral retropharyngeal node in a patient with metastatic nasopharyngeal carcinoma. *B*: Note the close proximity of the lateral retropharyngeal nodes to the lower cranial nerves below the base of the skull. (From Reede DL, Bergeron RT, Whelan MA, Cohen NL, Persky MS: Computed tomography of cervical lymph nodes. *RadioGraphics* 3:339–351, 1983.)

nasal fossae, sinuses and nasopharynx, oropharynx, palate, and middle ear. The efferent vessels carry lymph to the internal jugular chain (Montgomery, 1971).

### Anterior Cervical Nodes

Nodes in this chain are located in the anterior triangle of the neck between the two carotid sheaths. This lymph node chain has superficial and deep components. The superficial portion (anterior jugular nodes) follows the course of the anterior jugular veins and, therefore, is located superficially to the strap muscles. The deep component of the anterior cervical nodes consists of a number of lymph node chains that are named for their relationship to the major anterior midline structures: prelaryngeal, pretracheal (Delphian nodes), prethyroid, and lateral tracheal (paratracheal) (Fig. 14.8).

The afferent vessels to these nodes drain the infraglottic larynx and thyroid. On the left side, the efferent vessels carry lymph to the internal jugular chain and terminate in the thoracic duct and/or left anterior mediastinal nodes. On the

right side the efferent vessels terminate in nodes located at the jugular-subclavian junction, inferior node of the internal jugular chain, or highest intrathoracic node on the right (Rouviere, 1938).

### Lateral Cervical Nodes

Since these nodes serve as the common route of drainage for all of the major regional structures (including the nasopharynx, larynx, tongue, tonsils, and thyroid), pathology is commonly encountered in this lymph node chain (Last, 1978). Like the anterior cervical nodes, this group also has both a superficial and deep component. The superficial nodes in this group (*external jugular chain*) follow the course of the external jugular vein and are, therefore, located superficial to the sternocleidomastoid muscle (Fig. 14.9). The nodes located in the deep portion of this group have three components: internal jugular, spinal accessory, and transverse cervical chains. This subgroup of nodes forms a triangle of nodes that has components in both the anterior and posterior triangles (Fig. 14.1*B*). *This is the most important group of nodes to recognize in*

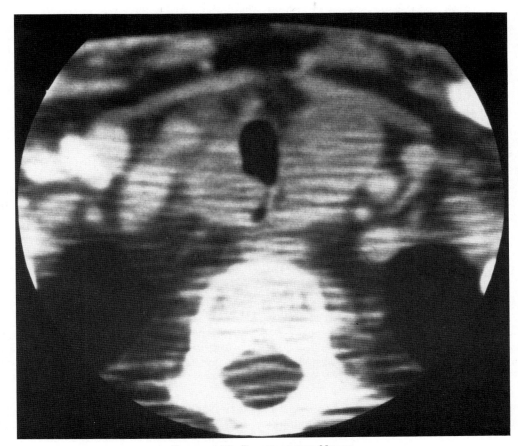

FIGURE 14.8. PARATRACHEAL NODES
Bilateral nonenhancing paratracheal nodes in this patient with Hodgkin's lymphoma are causing compression of the trachea. Note the intratracheal component on the right.

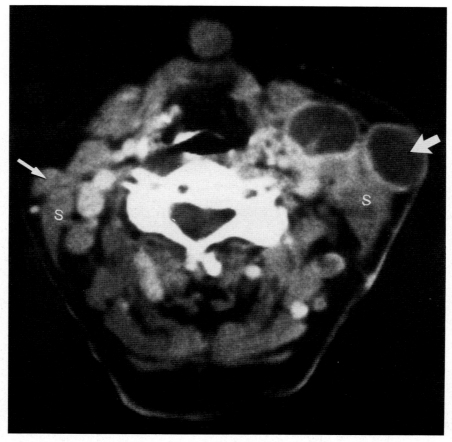

FIGURE 14.9. EXTERNAL JUGULAR NODES

Multiple enlarged lymph nodes are visible on this contrast CT scan. However, this scan demonstrates the location of the external jugular nodes (*arrows*). These nodes are located superficial to the sternocleidomastoid muscle (*s*) in close association with the external jugular vein. (Metastatic squamous cell carcinoma.)

*the neck* because they form a catch-basin for a high percentage of metastases from head and neck tumors.

The internal jugular nodes located in the anterior and posterior triangle of the neck follow the course of the internal jugular vein and are, therefore, located alongside and immediately beneath the anterior border of the sternocleidomastoid muscle. On CT, when these nodes are enlarged, they can be seen in close apposition to the carotid sheath structures (Fig. 14.10). They lie outside the sheath.

Following the course of the spinal accessory nerve, the spinal accessory chain crosses the posterior triangle obliquely, superior to inferior and anterior to posterior. On CT scans enlarged nodes in this group appear in the posterior triangle deep to the sternocleidomastoid muscle (Fig. 14.11). Low in the neck the sternocleidomastoid muscle migrates anteriorly, and the pos-

terior triangle nodes lie deep to the superficial layer of the deep cervical fascia, which constitutes the so-called roof of the posterior triangle. Normally the posterior triangle appears as a black, fat-filled cleft on CT scans except for a number of small structures of positive attenuation values caused by nerves, tiny inconsequential lymph nodes, and small nutrient vessels (Fig. 14.12).

The most superior extent of the internal jugular and spinal accessory chains joins some distance above the level of the hyoid bone. The largest node in this suprahyoid location is labeled the *jugulodigastric* node and is a member of the internal jugular chain. This node is located at the junction between the posterior belly of the digastric muscle and the internal jugular vein (that is, where this muscle crosses the anterior jugular vein). On CT scans the node is located anterior to the carotid sheath structures at or

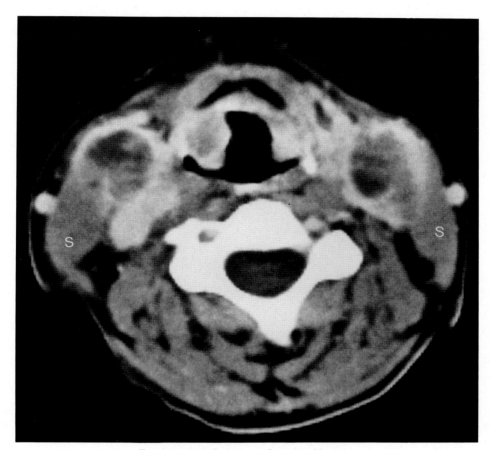

FIGURE 14.10. INTERNAL JUGULAR NODES

Bilateral enlarged low density nodes with thin enhancing rims are visible adjacent to the anterior border of the sternoclei-domastoid muscles (*s*). The left carotid sheath structures are not well visualized. The fascial planes abutting the lateral border of the carotid sheath structures are obliterated. Note the marked thickening of the epiglottis secondary to carcinoma. (Metastatic squamous cell carcinoma of the epiglottis.)

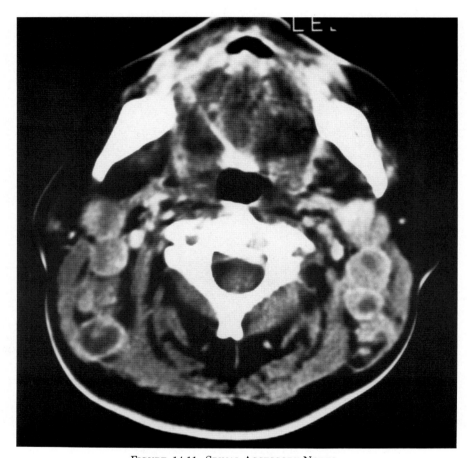

FIGURE 14.11. SPINAL ACCESSORY NODES

Multiple enlarged low density nodes with thick irregular rims of enhancement are demonstrated bilaterally in the internal jugular and spinal accessory chains. (Tuberculous adenitis.)

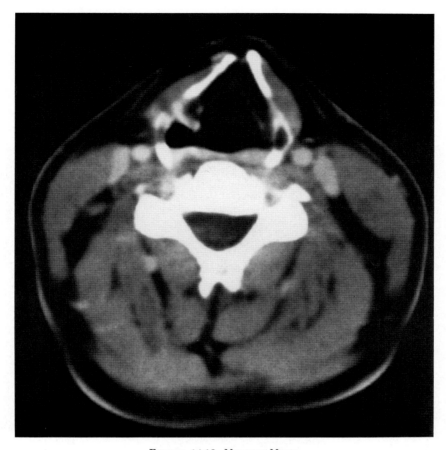

FIGURE 14.12. NORMAL NECK
The normal CT appearance of the posterior triangle is demonstrated on this contrast scan. Note the fat-filled area deep to the sternocleidomastoid muscles. A few small soft tissue densities can be seen deep to the right sternocleidomastoid muscle. These represent either small lymph nodes or nerves.

just above the level of the hyoid bone (Fig. 14.13). The relationship of this node to the hyoid bone on CT scans is variable and depends in part on the position of the chin at the time of examination and size of the node. If the chin is flexed, the node will appear in closer proximity to the hyoid bone than one would normally expect. Also, if the node is markedly enlarged, it may extend inferiorly to the level of the hyoid bone.

The transverse cervical chain follows the course of the transverse cervical artery in the inferior aspect of the posterior triangle. These nodes join the inferior extremes of the internal jugular and spinal accessory chains. These are termed the *supraclavicular* nodes (Fig. 14.14).

## TECHNIQUE

All scans are performed with intravenous contrast material unless the patient has a history of allergies. This enables one to distinguish blood vessels from other soft tissue structures, such as lymph nodes, muscles, and nerves. Several methods of contrast administration can be used. We prefer to infuse 300 ml of Reno-M-Dip over 15 min rather than inject a bolus because there is less likelihood of nausea and vomiting. Admit-

tedly, enhancement with the infusion technique is inferior to that with the bolus technique. When using this technique, scanning is started after approximately 150 ml are infused. As an alternative, a 50-ml bolus of contrast material can be given prior to the infusion to maximize the opacification of vascular structures. This modified bolus/infusion technique is particularly recommended when one is using a low resolution scan-

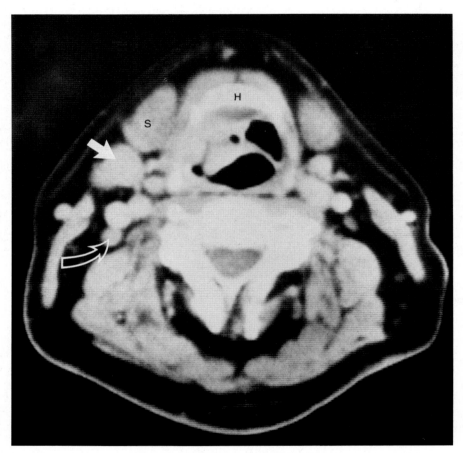

FIGURE 14.13. JUGULODIGASTRIC NODE

A contrast scan at the level of the hyoid bone (*H*) demonstrates an enlarged jugulodigastric node (*solid arrow*) posterior to the right submandibular gland (*S*). An enlarged spinal accessory node (*open arrow*) is also visible posterior to the right carotid sheath structures. Note the thickening of the right side of the epiglottis secondary to squamous cell carcinoma. (Metastatic squamous cell carcinoma of the epiglottis.)

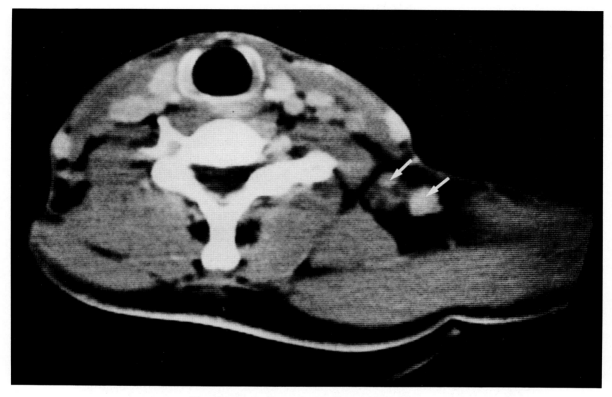

FIGURE 14.14. TRANSVERSE CERVICAL NODES

Several enlarged contrast-enhanced nodes are visible in the left supraclavicular area (*arrows*). Nodes are also present in the spinal accessory chains bilaterally. (Tuberculous adenitis.)

ner. In addition, one can begin scanning immediately after the bolus injection, thus decreasing the amount of time the patient is on the scanner.

Patient positioning is extremely important. To decrease the amount of overlap of suprahyoid and infrahyoid structures, the patient is positioned supine with the chin extended so that the horizontal ramus of the mandible is parallel to the x-ray beam. The gantry angle is positioned at 0°, and 5-mm thick contiguous cuts are obtained through the area of interest. During the actual scanning process the patient is asked not to swallow because it may cause a motion artifact. This precaution may not be necessary with the faster scanners.

## Pathology

One should have a working knowledge of the normal (gross and CT) anatomy as well as common pathological entities encountered in the neck before attempting to interpret scans of this area. Helpful reviews include the work of Mancuso et al. (1978), Reede et al. (1982a–c), and Miller and Norman (1979).

The current staging system used in evaluation of patients with head and neck neoplasms can be reviewed in the publication *Staging of Cancer of Head and Neck Sites and of Melanoma 1980*. This publication uses the TNM classification of malignant tumors, defining the extent of the primary tumor (T), the status of regional lymph nodes (N), and the presence of distant spread or metastasis (M).

CT is superior to other imaging modalities in the evaluation of patients with head and neck neoplasms because it allows one to determine both the extent of the primary lesion and the presence of regional node metastasis. It is well known that cervical lymph node metastasis in squamous cell carcinoma of the aerodigestive tract diminishes the cure rate (McGauran et al., 1961; Ballantyne, 1964; Spiro et al., 1974; Jesse, 1977; Jesse and Fletcher, 1977; Kalnins et al., 1977; Batsakis, 1979; Cachin et al., 1979). The cure rate decreases progressively as the extent of lymph node involvement increases from solitary ipsilateral nodes to multiple ipsilateral, solitary contralateral, and, finally, bilateral nodes (Spiro et al., 1974). Since the presence of nodal metastasis may alter the treatment plan, detection of such secondary involvement has paramount importance.

Traditionally, detection of nodal disease prior to surgery has relied upon physical examination. In a study performed by the clinicians at Roswell Park Memorial Institute, it was found that palpation of an enlarged node depended upon its location and consistency. In their experience in a neck of average size, the lower limit of palpability is approximately 0.5 cm for a superficial node as found in the submandibular and submental area and 1 cm for nodes in deeper areas (Sako et al., 1964). It is possible to detect both palpable and nonpalpable nodal disease with CT (Mancuso and Hanafee, 1981; Mancuso et al., 1981; Reede et al., 1982c). Based on the work of Mancuso et al. and that at our institution, the following conclusions regarding nodal disease as demonstrated by CT have been proposed:

1. In an area with lymph nodes, a mass with central lucency (other than fat), irrespective of size, is abnormal. This pattern of nodal disease can be seen in both neoplastic and inflammatory processes. If peripheral enhancement is present, this sign may be helpful in differentiating between the two. The peripheral enhancement seen in neoplastic disease is usually uniform in thickness and enhancement (Fig. 14.15). Peripheral enhancement seen in inflammatory disease tends to be thick and irregular (Fig. 14.16), particularly with tuberculous disease (Reede et al., 1982c). The CT appearance of a branchial cleft cyst (Fig. 14.17) or abscess may be similar to that of neoplastic nodal disease.

2. A nonenhancing mass with a diameter greater than 1.5 cm in an area of lymph nodes is abnormal. In the retropharyngeal chain abnormal nodes may be as small as 1 cm in size (Mancuso et al., 1983). Because reactive as well as neoplastic nodes may become enlarged (Figs. 14.18 and 14.19), enlargement is a potential source of false-positive CT diagnoses of neoplastic disease.

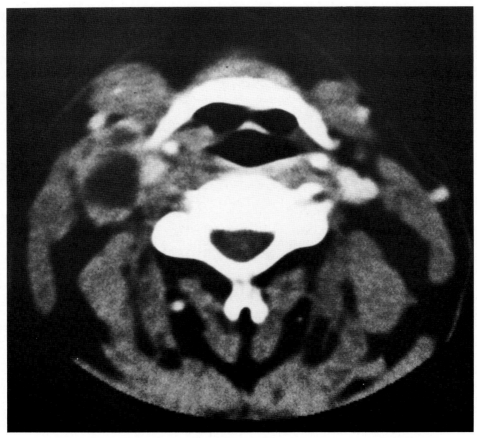

FIGURE 14.15. METASTATIC SQUAMOUS CELL CARCINOMA OF THE PIRIFORM SINUS
Several enlarged right internal jugular nodes with low density centers and thin peripheral rim enlargement are visible. The fascial planes adjacent to the carotid sheath structures are obliterated.

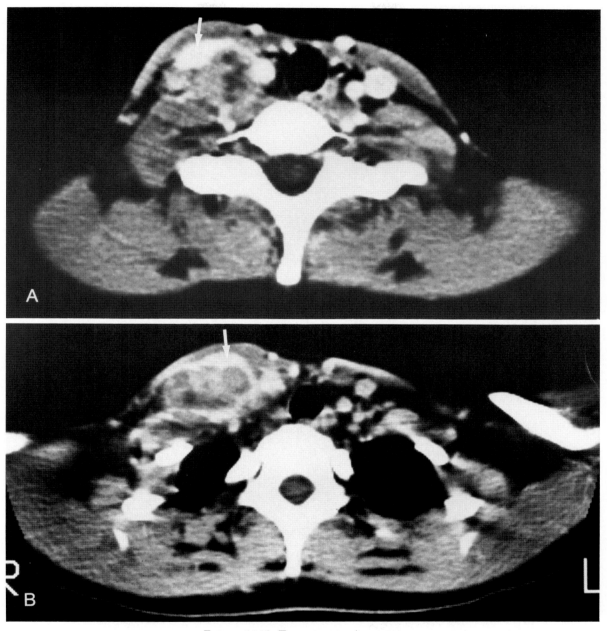

FIGURE 14.16. TUBERCULOUS ADENITIS

A low density mass with thick irregular enhancement is seen in the right posterior triangle. The fascial planes around this mass are obliterated except along the lateral border. Note the lateral displacement and compression of the internal jugular vein (*arrow*).

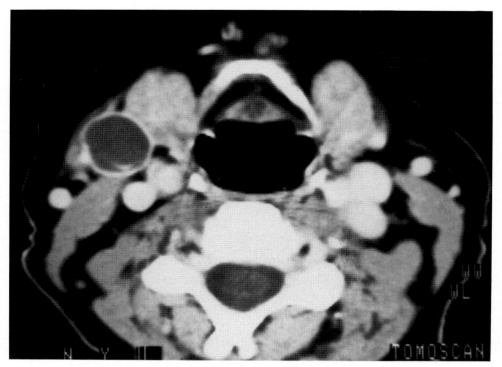

FIGURE 14.17. BRANCHIAL CLEFT CYST

A low density lesion with a thin rim of peripheral enhancement is seen adjacent to the anterior border of the sternocleido-mastoid muscle.

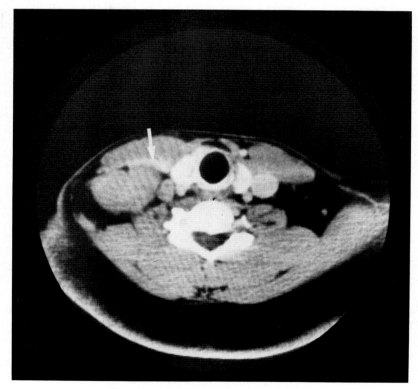

FIGURE 14.18. HODGKIN'S LYMPHOMA

Nonenhancing soft tissue masses are noted in the right posterior triangle (spinal accessory nodes). The fascial planes around the masses are preserved. The right internal jugular vein is compressed (*arrow*).

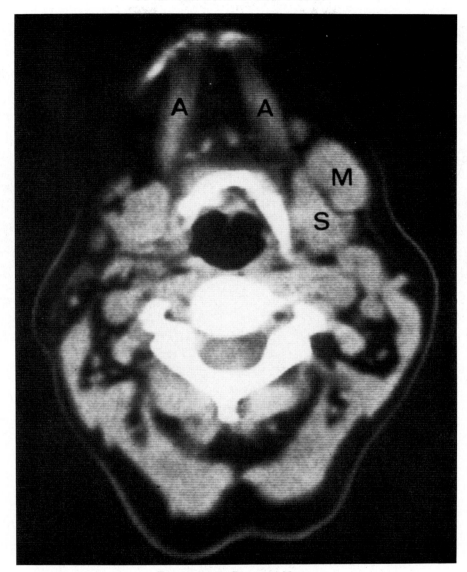

FIGURE 14.19. REACTIVE NODE

An enlarged submandibular node (*M*) is demonstrated in the left submandibular triangle. This node is separate from the submandibular gland (*S*). A few small submental nodes are visible between the anterior bellies of the digastric muscles (*A*).

3. Obliteration of fascial planes in the neck can be seen in the postoperative and postirradiation neck as well as in neoplastic and inflammatory processes. Therefore, obliteration of fascial planes around enlarged nodes is significant in the nonirradiated or nonoperated neck (Mancuso et al., 1981). In neoplastic disease this appearance indicates either direct extension of the primary disease into adjacent tissues or extranodal extension of disease beyond the lymph node capsule.

Relatively extensive obliteration of the fascial planes is seen in inflammatory processes (Figs. 14.16 and 14.20), while neoplastic disease tends to cause more focal obliteration. This finding is best demonstrated when metastatic disease is encountered in the internal jugular chain. In this area obliteration of fascial planes is usually more pronounced along the medial border of the nodes where they abut the carotid sheath structures (Figs. 14.10, 14.15, and 14.21) (Reede et al., 1982c).

4. Total or relatively uniform enhancement of an enlarged node is rarely encountered in noninflammatory disease.

5. Three or more contiguous, ill defined nodes

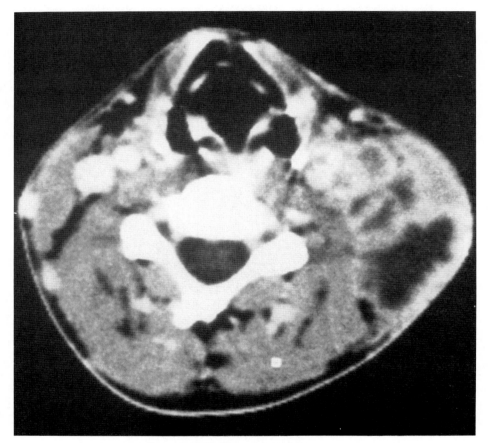

FIGURE 14.20. TUBERCULOUS ADENITIS
Multiple necrotic nodes with thick irregular rim enhancement are present in the left posterior triangle. The fascial planes around these nodes are obliterated except along the anterior border. Enhancement of the left sternocleidomastoid muscle is apparent.

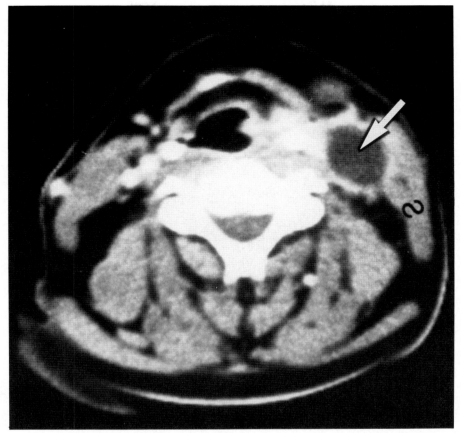

FIGURE 14.21. METASTATIC SQUAMOUS CELL CARCINOMA OF THE PIRIFORM SINUS
A low density node (*arrow*) with a thin rim of peripheral enhancement is visible along the anterior border of the left sternocleidomastoid muscle (*S*). The fascial planes adjacent to the carotid sheath structures are obliterated.

measuring 8–15 mm in diameter or greater suggests neoplastic disease. This may also be seen in non-neoplastic processes, however, and is another potential source of false-positive reading in patients with a head or neck neoplasm (Mancuso et al., 1981).

Because reactive and inflammatory nodes may be mistaken for neoplastic disease on CT, it is important to correlate observations with clinical history and physical findings. This will enable one to weigh properly the differential diagnosis of an enlarged node.

The number of clinically negative necks that are found to be pathologically positive upon radical neck dissection varies between 0–40% (Jesse et al., 1973; Nahum et al., 1977). In the appropriate clinical context (known primary head and neck tumor), designating cervical lymph nodes exceeding 1.5 cm in diameter on the CT scan as positive for metastatic disease has resulted in finding occult nodes in clinically negative necks in about 5% of patients in one series (Mancuso

et al., 1983). Using 1-cm nodes on the CT study as the criterion for positive disease converted 5 of 18 patients with clinically negative necks to $N_1$ disease in a report by Friedman et al. (1984). In their series of 50 operated necks, there were two false-positive and two false-negative CT interpretations.

## Occult Primary Neoplasm

Cervical metastasis may present without evidence of a primary neoplasm (occult primary). Approximately 5% of patients with cancer and 12% of patients with head and neck cancer present with a cervical mass as the sole presenting symptom (Simpson, 1980). If thyroid neoplasms are excluded, 90% of cervical masses in patients over the age of 40 are found to represent metastatic disease (Winegar and Griffin, 1973). The nasopharynx, piriform sinus, tonsillar fossa, and base of the tongue are the common sites of primary tumors in patients who present with cervical nodal metastases (Shaw, 1970; Jesse et

TABLE 14.1.
COMMON LOCATIONS FOR METASTATIC NODES BASED ON
THE LOCATION OF PRIMARY NEOPLASM

| Metastatic Site | Primary Site |
|---|---|
| Upper cervical nodes | Nasopharynx |
| | Base of tongue |
| | Tonsil |
| Mid- and lower jugular nodes | Larynx |
| | Pharynx |
| | Esophagus |
| | Thyroid |
| Midline or paratracheal nodes | Thyroid |
| | Larynx |
| | Pulmonary |
| Submandibular nodes | Tongue |
| | Floor of mouth |
| Supraclavicular nodes | May be metastatic from any part of the body, especially bronchi, breast, stomach, and esophagus |

al., 1973; Winegar and Griffin, 1973). The specific node group involved in metastasis as well as the tissue type may also give a clue to location of the primary lesion (Table 14.1).

If physical examination and routine imaging modalities fail to locate a primary site, CT may be helpful because it can detect submucosal disease when mucosal changes are absent. Additionally, CT can reveal areas that are technically difficult to evaluate by physical examination. Modifying the work-up as suggested by Mancuso and Hanafee (1981), we suggest the decision tree protocol found in Figure 14.22 for evaluation of these patients.

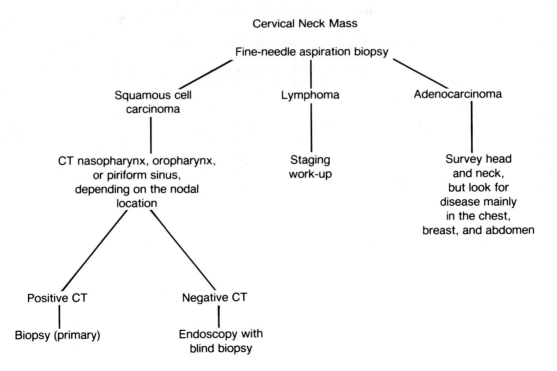

FIGURE 14.22. DECISION TREE FOR EVALUATION OF PATIENTS WITH METASTATIC CERVICAL NODE DISEASE AND AN
UNKNOWN PRIMARY TUMOR
(Modified from Mancuso and Hanafee, 1981.)

# REFERENCES

Ballantyne AJ: Significance of retropharyngeal nodes in cancer of the head and neck. *Am J Surg* 108:500–504, 1964.

Batsakis JG: *Tumors of the Head and Neck: Clinical and Pathological Considerations.* Baltimore, Williams & Wilkins, 1979.

Cachin U, Garnier HS, Micheau C, Marandas P: Nodal metastasis from carcinoma of the oropharynx. *Otolaryngol Clin North Am* 12:145–154, 1979.

Cornog JL, Gray SR: Surgical and clinical pathology of salivary gland tumors. In Rankow RM, Polayes IM (eds): *Diseases of the Salivary Glands.* Philadelphia, WB Saunders, 1976.

Feind CR: The head and neck. In Haagensen CD, Feind CR, Herter FP, Slanetz CA, Weinberg JA: *The Lymphatics in Cancer.* Philadelphia, WB Saunders, 1972.

Fisch VP, Sigel ME: Cervical lymphatic system as visualized by lymphography. *Ann Otol Rhinol Laryngol* 73:869–882, 1964.

Friedman M, Shelton V, Mafee M, Bellity P, Skolnik E: Metastatic neck disease, evaluation by computed tomography. *Arch Otolaryngol* 110:443–447, 1984.

Gruart FJ, Yoel J, Wagner A: Value of perilingual lymphography in cancer of the head and neck. *Am J Surg* 114:520–524, 1967.

Jesse RH: The philosophy of treatment of neck nodes. *Ear Nose Throat J* 56:58–63, 1977.

Jesse RH, Fletcher GH: Treatment of the neck in patients with squamous cell carcinoma of the head and neck. *Cancer* 39:868–872, 1977.

Jesse RH, Perez CA, Fletcher GH: Cervical lymph node metastasis from unknown primary cancer. *Cancer* 31:854–859, 1973.

Johner CH: The lymphatics of the larynx. *Otolaryngol Clin North Am* 3:439–450, 1970.

Kalnins IK, Leonard AG, Sako K, Razack MS, Shedd DP: Correlation between prognosis and degree of lymph node involvement in carcinoma of the oral cavity. *Am J Surg* 134:450–454, 1977.

Last RJ: *Anatomy Regional and Applied.* New York, Churchill Livingstone, 1978.

Mancuso AA, Hanafee WN: *The Radiographic Evaluation of Patients with Head and Neck Cancer.* Categorical Course in Radiation Therapy. Chicago, Radiological Society of North America, 1981.

Mancuso AA, Calcaterra TC, Hanafee WN: Computed tomography of the larynx. *Radiol Clin North Am* 16:195–208, 1978.

Mancuso AA, Maceri D, Rice D, Hanafee WN: CT of cervical lymph node cancer. *AJR* 136:381–385, 1981.

Mancuso AA, Harnsberger HR, Muraki AS, Stevens MH: CT of the cervical and retropharyngeal lymph nodes: normal anatomy, variants of normal, and applications in staging head and neck cancer. Part II. Pathology. *Radiology* 148:709–723, 1983.

Matoba N, Kikuchi T: Thyroidolymphography. *Radiology* 92:339–342, 1969.

McGauran MH, Bauer WC, Ogura JH: The incidence of cervical lymph node metastases from epidermoid carcinoma of the larynx and their relationship to certain characteristics of the primary tumor. *Cancer* 14:55–66, 1961.

Miller EM, Norman D: The role of computed tomography in the evaluation of neck masses. *Radiology* 133:145–149, 1979.

Montgomery RL: *Head and Neck Anatomy with Clinical Correlations.* New York, McGraw-Hill, 1981.

Montgomery WW: *Surgery of the Upper Respiratory System.* Philadelphia, Lea and Febiger, 1971.

Nahum AM, Bone RC, Davidson TM: The case for elective prophylactic neck dissection. *Laryngoscope* 87:588–599, 1977.

Reede DL, Bergeron RT: CT of cervical lymph nodes. *J Otolaryngol* 11:411–418, 1982.

Reede DL, Bergeron RT, McCauley DI: CT of the thyroid and of other thoracic inlet disorders. *J Otolaryngol* 11:349–357, 1982a.

Reede DL, Whelan MA, Bergeron RT: Computed tomography of the infrahyoid neck: normal anatomy. *Radiology* 145:389–395, 1982b.

Reede DL, Whelan MA, Bergeron RT: Computed tomography of the infrahyoid neck. Part II. Pathology. *Radiology* 145:397–402, 1982c.

Rouvière H: *Anatomy of the Human Lymphatic System* (translated by Tobias MJ). Ann Arbor, MI, Edwards Brothers, 1938.

Sachdeva HS, Chowdhary GC, Bose SM, Gupta BB, Wig JD: Thyroid lymphography. *Arch Surg* 109:385–387, 1974.

Sako K, Pradier RN, Marchetta FC, Pickren JW: Fallibility of palpation in the diagnosis of metastases to cervical nodes. *Surg Gynecol Obstet* 118:989–990, 1964.

Shaw HJ: Metastatic carcinoma in cervical lymph nodes with occult primary tumors: diagnosis and treatment. *J Laryngol Otol* 84:249–265, 1970.

Sigel ME: Cervical lymphangiography. In Paperrela MM, Shumrick DA (eds): *Otolaryngology.* Philadelphia, WB Saunders, 1980, vol 1.

Simpson GT: The evaluation and management of neck masses of unknown etiology. *Otolaryngol Clin North Am* 13:489–498, 1980.

Spiro RH, Alfonso AE, Farr HW, Strong EW: Cervical nodal metastasis from epidermoid carcinoma of the oral cavity and oropharynx. *Am J Surg* 128:562–567, 1974.

*Staging of Cancer of Head and Neck Sites and of Melanoma 1980.* Chicago, American Joint Committee on Cancer, 1980.

Winegar LK, Griffin W: The occult primary tumor. *Arch Otolaryngol* 98:159–163, 1973.

# 15

# *Percutaneous Lymph Node Biopsy*

JESUS ZORNOZA, M.D.

Small gauge needle aspiration biopsy has been practiced for many years, particularly in Europe, and has been utilized to assess both neoplastic and inflammatory disease processes in a number of organs (breast, lymph nodes, thyroid, salivary glands, lungs). During the 1960s, several Swedish authors presented reports that substantiated the diagnostic possibilities of this method (Eneroth and Zajicek, 1966; Frazen and Zajicek, 1966; Söderström, 1966; Zajicek et al., 1967; Engzell et al., 1971b).

Over the last several years, radiological localization of abdominal masses and lymph nodes has grown more precise because of the new imaging modalities, ultrasound and computed tomography (CT). Although the greater accuracy in diagnosis allows better determination of the extent of disease, some lesions remain dilemmas. For such problems and for therapeutic purposes, percutaneous aspiration of abdominal masses and lymph nodes is useful.

Since lymphangiography was introduced by Kinmonth in 1952, this procedure has experienced varying degrees of popularity. At the present time, lymphangiography is an accepted procedure for pretreatment evaluation of the extent of involvement in patients with lymphomatous diseases, but its value in staging patients with epithelial tumors remains controversial. At M. D. Anderson Hospital, lymphangiography is used to great advantage in the staging of carcinomas of the cervix, ovary, testicle, bladder, and prostate. Of the 1100 examinations performed by this method each year at this hospital, over half are in search of metastatic carcinoma.

The reported accuracy of lymphangiography varies considerably. Spellman et al. (1977) achieved a sensitivity of 57% and a specificity of 98% in patients with prostatic carcinoma. The accuracy rate in carcinoma of the cervix reported by Piver et al. (1971) was 87%. In a study of testicular carcinoma, Wallace and Jing (1970) showed an 88% accuracy.

Recognition of lymph node replacement by metastatic tumor is sometimes a problem, making the interpretation of lymphangiograms difficult. Strict diagnostic criteria should be used to prevent a high incidence of false-positive lymphangiograms. Proper criteria do not always assure accuracy, however, because metastasis is not the only possible cause of a filling defect in a lymph node. Similar changes may be seen in caseous fibrosis, fatty replacement, and conglomerate lymph nodes. All of these factors lower the clinical value of the examination.

CT allows only gross morphological evaluation of the nodes and can only define the size of the lymph node, not the internal architecture. It is a very precise method of guidance for percutaneous biopsy, however (Haaga and Alfidi, 1976).

The practice of percutaneous biopsy of the iliac and lumbar lymph nodes has enhanced the value of lymphangiography and CT. Ruttimann (1968) first used the paravascular approach, but he was unable to reach the para-aortic lymph nodes. Wallace et al. (1975) tested a similar technique in animals and cadavers and successfully biopsied the para-aortic lymph nodes. An obvious path to diagnosis is the direct percutaneous transabdominal approach by aspiration biopsy during fluoroscopy or CT (Gothlin, 1976; Zornoza et al., 1977d). Since then, several reports have confirmed the accuracy and safety of this method (Thomson et al., 1977; Wallace et al., 1977; Zornoza et al., 1977a–c; Berkowitz et al., 1978; Gothlin, 1978; Jaques, 1978; McLoughlin et al., 1978; Bonfiglio et al., 1979; Efremidis et al., 1979; Mennemeyer et al., 1979; Prando et al., 1979; Correa et al., 1980; Dunnick et al., 1980; Ennis and MacErlean, 1980; Gothlin and Holem, 1981; Zornoza, 1981; Edeiken-Monroe and Zornoza, 1982).

## EQUIPMENT

Image intensifier fluoroscopy is utilized in most transabdominal biopsies. Any fluoroscopic room equipped with an image intensification system can serve this purpose. Simultaneous fluoroscopy in two planes at right angles, when available, may prove more accurate in the exact localization of the point of the needle. In most cases, however, a single projection is satisfactory.

Fluoroscopy is preferred for filming when feasible, but CT provides the more precise guidance needed for localization of nonopacified small lesions and those deeply located in the retroperitoneal space. Also, larger needles can be used with CT because of its ability to localize the needle within the lesion accurately. Any CT scanner can be used to perform the biopsies although a control scan with a skin marker system facilitates localization of the needle puncture site relative to the lesion to be biopsied (Fig. 15.1).

Several different caliber small gauge needles have been utilized for aspiration biopsy of abdominal lesions. The needles are commercially available in lengths of 10, 15, and 20 cm. Those most commonly used have been 19 to 22 gauge needles (Fig. 15.2). In certain cases, 21 and 22 gauge needles are unsuitable for biopsy of lesions deeply located in the retroperitoneal space or in obese patients. Because of its flexibility, the needle bends when it is advanced through the anterior abdominal wall or the anterior portion of the retroperitoneal space. In such cases, a 19 gauge needle has been used because its greater rigidity allows better control.

The flexible steel needles are fitted with an inner stylet and have a bevel angle of 24°, which facilitates introduction as well as loosening of tissue fragments near the point of the needle when rotated. The needles can be fitted to different types of syringes for aspiration. Routinely, a disposable 12-ml plastic syringe is used. Through the use of disposable syringes, multiple aspirations can be made without dependence on a large supply of glass instruments.

## TECHNIQUE

Once the appropriate radiological examination has been performed to localize the lesion to be biopsied, the patient is placed on the examining table for the procedure. Biopsies are performed on outpatients and inpatients, and no fasting is required. The procedure rarely requires premedication. If a patient is anxious, 10 mg of diazepam are given intramuscularly. An anterior transabdominal approach is used for most biopsies; only biopsies of paravertebral masses call for a posterior approach.

When image intensifier fluoroscopy is used, a radiopaque object is positioned on the skin directly overlying the lesion to be biopsied. If a large tumor is present, the indicator should be located at the edge of the lesion. The center is frequently necrotic, and, although a large amount of aspirated material can be obtained, it usually contains no viable cells.

The skin and subcutaneous tissues down to the peritoneum are anesthetized locally with 2% lidocaine. A small incision with a surgical blade and separation of the tissues with a hemostat facilitate entry of the needle. At this point in the procedure, it is very important to maintain the needle on a straight path. A minimal deviation from the desired course ultimately will misplace the needle, which cannot be realigned by bending the hub portion of the needle. In such circumstances, it is necessary to withdraw the needle completely and readvance it. The position of the needle should be checked frequently under fluoroscopy to be sure of the desired vertical course.

If a 15- or 20-cm needle is used, one hand should advance the needle while the other stabilizes it at the skin. The needle should be advanced in small increments, and fluoroscopy should be performed after each advance. Manual control of the needle is preferable to the use of rubber-tipped hemostats to maintain stability.

Once the abdominal cavity has been entered, no resistance is met until the tip of the needle reaches the posterior parietal peritoneum. At this time, the patient may experience pain which can be alleviated by injection of a small amount of lidocaine. Small gauge needles (22–23 gauge) tend to bend at this point if they are advanced with a quick motion. Slight continuous pressure allows an easier passage of the needle through the anterior retroperitoneal fascia.

The introduction of the needle is time consuming. Because it is difficult for a patient to achieve a consistent degree of respiration and any abrupt respiratory movement is undesirable while the needle is in the abdominal cavity, the patient is allowed to breath normally during the procedure.

Often, increased resistance to the needle indicates that the mass lesion has been reached. The desired point to be biopsied also can be verified by oblique projections and biplane fluoroscopy or CT, whichever is being used to guide the procedure. Precision localization under CT guidance can be facilitated by injection of a small amount of contrast material during the biopsy procedure (Stephenson et al., 1979).

The site of biopsy will differ depending upon

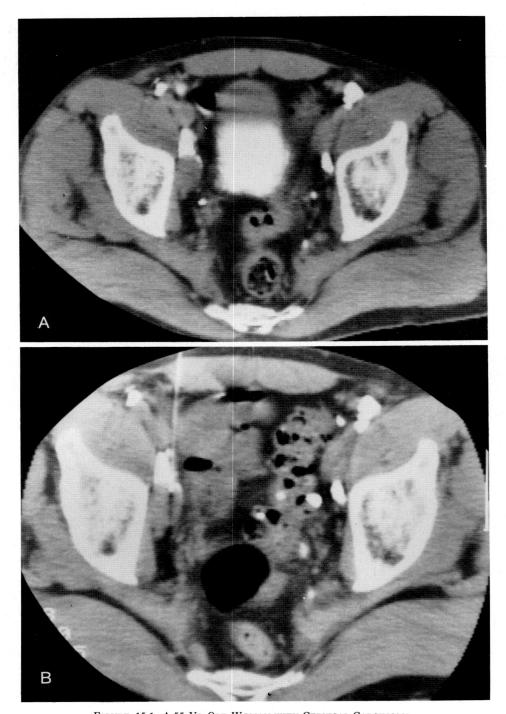

FIGURE 15.1. A 55-YR-OLD WOMAN WITH CERVICAL CARCINOMA

*A*: CT scan shows enlarged right external iliac node. *B*: CT scan demonstrates precisely the tip of the needle in the lymph node.

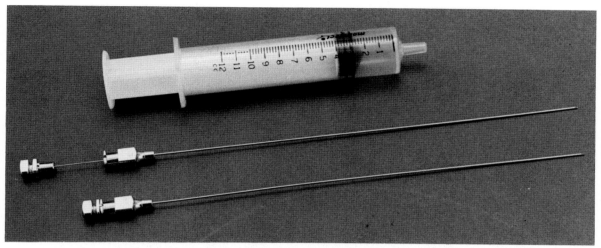

FIGURE 15.2. INSTRUMENTS FOR PERCUTANEOUS LYMPH NODE BIOPSY
Twenty-two gauge needle and 12-ml disposable plastic syringe.

the histological type of primary tumor. The most common lymphangiographic finding in carcinoma metastatic to the lymph nodes is a sharply defined, concave filling defect not traversed by lymphatics. The remaining, normally functioning portion of the node frequently shows a crescentic configuration representing a node partially replaced by tumor. Biopsy of the tissue adjacent to the crescentic area provides the best diagnostic yield. In lymphoma, the site of the biopsy is less critical because there is a more diffuse involvement. Care should be taken not to inject local anesthetic into the lymph node and thus disrupt the configuration of the lymphoid cells.

When the biopsy is performed under fluoroscopy, the patient is rotated slightly to both sides to determine the relative depth of the needle (Fig. 15.3). When the node is punctured, it will move in concert with the needle tip, indicating an accurate placement. Because the defects biopsied are usually small (1–2 cm), the needle should be moved very gently to detach material. Large excursions would yield an undesirable amount of blood and extranodal tissue. The presence of oil droplets in the aspirate demonstrates that a node previously opacified during lymphangiography has been punctured.

At the time of biopsy, the needle is rotated clockwise and counterclockwise around its longitudinal axis. This maneuver detaches cellular material near the needle point. After the needle has been rotated a few times, the stylet is removed, and a disposable 12-ml plastic syringe is attached to the hub. Suction is applied while the needle is gently moved up and down several times with approximately a 1-cm excursion. Suction is relieved when the aspiration has been completed; pressure in the syringe is then allowed to equalize before the needle is withdrawn from the lesion. This maneuver retains the tissue in the needle from which it can be ejected easily onto glass slides or into preservative solution. If suction continues during or after withdrawal of the needle, the material passes into the syringe, making retrieval more difficult. The same procedure is performed two or three times to obtain sufficient cytological material. After biopsy, patients are kept under observation for 2–3 hr without further radiographs unless required by special circumstances.

## INDICATIONS

The value of CT and lymphangiography has been enhanced by the advent of percutaneous biopsy of lymph nodes. Laparotomy and lymph node biopsy in conjunction with lymphangiography and CT are used in the pretreatment evaluation of patients with epithelial malignancies, Hodgkin's disease, and non-Hodgkin's lymphoma.

The percutaneous approach to para-aortic and pelvic lymph nodes represents a simple technique to confirm the presence of neoplasm, thereby determining the extent of disease and

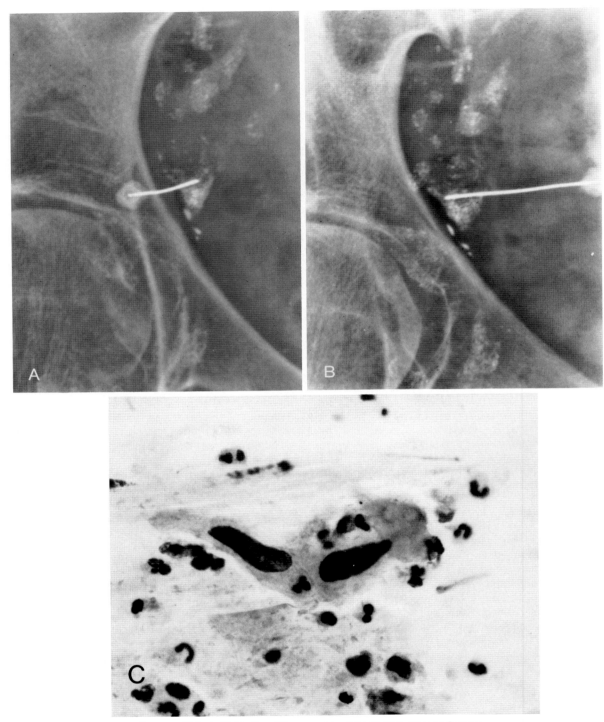

FIGURE 15.3. A 46-YR-OLD WOMAN WITH CARCINOMA OF THE CERVIX

Anteroposterior (A) and oblique (B) projections demonstrate the tip of the needle in replaced part of a right external iliac lymph node. C: Squamous cell carcinoma. Original magnification ×425.

facilitating treatment planning. If metastases are identified in the external iliac region of a patient with cervical carcinoma, then the irradiation portal is extended to L4. When metastatic disease is detected above that level, however, the irradiation field is extended to the diaphragm (Fletcher and Rutledge, 1971). Extensive surgical lymph node biopsy and large portal fields have a high incidence of complications. In such cases, percutaneous lymph node biopsy can confirm the presence of metastases, obviating the use of surgical biopsy (Fig. 15.4).

Because lymphangiographic contrast medium remains in the lymph nodes for a prolonged period of time, approximately 15 months, changes in the lymph nodes in response to treat-

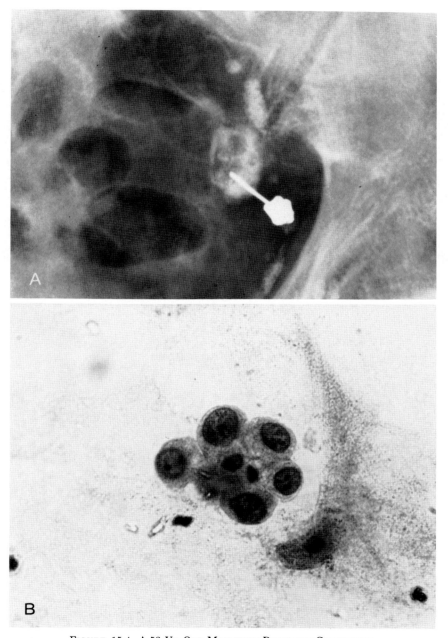

FIGURE 15.4. A 53-YR-OLD MAN WITH PROSTATE CARCINOMA
*A*: Needle in a small filling defect of external iliac lymph node. *B*: Metastatic adenocarcinoma. Original magnification ×425.

ment can be evaluated at varying intervals. When possible recurrent disease is noted, percutaneous biopsy offers the possibility of a tissue diagnosis, and a more appropriate treatment can be started (Fig. 15.5).

In patients with lymphoma in clinical remission, evaluation of residual disease is usually difficult (Zornoza et al., 1981). CT and ultrasound offer a good definition of the response to treatment. When chemotherapy should be continued or discontinued, however, a tissue diagnosis should be obtained to avoid unnecessary use of such toxic drugs.

On certain occasions, the nodal architectural changes in patients with carcinoma are most compatible with the configuration seen in lym-

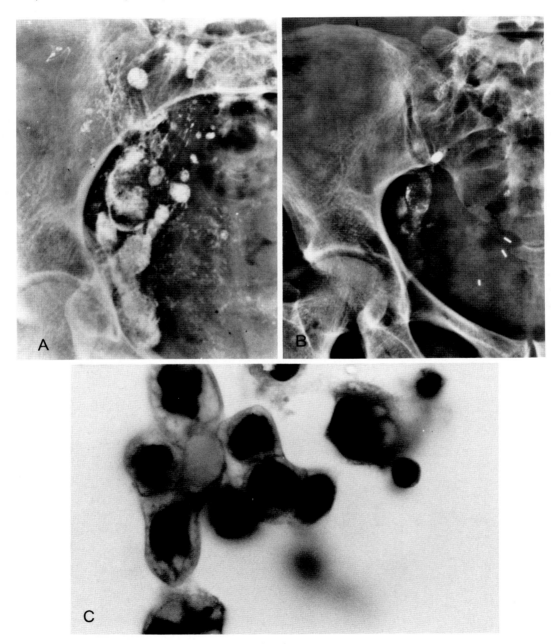

FIGURE 15.5. A 62-YR-OLD WOMAN WITH ENDOMETRIAL CARCINOMA

*A:* Lymphangiogram shows metastatic disease to right external iliac node. *B:* One year later, the lymph node remains abnormal. *C:* Metastatic adenocarcinoma. Original magnification ×1000.

phoma (Fig. 15.6). Percutaneous biopsy can provide the diagnosis of metastatic disease or of a second primary. Residual masses in the retroperitoneum in patients with lymphomas or testicular tumors need not represent viable tumor. Persistent masses should be biopsied to determine if they represent recurrent or sterilized tumor (Libshitz et al., 1983).

## RESULTS

Percutaneous biopsy of the lymph nodes in 107 patients was reported by Gothlin (1978). Ninety-five of the biopsies were successful, and 12 were failures. In a study by Bonfiglio et al. (1979), the correct diagnosis was obtained in 45 of 47 patients, and 11 of the biopsies were positive for malignant tumor. MacIntosh et al. (1979) and Thomson et al. (1977) reported similar results with no false-positive diagnoses and few false-negatives.

The results of percutaneous biopsy of lymph nodes in 363 patients are summarized in Table 15.1. There were 328 biopsies performed in patients with lymph node metastases and 35 in patients with lymphoma. The primary neoplasms in metastatic lymph nodes and their frequency of occurrence are presented in Table 15.2.

The biopsy was considered true-positive if a diagnosis of malignancy was obtained. A true-negative biopsy occurred when the aspiration did not reveal malignancy and surgery, autopsy, or clinical follow-up also failed to demonstrate tumor. When patients were lost to follow-up or when inadequate material and normal lymphoid tissue were obtained in the presence of a tumor, the biopsy was ruled inconclusive. A true-positive diagnosis was obtained from the results of 160 biopsies; 99 studies were true-negative; and 104 cases were inconclusive. The overall success rate was 71%. The relatively low success rate in this series is due mainly to the multiplicity of radiologists now performing the procedure; with fewer radiologists, greater skill and consistency in the performance of biopsies yield a consequent increase in the accuracy rate.

Biopsy results have yielded the correct diagnosis in 241 patients (73%) with metastatic carcinoma, while results for 87 (27%) have remained

TABLE 15.1.
RESULTS IN PERCUTANEOUS BIOPSY OF LYMPH NODES

| True-positives | Carcinoma | 155 |
|---|---|---|
| | Lymphoma | 5 |
| True-negatives | Carcinoma | 86 |
| | Lymphoma | 13 |
| Inconclusives or false-negatives | Carcinoma | 87 |
| | Lymphoma | 17 |
| | Total | 363 |

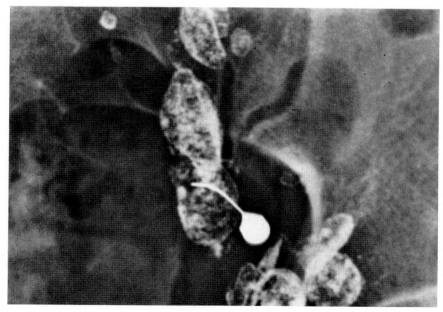

FIGURE 15.6. PATIENT WITH TRANSITIONAL CARCINOMA OF THE BLADDER
Lymphangiogram shows abnormally enlarged nodes. Percutaneous biopsy revealed large cell lymphoma.

TABLE 15.2.
PRIMARY NEOPLASMS IN METASTATIC LYMPH NODES

| | |
|---|---|
| Cervix | 169 |
| Prostate | 60 |
| Bladder | 48 |
| Testicle | 12 |
| Ovary | 9 |
| Endometrium | 7 |
| Melanoma | 5 |
| Vagina | 5 |
| Unknown | 4 |
| Urethra | 2 |
| Vulva | 2 |
| Ureter | 2 |
| Kidney | 1 |
| Lung | 1 |
| Synovial sarcoma | 1 |
| Total | 328 |

TABLE 15.3.
RESULTS IN PERCUTANEOUS BIOPSY OF LYMPH NODES:
CARCINOMA VERSUS LYMPHOMA

| 328 Carcinoma | Correct | 241 (73%) |
|---|---|---|
| | Incorrect | 87 (27%) |
| 35 Lymphoma | Correct | 18 (51%) |
| | Incorrect | 17 (49%) |

inconclusive. In patients with lymphoma, 18 biopsy specimens (51%) revealed adequate cytological material for a correct diagnosis, while 17 (49%) were inconclusive (Table 15.3). Correct diagnosis has been possible only in patients with histiocytic lymphoma or with Hodgkin's disease (Fig. 15.7). The results of aspiration biopsy of lymph nodes containing metastatic carcinoma were more successful than those of nodes involved by lymphoma, 73% as compared with 51%. Epithelial metastases, characteristically highly cellular and readily distinguishable from the normal cells of a lymph node (Berg, 1961), have been relatively easy to diagnose. It has been more difficult to diagnose lymphomas correctly, especially when specifying the histological type, although Drose and Zajicek (unpublished data) have achieved a definite diagnosis in 70% of patients with Hodgkin's disease involving superficial lymph nodes.

External iliac lymph nodes were biopsied in 247 patients, the common iliac nodes in 23 patients, and para-aortic lymph nodes in 93. There were 181 biopsy specimens (73%) from nodes in the external iliac region that yielded successful diagnoses, but 66 (27%) were inconclusive. Common iliac lymph nodes were correctly diagnosed in 16 patients (69%), and inconclusive results were obtained in 7 patients (31%). Para-aortic lymph node biopsies yielded a correct diagnosis in 62 patients (66%), but 31 (34%) were inadequate (Table 15.4). The lower success in the common iliac and para-aortic regions as compared to that in the external iliac is probably due to the difficulty in guiding the needle through the greater amount of tissue traversed at these levels.

Percutaneous abdominal mass biopsies have been performed in 300 patients, and a correct diagnosis was obtained in 83% (Fig. 15.8). Of the 25 patients with known lymphoma, a diagnosis was obtained in 18, and 7 remained inconclusive. Ten of 11 patients with an abdominal mass and an unknown primary were diagnosed as having lymphoma. Overall, a correct diagnosis of lymphoma was obtained in 78% of the cases. The higher success rate of biopsies of masses as compared with the results of lymph node biopsies in patients with lymphoma is due to the large size of the masses and the retrieval of more tissue by larger needles.

## COMPLICATIONS

The clinical value of a diagnostic procedure is limited by the frequency and severity of attendant complications. Transabdominal biopsy involves the passage of a needle through various abdominal organs, both solid and hollow. According to our experience and that of others, there is no need for serious apprehension with regard to bleeding or perforation provided the necessary precautions are taken and a careful technique is used. The only relative contraindications to the procedure are bowel dilatation and abnormal bleeding parameters. The establishment of strict aseptic conditions prevents infections, such as peritonitis, cholangitis, and abscess.

To date, no significant complications with this technique have been reported (Hancke et al., 1975; Holm et al., 1975; Smith et al., 1975; Goldstein et al., 1977; Evander et al., 1978; Ferrucci and Wittenberg, 1978; Goldstein and Zornoza, 1978; Gothlin, 1978; McLoughlin et al., 1978; Pereiras et al., 1978; Zornoza, 1981). No deaths have been related to the procedure, and the morbidity is minimal. In our experience, during the actual movement of the needle within the mass, about 15% of the patients complained of some

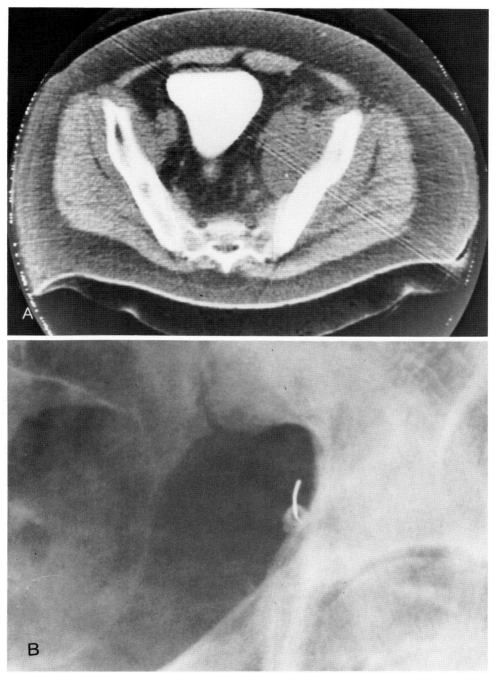

FIGURE 15.7. A 35-YR-OLD MAN WITH THE DIAGNOSIS OF HODGKIN'S DISEASE BUT WITHOUT CLINICAL EVIDENCE OF DISEASE

*A*: CT scan demonstrates a pelvic mass. *B*: Radiograph of the needle at the level of the mass. *C*: Hodgkin's disease. Reed-Sternberg cell. Original magnification ×665. (From Zornoza, 1981.)

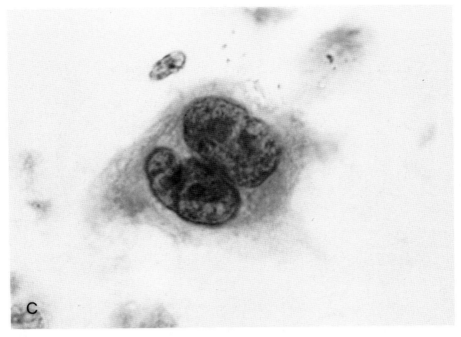

FIGURE 15.7C.

TABLE 15.4.
RESULTS IN PERCUTANEOUS BIOPSY OF LYMPH NODES
ACCORDING TO BIOPSY SITE

| | | |
|---|---|---|
| 247 External iliac | Correct | 181 (73%) |
| | Incorrect | 66 (27%) |
| 23 Common iliac | Correct | 16 (69%) |
| | Incorrect | 7 (31%) |
| 93 Para-aortic | Correct | 62 (66%) |
| | Incorrect | 31 (34%) |

pain or discomfort in the area of the biopsy. During biopsies performed at the para-aortic region, the patients complained of some pain or discomfort, usually when the needle was advanced through the anterior retroperitoneal fascia. Thomson et al. (1977) reported some pain when the capsule of the lymph node was penetrated during lymph node aspiration biopsy. During our biopsies of lymph nodes and of masses located in the pelvic rim or the external iliac region, a few of the patients experienced radicular pain radiating toward the leg. This was most likely due to some irritation of a nerve plexus, and withdrawal of the needle sufficed to relieve the discomfort.

Although the needle may traverse blood vessels, depending upon the biopsy location, only one case of a 200-ml hematoma has been reported (Holm et al., 1975). The blood collection was found at surgery 2 months after aspiration of a pancreatic pseudocyst. Occasionally, small

ecchymoses at the biopsy site have been found at the time of surgery (Goldman et al., 1977; McLoughlin et al., 1978). To assess the effect of needle biopsy on abdominal organs and to evaluate the potential occurrence of complications, an experimental study with animals was performed at our institution (Goldstein et al., 1977). Six healthy mongrel dogs were anesthetized, and multiple percutaneous biopsies, as well as biopsies directed into solid and hollow abdominal organs, were performed. The technique used in the study duplicated the clinical technique. Abdominal contents were inspected at laparotomy and at varying intervals up to 48 hr after the biopsies. The inspection yielded no significant findings. In most instances, it was impossible to identify the path of the needle. Bowel contents could not be expressed even with manual squeezing.

The risk of dissemination of tumor cells through the needle tract is important when the biopsy is performed on a lesion suspected of malignancy. To determine whether aspiration biopsy can promote the spread of tumor cells, Engzell et al. (1971a) conducted an investigation using 21 rabbits with artificially transplanted popliteal lymph node metastases. The efferent lymph and blood vessels were examined for the presence of carcinoma cells before and after the biopsy. In addition, fluid escaping from the needle tract was analyzed. The results of the

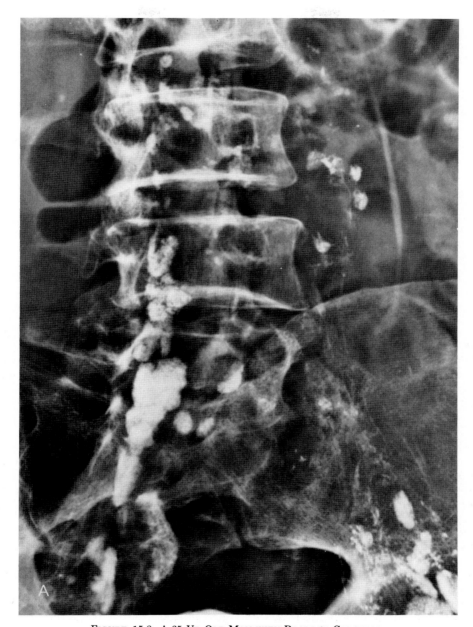

FIGURE 15.8. A 65-YR-OLD MAN WITH BLADDER CARCINOMA

*A*: Nonpacification of common iliac region by lymphangiography. *B*: Venogram shows irregular narrowing of left external iliac vein. Percutaneous biopsy revealed metastatic carcinoma.

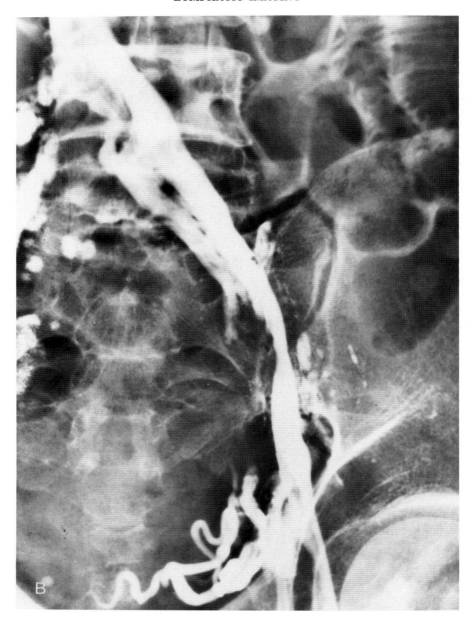

FIGURE 15.8*B*.

experiment demonstrated no evidence of tumor cells in either the lymphatic or blood vessels. In a few instances, carcinoma cells were found outside the lymph node.

The clinical significance of tumor cells escaping from lesions is difficult to evaluate because most tumors undergo therapeutic measures after the aspiration biopsy. Only a few cells enter the needle tract, and these are destroyed before they can give rise to local tumor growth. Occasionally, tumor growth along the needle tract has been reported (Crile and Hazard, 1951; Labardini and Nesbit, 1967; Wolinsky and Lischner, 1969; Berger et al., 1972; Desai and Woodruff, 1974; Ferrucci et al., 1979). In all but one case (Ferrucci et al., 1979), the needle used was a large cutting type.

## SUMMARY

Aspiration biopsy of abdominal neoplasms using small gauge needles has been shown to be a safe and accurate technique, increasingly accepted as a method for establishing tissue diagnosis without surgery. Laparotomy can be avoided in inoperable cases or in patients with recurrent disease, thus obviating the necessity for prolonged hospitalization of such patients.

## REFERENCES

Berg JW: The aspiration biopsy smear. In Koss LG, Durfee GR (eds): *Diagnostic Cytology and Its Histopathologic Bases.* Philadelphia, JB Lippincott, 1961.

Berger RL, Dargan EL, Huang BL: Dissemination of cancer cells by needle biopsy of the lung. *J Thorac Cardiovasc Surg* 63:430–432, 1972.

Berkowitz RS, Leavitt T Jr, Knapp RC: Ultrasound-directed percutaneous aspiration biopsy of periaortic lymph nodes in recurrence of cervical carcinoma. *Am J Obstet Gynecol* 131:906–908, 1978.

Bonfiglio TA, MacIntosh PK, Patten SF Jr, Cafer DJ, Woodworth FE, Kim CW: Fine needle aspiration cytopathology of retroperitoneal lymph nodes in the evaluation of metastatic disease. *Acta Cytol* 23:126–130, 1979.

Correa RJ Jr, Kidd CR, Burnett L, Brannen GE, Gibbons RP, Cummings KB: Percutaneous pelvic lymph node aspiration in carcinoma of the prostate. *J Urol* 126:190–191, 1980.

Crile G Jr, Hazard JB: Classification of thyroiditis with special reference to the use of needle biopsy. *J Clin Endocrinol* 11:1123–1127, 1951.

Desai SG, Woodruff LM: Carcinoma of prostate. Local extension following perineal needle biopsy. *Urology* 3:87–88, 1974.

Dunnick NR, Fisher RI, Chu EW, Young RC: Percutaneous aspiration of retroperitoneal lymph nodes in ovarian cancer. *AJR* 135:109–113, 1980.

Edeiken-Monroe BS, Zornoza J: Carcinoma of the cervix: percutaneous lymph node aspiration biopsy. *AJR* 138:655–657, 1982.

Efremidis SC, Pagliarulo A, Dan SJ, Weber HN, Dillon RN, Nieburgs H, Mitty HA: Post-lymphangiography fine needle aspiration lymph node biopsy in staging carcinoma of the prostate: preliminary report. *J Urol* 122:495–497, 1979.

Eneroth CM, Zajicek J: Aspiration biopsy of salivary gland tumors. III. Morphologic studies on smears and histologic sections from 368 mixed tumors. *Acta Cytol* 10:440–454, 1966.

Engzell U, Esposti PL, Rubio C, Sigurdson A, Zajicek J: Investigation on tumor spread in connection with aspiration biopsy. *Acta Radiol [Diagn] (Stockh)* 10:385–398, 1971a.

Engzell U, Jakobsson PA, Sigurdson A, Zajicek J: Aspiration biopsy of metastatic carcinoma in lymph nodes of the neck. A review of 1101 consecutive cases. *Acta Otolaryngol* 72:138–147, 1971b.

Ennis MG, MacErlean DP. Percutaneous aspiration biopsy of abdomen and retroperitoneum. *Clin Radiol* 31:611–616, 1980.

Evander A, Ihse I, Lunderquist A, Tylen U, Akerman M: Percutaneous cytodiagnosis of carcinoma of the pancreas and bile duct. *Ann Surg* 188:90–92, 1978.

Ferrucci JT, Wittenberg J: CT biopsy of abdominal tumors: aids for lesion localization. *Radiology* 129:739–744, 1978.

Ferrucci JT, Wittenberg J, Margolies MN, Carey RW: Malignant seeding of the tract after thin-needle aspiration biopsy. *Radiology* 130:345–346, 1979.

Fletcher GH, Rutledge FN: Carcinoma of uterine cervix. In Deeley TJ (ed): *Modern Radiotherapy: Gynecological Cancer.* London, Butterworths, 1971.

Franzen S, Zajicek J: Aspiration biopsy in diagnosis of palpable lesions of the breast. Critical review of 3,479 consecutive biopsies. *Acta Radiol [Diagn] (Stockh)* 7:241–262, 1966.

Goldman ML, Naib ZM, Galambos JT, Rude JC III, Oen KT, Bradley EL III, Salam A, Gonzalez AC: Preoperative diagnosis of pancreatic carcinoma by percutaneous aspiration biopsy. *Dig Dis* 22:1076–1082, 1977.

Goldstein HM, Zornoza J: Percutaneous transperitoneal aspiration biopsy of pancreatic masses. *Dig Dis* 23:840–843, 1978.

Goldstein HM, Zornoza J, Wallace S, Anderson JH, Bree RL, Samuels BI, Lukeman JM: Percutaneous fine needle aspiration biopsy of pancreatic and other abdominal masses. *Radiology* 123:319–322, 1977.

Gothlin JH: Post-lymphographic percutaneous fine needle biopsy of lymph nodes guided by fluoroscopy. *Radiology* 120:205–207, 1976.

Gothlin JH: Percutaneous transperitoneal fluoroscopy-guided fine-needle biopsy of lymph nodes. *Acta Radiol [Diagn] (Stockh)* 20:660–664, 1978.

Gothlin JH, Holem L: Percutaneous fine-needle biopsy of radiographically normal lymph nodes in the staging of prostatic carcinoma. *Radiology* 141:351–354, 1981.

Haaga JR, Alfidi RJ: Precise biopsy localization by computed tomography. *Radiology* 118:603–607, 1976.

Hancke S, Holm HH, Koch F: Ultrasonically guided percutaneous fine needle biopsy of the pancreas. *Surg Gynecol Obstet* 140:361–364, 1975.

Holm HH, Pedersen JF, Kristensen JK, Rasmussen SN, Hancke S, Jensen F. Ultrasonically guided percutaneous puncture. *Radiol Clin North Am* 13:493–503, 1975.

Jaques PF, Staab E, Richey W, Photopulos G, Swanton M: CT-assisted pelvic and abdominal aspiration biopsies in gynecological malignancy. *Radiology* 128:651–655, 1978.

Kinmonth JB: Lymphography in man. *Clin Sci* 11:13–29, 1952.

Labardini MM, Nesbit RM: Perineal extension of adenocarcinoma of the prostate gland after punch biopsy. *J Urol* 97:891–893, 1967.

Libshitz HI, Jing BS, Wallace S, Logothetis CJ: Sterilized metastases: a diagnostic and therapeutic dilemma. *AJR* 140:15–19, 1983.

MacIntosh PK, Thomson KR, Barbaric ZL: Percutaneous transperitoneal lymph node biopsy as a means of improving lymphographic diagnosis. *Radiology* 131:647–649, 1979.

McLoughlin MJ, Ho CS, Langer B, McHattie J, Tao LC: Fine needle aspiration biopsy of malignant lesion in and around the pancreas. *Cancer* 41:2413–2419, 1978.

Mennemeyer R, Bartha M, Kidd CR: Diagnostic cytology and electron microscopy of fine needle aspirates of retroperitoneal lymph nodes in the diagnosis of metastatic pelvic neoplasms. *Acta Cytol* 23:370–373, 1979.

Pereiras RV, Meirers W, Kunhardt B, Troner M, Hutson D,

Barkin JS, Viamonte M: Fluoroscopically guided thin needle aspiration biopsy of the abdomen and retroperitoneum. *AJR* 131:197–202, 1978.

Piver SM, Wallace S, Castro JR: The accuracy of lymphangiography in carcinoma of the uterine cervix. *AJR* 111:278–283, 1971.

Prando A, Wallace S, VonEschenbach AC, Jing BS, Rosengreen JE, Hussey DH: Lymphangiography in staging of carcinoma of the prostate. *Radiology* 131:641–645, 1979.

Ruttimann A: Iliac lymph node aspiration biopsy through paravascular approach; preliminary report. *Radiology* 90:150–152, 1968.

Smith EH, Bartrum RJ Jr, Chang YC, D'Orsi CJ, Lokick J, Abbruzzese A, Dantono J: Percutaneous aspiration biopsy of the pancreas under ultrasonic guidance. *N Engl J Med* 292:825–828, 1975.

Söderström N: *Fine-Needle Aspiration Biopsy Used as a Direct Adjunct in Clinical Diagnostic Work.* Stockholm, Almqvist & Wiksell, 1966.

Spellman MC, Castellino RA, Ray GR, Pistenna DA, Bagshaw MA: An evaluation of lymphography in localized carcinoma of the prostate. *Radiology* 125:637–644, 1977.

Stephenson TF, Mehnert PJ, Marx AJ, Boger JN, Moyo LR, Balaji MR, Nadajara N: Evaluation of contrast markers for CT aspiration biopsy. *AJR* 133:1097–1100, 1979.

Thomson KR, House AJS, Gothlin JH, Dolan TE: Percutaneous lymph node aspiration biopsy: experience with a new technique. *Clin Radiol* 28:329–332, 1977.

Wallace S, Jing BS: Lymphangiographic diagnosis of nodal metastases from testicular malignancies. *JAMA* 213:94–96, 1970.

Wallace S, Schwartz PE, Anderson JH, Gianturco C, Luna MA, Smith JP: A feasibility study for percutaneous retroperitoneal lymph node biopsy. *AJR* 125:234–239, 1975.

Wallace S, Jing BS, Zornoza J: Lymphangiography in the determination of the extent of metastatic carcinoma. *Cancer* 39:706–718, 1977.

Wolinsky H, Lischner MW: Needle tract implantation of tumor after percutaneous lung biopsy. *Ann Intern Med* 71:359–362, 1969.

Zajicek J, Franzen S, Jakobsson P, Rubio C, Unsgaard B: Aspiration biopsy of mammary tumors in diagnosis and research. A critical review of 2,200 cases. *Acta Cytol* 11:169–175, 1967.

Zornoza J: Abdomen. In *Percutaneous Needle Biopsy.* Baltimore, Williams & Wilkins, 1981.

Zornoza J, Handel P, Lukeman JM, Jing BS, Wallace S: Percutaneous transperitoneal biopsy in urologic malignancies. *Urology* 9:395–398, 1977a.

Zornoza J, Jonsson K, Wallace S, Lukeman JM: Fine needle aspiration biopsy of retroperitoneal lymph nodes and abdominal masses: an updated report. *Radiology* 125:87–88, 1977b.

Zornoza J, Lukeman JM, Jing BS, Wharton JT, Wallace S: Percutaneous retroperitoneal lymph node biopsy in carcinoma of the cervix. *Gynecol Oncol* 5:43–51, 1977c.

Zornoza J, Wallace S, Goldstein HM, Lukeman JM, Jing BS: Transperitoneal percutaneous retroperitoneal lymph node aspiration biopsy. *Radiology* 122:111–115, 1977d.

Zornoza J, Cabanillas FF, Altoff TM, Ordonez N, Cohen MA: Percutaneous needle in abdominal lymphoma. *AJR* 136:97–103, 1981.

# 16

# *Complications*

MELVIN E. CLOUSE, M.D.

Lymphography, like all procedures that introduce a foreign substance into the body, is associated with complications. The major complications of lymphography are caused by the vital dyes and contrast materials rather than technique. The ideal contrast material—one that has no negative side effects and gives sharp delineation of lymph vessels and nodes for a period of time—is not yet available. Initially, water-soluble contrast media such as Cholegraphin were used (Tjernberg, 1956). Node detail was inadequate with these media, however, because they are diluted during passage through the lymphatic system. Ethiodol, a fat-soluble contrast agent, is the contemporary agent of choice: it offers sharp delineation and remains in the lymph nodes for several months (permitting follow-up of progressive lymph node changes). Ethiodol also has negative side effects, however.

## Body Distribution of Ethiodol

Ethiodol passes from the lymph vessels into the venous system via the thoracic duct or by lymphaticovenous communications (usually caused by lymphatic obstruction peripheral to the thoracic duct). The lower the obstruction in the lymphatic system, the greater the chance of more oil entering the venous system, passing into the lungs, and thus increasing the severity of pulmonary oil emboli.

Koehler et al. (1964) studied the body distribution of Ethiodol in dogs. After 3 days the oil was concentrated in the lungs (50%), lymphatic system (25%), bone (4.2%), muscle (3.9%), brain (0.38%), and kidney (0.2%). The concentration in the lungs decreased to 9.8% after 17 days while that retained in lymph nodes remained almost constant at 20%. These figures are not directly applicable to humans because the number of iliac and retroperitoneal lymph nodes in the dog is considerably less than in humans.

On whole body scans performed after intraaortic injection of [131]I Ethiodol, Threefoot (1968) found the major portions in the liver, lungs, and kidneys. This finding suggests that these organs

have a more effective filter for oil than the other organs and peripheral regions. Further studies by Threefoot showed that 75–90% of the iodine in venous blood during the first 2 days was in the lipid form in the plasma. The iodine was redistributed in the plasma to lipid and aqueous states as well as being adhered to the red cells. After 9 days almost all of the plasma iodine was in the aqueous state. The iodine was excreted by the kidneys in this form with approximately 90% being recovered in 3 weeks. The fate of the lipid portion of the molecule is not completely known, but it is probably degraded by beta oxidation.

## Pulmonary Oil Emboli

Because the lymphatics drain directly into the venous system, oil embolization occurs to a degree in every patient examined, but the amount of pulmonary oil embolization is difficult to determine. Even when constant amounts of contrast material are injected, variations occur in the amount retained in the nodes, the size and number of nodes, and the presence or absence of lymphaticovenous communications. Ethiodol can be identified in only 19–55% of routine postlymphography chest films (Bron et al., 1963; Wallace, 1965; Clouse et al., 1966) (Fig. 16.1). At postmortem in dogs Abrams et al. (1968) have found considerable amounts of Ethiodol in small pulmonary arteries that were not visible on the chest radiographs. Ethiodol can be differentiated from neutral fat in the tissues using brilliant cresyl blue and silver nitrate stain (Felton, 1952; Hallgrimsson and Clouse, 1965).

Pulmonary oil embolization usually does not produce clinical symptoms unless there is underlying cardiopulmonary pathology, excess amounts of contrast material are given (over 14–16 ml of Ethiodol), patent lymphaticovenous communications shunt more oil to the lungs, or the patient is hypersensitive to the oil. Fraimow et al. (1966) noted a decrease in diffusion capacity 2–24 hr after injection with a beginning of return to normal in 48 hr. Gold et al. (1965) also reported a decrease in diffusion capacity, pul-

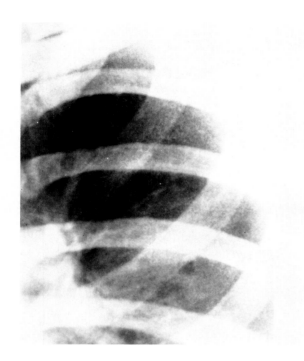

FIGURE 16.1. ETHIODOL
Left upper lung field 24 hr after injection of 7 ml of
Ethiodol into lymphatics of each lower extremity. Fine stippled densities indicate embolized Ethiodol. The patient was
asymptomatic.

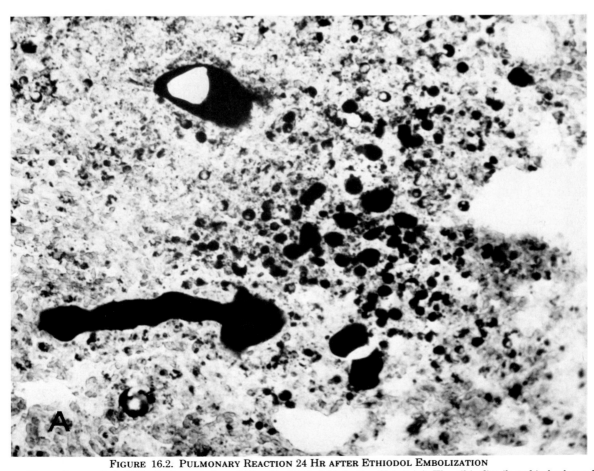

FIGURE 16.2. PULMONARY REACTION 24 HR AFTER ETHIODOL EMBOLIZATION

*A.* Photomicrograph (×290) of guinea pig lung 24 hr after Ethiodol injection (fat stain). The oil is distributed in both small
arterioles and alveoli.

monary capillary blood volume, and lung compliance without any clinical symptoms of pulmonary oil emboli. Gold et al. attributed the abnormality in diffusion capacity to a decrease in pulmonary capillary blood volume produced by oil emboli. Fraimow et al., however, believe it is caused by both a decrease in capillary blood volume and an inflammatory reaction in the alveolocapillary space. White et al. (1973) could not demonstrate an abnormality in the forced expiratory volume in 1 and 2 sec or vital capacity 1 month after lymphography. They concluded that only patients with severe lung disease would require careful assessment before lymphography.

To study the fate of Ethiodol in the lungs and the pulmonary reaction, 0.1 ml of Ethiodol was given intravenously to 0.4- and 0.5-kg guinea pigs. The animals were sacrificed 24 hr to 32 days after injection. Ethiodol was not visible roentgenographically after 12 days, but it was found microscopically in considerable amounts even after 32 days. The animal sacrificed at 24 hr showed Ethiodol in small pulmonary arteries as well as extravasation of serum and Ethiodol into the alveoli surrounded by large numbers of neutrophils and lymphocytes (Fig. 16.2). Histiocytes were present within 48 hr (Fig. 16.3), and after 8 days these predominated over the acute inflammatory response (Fig. 16.4).

The acute inflammatory response gradually regressed so that in 32 days there was clearing of most of the alveolar exudate and lipid material. Alveolar walls remained thickened by proliferation of capillary endothelium and alveolar lining cells. The remaining Ethiodol was scattered throughout the blood vessels of the lung with isolated oil granulomata (Fig. 16.5).

Ethiodol was demonstrated in pulmonary arteries and capillaries of four patients dying from causes unrelated to lymphography 1–33 days after lymphography. An endothelial reaction consisting of histiocytic cells was identified

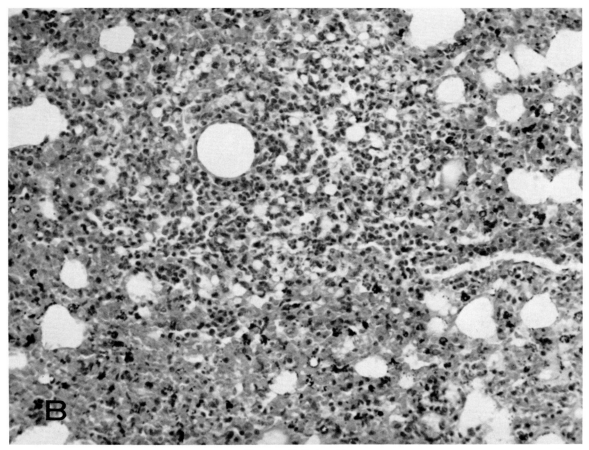

FIGURE 16.2. (cont.)

*B.* Photomicrograph (×290) of guinea pig lung 24 hr after Ethiodol injection (hematoxylin and eosin stain). Acute inflammatory infiltrate surrounding globules of oil (clear spaces).

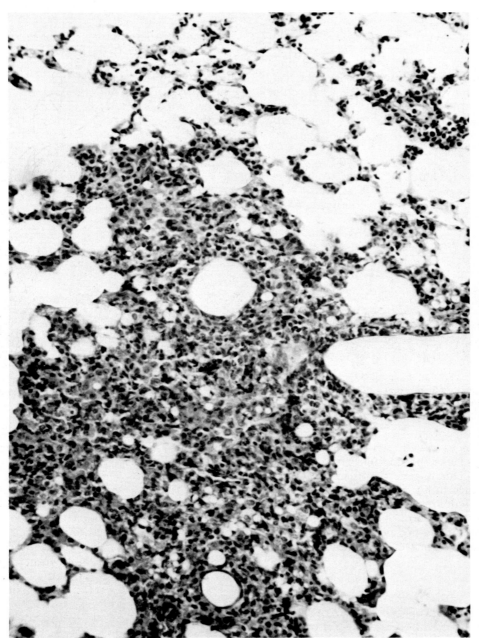

FIGURE 16.3. PULMONARY REACTION 48 HR AFTER ETHIODOL EMBOLIZATION

Photomicrograph (×255) of guinea pig lung 48 hr after Ethiodol injection (hematoxylin and eosin stain). Histiocytes now predominate over lymphocytes and neutrophiles. Oil is seen as clear spaces within infiltrate.

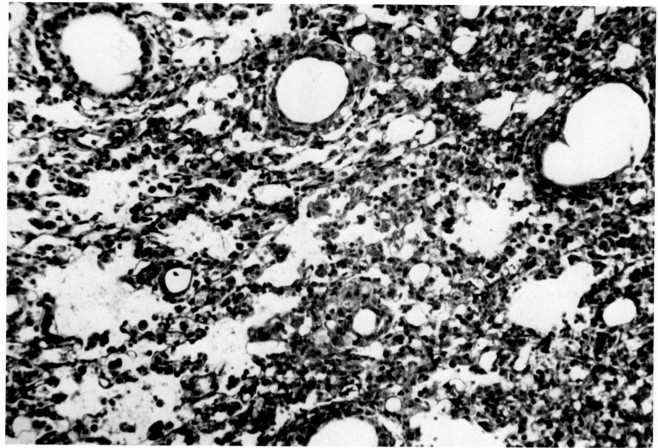

FIGURE 16.4. PULMONARY REACTION 8 DAYS AFTER ETHIODOL EMBOLIZATION
Photomicrograph (×255) of guinea pig lung 8 days after Ethiodol injection. Oil granulomas are seen as clear spaces surrounded by giant cells and large histiocytes.

within the lipid-containing vessels. These inflammatory changes presumably regressed without serious sequelae or the amount of oil reaching the lungs did not damage a significant number of alveolocapillary units. Schaffer et al. (1963) reported no Ethiodol in pulmonary capillaries in patients autopsied several months after lymphography. There have not been reports of significant long term effects of pulmonary oil embolization.

## Pneumonia

The incidence of oil pneumonitis is probably greater than is reported because it is not usually life threatening. Patients with pneumonia usually spike a temperature of 101–104° within 6–12 hr after the injection. Roentgenograms of the chest in these patients show diffuse oil emboli as soft discrete nodular densities throughout both lungs (Fig. 16.6). Fever gradually subsides within

4–5 days, and the pulmonary infiltrate resolves within 5–7 days. Pneumonia has been reported in five of 108 consecutive examinations (4.6%) (Clouse et al., 1966) and 2.8% (Kutarna et al., 1972). In a survey of 32,000 examinations, Koehler (1968) found an incidence of 1:2500 but believed it was much higher.

Pulmonary edema, infarction, and cardiovascular collapse associated with dyspnea, cyanosis, and pleuritic chest pain have been reported. These reactions are life threatening and require oxygen, vasopressors, and digitalis (Fuchs, 1962; Schaffer et al., 1962; Bron et al., 1963).

## Neurologic Complications

Cerebral complications after lymphography are rare. Twenty-two cases have been reported in the world literature (Nelson et al., 1965; Boudin et al., 1967; Cardis, 1967; Colette, 1967; Gerest et al., 1967; Gruwez, 1967; Koehler, 1968;

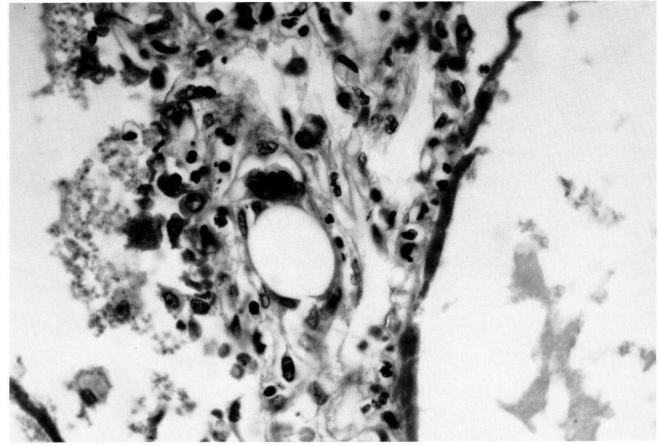

FIGURE 16.5. HUMAN LUNG 11 DAYS AFTER LYMPHOGRAPHY

Photomicrograph (×725) of human lung 11 days after lymphography. Oil granuloma represented by a clear space with surrounding foreign body giant cells.

Collard et al., 1969; Collard and Noel, 1969; Davidson, 1969; Rasmussen, 1970; Okuda et al., 1971; Veyssier et al., 1971; Gerhard and Brolsch, 1972; Moskowitz et al., 1972; Sviridov, 1972). Three of these were fatal (Nelson et al., 1965; Gruwez, 1967; Gerhard and Brolsch, 1972). Nelson et al. reported the first fatality after injecting 20 ml of Ethiodol into each lower extremity. Gerhard and Brolsch reported a patient who received 15 ml of Lipiodol, but the patient had received irradiation for lymphoma. These patients experienced mental confusion, disorientation, motor weaknesses or paralysis, and coma. Rasmussen (1970) and Jay and Ludington (1973) reported temporary blindness in association with other cerebral symptoms of oil emboli in two patients. Both recovered completely within 6 weeks.

Ethiodol may short-circuit the lung filter via intracardiac shunts, pulmonary arteriovenous fistulae, and possibly shunts within a lung tumor. Lymphaticovenous communications may also allow excess contrast material to reach the lung and overload its filter system. Animal experiments by Davidson (1969) suggest that radiation to the lung impairs the filter mechanism, presumably by capillary damage. This allows more oily contrast media to pass into the arterial circuit and become peripheral emboli.

## Hypersensitivity

### Patent Blue Dye

Hohenfellner and Ludvik (1964) reported the first patient having an allergic reaction to patent blue violet dye. Since then approximately 32 cases have been reported (Collard and Colette, 1967; Gruwez, 1967; Sieber, 1968; Mortazavi and Burrows, 1971). The true incidence is difficult to ascertain. Mortazavi and Burrows reported three cases in a series of 120 lymphograms. Two of

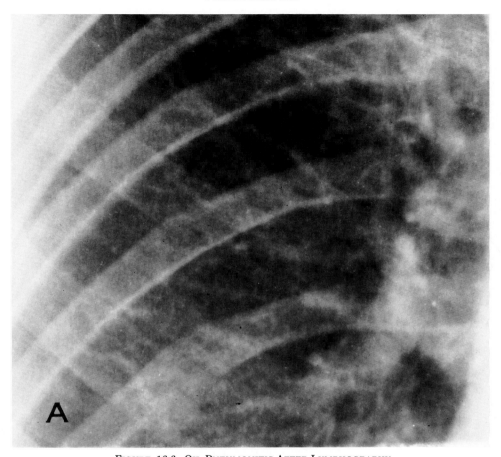

FIGURE 16.6. OIL PNEUMONITIS AFTER LYMPHOGRAPHY

*A.* Chest normal on a 42-yr-old female who had lymphography (7 ml of Ethiodol injected into each extremity) for carcinoma of the vulva.

their patients had negative skin tests to Xylocaine. Kropholler (1967), who does not mix patent blue with Xylocaine, reported six cases in 400 lymphograms. These reports suggest that the true incidence is much more common than originally reported, probably near 1%.

The allergic reaction usually manifests itself within minutes after injection by urticaria and blue wheals stained by blue serum from the dye. The reaction may require only subcutaneous epinephrine or intravenous antihistamines. More severe reactions may lead to bronchospasm; periorbital, glossal, and laryngeal edema; and hypotension. In such patients epinephrine, intravenous hydrocortisone, vasopressors, or tracheal intubation with respiratory assistance may be necessary. Death has not been reported.

Sokolowski and Engeset (1974) have reported marked cellular death and lymphocyte depletion in lymph nodes of dogs whose efferent vessels were ligated prior to the injection of patent blue

violet dye. Similar but less severe changes were noted in nodes, the efferent vessels of which were not ligated. These changes have not been reported in humans and probably are not clinically significant. The lymph nodes observed in humans almost always have superimposed inflammatory changes secondary to Ethiodol, however.

### Ethiodol

Allergic reactions to the oily contrast media are sometimes difficult to evaluate because of the normal reaction of the lung to oil and superimposed pneumonia (which is probably always present even though it is not detected roentgenographically). Koehler (1968) reported an incidence of one in 800 lymphographies. Bray et al. (1970) reported two cases of Loeffler's syndrome in a series of 88 lymphograms. Symptoms began at 2 and 6 days after lymphography and were characterized by chills, fever, slight cyanosis, and

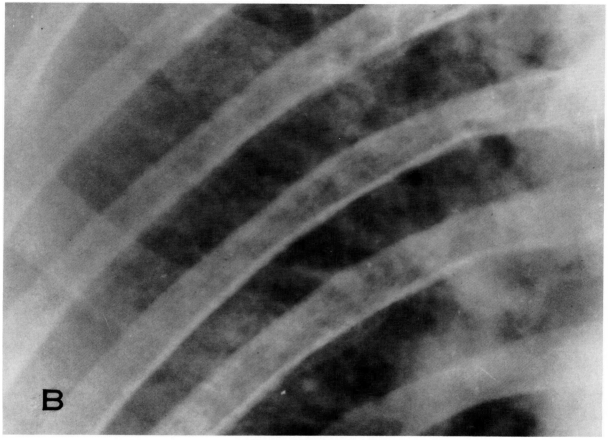

FIGURE 16.6. (*cont.*)

*B.* The patient's temperature was 102° 6 hr after injection. She was slightly dyspneic with no cough, chest pain, or cyanosis. Chest roentgenogram 48 hr after injection revealed multiple small soft nodular densities in both lungs.

blood-streaked sputum with eosinophiles. The white blood cell count demonstrated 22% and 6% eosinophilia. The syndrome slowly cleared spontaneously.

Wiertz et al. (1971) reported a case of intrapulmonary hemorrhage and anemia occurring 5 days after lymphography. Dyspnea and hemoptysis were combined with a drop in the hematocrit from 43% to 28% over a 3-day period. The reaction did not impair pulmonary functions seriously and the lungs cleared spontaneously after 1 week. Kohler et al. (1969) reported nine cases in a series of 1000 lymphangiograms using 7–8 ml of ultrafluid Lipiodol for the lower extremities and 3–4 ml for the arm. This large series suggests that allergy to the contrast material approaches 1%.

## Cardiac

No cardiac fatalities have been reported, but Leitsmann and Dietzsch (1972) reported abnormal electrocardiogram changes in 12 of 25 patients undergoing lymphography. The abnormalities were S-T segment depression and T wave flattening.

## Minor Complications

Fever may occur as an isolated complication. The patient may experience one transient temperature elevation 6–18 hr after lymphography. This may be caused by pyrogens entering the lymphatics or, more likely, Ethiodol. This complication is missed when lymphograms are done as an outpatient procedure, but it is not significant.

Patients may also experience a low grade temperature (99–101°) with gradual return to normal after 3–4 days. Although it cannot be documented radiographically, this probably is a low grade oil pneumonitis or generalized low grade inflammatory reaction to the contrast material. Only symptomatic treatment is required.

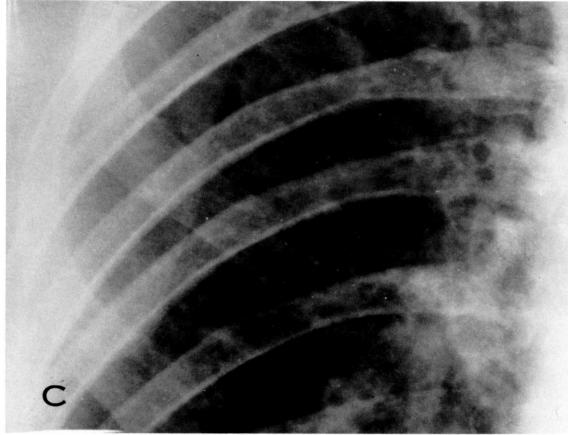

FIGURE 16.6. (*cont.*)

*C.* The patient experienced daily temperature elevations gradually decreasing to normal over a 4-day period. Chest roentgenogram shows almost complete clearing after 9 days.

Delayed wound healing, which can be treated with warm saline soaks, occurs in a few patients. Lymphangitis and wound infection rarely develop but do respond to antibiotics and warm saline soaks.

## REFERENCES

Abrams HL, Takahashi M, Adams DF: Clinical and experimental studies of pulmonary oil embolism. *Cancer Chemother Rep* 52:81, 1968.

Boudin G, Pepin B, Vernant J-C: Manifestations neuropsychiatriques au decors d'une lymphographie. *Bull Soc Med Hop Paris* 118:1027, 1967.

Bray DA, Brown CH, Herdt JR, DeVita VT: Loeffler's syndrome as a complication of bipedal lymphangiography. *JAMA* 214:369, 1970.

Bron KM, Baum S, Abrams HL: Oil embolism in lymphangiography. Incidence, manifestations, and mechanisms. *Radiology* 80:194, 1963.

Cardis R: Lymphography, panel discussion. II. A. Complications and accidents. In *Progress in Lymphology: Proceedings of the International Symposium on Lymphology, Zurich, Switzerland, July 19–23, 1966.* Stuttgart, Georg Thieme Verlag, 1967, p 323.

Clouse ME, Hallgrimsson J, Wenlund PE: Complications following lymphography with particular reference to pulmonary oil embolization. *Am J Roentgenol Radium Ther Nucl Med* 96:972, 1966.

Colette JM: Lymphography, panel discussion. II. A. Complications and accidents. In *Progress in Lymphology: Proceedings of the International Symposium on Lymphology, Zurich, Switzerland, July 19–23, 1966.* Stuttgart, Georg Thieme Verlag, 1967, p 323.

Collard M, Colette JM: Les modalities cliniques de l'allergie au bleu patente violet. *J Belge Radiol* 50:407, 1967.

Collard M, Leroux G, Noel G, Declercq A: L'embolie cerebrale graisseuse diffuse: complication de la lymphographie lipiodolee. *J Radiol Electrol Med Nucl* 50:793, 1969.

Collard M, Noel G: Embolies cerebrales graisseuses, complication de l'exame l'esamen lymphographique au lipiodol. *Acta Neurol Belg* 69:419, 1969.

Davidson JW: Lipid embolism to the brain following lymphography. Case report and experimental study. *Am J*

*Roentgenol Radium Ther Nucl Med* 105:763, 1969.

Felton EL II: A method for the identification of Lipiodol in tissue sections. *Lab Invest* 1:3, 1952.

Fraimow W, Wallace S, Lewis P, Greening RR, Cathcart RT: Changes in pulmonary function due to lymphangiography. *Radiology* 85:231, 1966.

Fuchs WA: Complications in lymphography with oily contrast media. *Acta Radiol* 57:427, 1962.

Gerest F, Rouves L, Maleysson M, Saint-Paul J: Encephalopathie a semeiologie psychiatrique consecutive a une lymphographie. *Lyon Med* 218:1435, 1967.

Gerhard L, Brolsch C: Morphology of the central nervous system with Lipiodol following lymphography. *Verh Dtsch Ges Sch Path* 56:401, 1972.

Gold WM, Youker J, Anderson S, Nadel JA: Pulmonary function abnormalities after lymphangiography. *N Engl J Med* 273:519, 1965.

Gruwez J: Lymphography, panel discussion II. A. Complications and accidents. In *Progress in Lymphology: Proceedings of the International Symposium on Lymphology, Zurich, Switzerland, July 19–23, 1966.* Stuttgart, Georg Thieme Verlag, 1967, p 322.

Hallgrimsson J, Clouse ME: Pulmonary oil emboli after lymphography. *Arch Pathol* 80:426, 1965.

Hohenfellner R, Ludvik W: Die Lymphographie in der Urologischn diagnostik. *Urologe [A]* 3:87, 1964.

Jay JC, Ludington LG: Neurologic complications following lymphangiography. Possible mechanism and a case of blindness. *Arch Surg* 106:863, 1973.

Koehler PR: Complications of lymphography. *Lymphology* 1:116, 1968.

Koehler P, Meyers WA, Skelley JF, Schaffer B: Body distribution of Ethiodol following lymphography. *Radiology* 82:866, 1964.

Kohler I, Platzbecker H, Fritz H: Komplikationen bei de oligen Lymphographie—ein bericht uber 1000 lymphographische Untersuchungen. *Cesk Radiol* 23:48, 1969.

Kropholler RW: Lymphography, panel discussion. II. A. Complications and accidents. In *Progress in Lymphology: Proceedings of the International Symposium on Lymphology, Zurich, Switzerland, July 19–23, 1966.* Stuttgart, Georg Thieme Verlag, 1967, p 306.

Kutarna A, Hanecka M, Saskova B, Javorkova J: Lung complications following lymphographies with iodinated poppyseed oil. *Bratisl Lek Listy* 58:581, 1972.

Leitsmann H, Dietzsch J: Electrocardiographic changes following lymphography. *Zentralbl Gynaekol* 14:1392, 1972.

MacDonald JS, Wallace E: Lymphangiography in tumors of the kidney, bladder and testicle. *Br J Radiol* 38:93, 1965.

Mikol J, Bousser MG, Grellet F, Chomette G, Sors C, Garcin R: Paraplegie au cours d'une lymphographie chez une malade atteinte d'un reticulosarcome glanglionnaire cervical; etude anatomo-clinique. *Ann Med Interne (Paris)* 121:355, 1970.

Mortazavi SH, Burrows BD: Allergic reaction to patent blue dye in lymphography. *Clin Radiol* 22:389, 1971.

Moskowitz G, Chen P, Adams DF: Lipid embolization to the kidney and brain after lymphography. *Radiology* 102:327, 1972.

Nelson B, Rush EA, Takasugi M, Wittenberg J: Lipid embolism to the brain after lymphography. *N Engl J Med* 273:1132, 1965.

Okuda K, Matsuo H, Adachi M: Side effect of lymphography with special reference to pulmonary and cerebral embolism. *Rinsho Hoshasen* 16:979, 1971.

Rasmussen KE: Retinal and cerebral fat emboli following lymphography with oily contrast media. *Acta Radiol (Diagn)* 10:199, 1970.

Schaffer B, Gould RJ, Wallace S, Jackson L, Iuker M, Leherman PR, Felten TR: Urological application of lymphangiography. *J Urol* 87:91, 1962.

Schaffer B, Koehler PR, Daniel RC, Wohl GT, Rivera E, Meyers WA, Skelley JF: A critical evaluation of lymphangiography. *Radiology* 80:917, 1963.

Sieber F: Incidents after the subcutaneous instillation of patent blue (Patent blau) for lymphography. *Med Bild* 11:102, 1968.

Sokolowski J, Engeset A: The toxic effect of patent blue violet on rat lymph node lymphocytes. *Lymphology* 7:28, 1974.

Sviridov NK: Embolia mazga posle limfografii. *Khirurgiia (Mosk)* 48:145, 1972.

Threefoot SA: Pulmonary hazards of lymphography. *Cancer Chemother Rep* 52:107, 1968.

Tjernberg B: Lymphography as an aid to examination of lymph nodes. *Acta Soc Med Upsalien* 61:207, 1956.

Veyssier P, et al: Embolie grasseuse cerebrale and lymphographie. *Ann Med Interne (Paris)* 122:1127, 1971.

White RJ, Webb JAW, Tucker AK, Foster KM: Pulmonary function after lymphography. *Br Med J* 4:775, 1973.

Wiertz LM, Gagnon JH, Anthonisen NR: Intrapulmonary hemorrhage with anemia after lymphography. *N Engl J Med* 285:1364, 1971.

# Index

## A

Abrams HL, 58, 62, 89, 204, 267, 511
Ackerman T, 162
Adair TH, physiology, 120–141
Adrenal lymphatics, 81, 183
Akisada M, 236
Albrecht A, 235, 236
Albumin disappearance curves, in lymphedema, 151
Allen EV, 142
Allenby F, 154
Allergy to foods, and mesenteric lymphatic malformation, 201–202
Anatomy, lymphatic, 15–94, 472–485. *See also specific lymphatic structures*
Anderson KC, 99
Angiosarcoma, 164
Ann Arbor classification for lymphoma, 96, 265
Aortic lymphatics. *See* Para-aortic lymphatics
Aortography, in retroperitoneal fibrosis, 230
Arger PH, 230
Arnulf G, 144
Arthritis, 224
Arts V, 116
Ascites
  chylous, 161
  in ovarian carcinoma, 342, 343
Asellius G, 1, 8
Axilla
  carcinoma, 102–103
  lymphatic anatomy, 90–91, 398

## B

Bacsa S, 235
Bagshaw MA, 343
Bartels P, 305
Bartholin T, 1, 7
Bassani G, 240
Baum H, 168
Bennett MH, 253, 257
Benson KH, 383
Bergeron RT, cervical nodes, 472–495
Bergquist L, 101
Biligrafin, 12, 14
Biopsy, percutaneous, 496–510
  complications, 504–508
  equipment, 496–497
  indications, 499–503
  small intestine, 190
  solid tumor diagnosis, 297
  technique, 497–499
Bladder, urinary
  carcinoma, 105, 209, 295, 368, 371–378
  CT appearance, 376–378
  lymphatics, 50, 368–371
  lymphographic appearance, 371–378
Blalock A, 162, 165
Blaudow K, 235, 236

Boerhaave H, 12
Bone
  lymphatics, 195–196, 424
  lymphoma, 429–437
  tumors, 424–429
Bonfiglio TA, 503
Bottcher J, 236
Bray DA, 517
Breast
  carcinoma, 101, 102–104, 106, 389–397, 399–400
  consequences of surgery, 144, 149, 156, 157, 160
  CT appearance, 400, 466
  lymphatic drainage, 397–399
  lymphographic appearance, 118, 399–400
  scintigraphic appearance, 102–104
  thoracic metastases from, 452, 466
  *See also* Mammary lymphatics
Brice M, II, 376
Brill NE, 264
Broder S, 248, 255
Brolsch C, 516
Bron KM, 169
Bronchial lymphatics, drainage, 106
Bronskill MJ, 101
Brucellosis, 236
Bruun S, 115
Buffalo hump, in lymphedema, 145
Burke JF, 12
Burkitt D, 264
Burkitt's lymphoma, 249, 251, 257
Burn JI, 143
Burns, causing edema, 136
Burrows BD, 112, 516
Busch FM, 348
Bussey HJR, 386
Butler JJ, 228

## C

Calnan J, 143
Camiel MR, 165
Cannulation of lymphatics, 114–115
Capillaries, lymphatic, 120
  anatomy, 17
  contractions, 131–132
  filtration, 122–123, 133
  permeability, 123–127, 136
  pressure, 136
  pumps, 130–132, 133
Carcinoma, 290–450
  genitourinary, 348–385
  gynecologic, 321–348
  imaging techniques, 290–297
  mechanism of lymphatic metastasis, 297–305
  modes of lymphatic metastasis, 305–321
  squamous cell, 106
  *See also specific organ or type*
Carvalho R, 12
Casley-Smith JR, 12
Castellino RA, 268, 365, 383
Catovsky D, 255

Cavography. *See* Venography
Celiac lymphatics, 71, 106
Cervical (neck) lymphatics, 91, 472–495
  anatomy, 106, 472–485
  CT appearance, 487–493
  examination technique, 91, 485–487
  in cisterna chyli malformations, 183
  metastasis, 476, 493–494, 452
  size, 488
Cervix, uterine, 321–327
  biopsy of metastases, 501
  carcinoma, 105, 172, 296–297, 310, 321–327
  CT appearance, 325–327
  lymphatics, 52, 106, 322–323
  lymphographic appearance, 323–327, 496
Charles H, 158
Charles procedure, for lymphedema, 158
Chemotherapy, 265, 302, 502
Chiappa S, 55, 348
Chilvers AS, 156
Cholegraphin, 511
Chondrosarcoma, 424–429
Chylarthrosis, in mesenteric malformations, 183
Chyloma, 182
Chylopericardium, 188, 200
Chyloperitoneum, 182, 192–194
Chylorrhea, 182, 195
Chylothorax, 162, 186, 198–200
Chylous syndromes, 161–163
Chyluria, 162–163, 183, 196–198
Cisterna chyli
  discovery of, 1, 89
  malformations of, 180–188
Clementz B, 116
Clodius L, 157
Cloquet, node of. *See* Rosenmüller, node of
Clouse ME
  anatomy, 15–94
  benign nodal disease, 224–242
  complications of lymphography, 511–520
  history, 1–14
  interpretation, 203–223
  lymphoma, 264–289
  obstruction and collateral flow, 165–169
  technique of lymphography, 111–119
Coefficient of capillary filtration, 122
Collagen diseases, lymphographic appearance, 209
Collargol, 12
Collaterals, lymphatic
  in carcinoma, 301, 310, 358
  in mesenteric lymphatic malformations, 180, 182
  in obstruction, 165–167
  in upper extremity edema, 403–408
Collins RD, 243
Computed tomography. *See* Tomography, computed

Contiguity theory, 265
Contrast material, 12–14, 21, 115–116
Cook FE, 348
Cook PL, 165
Copeland EM, 386
Crampton AR, 144, 160
Craven CE, 165
Crile G, Jr, 386
Cruikshank W, 1, 7, 12
Cunningham JB, 165
Cusick H, 116
Cyst, chylous, 182, 198–200

D

Damascelli B, 114
Das SK, 157
Davidson JD, 176
Davidson JW, 516
Davis HK, 89
Decision trees, 284–287, 494
Dellon AL, 158
Dermal flap, in lymphedema, 157–158
DeRoo T, 114, 116
Diaphragmatic nodes, 82, 463–466
Dietsch J, 518
Dionne L, 103
Ditchek T, 118
Dorfman RF, 256
Doss LL, 112
Douglas B, 332, 342
Drinker, Cecil K, 1, 12, 162
Dukes CE, 386
Dunnick NR, 360
Dyes, vital, 111–112, 516–517. See also
        specific dyes
Dysglobulinemia, 249, 250, 257, 258

E

Edeiken-Monroe B, 327
Edema. See Lymphedema
Edwards CL, 96
Ege GN, 100, 101, 102, 103
Elephantiasis, 190, 201
Ellert J, 389
Embolization of oil, 511–515
Endometrium, carcinoma of, 295, 327
Engeset A, 115, 240, 349, 517
Engzell U, 506
Enteropathy, protein-losing, 182,
        190–192
Epstein AL, 256
Esophagography, 453–466, 468
Esophagus, carcinoma of, 106, 440–441
Esterly JR, 147
Ethiodol, 115–116, 118, 511–518
Eustace PW, 148, 149
Eustachius, 1
Evans blue dye, 180, 189
Exercise, effect on lymph flow, 128
Extremites
    abnormalities, 142–176
    anatomy, lower, 21–28
    anatomy, upper, 90–91
    lymphographic filling, 22
    scintigraphic appearance, 103
    See also Lymphedema

F

Facial nodes, 477
Faling LJ, 469
Fallopian tubes, 51–52
Feins NR, 160
Fibrolipoma, 63, 233
Fibrosarcoma, 416, 423–424
Fibrosis
    in chyluria, 162
    in lymphedema, 154, 155
    retroperitoneal, 176, 230–232
Filaria parasite
    causing chyluria, 162
    causing lymphedema, 144, 150, 160
Filly R, 455, 459
Filming, for lymphography, 116–118
Fisch U, 90
Fischer HW, 116
Fistula, lymphatic, 172
Floating aorta sign, 294
Fluid, interstitial
    anatomy, 120–121
    formation, 121–123, 128
    pressure, 132, 133, 134–135, 137
    protein, 125–127
Fluoroscopy, 200, 496–497
Foaminess
    grades of, 204–205, 267
    normal, 43–46, 62
Földi M, 171
Fonkalsrud EW, 160
Fornier AM, 224
Fosburg RG, 469
Fraimow W, 511, 513
Friedman E, 292
Friedman M, 493
Frommhold H, 89
Fuchs WA, 29, 89, 165, 324, 343
Fuks J, 99
Fuks Z, 256
Funaoka S, 12
Fussek H, 383
Fyfe NC, 143

G

Gallium-67, 95–101, 453, 469–470
Gammopathy, IgM, 257
Gamsu G, 459
Ganel A, 144
Gangolli SD, 112
Gastroduodenal lymph nodes, 71
Genitourinary tract
    lymphatics, 48–56
    thoracic metastasis, 452
    tumors, 348–385
    See also specific organs
George P, 144, 149
Gerhard L, 516
Gerota D, 12
Gerota's fascia, lymphatics, 48
Gerteis W, 324
Gilbert R, 265
Gilchrist MR, 116
Gillies procedure, in lymphedema, 157
Glick AD, 256
Gold WM, 511, 513
Gold-198 colloid, 100, 101, 102, 104
Goldsmith HS, 157

Golimbu M, 383
Gong-Kang H, 157
Good RA, 244
Gooneratne BWM, 144
Goplerud DR, 325
Gothlin JH, 503
Granulomatous diseases, 209, 235–240,
        476. See also specific types
Gregl A, 236
Gross R, 162
Gruart FJ, 118
Guyton AC, physiology, 120–141

H

Hall JG, 240
Hammond JA, 325
Hanafee WN, 494
Handley WS, 156
Hanks GE, 343
Hansen JA, 244
Harrison DA
    anatomy, 15–94
    interpretation, 203–223
Harvey RF, 157
Harvey W, 1
Hashimoto's disease, 258
Hayes RL, 96
Heart
    complications due to lymphography,
        518
    in disease, 106
    in lymphedema, 146
    in protein-losing enteropathy, 176
    in pulmonary chyle reflux, 200–201
    lymphatic drainage, 106
Heidenhain R, 12
Heineke H, 240
Hellman S, 96
Henriksen E, 292
Hepatic lymphatics, 69–71, 182
Herman PG, 29
Herman T, 99
Herophilus, 8
Hilar nodes, 466
Hirsh JI, 112
His W, 8, 51
Histiocytoma, 429
Histoplasmosis, 236
Historical considerations, 1–14
Hodgkin's disease. See Lymphoma
Hodgkin, Thomas, 264
Hohenfellner R, 516
Holsten DR, 240
Homans J, 160
Hoopes JE, 158
Howland WJ, 114
Hreschyshyn MM, 14
Hudack S, 14, 111, 112
Hughes JH, 144, 160
Hunter, William, 1, 12
Huntington GS, 16
Hygroma, cystic, 164
Hyperlipidemia test, 180, 188–189, 198
Hyperplasia
    follicular, 62
    mediastinal, 228–230
    reactive, 205, 227–228
Hypersensitivity to lymphographic oils

and dyes, 517–518
Hypogastric nodes, 38, 101. 293. 323.
  *See also* Iliac lymphatics
Hypoproteinemia, in mesenteric
  lymphatic malformation, 201

I

Iliac (pelvic) lymphatics, 29–47
  anatomy, 29–47
  CT appearance, 293
  in carcinoma of vulva, 344
  in mesenteric malformations, 182–183
  in ovarian carcinoma, 337–342, 344
  in prostate carcinoma, 382
  lymphographic appearance, 305
  scintigraphic appearance, 101, 105–106
  size, 15, 204, 212
Immunosuppression, and immunoblastic sarcoma, 257–258
Infection, lymphographic appearance, 209
Inflammation, nodal, 224–226. *See also*
  *specific inflammatory diseases*
Inguinal lymphatics
  anatomy, 23–29
  in carcinoma of vulva, 344
  in ovarian carcinoma, 337, 343
  lymphographic interpretation, 205
  size, 15, 204, 212
Injectors, for lymphography, 116
Interstitium, anatomy, 120–121
Intestine, 71, 106, 386–389. *See also*
  Mesenteric lymphatics
Iodopin, 115
Iriarte P, 114
Isosulfan blue, 111, 112
Ito Y, 97
Ivanov GF, 171

J

Jackson BT, 64
Jaffe ES, 256
Jamieson CW, 161
Javadpour N, 360
Jay JC, 516
Jewett HJ, 371
Jing B-S, 114, 116, 167, 496
  interpretation, 203–223
  solid tumors, 290–450
Joduron, 12
Jones SE, 99
Jossifow GM, 12
Jugular nodes, in esophageal car-
  cinoma, 441
Juxta-aortic lymphatics. *See* Para-aor-
  tic lymphatics

K

Kademain MT, 332
Kampmeier OF, 16
Kapdi CC, 112
Kaplan HS, 256, 265, 266, 274
Kaspar Z, 144, 151
Kay DN, 96–97
Kett K, 118
Kidney, in lymphoma, 274. *See also*
  Renal lymphatics.

Kiel classification of lymphomas, 243
Kienle J, 236
Kikuchi T, 118
Kinmonth JB, 13, 15, 21, 64, 111, 142, 144, 146, 147, 148, 149, 150, 156, 157, 158, 161, 496
Klippel-Trenaunay syndrome, 190
Koehler RP, 116, 511, 517
Kohler I, 518
Kojima M, 247, 256
Kolbenstvedt S, 324
Kondoleon E, 156
Koss JC, 376
Kountz SI, 143
Kreel L, 144, 149, 389
Kropholler RW, 114, 517
Kumita, 48

L

Lackner K, 360
Lacunar nodes, 29
Lagasse LD, 324
LaMarque JL, 236
Langhammer H, 96
Laparotomy, 96, 189
Laplante M, 376
Larson DL, 170, 171
Larson NE, 144, 160
Larson SM, 469
Larynx, lymphatic drainage, 106
Lawrentjew AP, 7
Leak LV, 12
Lee FC, 162
Lee JK, 360
Lee KF, 114
Left aortic chain, 59, 64–68
Leiomyosarcoma, 416, 423–424
Leitsmann H, 518
Lennert K, 256
Lenzi M, 240
Leukemia, 97, 254
Levine GD, 256
Lewis TR, 162
Lichenification, in lymphedema, 145
Lien HH, 363, 365
Lipectomy, in lymphedema, 160
Lipiodol, 12, 115, 118, 189
Liposarcoma, 416, 423–424
Liver, 95, 126. *See also* Hepatic
  lymphatics
Ludington LG, 516
Ludvik W, 516
Ludwig, 12
Lukes RJ, functional pathology of lym-
  phoma, 243–263
Lukes-Butler classification of lympho-
  mas, 249, 252
Lukes-Collins classification of lympho-
  mas, 264
Lumbar lymphatics, 59–64, 182–183
Lung
  carcinoma, 440, 451–452, 455–466
  diagnostic work-up, 466–469
  scintigraphic appearance, 95, 97, 106
  *See also* Pulmonary lymphatics;
    Bronchial lymphatics
Lupus erythematosis, 257–258

Lymph, 120–141
  definition, 123
  edema, 135–138
  flow, 120–123, 132–134, 136
  fluid pressure, 134–135
  fluid protein, 125–126
  formation, 12, 123–125
  movement, 127–132
  volume, 133–134
Lymph nodes
  CT appearance, 15, 212
  development of, 16
  discovery of, 8
  in benign disease, 224–242
  in lymphedema, 142
  lymphographic appearance, 18–21, 29, 203–212
  mechanisms of metastasis, 297–305
  modes of metastasis, 305–321
  scintigraphic appearance, 101
  *See also specific lymphatics and spe-*
    *cific diseases*
Lymph vessels
  anatomy, 17–18, 121
  contractions, 129–130
  discovery of, 1
  in lymphedema, 142
  neoplasms of, 164
  obstruction, 165–176
  permeability, 124
  pressure, 128–129
  proliferation, 137
  pumps, 127–132, 133
  *See also specific anatomic area;* Cap-
    illaries, lymphatic; Prelympha-
    tics
Lymphadenopathy, lipoplastic, 233–235
Lymphangiectasia, primary, 174–176
Lymphangiectomy, 160, 194
Lymphangiography. *See* Lymphography
Lymphangioma, 164
Lymphangiomatosis of bone, 436–437
Lymphangitis, in lymphedema, 145, 155
Lymphatic system, 8, 12, 16–17, 125.
  *See also specific anatomic area*
Lymphaticovenous communication, 167, 310
Lymphazurin. *See* Isosulfan blue
Lymphedema, 135–138, 142–160
  causes, 136
  classification, 142
  clinical considerations, 144–147
  definition, 135
  etiology, 142–144
  evaluation methods, 147–153
  formation of fluid, 121
  genital, 160–164, 201
  interstitial pressure, 132, 133, 135–136
  lymphographic appearance, 142, 147–151
  safety factors, 137–138
  treatment, nonsurgical, 153–156
  treatment, surgical, 156–160
  upper extremity, 103, 403–408
Lymphocele, 172

Lymphochromea, in mesenteric malfor-
    mations, 182, 189–190
Lymphocytes, 243–263
    B cells, 246–247, 250–251
    in lymphoma, 248–253
    systems, 244–245
    T cells, 247–248, 249–250
    transformation, 245–246
Lymphography
    breast, 118
    cervical, 91, 472
    mesenteric, 180–191
        findings, 181–186, 190–191, 197
        technique, 180, 189–190
    pedal
        accuracy, 15, 205, 274–283, 321, 496
        advantages, 15
        cannulation, 114–115
        complications, 511–520
        contraindications, 111
        contrast material, 115–116
        disadvantages, 15
        exposure of lymphatics, 112–114
        filming, 62, 116–118
        follow-up, 118
        history of, 12–14
        injectors, 116
        interpretation, 203–212, 290–292
        preparation of patient, 111
        technique, 111–118
        vital dyes, 111–112
        See also specific diseases
    radionuclide, 95–110. See also specific
        diseases
    testicular, 56, 348–349
    thyroid, 118
    upper extremity, 90–91, 389–397,
        399–400
Lymphoma, 248–261, 264–289,
    455–466, 511–520
    classification, 96, 248–253
    clinical and morphological correla-
        tions, 256–259
    diagnosis and follow-up
        accuracy, 274–283
        biopsy, 499–502, 504
        CT, 212, 266, 269–274, 280–287, 502
        decision tree, 284–287
        lymphography, 62, 96, 99–100,
            205–212, 267–268, 274–287
        other techniques, 266
        scintigraphy, 96–97, 99, 106, 266
        ultrasonography, 267, 502
    histologic appearance, 248–253, 258
    history, 264–265
    immunology and morphology,
        244–248
    pathogenesis, 264–265
    presentation, 96
    sites
        abdomen, 264–289
        bone, 429–436
        cervical (neck) area, 476
        retroperitoneum, 264–289
        thorax, 452, 455–466, 469–470
    staging, 96–97, 265
    survival, 265
    symptoms, 265

    therapy, 265
    working formulation, 259
Lymphoscintigraphy, 101–106. See also
    specific diseases

M

MacIntosh PK, 503
Macroglobulinemia, 249, 250, 257, 258
Malabsorption syndromes, causing
    edema, 136
Malek P, 14
Mammary lymphatics
    anatomy, 82–83, 398–399, 466
    in breast carcinoma, 400
    in lymphatic malformations, 183, 185
    lymphoscintigraphy, 102–104
Mancuso AA, 472, 487, 488, 494
Mandi L, 235
Manson P, 162
Marcille M, 51, 336, 343
Marglin SI, 268, 365
Marshall VF, 371
Mascagni P, 12
Mason DY, 247, 254
Mastoid nodes, 476
Mathe G, 258
Matoba N, 118
Mayerson P, 168
Mayes GB, 389
McClure CFW, 16
McClure S, 233
McCort JJ, 88
McCready RV, 96–97
McHale NG, 129
McKusick KA, radionuclide lympho-
    graphy, 95–110
McLoud TC, thoracic imaging, 451–471
McMaster PD, 14, 111, 112
Measles, 224
Mediastinal lymphatics, 451–466
    anatomy, 82–85, 453–466
    CT appearance, 451–452
    hyperplasia of, 228–230
    in lung carcinoma, 451–452
    in lymphatic malformations, 186
    in lymphoma, 452
    in ovarian carcinoma, 343
Megalymphatics, in lymphedema, 148
Melanoma
    CT appearance, 416
    lymphatic effects, 310, 411
    lymphographic appearance, 411–416
    metastasis, 452, 476
    scintigraphic appearance, 101,
        104–105
    surgical planning, 101
Mesenteric lymphatics, 180–202
    anatomy, 79–81
    clinical aspects, 190–202
    examination of, 188–190
    lymphangiectasia, 174
    malformations of, 180–202
    pathophysiology, 181–188
Meyer JE, 103
    thoracic imaging, 451–471
Milanov NO, 157
Miller EM, 487
Miller TA, 160

Millett YL, 257
Milroy WF, 146
Milroy's disease, 146–147, 201
Monoclonal antibodies, 106
Mononucleosis, 246
Morehead R, 233
Morgan CL, 376, 383
Morris B, 240
Mortazavi SH, 112, 516
Mueller PR, 272
Munzenrider JE, 103
Musumeci R, 342, 343
Mycosis fungoides, 248–250, 255–258
Myeloma, 254, 429

N

Naidich DP, 469
Nasopharynx, carcinoma, 437
Nathwani BN, 255
Negus D, 143
Nelson B, 516
Nephrosis, 136
Neuroblastoma, 441
Ngu VA, 23
Nielubowicz J, 156, 157
Norman D, 487
Nossal GJV, 246
Nuck, Anton, 1, 12
Nutrition, in edema, 136

O

Oberling C, 264
O'Brien BM, 157
Obturator node, 29, 293, 305
Obstruction, 165–176
Occipital nodes, 472–476
O'Connor FW, 162
O'Donnell TF, Jr, abnormal peripheral
    lymphatics, 142–179
Ohnuma T, 258
Olin T, 116
Olszewski W, 142, 156, 157
Omental transposition, in
    lymphedema, 157
O'Reilly K, 156
Ormond JK, 230
Osborne DR, 469
Ottoviani, 171
Ovaries, 335–344
    carcinoma, 295, 335–344
    CT appearance, 343–344
    lymphatics, 51, 335–337
    lymphographic appearance, 105–106,
        337–343

P

Pancreatic lymphatics, 76–78, 182
Pancreatitis, lymphatic obstruction in,
    176
Panniculitis, retroperitoneal, 232
Panning WP, 116
Pappenheimer JR, 17
Para-aortic lymphatics
    anatomy, 56–69
    CT appearance, 293–294
    in bladder carcinoma, 377–378
    in esophageal carcinoma, 441
    in ovarian carcinoma, 337–344

in prostate carcinoma, 382
lymphographic appearance, 205
size, 15, 204, 212
Paracaval nodes, 60–61, 64
Paratracheal lymphatics
anatomy, 455–460
in lymphatic malformations, 186
in malignant disease, 451
Parietal intrathoracic lymphatics, 81–82
Parker BR, 228, 342
Parotid nodes, 476
Patel AR, 144, 150, 160
Patent blue violet dye, 13, 111, 112, 516–517
Pecquet J, 1
Pecquet, cistern of, 182, 184, 192, 194
Pelvic lymphatics. See Iliac lymphatics; or specific pelvic organ
Pelvis, 101, 105–106, 295–296. See also specific organs
Penis, 383, 385–386
Periaortic lymphatics. See Para-aortic lymphatics
Peritracheal lymphatics. See Para-tracheal lymphatics
Pfahler GG, 12
Pirogow, node of. See Rosenmüller, node of
Piver SM, 496
Platzbekder H, 235
Plentl A, 292
Poliomyelitis, 224
Politowski M, 157
Pomerantz M, 175
Pores, Pappenheimer's, 17
Prelymphatics, 120, 124, 310
Pressman JJ, 168
Prostate
carcinoma, 105, 295, 378, 379–383
CT appearance, 383
lymphatics, 50–51, 378–379
lymphographic appearance, 379–383, 496
Protein, in edema, 136
Pruritis, in lymphedema, 145
Puckett CL, 157
Puckett J, 156
Pulmonary lymphatics
anatomy, 85–88
in chylous reflux, 200–201
in lymphatic malformations, 186–188
Pump, lymphatic. See Lymph vessels
Pusey WA, 265
Pyelography. See Urography

R

Radioactive albumin studies. See Albumin disappearance curves
Radiography
in lung carcinoma, 466
in lymphoma, 266, 470
in mediastinal lymphadenopathy, 453–466, 470
Radionuclide studies, 95–110. See also specific diseases and radioisotopes

Radiotherapy
effect on tissues, 240, 302, 327
for lymphoma, 265
planning, 101, 103–104, 327, 501
Randolph J, 162, 163
Rappaport classification of lymphomas, 258, 264
Rappaport H, 96, 243, 244
Rasmussen KE, 516
Rauste J, 235
Reed, Dorothy, 264, 265
Reed-Sternberg cell, 246, 250, 252
discovery of, 264
prevalence in Hodgkin's disease, 96
Reede DL, cervical nodes, 472–495
Reflux, chylous, in mesenteric malformations, 182–183, 200–201
Reichert FL, 165
Reiffenstuhl G, 324
Renal lymphatics, 48, 183
Respiration, effect on lymph flow, 127–128
Reticulosarcoma, 429
Retrocrural nodes, 15, 29, 212
Retropharyngeal nodes, 478–480
Rhabdomyosarcoma, 349, 416, 423–424
Richter syndrome, 256
Rim sign, 292, 301
Robbins LL, 88
Roddie IC, 129
Rosenberg SA, 265
Rosenberger A, 89
Rosenmüller, node of, 26, 28, 29, 38
Rouvière H, 12, 29, 47, 56, 71, 76, 79, 81, 90, 348, 451, 452, 453, 472
Rudbeck, Olaf, 1, 7
Rummelhardt H, 383
Ruttimann A, 496
Ruttner JR, 224, 228
Ruysch, Frederick, 8
Rye classification of lymphomas, 96, 249, 252–253

S

Sabin, Florence, 16
Sandwich sign, 272
Sarcoid, 476
Sarcoidosis, 209–212, 235–236
Sarcoma, 423–429
bone, 424–429
Ewing's, 424–429
immunoblastic, 248, 250, 251–252, 256, 257–258
Kaposi's, 164, 416, 423–424
nodular sclerosing lymphosarcoma, 257
reticulum cell, 212
soft tissues, 416, 423–424
Sawney CP, 158
Scanlon GT, 118
Schaffer B, 515
Scharkoff T, 235, 236
Schmidt KR, 150
Schnyder PA, 459
Scintigraphy. See Lymphoscintigraphy
Scrotectomy, in lymphedema, 160
Seiler RG, 324
Seminal vesicles, lymphatics, 51

Seminoma, 349, 365
Servelle M, 12–13, 161
mesenteric malformations, 180–202
Sézary's syndrome, 245, 248, 249–250, 255, 256–258
Shammas HJ, 148
Shanbrom E, 115, 169
Shevland JE, 468
Shimkin PM, 175
Sigurjonsson K, 112
Silver D, 156
Silvester CF, 168
Sistrunk WE, 156
Sjögren's syndrome, 258
Skin, 411, 408
Smalley RH, 235
Smith EB, 240
Smith RO, 129
Sokol GH, 111
Sokolowski J, 517
Spaces, perineural and perivascular, 170–171
Spellman MC, 383, 496
Spleen, 96–97
Splenectomy, in lymphoma, 96
Splenic nodes, 76–78
Spondylitis, 224
Stahr H, 48
Starling EH, 12, 121
Starling forces, 121–122, 125, 135, 137
Starvation, causing edema, 136
Stein H, 255
Sternberg C, 264
Stevens RC, 114
Stoppani F, 12–13
Storen EJ, 172
Strickstrock KH, 236
Strong GH, 371
Subcarinal nodes, 460–463
Subfascial lymphatic system of lower extremities, 23
Sublingual nodes, 478
Submandibular nodes, 477
Submental nodes, 478
Sullivan DC, 104
Superficial prefascial lymphatic system of lower extremities, 22–23
Supraclavicular nodes, 337, 343, 399, 441
Suramo L, 236
Symmers D, 264
Syphilis, 236

T

Takahashi M, 58, 62, 165, 204, 267
Takashima T, 176
Takekoshi N, 176
Tallroth K, 423, 429
Tapper RI, 161
Taylor CR, 247, 254
Taylor GW, 144
Technetium-99m, 97, 99, 101–106
Tegtmeyer CJ, 114
Teneff S, 12–13
Testes, 348–368
biopsy, 503
carcinoma of, 52–53, 56, 101, 209, 349–368

Testes—*continued*
  CT appearance, 360–368
  embryology, 348
  lymphatics, 52–53, 348–349
  lymphographic appearance, 349–368,
    496
Thompson N, 157
Thompson procedure, in lymphedema,
  157
Thomson KR, 503, 506
Thoracentesis, in chylothorax, 162
Thoracic duct
  anatomy, 17, 88–90
  discovery of, 1
  embryology, 16, 89
  in chyluria, 162
  lymphographic appearance, 305
  obstruction, 310
Thoracic lymphatics, 81–90, 183–188,
  452
Thorotrast, 12–14
Threefoot SA, 116, 169, 511
Tjernberg B, 224
TNM staging system
  for lung cancers, 451
  for neck cancers, 487
Tomography, computed (CT)
  accuracy, 15, 274–283
  advantages, 15
  cervical, 472–495
  disadvantages, 15
  guiding biopsy, 497
  interpretation,   212–222,   268–269,
    292–295
  retroperitoneal, 268–274
  technique, 15–16, 268
  thoracic (mediastinal), 451–470
  *See also specific diseases*
Tomography, linear
  in lung carcinoma, 466–469
  in lymphoma, 266
  in mediastinal lymphadenopathy,
    453–466
Tong ECK, 114

Tonometry, tissue measurement, 153
Toth LM, 154
Trachea, 106. *See also* Paratracheal
  lymphatics
Trowell OA, 240
Tsunoda R, 247
Tuberculosis, 209–212, 236, 476, 488
Turner AF, 114
Turner DA, 97
Turner's syndrome, in lymphedema,
  146

U

Ujiki GT, 240
Ultrasonography
  in chylopericardium, 200
  in lymphoma, 267, 280, 502
  in solid tumor, 295–296
Ureteral lymphatics, 48–50
Urografin, 12, 14
Urography (pyelography)
  in chyluria, 162
  in lymphoma, 266
  in retroperitoneal fibrosis, 230
  in solid tumor, 296–297
Uterine corpus, 52, 327–335

V

Vagina, lymphatics, 52
Van Den Brenk HAS, 240
Van der Mollen HR, 154
Van Horne J, 1
Vasa serosa, 12
Vasko JS, 161
Venography, 230, 266, 297
Verrucose formations, 195
Vessels, lymphatic. *See* Lymph vessels
Viamonte M, 114, 116, 224, 235, 236
Vieussens R, 12
Virchow R, 12, 240
Virchow-Robbins space, 170
Visceral lymphatics
  abdominal, 69–81
  thoracic, 83–85

Vitek J, 144, 151
Von Recklinghausen FD, 12

W

Waldenström's macroglobulinemia,
  249, 250, 257, 258
Waldeyer's tonsillar ring, 91
Waldmann TA, 175
Wallace S, 14, 116, 167, 169, 171, 496
  interpretation, 203–223
  solid tumors, 290–450
Walsh JW, 325, 376
Weichert RF, 161
Weissleder H, 236
Weston BV, 135
White RJ, 513
Whitley NO, 325
Wiederhielm CA, 135
Wiertz LM, 518
Wiljasalo M, 62, 224
Williams RD, 360
Wirth W, 89
Wolfel DA, 169, 233
Wrisberg H, 7
Wücherer O, 162
Wutzer CW, 168

X

Xeroradiography, 153

Y

Yam LT, 254
Yoffey JM, 162
Youker JE, 114

Z

Zalar J, 236
Zeissler RM, 154
Zelikovski A, 155
Zheutlin N, 115, 169
Zornoza J, 327, 389
  nodal biopsy, 496–510
Zuppinger A, 165